HANDBOOK OF SELF-KNOWLEDGE

HANDBOOK OF SELF-KNOWLEDGE

edited by
**Simine Vazire
Timothy D. Wilson**

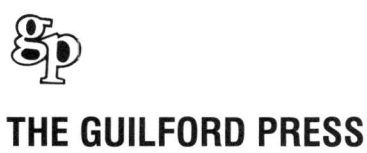

THE GUILFORD PRESS
New York   London

© 2012 The Guilford Press
A Division of Guilford Publications, Inc.
72 Spring Street, New York, NY 10012
www.guilford.com

All rights reserved

No part of this book may be reproduced, translated, stored in a retrieval system, or transmitted, in any form or by any means, electronic, mechanical, photocopying, microfilming, recording, or otherwise, without written permission from the publisher.

Printed in the United States of America

This book is printed on acid-free paper.

Last digit is print number: 9 8 7 6 5 4 3 2 1

Library of Congress Cataloging-in-Publication Data

Handbook of self-knowledge / edited by Simine Vazire, Timothy D. Wilson.
    p. cm.
  Includes bibliographical references and index.
  ISBN 978-1-4625-0511-1 (hardcover)
  1. Self-perception. 2. Subconsciousness. 3. Personality (Theory of knowledge). I. Vazire, Simine. II. Wilson, Timothy D.
  BF697.5.S43H364 2012
  155.2—dc23
                                                              2011049298

About the Editors

Simine Vazire, PhD, is Assistant Professor of Psychology at Washington University in St. Louis. Her research examines how well people know their own personalities and behavior, and how well people know the impressions they make on others. Dr. Vazire has received the SAGE Young Scholar Award from the Foundation for Personality and Social Psychology, the Early Career Award from the International Society for Self and Identity, and the Outstanding Faculty Mentor Award from Washington University in St. Louis.

Timothy D. Wilson, PhD, is Sherrell J. Aston Professor of Psychology at the University of Virginia. He has conducted research in the areas of self-knowledge, happiness, social cognition, and using social psychological principles to solve personal and social problems. Dr. Wilson is a recipient of the All-University Outstanding Teacher Award and the Distinguished Scientist Award from the University of Virginia and is an elected member of the American Academy of Arts and Sciences.

Contributors

Jonathan M. Adler, PhD, Department of Psychology, Franklin W. Olin College of Engineering, Needham, Massachusetts

Mitja D. Back, PhD, Department of Psychology, University of Münster, Münster, Germany

Galen V. Bodenhausen, PhD, Department of Psychology, Northwestern University, Evanston, Illinois

Maarten W. Bos, PhD, Department of Negotiation, Organizations and Markets, Harvard Business School, Boston, Massachusetts

Pablo Briñol, PhD, Department of Psychology, Universidad Autónoma de Madrid, Madrid, Spain

Erin Buckels, BA, Department of Psychology, University of British Columbia, Vancouver, British Columbia, Canada

Erika N. Carlson, MA, Department of Psychology, Washington University in St. Louis, St. Louis, Missouri

Jason Chin, PhD, Faculty of Law, University of Toronto, Toronto, Ontario, Canada

Gerald L. Clore, PhD, Department of Psychology, University of Virginia, Charlottesville, Virginia

Ap Dijksterhuis, PhD, Behavioral Science Institute, Radboud University Nijmegen, Nijmegen, The Netherlands

Elizabeth W. Dunn, PhD, Department of Psychology, University of British Columbia, Vancouver, British Columbia, Canada

David Dunning, PhD, Department of Psychology, Cornell University, Ithaca, New York

Jennifer Fillo, BS, Department of Psychology, University of Minnesota, Minneapolis, Minnesota

Bertram Gawronski, PhD, Department of Psychology, University of Western Ontario, London, Ontario, Canada

Katherine E. Hansen, MA, Department of Psychology, Princeton University, Princeton, New Jersey

Daniel Hart, PhD, Center for Children and Childhood Studies, Camden College of Arts and Sciences, Rutgers, The State University of New Jersey, Camden, New Jersey

Erik G. Helzer, MA, Department of Psychology, Cornell University, Ithaca, New York

Galit Hofree, MA, Department of Psychology, University of California, San Diego, La Jolla, California

Larry L. Jacoby, PhD, Department of Psychology, Washington University in St. Louis, St. Louis, Missouri

Colleen M. Kelley, PhD, Department of Psychology, Florida State University, Tallahassee, Florida

David A. Kenny, PhD, Department of Psychology, University of Connecticut, Storrs, Connecticut

Kostadin Kushlev, MA, Department of Psychology, University of British Columbia, Vancouver, British Columbia, Canada

Mark R. Leary, PhD, Department of Psychology and Neuroscience, Duke University, Durham, North Carolina

Nira Liberman, PhD, Department of Psychology, Tel Aviv University, Tel Aviv, Israel

Matthew D. Lieberman, PhD, Department of Psychology, University of California, Los Angeles, Los Angeles, California

M. Kyle Matsuba, PhD, Department of Psychology, Kwantlen Polytechnic University, Surrey, British Columbia, Canada

Michael Mrazek, BA, Department of Psychological and Brain Sciences, University of California, Santa Barbara, Santa Barbara, California

John Myers, MS, Department of Psychology, University of Minnesota, Minneapolis, Minnesota

Thomas F. Oltmanns, PhD, Department of Psychology, Washington University in St. Louis, St. Louis, Missouri

Delroy L. Paulhus, PhD, Department of Psychology, University of British Columbia, Vancouver, British Columbia, Canada

Richard E. Petty, PhD, Department of Psychology, Ohio State University, Columbus, Ohio

Abigail D. Powers, MA, Department of Psychology, Washington University in St. Louis, St. Louis, Missouri

Emily Pronin, PhD, Department of Psychology, Princeton University, Princeton, New Jersey

Richard W. Robins, PhD, Department of Psychology, University of California, Davis, Davis, California

Michael D. Robinson, PhD, Department of Psychology, North Dakota State University, Fargo, North Dakota

Jonathan Schooler, PhD, Department of Psychology, University of California, Santa Barbara, Santa Barbara, California

Roberta A. Schriber, MA, Department of Psychology, University of California, Davis, Davis, California

Contributors

Oliver C. Schultheiss, PhD, Department of Psychology and Sport Sciences, Friedrich-Alexander University, Erlangen, Germany

Jeffry A. Simpson, PhD, Department of Psychology, University of Minnesota, Minneapolis, Minnesota

Sanjay Srivastava, PhD, Department of Psychology, University of Oregon, Eugene, Oregon

Alexandra Strasser, DPhil, Faculty of Psychology, Technical University of Munich, Munich, Germany

Michael J Strube, PhD, Department of Psychology, Washington University in St. Louis, St. Louis, Missouri

Kaitlin Toner, MA, Department of Psychology and Neuroscience, Duke University, Durham, North Carolina

Yaacov Trope, PhD, Department of Psychology, New York University, New York, New York

Simine Vazire, PhD, Department of Psychology, Washington University in St. Louis, St. Louis, Missouri

Cheryl J. Wakslak, PhD, Department of Management and Organization, Marshall School of Business, University of Southern California, Los Angeles, California

Timothy D. Wilson, PhD, Department of Psychology, University of Virginia, Charlottesville, Virginia

Piotr Winkielman, PhD, Department of Psychology, University of California, San Diego, La Jolla, California

Contents

1. Introduction — 1
Simine Vazire and Timothy D. Wilson

PART I. THE ORIGINS AND NATURE OF SELF-KNOWLEDGE

2. The Development of Self-Knowledge — 7
Daniel Hart and M. Kyle Matsuba

3. Self-Insight from a Dual-Process Perspective — 22
Bertram Gawronski and Galen V. Bodenhausen

4. Referential Processing and Competence as Determinants of Congruence between Implicit and Explicit Motives — 39
Oliver C. Schultheiss and Alexandra Strasser

5. Self-Knowledge: From Philosophy to Neuroscience to Psychology — 63
Matthew D. Lieberman

6. Blind Spots to the Self: Limits in Knowledge of Mental Contents and Personal Predispositions — 77
Jason Chin, Michael Mrazek, and Jonathan Schooler

7. Other People as a Source of Self-Knowledge — 90
Sanjay Srivastava

8. Self-Knowledge: An Individual-Differences Perspective — 105
Roberta A. Schriber and Richard W. Robins

PART II. DOMAINS OF SELF-KNOWLEDGE

9. Knowing Our Personality — 131
Mitja D. Back and Simine Vazire

10. Knowing Our Attitudes and How to Change Them — 157
Pablo Briñol and Richard E. Petty

11. Self-Knowledge, Unconscious Thought, and Decision Making — 181
Maarten W. Bos and Ap Dijksterhuis

12. Knowing Our Emotions: How Do We Know What We Feel? — 194
Gerald L. Clore and Michael D. Robinson

13. On (Not) Knowing and Feeling What We Want and Like — 210
Galit Hofree and Piotr Winkielman

14. Partner Knowledge and Relationship Outcomes — 225
Jeffry A. Simpson, Jennifer Fillo, and John Myers

15. Meta-Accuracy: Do We Know How Others See Us? — 242
Erika N. Carlson and David A. Kenny

16. Knowing Our Pathology — 258
Thomas F. Oltmanns and Abigail D. Powers

PART III. KNOWING OUR PAST AND FUTURE SELVES

17. Affective Forecasting: Knowing How We Will Feel in the Future — 277
Kostadin Kushlev and Elizabeth W. Dunn

18. Past Selves and Autobiographical Memory — 293
Colleen M. Kelley and Larry L. Jacoby

19. Self-Conceptualization, Self-Knowledge, and Regulatory Scope: A Construal-Level View — 310
Cheryl J. Wakslak, Yaacov Trope, and Nira Liberman

20. Sitting at the Nexus of Epistemological Traditions: Narrative Psychological Perspectives on Self-Knowledge — 327
Jonathan M. Adler

Contents

PART IV. MOTIVES AND BIASES IN SELF-KNOWLEDGE

21. Illusions of Self-Knowledge   345
Katherine E. Hansen and Emily Pronin

22. Classic Self-Deception Revisited   363
Delroy L. Paulhus and Erin Buckels

23. On Motivated Reasoning and Self-Belief   379
Erik G. Helzer and David Dunning

24. From "Out There" to "In Here": Implications of Self-Evaluation Motives for Self-Knowledge   397
Michael J Strube

25. Reducing Egoistic Biases in Self-Beliefs   413
Mark R. Leary and Kaitlin Toner

Author Index   429

Subject Index   449

HANDBOOK OF SELF-KNOWLEDGE

CHAPTER 1
Introduction

SIMINE VAZIRE
TIMOTHY D. WILSON

The importance of self-knowledge is a common theme in ancient and modern literature, was carved in stone at the Greek oracle in Delphi, and is stressed by many religions and philosophical schools of thought (not to mention the self-help industry). Until recently, however, it has not been a central topic in psychological science. There are no journals on the topic, no professional societies organized to study it, and few college courses that teach it. There are many reasons for this, including the long shadow of psychoanalysis and the desire of psychological researchers to move away from it, and difficult methodological problems with studying self-knowledge.

It seems, however, that the study of self-knowledge is making a comeback. What's more, this revival can be seen across all branches of psychology. In social psychology, researchers are examining topics such as self-insight and self-awareness, the limits and dangers of introspection, unconscious thought, implicit biases, and the accuracy of people's predictions about their future feelings and behaviors. In personality psychology, researchers are examining the validity of self-assessment, the process and outcome of self-perception, how people construct a coherent self-narrative, and the extent to which other people know us better than we know ourselves. In cognitive psychology, researchers are studying metacognition (people's beliefs about the workings of their own mind), as well as the accuracy of people's memories about the past and how they think about the future. In developmental psychology, researchers are examining how children acquire an understanding of their own and other people's minds. In clinical psychology, researchers are studying repression, people's knowledge of their own personality disorders, and alexithymia, the tendency to fail to recognize one's own emotions. Finally, neuroscientists are examining the brain regions uniquely associated with self-perception. Across all of these fields, dual-process theories are gaining popularity, and researchers are developing methods for measuring self-processes that reside outside of conscious awareness (e.g., implicit attitudes, nonconscious thought, implicit personality, and implicit motives).

These developments have led to a rich network of findings about the strengths and limits of self-knowledge, the structure of self-knowledge, and the function of self-knowledge. However, there is little communication among researchers working in different disciplines. The goal of this handbook is to bring together these areas of research and show that they belong under a common tent, thereby defining a new interdisciplinary area in psychology. We see self-knowledge as a topic with great potential. First, as noted, the topic bridges areas of psychology that have traditionally had little contact. Even social and personality psychology, which are usually considered part of the same subfield, have suffered from lack of communication and collaboration. By bringing together excellent research from both sides of this divide, we hope this handbook will make it clear that they have much in common, and that there is much potential for cross-fertilization of ideas. Second, research on self-knowledge has the potential to stimulate the public's interest in psychological science by serving as an example of how rigorous psychological research can help satisfy laypeople's thirst for knowledge that is directly applicable to their everyday lives. Many of the chapters in this book tackle questions about which human beings are naturally curious (e.g., Do some people know themselves better than others? Can we not know what we're feeling?).

What makes self-knowledge different from other, related areas of research? The study of the self is not new, and there is a very large and active community of researchers studying self-schemas, self-concepts, self-views, self-esteem, self-regulation, self-consciousness, and many other self topics. All of these are relevant to the study of self-knowledge, but self-knowledge has one feature that sets it apart from these other areas of research: its emphasis on the accuracy of self-views. Historically, research on the self examines how self-views and self-beliefs shape behavior, thoughts, and feelings, without asking whether these self-views track reality. What sets self-knowledge research apart from the rest of self research is the examination of the accuracy of self-views.

The focus on accuracy inherent to self-knowledge research has opened new research topics, such as self-deception, self-enhancement, affective forecasting, meta-perception, metacognition, and implicit cognition. The concept of accuracy or inaccuracy in self-views also adds a new dimension to research in almost every area of psychology. The extent to which people have insight into their own feelings, attitudes, motives, behaviors, traits, personal histories, relationships, mental processes, and reputations has important consequences. Self-knowledge in these domains likely influences important outcomes such as happiness, interpersonal relationships, and personal achievement. Furthermore, self-knowledge is relevant to fundamental human capacities such as agency, self-regulation, decision making, and perhaps even moral responsibility. If people lack self-knowledge, it might be difficult for them to exert control over their lives, make good decisions, exercise their values, and be fully responsible for their actions.

There are challenges in studying the accuracy of self-views. Evaluating accuracy requires a criterion against which to measure people's beliefs. In some domains (e.g., people's beliefs about how others view them—their reputations), this is fairly straightforward (i.e., collecting observer reports). In other domains, however, obtaining a valid measure of "reality" is more difficult. What are objective measures of people's traits, emotions, attitudes, or thoughts? While there will always be some controversy about appropriate criterion measures for these constructs, new methods have greatly improved our ability to assess these constructs without relying on self-reports. For example, implicit measures allow researchers to access mental processes that may not be accessible to consciousness (in this volume, see Chapter 3 by Gawronski & Bodenhausen and Chapter 4 by Schultheiss & Strasser), and behavioral observation tools allow researchers to unobtrusively record objective, naturalistic behavior (Mehl & Pennebaker, 2003; see also Chapter 9 by Back & Vazire and Chapter 14 by Simpson, Fillo, & Myers, this volume). As technology and methods continue to develop, opportunities to obtain criterion measures, and assess self-knowledge across a broad range of domains, will only grow.

We see many hopeful signs that self-knowledge is gaining traction as a vibrant, rigorous area of research. The chapters in this handbook highlight some of the very best and newest research in this area, and we hope they will spur even more people to pursue this topic. We expect that some readers, like some of the authors in this handbook, will realize that they have been studying self-knowledge for years without labeling it as such.

We have organized the book into four parts. The first part explores the origins and nature of self-knowledge, including the ontological development of self-knowledge (Chapter 2 by Hart & Matsuba), the mental processes underlying self-knowledge (Chapter 3 by Gawronski & Bodenhausen; Chapter 4 by Schultheiss & Strasser; and Chapter 6 by Chin, Mrazek, & Schooler), biological bases of self-knowledge (Chapter 5 by Lieberman), the social processes involved in self-knowledge (Chapter 7 by Srivastava), and individual differences in self-knowledge (Chapter 8 by Schriber & Robins). The purpose of this section is to examine the biological, mental, and social structures that make self-knowledge possible. The second part explores specific domains of self-knowledge, including people's knowledge of their own traits (Chapter 9 by Back & Vazire), attitudes (Chapter 10 by Briñol & Petty), thoughts (Chapter 11 by Bos & Dijksterhuis), emotions (Chapter 12 by Clore & Robinson), desires (Chapter 13 by Hofree & Winkielman), relationships (Chapter 14 by Simpson et al.), reputations (Chapter 15 by Carlson & Kenny), and pathologies (Chapter 16 by Oltmanns & Powers). The purpose of this section is to examine the bright spots and blind spots in self-knowledge across psychological functions. How good are people at knowing how they act, feel, think, and connect with others? The third part explores self-knowledge of past and future selves. Its purpose is to examine the role of time in self-knowledge—how accurate people are at predicting their future psychological states (Chapter 17 by Kushlev & Dunn) or recalling their past ones (Chapter 18 by Kelley & Jacoby). Does thinking about ourselves in the past or future influence the accuracy of our self-views (Chapter 19 by Wakslak, Trope, & Liberman)? How important is accuracy in constructing a life narrative (Chapter 20 by Adler)? Finally, the fourth part explores motives and biases that influence self-knowledge. Its purpose is to highlight the motivational obstacles to accurate self-perception (Chapter 21 by Hansen & Pronin; Chapter 22 by Paulhus & Buckels; Chapter 23 by Helzer & Dunning) and how they might be overcome (Chapter 24 by Strube; Chapter 25 by Leary & Toner).

Although the chapters illustrate the considerable progress that has been made in the study of self-knowledge, they also highlight the many questions that remain. For example, readers will encounter a lively debate over the question of whether it is beneficial to engage in self-enhancement, or whether it is best to have accurate views of one's traits and abilities (see Chapters 8, 9, 20, 22, and 25). Exactly what is assessed by implicit measures of attitudes and motives? Chapter 3 by Gawronski and Bodenhausen, Chapter 4 by Schultheiss and Strasser, and Chapter 10 by Briñol and Petty go a long way toward answering this question, but important issues remain unresolved. Although methodological advances are discussed in virtually all chapters, vexing questions remain about the best criteria by which to judge the accuracy of self-views.

Nonetheless, it is safe to say that the study of self-knowledge has become a vibrant cross-disciplinary subfield of psychology. During the Watergate hearings, Senator Howard Baker famously asked about President Nixon, "What did he know and when did he know it?" The present chapters go a long way toward answering a similar question about the self: "What do we know about ourselves and how do we know it?" We believe that readers are in for a treat and will find much to get excited about in this volume.

REFERENCE

Mehl, M. R., & Pennebaker, J. W. (2003). The sounds of social life: A psychometric analysis of students' daily social environments and natural conversations. *Journal of Personality and Social Psychology, 84,* 857–870.

PART I
THE ORIGINS AND NATURE OF SELF-KNOWLEDGE

CHAPTER 2

The Development of Self-Knowledge

DANIEL HART
M. KYLE MATSUBA

To "know thyself," the ancient Greeks maintained, is fundamental for virtue. The person with self-knowledge is equipped to make decisions serving the self's true interests and can sidestep the temptations that deflect one from flourishing and achieving wisdom. Contemporary Western thought continues to enshrine self-knowledge, as it is seen as essential for ethical and meaningful life (e.g., Williams, 1995). Choices concerning careers and relationships, common knowledge suggests, are best made in awareness of the self's talents, qualities, and aspirations. The centrality of self-knowledge is the foundation for popular measures of values, interests, and personality; adolescents and young adults take career-related inventories in order to choose appropriate jobs in light of their real interests; managers seek insight into their personality types in order to choose the techniques that will be most effective in managing employees, and so on.

Self-knowledge might well serve these ends and many more; to prize it, however, does not ensure that its meaning is well understood. One reason this is so is that both "self" and "knowledge" are immensely more complicated than ordinarily realized. Before embarking on an account of how self-knowledge develops—the central goal of this chapter—it is necessary to identify the complexities inherent in the constructs of knowledge and self.

Knowledge and the Nature of the Self

Knowledge

Three conditions are prerequisite to the judgment that a person has knowledge (Scheffler, 1983; Steup, 2008). First, the proposition embodying the knowledge must be *true*. The complexities of determining the truth value of a proposition are increased when the self is the object of knowledge, a point discussed at greater length in the next section. It suffices for the discussion here to note that *self-knowledge*—the true beliefs one has about one's self—is only a subset of the ideas and beliefs an individual has about the self, and given the difficulty of ascertaining the truth value of propositions, it seems likely that self-knowledge is difficult to assess. Second, knowledge must be *justified* (Scheffler, 1983; Steup, 2008). This means that for a proposition to constitute knowledge, it must be validated using processes known to track truth. Finally, knowledge requires *belief* in a proposition (Scheffler, 1983; Steup, 2008). To know requires an attitude of commitment to and investment in a truthful, justified proposition. Most often, propositions about the self arouse self-concern from which commitment and investment can be inferred.

Self

Components

Self-knowledge is difficult to acquire because *the self* refers not to a single object but to a loose collection of experiences, memories, propositions, and theories. Conceptual distinctions about the self made by William James more than 100 years ago remain insightful today. For James, the self results from consciousness. In his terms, "a man's self is the sum total of all that he can call his" (James, 1890/1998, p. 291). Three implications flow from this claim. The first of these is that in order for there to be a self, some faculty for reflection must exist; there must be a capacity for self-consciousness. Second, the notion of "all that he can call his" suggests that the individual is the final arbiter on what is to be considered part of the self. Third, the notion of "all that he can call his" suggests proprietary interests in elements included within the self, what can be referred to as *self-identification*. Reflecting upon the self is frequently accompanied by self-awareness, what James called a "unique kind of interest" (1890/1998, p. 289) and emotional involvement in specific elements associated with the self with which we identify.

Two components relate to the self. First, there are *personal memories*, memories that an individual considers to define the self and that are linked to particular times and locations. While Freud acknowledged that some younger children were capable of reporting a sequence of personal memories, he claimed that "in many cases [it is] only after the tenth year . . . that our lives can be reproduced in memory as a connected chain of events" (cited in Ross, 1991, p. 224). Second, people form representations and generalizations about the self, such as the self's appearance (e.g., "I am tall"), capabilities (e.g., "I'm a good dancer"), relationships (e.g., "I'm a good friend") and other psychological characteristics (e.g. "I'm smart and perceptive"). While infants do not have such representations of self, Neisser (1991) argues that they at least have "implicit self" representation growing through interactions with others and with their physical environment. By *implicit self*, Neisser is referring to infants' perceptual awareness of self.

However, autobiographical memories and representations by themselves would constitute only a collection of self-characteristics without the sense of integration provided by a *theory* or *narrative of self*. Theories of self provide persons with a framework within which personal memories and representations can be evaluated, weighted for importance to the self, and aligned with other characteristics of self.

Which Components Allow for Knowledge?

Not all the components of self genuinely allow for knowledge. For example, an individual may provide different narratives of the self at different times and in different locations, and it may be difficult to judge one of the narratives to be true and the others to be false (see also Adler, Chapter 20, this volume). Similarly, it is difficult to assign truth value to boundaries of self-identification. A child who identifies fiercely with a doll and consequently judges injury to the doll to be an injury to self is including within the self an object that ordinary adults would not see as part of the self; nonetheless, it is difficult to judge that the child is mistaken in seeing the doll as an extension of self. This is because we ordinarily grant authority to the individual to determine which experiences elicit the "unique kind of interest" noted by James that defines the boundaries of self (for a philosophical discussion of the issue of first-person authority, see Davidson, 1984).

Self-knowledge is largely possible in the domains of personal memories and representations (see also Kelley & Jacoby, Chapter 18, this volume). We generally believe that children can be correct or mistaken, at least to an important degree, in their memories for important events and in their generalizations about themselves. In a later section, we sketch developmental trends in each of these components.

Three Traditional Developmental Perspectives on Self-Knowledge

Most grand theories of development have attended, to one degree or another, to the origins of self-knowledge. Neopsychoanalytic theories posit that powerful emotions and needs dominate psychological functioning and provide the landscape within which self-knowledge is obtained. Ausubel (1949) proposed that infants believe themselves to be powerful (*infantile omnipotence*) because their needs—for nutrition, for example—are satisfied shortly after these needs are experienced. It is, of course, parents who satisfy these needs; however, in infancy, parents are viewed as extensions of self, subject to volitional control. As infants age, however, they recognize that parents are separate individuals who choose to minister to their infants' needs. This insight brings with it, Ausubel argues, self-devaluation as infants realize that they are dependent on others rather than omnipotent. Infants accommodate to this realization by identifying, at least loosely, with their competent parents.

One stream of cognitive developmental theory has followed Baldwin in imagining that imitation is the motor for early self-knowledge development. Baldwin (1906) argued that the self evolved largely as a result of social imitation. Baldwin noted that human infants are born without most of the skills necessary for survival and must acquire these skills by imitating appropriate models. As Baldwin described it:

> All were born helpless; all have been educated. Each has been taught; each is to become a teacher. Each learns new things by doing what he sees others do; and each improves on what the other does only by doing what he has already learned. (pp. 79–80)

Through imitation, the infant and child's self emerges and is influenced in predictable ways. First, the process of imitation results in structural commonalities between representations of self and other. Second, imitation reveals to the individual the prominence of volition in the experience of self.

The first stage in the sequence was called by Baldwin the *projective stage*. Baldwin (1906) argued that from birth infants are equipped to distinguish between persons and other objects in the world, and are particularly interested in the former. As infants focus their attention on others, they recognize that these others perform interesting actions, and they seek to emulate these behaviors. These nascent efforts to imitate result in the recognition that self and other differ: While the self's actions may resemble visually the actions of another, only the self's actions are accompanied by the experience of volition. This recognition demarcates the onset of the *subjective stage* in self development. Eventually, the child recognizes that if the self and other perform similar actions, then self and other probably have similar experiences accompanying those actions. That is, the sense of volition that accompanies the self's actions is probably experienced by others when they act; more generally the other's conscious experience is probably much like the self's: "Other people's bodies, says the child to himself, have experiences *in them* such as mine has. They are also me's" (p. 14). This discovery is the defining feature of Baldwin's ejective stage, and allows the child to empathize with others (because the child now understands that others experience emotional states similar to the self's).

A final mechanism of self-knowledge is *social attunement*, where knowledge of the self is acquired through inferring what others believe of the self. This mechanism has its roots in symbolic interactionism, particularly in the work of George H. Mead (1934). Mead argued that communication facilitates self-reflection: "The importance of what we term 'communication' lies in the fact that it provides a form of behavior in which the organism or the individual may become an object to himself" (p. 138). Mead suggested that early in the development of self-consciousness, the child mentally assumes specific perspectives—that of the mother, that of the father, that of the peer, and so on—from each of which the self is viewed differently; consequently, the child discerns little unity in the self and experiences the self differently across roles. This leads to role-specific behavior:

> The child is one thing at one time and another at another, and what he is at one moment does not determine what he is at another. That is both the charm of childhood as well as its inadequacy. You cannot count on the child; you cannot assume all the things he does are going to determine what he will do at any moment. He is not organized into a whole. (p. 159)

With extensive social experience in groups and in networks of relationships, the child develops the ability to infer commonalities among the various perspectives he or she imaginatively assumes, and acquires a fully developed self:

> Full development of the individual's self is constituted not only by an organization of these particular individual attitudes, but also by an organization of the social attitudes of the generalized other or the social group as a whole to which he belongs. (p. 158)

It is only in this last stage of self-development that the individual acquires sufficient self-coherency to be able to act consistently across contexts.

Three points of agreement can be noted in these accounts. The first is that in the first two accounts, agency, or the experience of volition, plays a central role in the emergence of self-knowledge. Infants learn that they cannot control others, Ausubel

The Development of Self-Knowledge

(1949) notes, and Baldwin (1906) suggests that infants identify experiences of volition that arise with actions of the self but do not intrude into consciousness when visually identical actions are performed by the self. Second, both Ausubel and Baldwin focus their accounts on the developmental acquisition of knowledge of the self's boundaries, which suggests each believed that distinguishing self from nonself is an achievement dependent upon considerable experience with an interpersonal world. Finally, all three points view early self-knowledge as emerging in interactions with others. The argument that self-knowledge emerges in a social context has become a fundamental tenet of many theories of self and remains influential today (e.g., Fogel, 1993, 1995; Lewis, 1999; Neisser, 1991; Stern, 1985).

Contemporary Directions on the Development of Self-Knowledge

One notable trend of the last 20 years is that research on the self has focused on perceptual and cognitive mechanisms that may give rise to self-knowledge. As we reviewed, traditional approaches—the neopsychoanalytic, cognitive-developmental, symbolic interactionist paradigms—noted in the previous section have emphasized the gradual construction of self-boundaries through social interaction, yet have not been specific about the underlying mechanisms. However, with methodological and technological advances, modern-day researchers highlight the critical roles that specific perceptual, cognitive, and biological brain-based mechanisms play in self-knowledge development, and how these dynamically interact with objects and people in our world. We briefly review some of this research below.

Imitation

Infant imitation in an important area of inquiry as it relates to the development of self-knowledge. Imitation requires an active mapping between the self and other. Specifically, infants are beginning to detect the similarities between their actions and those of others. Through reciprocal imitation infants are also focusing their attention on and learning from others. Meltzoff and Williamson (2010) argue that imitation is foundational to the development of later social-cognitive milestones such as the mastery of theory of mind, where children use their own self-experiences in order to understand those of others.

The discovery of *mirror neurons* has drawn renewed attention to imitation as a means of obtaining information about the self. Mirror neurons are found in humans in great density at the posterior edge of the frontal lobes and the anterior portion of the parietal lobes (Iacoboni & Dapretto, 2006), and have the unique property of being activated nearly equally by an action performed by the self and the same action performed by another. For example, the hand reaching for an object might cause a mirror neuron to fire; watching another reach for the object causes the same discharge in the same neuron. Mirror neurons consequently contribute to the causal understanding of how imitation of shared experiences occur, although they alone are not sufficient. Nevertheless, the research on mirror neurons has led to further brain imaging studies that have revealed shared neural circuitry for the observation and execution of acts in later adulthood (Iacoboni, 2005).

Perceptual Mechanisms

Rochat and Hespos (1997) focused on identifying the perceptual origins of self-knowledge. They reported that newborns are able to discriminate between double-touch (i.e., where they touched themselves) and single-touch stimulation (i.e., an external object touched them) to the cheek. At 3 months, infants are able to discriminate between unfamiliar and familiar (i.e., how they typically view their legs given the proprioceptive calibration of the head to body) views of their leg motions through online video feeds looking longer at the former over the latter (Rochat & Morgan, 1995). Hence, these results provide evidence that infants have an early perceptual sense of their own physical bodies that may be the precursor to an explicit conceptual sense of self.

Ehrsson, Spence, and Passingham (2004) demonstrated one illusion concerning the self's boundaries that is an example of the trend toward brain-based perceptual capacities in the study of self. Adult participants were seated at a table on which a prosthetic hand was visible; their own hands were occluded from view. With participants viewing the prosthetic hand, identical locations on the prosthetic hand and on their hidden hands were stimulated, creating the illusion that the prosthetic hand belonged to the self. This illusion illuminates the powerful roles of perception in defining the boundaries of self. In a later study (Ehrsson, Holmes, & Passingham, 2005), the illusion was found to be associated with activity in areas of the brain known to be important for integrating information from different senses.

The importance of sensory integration for the sense of self is evident in another illusion involving visual afterimages, the dim photograph-like images perceptible for seconds after brief exposures to very bright lights. If participants are looking at their hands when exposed to very bright light, the afterimages they see include their hands. However, if they move their hands after exposure to the flash of light, the representations of their hands in the afterimages disappears (Carlson, Alvarez, Wu, & Verstraten, 2010). This phenomenon demonstrates that there are connections between visual images and motor experiences of self. Particularly interesting is the finding that if an individual is holding an object with a hand, and the hand and object move following exposure to a bright light, the resulting afterimage evidences deterioration of the sensation of the hand and object. However, if the object is not held but is near the hand, and then is moved mechanically following exposure to the light, the afterimage shows no deterioration specific to the object. This suggests a held object that moves in concert with the hand is incorporated into the representation of self (Carlson et al., 2010). Like the research described earlier, the findings from research on afterimages suggest that the boundaries of self can be extended to include inanimate objects as a result of perceptual cues.

One way of interpreting this set of findings is to suggest that powerful sensory cues, or environmental affordances allow for distinctions between self and nonself at very early ages. Bremner, Holmes, and Spence (2008) argue that infants have very good knowledge of space relations within short distances of the self, with this understanding of spatial relations constructed upon the self's actions and body schema. This early understanding, based on the self's orientation to its immediate environment, is complemented by a more slowly developing understanding of spatial relations that exist outside the immediate, peripersonal space of the child.

Statistical Sensitivity

Research on social cognition in young children suggests that infants and preschoolers are able to make inferences about others based on statistical inferences. Kushnir, Xu, and Wellman (2010) asked toddlers (20 months of age, on average) to observe adults pulling toys out of clear plastic boxes. In one box, the target toy (either a frog or duck) was present in the box in the ratio of 31:7 (majority condition), and in the other box the target toy was in the minority (7:31). Toddlers observed the adult withdraw the same toy from the same box on five successive trials. Next, the experimenter asked the toddler to select a toy of his or her choosing and deliver it to the experimenter. Infants who observed the experimenter choose the target toy from the box in which the target toy was in the minority were more likely to choose that toy to deliver to the experimenter than were toddlers who watched the experimenter choose the target toy from the box in which the target toy was in the majority. The inference is that this occurs because toddlers can easily infer a preference for the target toy with the experimenter's repeated withdrawal of that toy, and that it is unlikely to reflect a random selection (the experimenter is unlikely to be withdrawing the target toy on five successive draws from a box in which there are many other types of toys, unless the experimenter is *selecting* the target toy; random selection could be occurring, however, when the experimenter selects the target toy on five successive draws when the target toy is in the majority). This study reveals that older infants are able to make inferences about others based on statistical information concerning the likelihood of different information. The findings do not pertain directly to self-knowledge; however, it seems possible that if older infants can make use of statistical information to make judgments about others, they can do so to make judgments about themselves.

Awareness of Capacities

Studies by Kagan (1981) and Richman and colleagues (1983) suggest that toddlers develop knowledge of their capabilities at about the same time that mark-directed behavior is first exhibited, such as being able to touch a rouge mark on their nose when gazing upon the self in a mirror. Researchers modeled both simple and complex actions to infants of a variety of ages, and found that a common response in infants 18–22 months of age was to imitate the simple actions but to exhibit distress and refuse to imitate after observing the complex actions. Kagan and Richman and colleagues inferred from this pattern that infants at this age were aware of their own capabilities, recognized the implicit demand to imitate the actions of the experimenter, and did so if they were able, but they reacted negatively to invitations to imitate actions that they knew exceeded their capabilities. In other words, toddlers have knowledge of the self's abilities.

Memory Maturation

One of the central achievements of the study of early cognitive development has been the demonstration that many skills long thought to emerge in middle childhood are in fact present even at young ages. Research on memory has illuminated that young infants are capable of not only recognition memory—a capacity long known to exist in infants—but also semantic and episodic memory (Hayne, 2004), the latter two forms of memory referring to the retention of explicit facts and events. However, while even young infants have these different memory capacities, early memory is characterized by high rates of forgetting, lack of detail, and an extremely limited accessibility to recall, with all these limitations diminishing dramatically over early childhood (Hayne, 2004). With the dynamic development of many interrelated cognitive systems, including language, memory, self and other forms of mental representations, and differing forms of narrative experiences, personal memories are believed to take shape in the fourth year of life (Nelson & Fivush, 2004). Moreover, personal memories, of the type important for self-knowledge, may draw upon neural circuits dependent upon a level of maturation in the frontal lobes not reached until approximately 4 years of age (Levine, 2004). Contemporary research, then, suggests that very early personal memories are likely to be short-lived and inaccessible, with major improvements occurring in the third and fourth years of life.

A Common Neural Basis to the Self

Recently, Spreng, Mar, and Kim (2009) have argued that an early developing neural system is responsible for different types of behaviors involving the self and the understanding of others' minds. This claim is important in several respects. First of all, it suggests a set of specific neural circuits, based in the medial prefrontal, medial temporal, and medial and lateral parietal regions of the brain, that generate phenomena of interest to scientists interested in self- and social cognition. Second, the idea that there is a single *self-projection* system of the brain responsible for self- and social cognition suggests that phenomena traditionally considered to be independent of each other—for example, the ability to attribute beliefs and thoughts to others (the focus of research for developmental and comparative researchers studying theory of mind), early autobiographical memories, the navigation of the self through space, and so on—are in fact united by their common neural and psychological processes. The idea that a single set of neural circuits regulates disparate kinds of actions and judgments is deeply provocative; while further work is necessary to explore the value of this idea for understanding self-knowledge development, it is in our view promising and suggests that researchers interested in the development should consider the possibility that self-knowledge incorporates inferences about the minds of others and the location of the self in physical space.

Social Attunement

While it is certainly true that inferring the perspectives of others toward the self can lead to self-knowledge, as Mead (1934) pointed out, it need not always do so (see also Srivastava, Chapter 7, this volume). As Vazire (2010) has pointed out, the perspectives of others—even once integrated in the form Mead suggests constitutes the apex of development—do not necessarily lead to self-knowledge. There are facets of the self with which others may not be concerned or they may lack relevant information. For example, Vazire has demonstrated that adults typically have more accurate insights into their own emotion tones than into the moods of others. Little is known about the developmental course of children's sensitivity to the value of the perspectives of others for gaining self-knowledge, though it seems likely that this development occurs over the course of childhood and adolescence.

Developmental Sequencing of Knowledge Acquisition Processes

This brief overview of mechanisms of self-knowledge reflects our hypothesized developmental ordering. We propose that mechanisms for deriving information about the self from imitation and perception are probably present at birth and are operational in the first year of life. Perhaps because the phenomena corresponding to these mechanisms are recently discovered, very little is known about how these mechanisms relate specifically to the emergence of a sense of self and its later development. In our view, these mechanisms offer rich opportunities for exploring the early development of self-knowledge.

The ability to draw upon statistical generalizations, successes and failures, personal memories, and the perspectives of others may not be present at birth, and may develop more slowly, perhaps well into adolescence. Little is known about either the trajectories of development in these mechanisms or their interactions with each other. One can imagine statistical information about the self and personal memories may yield different representations of self, and the reconciliation of these different kinds of information may assume a different form in adolescence than in childhood. There have been attempts to find common neurological bases for these cognitive capacities that are promising avenues of exploration in our understanding of self-knowledge development.

Finally, the contemporary research reviewed in this section suggests that self-knowledge is unlikely to be the result of a single insight derived from one social process, as postulated by Ausubel, Baldwin, and Mead; instead, we and others suggest that notions of self arise from a range of social, perceptual, cognitive, and biological processes dynamically interacting. Because these processes follow independent developmental trajectories, and correspond to different facets of self, it is unlikely that they yield a tightly integrated set of propositions concerning the self.

Development in Self-Knowledge

The sequencing of mechanisms of self-knowledge development is in correspondence with some of the most important findings on the development of self-knowledge. Space limitations preclude a thorough review of this literature; in this section, we limit our discussion to the diversity of findings and their relations to the mechanisms of self-knowledge. As noted earlier, only representations of self and personal memories are well characterized in terms of knowledge, and our review is limited to these facets of the self.

Representations

Physical Representations of Self

We proposed that perceptual and cognitive mechanisms for acquiring information about the body are present early in development. Perhaps not surprisingly, therefore, some of the most compelling early evidence for self-knowledge concerns physical characteristics of self. While there are clear signs of implicit self-knowledge in early infancy, as we reviewed earlier, evidence of explicit self-representation does not emerge until later. The best evidence for self-knowledge in infancy and early childhood makes use of the mirror self-recognition task. To briefly summarize it (for descriptions, see Amsterdam, 1972; Lewis & Brooks-Gunn, 1979), infants are first placed in front of a mirror and their behavior is observed; this serves as a baseline against which to judge infants' behavior in subsequent trials. Next, the mirror is turned away and the infant's face is surreptitiously marked with rouge on the ear or nose. The infant is once again seated in front of a mirror, and behavior is observed once again. At approximately 18 to 24 months of age, a human infant in this second episode shows *mark-directed behavior* by touching the rouge on its face, which it can only see by inspecting its image in the mirror.

Several facets of mark-directed behavior are relevant. First, the behavior indicates self-reflection because infants focus attention on representations of themselves in the mirror. Second, mark-directed behavior is an indication of identification with the image; the infant knows that the image marred with rouge is of him- or herself, and is sufficiently disturbed by the anomaly in the self's typical appearance to explore it tactually. Finally, mark-directed behavior is a demonstration that infants have constructed representations of their physical appearances, and have some knowledge of what their faces typically look like—and know that their faces typically do not have rouge on them (interestingly, this capability seems to depend little on the amount of exposure to mirrors, as it develops at about the same age even in infants with relatively little exposure of reflective surfaces; Priel & de Schonen, 1986).

Knowledge of the self's physical characteristics continues to develop into the third year of life. Brownell, Zerwas, and Ramani (2007) encouraged children between 17 and 30 months of age to attempt tasks that tapped knowledge of the self's characteristics. For example, children were encouraged to put on hats that were too small for their heads, and to crawl through an opening with two doors, one of which was too small for them to pass through. The number of errors—attempts to perform actions made impossible by the size or location of their bodies and appendages—was recorded. Brownell and colleagues found that the number of errors decreased with age, suggesting that children were developing more accrate representations of their bodies. In a second study, Brownell, Nichols, Svetlova, Zerwas, and Ramani (2010) asked children to place stickers on body locations modeled by an experimenter. Children who could correctly place a sticker on their elbows and 11 other locations, when a similar action was modeled by the experimenter, were judged to have knowledge of the location of various body parts and their locations. As children grew older, their ability to correctly locate the stickers increased.

Mark-directed behavior also occurs at about the same time that toddlers learn to appreciate the effects that their bodies' locations have on other objects. Moore, Mealiea, Garon, and Povinelli (2007) asked toddlers to push small carts with mats attached to the back. Toddlers pushing from directly behind the carts would stand on the mat and would then be unable to move the carts. Older toddlers (21 months of age) were more likely than younger toddlers (15 months of age) to solve the problem and push the cart from the side. Moore and colleagues interpreted this trend to indicate development in knowledge of the self's body in relation to the world.

Representations of Capabilities

As mentioned, studies by Kagan (1981) and his colleagues (Richman et al., 1983) suggest that toddlers have knowledge of the self's abilities. Over the next several years, children's success in reaching a standard continues to develop. Stipek, Recchia, McClintic, and Lewis (1992) studied affective responses to success and failure in children between 2 and 5 years of age. Although the findings weren't entirely consistent for expressions of positive emotion, the authors found that older children expressed more negative emotion than did younger children in response to failures. This suggests that older children were more likely to understand that they had failed on the task, and that the failure reflected poorly on the self's capabilities.

Hart and Matsuba (2007) and Lewis (2007) have highlighted the importance of the self in the development of self-conscious emotions such as pride, guilt, and shame. Lewis was able to demonstrate 3-year-olds' experiences of shame or pride relative to their failure or success at a task, but that these experiences were also dependent on children's attentional focus (i.e., being task-oriented vs. performance/self-oriented). Those children who were task-focused experienced relatively little shame when they failed an easy task, attributing most of their failure to the task and away from the self. In contrast, those children who were performance-focused experienced significantly more shame when they failed the same easy task, attributing their failure more to themselves. These findings further illustrate the link between self and emotional development.

One of the most frequently studied areas of self-evaluation is academic achievement. In a series of studies, Marsh and his colleagues (e.g., Marsh, Köller, & Baumert, 2001) studied adolescents' judgments regarding their academic abilities in the context of classmates' academic abilities. The general pattern found across countries is that adolescents' judgments of their own academic abilities rest most heavily on their achievements in their classes, as indexed by the grades they receive for their academic work: Adolescents receiving high grades for their academic work judge themselves to be talented academically. However, judgments about the self's abilities also depend in part on the success of classmates. The average achievement level for an adolescent's classmates is *inversely* associated with judgments of the self's abilities. This is the big fish–little pond effect. One's judgments about the self's academic abilities are most positive when one's classmates are weak students, and least favorable when one's peers are high-achieving students. This well-studied effect shows little relationship to age through adolescence (e.g., Marsh, Kong, & Hau, 2000) and is found in a variety of the world's cultures (Seaton, Marsh, & Craven, 2009). The big fish–little pond effect also illustrates the difficulty of obtaining self-knowledge of one's academic ability because it does depend on context and an adolescent's cognitive abilities to understand the self in this context.

Personal Memories

Memories of personally meaningful events are important constituents of the sense of self. To some degree, memories can be characterized as accurate or inaccurate, and consequently can be judged to be truthful or not. Adolescents and adults have few personal memories for their lives prior to the age of 4 or 5. However, infants and young children do form personal memories that are retained for short periods of time and, with rehearsal, can be retained over longer periods of time (Hartshorn, 2003). In one fascinating study, Wang (2008) asked mothers of 3-year-olds for two relevant events for their children that had occurred in the previous 2 months. Children then were questioned about these events. Wang followed the children longitudinally, using the same procedure at testing times 6 and 19 months subsequent to the initial assessment. At each assessment, children were also asked to identify situations that produced different types of emotions in order to measure their knowledge about emotions. As children aged, their ability to provide accurate details of personal memories increased. Wang found that the ability to provide accurate details in personal memories seems dependent, in part, upon children's knowledge of emotions.

There is evidence as well that, with age, children become better able to distinguish between personal memories of real events and false memories. *False memories* are memories for events not experienced by the individual. Children's false memories have frequently been studied. Oftentimes in this kind of research an experimenter proposes to a child that he or she experienced an event that never occurred, with the goal of determining whether the child will report the never-experienced event as a memory. In various studies, children have been asked to remember events they never actually experienced, such as medical mishaps, separation from parents, and physical pain. Generally, but not always, the evidence indicates that older children are more accurate than younger children in discerning real memories from false ones (Brainerd, Reyna, & Ceci, 2008).

Conclusions

Acquiring knowledge about the self is made difficult by the multiple facets of self, several of which are difficult to align with standards of knowledge. For example, self-identification and theories or narratives of self seem to exist apart from knowledge. Consider self-identification: Because we usually judge that individuals are the final arbiters of what is, and what is not, included in the self, people generally cannot be wrong about some aspects of the self. Theories and narratives of self seem to be impervious to evidence; it would be difficult to judge, for example, that the stories people tell about themselves after psychotherapy are in some important way more "true" than they were before experiencing psychotherapy (see also Adler, Chapter 20, this volume).

Contemporary cognitive and developmental research suggests that self-knowledge—concerning facets of self for which knowledge is possible—likely rests upon a variety of perceptual, cognitive, biological, and social processes that dynamically interact as infants and children actively explore their world. As a consequence, traditional theories that emphasize the developmental acquisition of fundamental insights regarding the self relative to social interactions must be complemented with new findings suggesting the early emergence of knowledge of the body and its properties.

New research on mechanisms that contribute to self-knowledge provides fascinating opportunities to explore how children acquire early self-knowledge, and how this self-knowledge might develop. The opportunities for synthesizing insights from disciplines traditionally isolated from each other—neuroscience, cognitive psychology, social/personality psychology, developmental psychology—for the study of the development of self-knowledge have never been richer.

REFERENCES

Amsterdam, B. (1972). Mirror self-image reactions before age two. *Developmental Psychobiology, 5*(4), 297–305.

Ausubel, D. P. (1949). Ego-development and the learning process. *Child development, 20*, 173–190.

Baldwin, J. M. (1906). *Social and ethical interpretations in mental development* (4th ed.). New York: Macmillan.

Brainerd, C. J., Reyna, V. F., & Ceci, S. J. (2008). Developmental reversals in false memory: A review of data and theory. *Psychological Bulletin, 134*(3), 343–382.

Bremner, A. J., Holmes, N. P., & Spence, C. (2008). Infants lost in (peripersonal) space? *Trends in Cognitive Sciences, 12*(8), 298–305.

Brownell, C. A., Nichols, S. R., Svetlova, M., Zerwas, S., & Ramani, G. (2010). The head bone's connected to the neck bone: When do toddlers represent their own body topography? *Child Development, 81*(3), 797–810.

Brownell, C. A., Zerwas, S., & Ramani, G. B. (2007). "So big": The development of body self-awareness in toddlers. *Child Development, 78*(5), 1426–1440.

Carlson, T. A., Alvarez, G., Wu, D., & Verstraten, F. A. (2010). Rapid assimilation of external objects into the body schema. *Psychological Science, 21*(7), 1000–1005.

Davidson, D. (1984). First person authority. *Dialectica, 38*(2–3), 101–111.

Ehrsson, H. H., Holmes, N. P., & Passingham, R. E. (2005). Touching a rubber hand: Feeling of body ownership is associated with activity in multisensory brain areas. *Journal of Neuroscience, 25*(45), 10564–10573.

Ehrsson, H. H., Spence, C., & Passingham, R. E. (2004). That's my hand!: Activity in premotor cortex reflects feeling of ownership of a limb. *Science, 305*, 875–877.

Fogel, A. (1993). *Developing through relationships: Origins of communication, self and culture*. Hemel Hempstead, UK: Harvester Press.

Fogel, A. (1995). Relational narratives of the prelinguistic self. In P. Rochat (Ed.), *The self in infancy: Theory and research* (pp. 117–140). Amsterdam: Elsevier.

Hart, D., & Matsuba, M. K. (2007). The development of pride and moral life. In J. L. Tracy, R. W. Robins, & J. P. Tangney (Eds.), *The self-conscious emotions: Theory and research* (pp. 114–133). New York: Guilford Press.

Hartshorn, K. (2003). Reinstatement maintains a memory in human infants for 1½ years. *Developmental Psychobiology, 42*, 269–282.

Hayne, H. (2004). Infant memory development: Implications for childhood amnesia. *Developmental Review, 24*(1), 33–73.

Iacoboni, M. (2005). Neural mechanisms of imitation. *Current Opinion in Neurobiology, 15*, 632–637.

Iacoboni, M., & Dapretto, M. (2006). The mirror neuron system and the consequences of its dysfunction. *Nature Reviews Neuroscience, 7*(12), 942–951.

James, W. (1998). *Principles of psychology*. Chicago: University of Chicago Press. (Original work published 1890)

Kagan, J. (1981). *The second year: The emergence of self-awareness*. Cambridge, MA: Harvard University Press.

Kushnir, T., Xu, F., & Wellman, H. M. (2010). Young children use statistical sampling to infer the preferences of other people. *Psychological Science, 21*(8), 1134–1140.

Levine, B. (2004). Autobiographical memory and the self in time: Brain lesion effects, functional neuroanatomy, and lifespan development. *Brain and Cognition, 55*(1), 54–68.

Lewis, M. (1999). Social cognition and the self. In P. Rochat (Ed.), *Early social cognition: Understanding others in the first months of life* (pp. 81–100). Mahwah, NJ: Erlbaum.

Lewis, M. (2007). Self-conscious emotional development. In J. L. Tracy, R. W. Robins, & J. P. Tangney (Eds.), *The self-conscious emotions: Theory and research* (pp. 134–149). New York: Guilford Press.

Lewis, M., & Brooks-Gunn, J. (1979). *Social cognition and the acquisition of self.* New York: Plenum.

Marsh, H. W., Köller, O., & Baumert, J. (2001). Reunification of East and West German school systems: Longitudinal multilevel modeling study of the big fish–little pond effect on academic self-concept. *American Educational Research Journal, 38*(2), 321–350.

Marsh, H. W., Kong, C. K., & Hau, K. T. (2000). Longitudinal multilevel modeling of the Big Fish Little Pond effect on academic self-concept: Counterbalancing social comparison and reflected glory effects in Hong Kong high schools. *Journal of Personality and Social Psychology, 78,* 337–349.

Mead, G. H. (1934). *Mind, self and society.* Chicago: University of Chicago Press.

Meltzoff, A. N., & Williamson, R. A. (2010). The importance of imitation for theories of social-cognitive development. In J. G. Bremner & T. D. Wachs (Eds.), *Infant development* (2nd ed., Vol. 1., pp. 345–364). West Sussex, UK: Wiley-Blackwell.

Moore, C., Mealiea, J., Garon, N., & Povinelli, D. J. (2007). The development of body self-awareness. *Infancy, 11*(2), 157–174.

Neisser, U. (1991). Two perceptually given aspects of the self and their development. *Developmental Review, 11,* 197–209.

Nelson, K., & Fivush, R. (2004). The emergence of autobiographical memory: A social cultural developmental theory. *Psychological Review, 111,* 486–511.

Priel, B., & de Schonen, S. (1986). Self-recognition: A study of a population without mirrors. *Journal of Experimental Child Psychology, 41*(2), 237–250.

Richman, C. L., Novack, T., Price, C., Adams, K. A., Mitchell, D., Reznick, J. S., et al. (1983). The consequences of failing to imitate. *Motivation and Emotion, 7,* 157–167.

Rochat, P., & Hespos, S. J. (1997). Differential rooting response by neonates: Evidence for an early sense of self. *Early Development and Parenting, 6,* 105–112.

Rochat, P., & Morgan, R. (1995). Spatial determinants in the perception of self-produced leg movements by 3–5 month old infants. *Developmental Psychology, 31,* 626–636.

Ross, B. M. (1991). *Remembering the personal past: Descriptions of autobiographical memory.* New York: Oxford University Press.

Scheffler, I. (1983). *Conditions of knowledge: An introduction to epistemology and education.* Chicago: University of Chicago Press.

Seaton, M., Marsh, H. W., & Craven, R. G. (2009). Earning its place as a pan-human theory: Universality of the Big Fish–Little Pond effect across 41 culturally and economically diverse countries. *Journal of Educational Psychology, 101*(2), 403–419.

Spreng, R. N., Mar, R. A., & Kim, A. S. N. (2009). The common neural basis of autobiographical memory, prospection, navigation, theory of mind, and the default mode: A quantitative meta-analysis. *Journal of Cognitive Neuroscience, 21,* 489–510.

Stern, D. (1985). *The interpersonal world of the infant.* New York: Basic Books.

Steup, M. (2008). The analysis of knowledge. In E. N. Zalta (Ed.), *The Stanford encyclopedia of philosophy.* Stanford, CA: Stanford University Press. Retrieved from *http://plato.stanford.edu/archives/fall2008/entries/knowledge-analysis.*

Stipek, D., Recchia, S., McClintic, S., & Lewis, M. (1992). Self-evaluation in young children. *Monographs of the Society for Research in Child Development, 57*(1), 1–95.

Vazire, S. (2010). Who knows what about a person?: The self–other knowledge asymmetry (SOKA) model. *Personality Processes and Individual Differences, 2*, 281–300.

Wang, Q. (2008). Emotion knowledge and autobiographical memory across the preschool years: A cross-cultural longitudinal investigation. *Cognition, 108*(1), 117–135.

Williams, B. (1995). Ethics. In A. C. Grayling (Ed.), *Philosophy: A guide through the subject* (pp. 545–582). Oxford, UK: Oxford University Press.

CHAPTER 3

Self-Insight from a Dual-Process Perspective

BERTRAM GAWRONSKI
GALEN V. BODENHAUSEN

Many cultures consider self-insight an important virtue for a fulfilled and authentic life (Wilson & Dunn, 2004). Challenging the feasibility of this enterprise, however, research in psychology has uncovered a plethora of obstacles that can undermine accurate self-knowledge, many of which are reviewed in this handbook. This chapter provides a conceptual analysis of these obstacles from a dual-process perspective. Over the past decades, dual-process approaches have provided theoretical guidance for virtually all areas of psychology, offering conceptual integrations of existing evidence and novel predictions of previously undetected phenomena (for a review, see Gawronski & Creighton, in press). Yet, despite their popularity, there have been few attempts to analyze the mental underpinnings of self-knowledge from a dual-process perspective (for a notable exception, see Epstein, 1994). The main goal of this chapter is to fill this gap.

Toward this end, we refrain from providing an exhaustive review of specific dual-process theories. Instead, we use the common foundation of dual-process theories—the distinction between automatic and controlled processes—to illustrate the range and the limits of people's insights into the causes, the contents, and the effects of their mental associations. Our focus on mental associations is based on recent definitions of major social-psychological constructs as associations between two concepts in memory (e.g., Greenwald et al., 2002). For example, the construct of *attitude* has been defined as the mental association between an object and its evaluation (Fazio, 1995). Correspondingly, *self-esteem* can be defined as the association between the self and its evaluation, just as *prejudice* can be defined as the association between a social group and its evaluation (Greenwald et al., 2002). With regard to nonevaluative constructs, *self-concept* can be defined as the association between the self and its attributes (e.g., self–extraverted), just as *stereotypes* can be conceptualized as associations between a social category and stereotypical attributes (e.g., women–warm). At a more complex level, goals can be conceptualized as a combination of two associations, namely, an association between means and an end-state (Kruglanski et al., 2002), and an additional association between the end-state and its evaluation (Custers & Aarts, 2005). In the following sections, we first discuss the notion of automaticity and control as the common foundation of dual-process theories. Expanding on this discussion, we then outline various implications of this distinction for people's insights into the causes, the contents, and the effects of their mental associations, including attitudes, prejudices, stereotypes, self-esteem, self-concepts, and goals.[1]

Automaticity and Control

Dual-process theories have their roots in the assumption that mental processes can be characterized on the basis of whether they operate in an automatic or controlled fashion. The defining features of automatic processes are that (1) they do not involve conscious awareness; (2) they do not require a person's intention to be started; (3) they operate even under limited cognitive resources; and (4) they cannot be stopped or altered voluntarily. Conversely, controlled processes (1) operate under conscious awareness; (2) require a person's intention to be started; (3) fail to operate when cognitive resources are limited; and (4) can be stopped or altered voluntarily (Bargh, 1994; Moors & De Houwer, 2006). As we outline below, all of these features play a significant role for specific aspects of self-insight. Yet the most important characteristic for the current analysis is the first one: conscious awareness. With regard to people's insight into their mental associations, the object of awareness can be further divided into three different components: (1) awareness of the causes of one's mental associations, (2) awareness of the contents of one's mental associations, and (3) awareness of the effects of one's mental associations (Gawronski, Hofmann, & Wilbur, 2006). Specifically, individuals may or may not know why they have certain mental associations; they may or may not know that they have certain kinds of mental associations; and they may or may not know how their mental associations influence their behavior (see Figure 3.1).

Insight into the Causes of One's Mental Associations

Inaccurate beliefs about the causes of one's mental associations can have significant consequences if judgments and decisions are based on these beliefs. For example, Wilson argued that people are often unaware of the true causes of their preferences (e.g., Wilson, Dunn, Kraft, & Lisle, 1989). Thus, when analyzing reasons for their preferences, people tend to rely on reasons that are accessible and easy to communicate. Yet these reasons do not always reflect the true causes of their preferences, leading them to shift their preferences toward those that are in line with the generated reasons. To the extent that these momentarily constructed preferences are taken as a basis for choices and decisions, the quality of these decisions can be suboptimal in terms of subjective (e.g., Wilson et al., 1993) and objective (e.g., Wilson & Schooler, 1991) standards. In a study by Wilson and colleagues (1993), for example, participants were

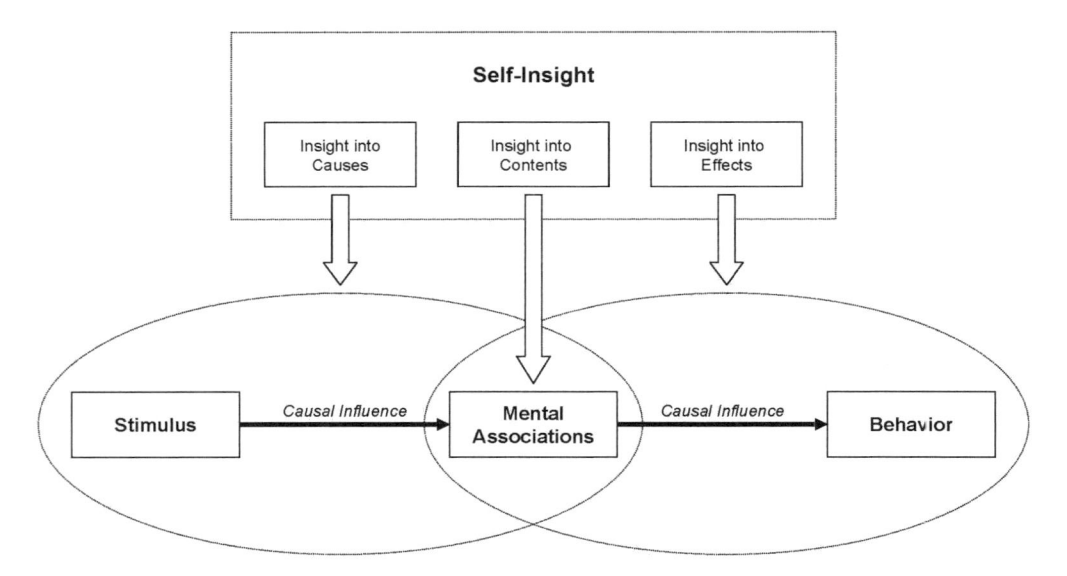

FIGURE 3.1. Different components of self-insight pertaining to the causes, contents, and effects of one's mental associations.

asked to choose between two kinds of posters. Half of the participants were additionally asked to think about reasons for their preference; participants in a control group were not asked to think about reasons. Those who were asked to think about reasons not only showed different preferences compared with those who were not asked to think about reasons but they were also less satisfied with their choice when they were contacted 3 weeks after the study.

From a theoretical perspective, accurate knowledge of the causes of one's mental associations requires awareness of three distinct components: (1) the causally relevant stimuli; (2) the mental associations themselves; and (3) the causal relation between the two (see Figure 3.1). Thus, insight into the causes of one's mental associations will be limited if people lack awareness of any one of these components.

Unawareness of Causally Influential Stimuli

In many cases, our mental associations are the product of conscious learning processes, for example, when we read a newspaper article about unhealthy ingredients of certain food products (*propositional learning*). Yet, in other cases, new associations are formed unintentionally outside of conscious awareness (*associative learning*). For example, research on evaluative conditioning (EC) has shown that repeated pairings of a formerly neutral conditioned stimulus (CS) with a positive or negative unconditioned stimulus (US) lead to changes in the evaluation of the CS in line with the valence of the US (for a meta-analysis, see Hofmann, De Houwer, Perugini, Baeyens, & Crombez, 2010). A common interpretation of these effects is that the CS–US pairings create a mental association between the CS and the US in memory (e.g., Gawronski & Bodenhausen, 2006, 2011). As a result, encountering the CS at future occasions activates the representation of the US, thereby producing an evaluative response to the CS that matches the one to the US (e.g., Baeyens, Eelen, Van den Bergh, & Crombez, 1992; Walther, Gawronski, Blank, & Langer, 2009). Importantly, some studies have shown EC effects even when the CS–US pairings involved subliminal presentations of the CS (e.g., Dijksterhuis, 2004; Gawronski & LeBel, 2008; Knight, Nguyen, & Bandettini, 2003) or the US (e.g., De Houwer, Hendrickx, & Baeyens, 1997; Krosnick, Betz, Jussim, & Lynn, 1992; Rydell, McConnell, Mackie, & Strain, 2006). These results suggest that mental associations can be formed without awareness of the relevant stimuli, implying that people can have mental associations without knowing their causal origin.

Whereas research on EC is concerned with the *formation* of mental associations, priming effects refer to the *activation* of existing associations. Similar to EC research using subliminal presentations of the CS or the US, a large body of research shows that subliminal presentations of stimuli can activate mental associations in memory (e.g., Wittenbrink, Judd, & Park, 1997). One of the most prominent examples in this regard is Devine's (1989) research on automatic and controlled processes in prejudice and stereotyping. In her study, participants were subliminally primed either with evaluatively neutral words or with words related to the stereotype of African Americans, and then read a brief story about a target who behaved ambiguously (cf. Bargh & Pietromonaco, 1982). Results showed that the behavior of the target was interpreted more negatively when participants were primed with the stereotype of African Americans than when they were primed with neutral words. Applied to the present question, these results suggest that participants had particular thoughts while reading the description of the behavior without being aware of the stimuli that were responsible for these thoughts. As a result, they misattributed their thoughts to the behavior of the target, thereby leading to more negative interpretations of the ambiguous behavior when they were primed with the stereotype of African Americans.

Similar effects have been found for the unconscious activation of goals. For example, Ferguson (2008) subliminally primed participants with words related to the goal of being thin or neutral control words that were unrelated to the goal of being thin. Afterwards, all participants completed a measure of automatic evaluations of diet-related words. Participants in the control condition showed relatively neutral responses to the diet-related words regardless of their dieting skills (which were assessed prior to the study). In contrast, participants in the goal-priming condition showed positive responses to the diet-related words when their dieting skills were high, but negative responses when their dieting skills were low. As with Devine's (1989) research, these results suggest that goals can be activated by goal-related stimuli without conscious awareness of these stimuli.

Unawareness of Causal Link

In many situations, people are consciously aware of the momentarily present stimuli, but they may not be aware of the causal impact of these stimuli on their mental associations. For example, research on EC effects often uses procedures with supraliminal presentations, in which participants are consciously aware of both the CS and the US. Yet when subsequently asked to report which CS was paired with which US, participants are sometimes unable to identify correctly the specific CS–US contingencies.

Even though EC effects tend to be larger when participants have conscious knowledge of the relevant CS–US pairings (for a meta-analysis, see Hofmann et al., 2010), a considerable body of research has found significant EC effects in the absence of contingency awareness (e.g., Baeyens, Eelen, & Van den Bergh, 1990; Olson & Fazio, 2001; Sweldens, Van Osselaer, & Janiszewski, 2010; Walther & Nagengast, 2006). Given that CS–US contingencies represent an important component in the causal link that is responsible for the newly formed associations, these results suggests that people can have mental associations without being aware of the causal link between their mental associations and consciously encoded stimuli.

Similar considerations apply to the activation of existing associations in priming effects. Instead of presenting the causally effective prime stimuli subliminally, many studies use procedures in which participants are consciously aware of the relevant primes. Yet they often remain unaware of the causal impact of the prime stimuli on their thoughts and behavior. For example, to activate the stereotype of older adults, Bargh, Chen, and Burrows (1996) used a scrambled-sentence task that was described as a test of language proficiency. For half of the participants, the task included words related to the older adults stereotype (e.g., *retired*). For the remaining half, the task included neutral words unrelated to the older adults stereotype (e.g., *thirsty*). The well-known finding is that participants walked slower down the hall at the end of the study when they were primed with stereotype-related words than when they were primed with stereotype-unrelated words. Note that in this task participants were fully aware of the words that were supposed to activate the stereotype of older adults. However, when participants were asked whether they thought that the words in the scrambled-sentence task might have affected them in any way, none of them believed that the words had any impact on their thoughts and behavior.

Similar procedures have been used in research on goal pursuit. For example, in Bargh, Gollwitzer, Lee-Chai, Barndollar, and Trötschel's (2001) seminal demonstration of unconscious goal priming, participants completed a word-search puzzle that included either words related to a high-performance goal (e.g., *succeed*) or neutral words that were unrelated to performance (e.g., *carpet*). Results showed that participants primed with performance-related words showed enhanced performance on a subsequent task compared with participants primed with neutral words. As with Bargh and colleagues' (1996) scrambled-sentence task, participants in this study were consciously aware of the words that were presented in the word-search puzzle. However, none of them thought that the words influenced their motivation or performance in the subsequent task. In other words, participants were consciously aware of the stimuli that influenced their momentary goals, but they were unaware of the causal impact these words had on their goals.

Unawareness of Mental Associations

A common interpretation in research on priming effects is that participants are not aware of the primed associations when these associations have been activated outside of conscious awareness. For example, in the literature on unconscious goal priming, it is often assumed that participants are not aware of their momentary goals if they (1) are not aware of the stimuli that activated these goals (e.g., Ferguson, 2008) or (2) are not aware of the causal impact of consciously perceived stimuli on their momentary goals (e.g., Bargh et al., 2001). This may well be true, but it is important to note that awareness of one's goals per se is conceptually distinct from awareness of the stimuli that influence one's goals, or awareness of the impact of these stimuli on one's goals. To establish empirically the unconsciousness of a goal, one would have to ask participants about their momentary goals rather than about the stimuli used to activate the goal or the perceived causal impact of these stimuli. Unfortunately, such measures are rarely included in research on unconscious goal pursuit, which makes inferences about the unconsciousness of the relevant goals premature (for a notable exception, see Bar-Anan, Wilson, & Hassin, 2010). This problem also applies to studies in which participants are asked about their goal-related behavior. For example, in a study by Bargh and colleagues (2001), participants were primed with cooperation-related words or neutral control words. Results showed that participants in the goal-priming condition showed more cooperation in a subsequent resource dilemma task compared with participants in the control condition. Yet participants' self-reports on how much they cooperated during the dilemma task were unrelated to their actual cooperation. In a strict sense, these findings show that participants' self-perceptions of their own behavior often deviate from their actual behavior. However, they remain silent about whether participants were aware or unaware of the primed goal. Again, to establish the unconsciousness of the goal per se, one would have to ask participants about the goal itself (e.g., "How important is it for you to cooperate during the task?"), not about their retrospective self-perception of their behavior. After all, there is an important difference between not knowing that one has a particular goal and having inaccurate perceptions of one's behavior.

To be fair, it is important to note that these issues seem less controversial in research on unconscious aspects of associative learning, in which the (un)consciousness of the resulting association is rarely conflated with (un)conscious aspects of the learning process that is responsible for this association. For example, most studies on EC effects assess evaluative representations by means of self-report measures that simply ask participants how much they like or dislike the CS (cf. Hofmann et al., 2010). In these studies, the relevant evaluative association is assumed to be consciously accessible even when certain aspects of the learning process that led to this association remain outside of conscious awareness (e.g., subliminal presentation of the stimuli, lack of contingency awareness). The important message is that unawareness of the relevant stimuli or the causal effect of these stimuli does not say anything about people's awareness of the relevant mental associations. The latter question is discussed in more detail in the following section.

Insight into the Contents of One's Mental Associations

One of the most central questions in the context of self-insight is whether people can have certain kinds of mental associations without being aware that they have these associations. In other words, is it possible that people have unconscious attitudes, unconscious prejudices, unconscious self-esteem, unconscious stereotypes, unconscious self-concepts, or unconscious goals (cf. Blanton & Jaccard, 2008; Buhrmester, Blanton, & Swann, 2011)? As illustrated in Figure 3.1, insight into the contents of one's mental associations—including the relevant concepts and the associative links between them—not only constitutes a key component in its own right, but also represents a central part in people's insight into the causes and the effects of their mental associations. If one is unaware of the existence of a particular mental association, it is logically impossible to know where this association is coming from and what effects it has on one's behavior.

In the dual-process literature, there are two classes of theories that make different assumptions about conscious and unconscious mental contents. Whereas some theories assume that conscious and unconscious contents are based on distinct memory structures that operate independently (e.g., Banaji, 2001; Rydell & McConnell, 2006), other theories assume that conscious and unconscious contents are based on the same memory structures, with unconscious contents being characterized by activation levels that do not pass the threshold of conscious awareness (e.g., Gawronski & Bodenhausen, 2006; Strack & Deutsch, 2004). Even though the debate between dual-representation and single-representation theories seems difficult to resolve on empirical grounds (Greenwald & Nosek, 2009), it is often assumed that unconscious associations can be captured with implicit measurement procedures, such as sequential priming tasks (e.g., Fazio, Jackson, Dunton, & Williams, 1995; Payne, Cheng, Govorun, & Stewart, 2005; Wittenbrink et al., 1997) and the Implicit Association Test (IAT; Greenwald, McGhee, & Schwartz, 1998). A common assumption in this research is that explicit self-report measures tap mental contents that are consciously accessible, whereas implicit measures provide access to associations that are introspectively inaccessible.

Of course, implicit measures do not presuppose introspective access for the assessment of mental contents. However, whether the mental contents captured by implicit measures are indeed unconscious is an empirical question that has to be tested as such (De Houwer, Teige-Mocigemba, Spruyt, & Moors, 2009). A frequently cited finding in support of the unconsciousness claim is that implicit and explicit measures often show rather low correspondence (Banaji, 2001). Yet further scrutiny of the available evidence suggests that the mental associations assessed by implicit measures are indeed consciously accessible, and that various other factors account for the frequently obtained dissociations between implicit and explicit measures (Fazio, 2007; Gawronski et al., 2006). In the domain of attitudes, for example, several studies have shown that implicit and explicit measures show rather high correspondence if participants focus on their gut feelings when reporting an evaluation (e.g., Banse, Seise, & Zerbes, 2001; Gawronski & LeBel, 2008; Hofmann, Gawronski, Gschwendner, Le, & Schmitt, 2005; Ranganath, Smith, & Nosek, 2008; Scarabis, Florack, & Gosejohann, 2006; Smith & Nosek, 2011). These results are difficult to reconcile with the claim that implicit measures tap mental associations that are generally inaccessible to introspection. Yet they are in line with dual-process theories that assume implicit measures tap spontaneous gut responses resulting from mental associations that are activated unintentionally upon the encounter of an attitude object (for a review, see Hofmann, Gschwendner, Nosek, & Schmitt, 2005). These gut responses, in turn, may serve as a basis for explicit judgments, unless the individual is motivated and able to deliberate on individual attributes of the object (Fazio, 2007) or the gut response is inconsistent with other momentarily considered information (Gawronski & Bodenhausen, 2006, 2011).

Even though the available evidence is consistent with dual-process accounts that emphasize other features of automaticity rather than the notion of awareness (e.g., intentionality, controllability; for a discussion, see Payne & Gawronski, 2010), it is worth noting that correspondence between implicit and explicit measures may be the result of at least three processes that have different implications for people's insight into the contents of their mental associations (see Hofmann & Wilson, 2010). First, it is possible that people have direct introspective access to their mental associations. In this case, there would be no a priori limits to people's ability to know their mental associations, and any lack of knowledge may be regarded as the product of insufficient motivation to introspect on one's associations. Second, there may be cases in which people have no direct access to their mental associations, but they may have indirect access through the subjective experiences that result from these associations. In such cases, people would have indirect access to contents that elicit subjective experiences (e.g., evaluative associations that elicit affective gut feelings), but there could be limits to the ability to know contents that do not elicit subjective experiences (e.g., purely semantic associations that do not elicit any feelings). Third, there may be cases in which people have no direct access to their associations, but they may have indirect access through self-perceptions of the behaviors that result from these associations (Bem, 1972). As with the first case, there would be no a priori limits to people's ability to know their mental associations, although knowledge of mental contents may be limited either when people fail to pay attention to their behavior (Carver & Scheier, 1981; Wicklund, 1975) or when their subjective interpretation of their behavior is biased (Jones & Nisbett, 1972). Yet what is essentially required is that people have accurate theories about what kinds of behaviors are caused by what kinds of associations. We return to the question of naive theories in the section on insights into the effects of mental associations.

Another important question in the context of attitudes concerns the correspondence between people's beliefs about what they like or dislike and their actual evaluative responses. Drawing on the distinction between implicit and explicit measures, one could argue that implicit measures capture people's actual responses to an attitude object, whereas explicit measures tap people's beliefs about what they like or dislike. From this perspective, correspondence between the two would indicate that people's beliefs about their attitudes are accurate, whereas dissociations between the two kinds of measures would indicate inaccurate self-beliefs. Even though this conceptualization resonates with interpretations of implicit measures as a window to people's "true self," we propose that self-beliefs and actual evaluative responses are rooted in two distinct types of mental associations, both of which could be assessed with implicit measures. Whereas self-beliefs could be considered as a particular aspect of one's self-concept, involving mental links between the self and the attribute of liking or disliking a particular object (e.g., an association between the concepts *self* and *liking baseball*), actual evaluative responses are presumably rooted in mental links between the object and positive or negative characteristics of that object (e.g., an association between the concepts *baseball* and *fun*). From this perspective, implicit measures may be designed to tap either one or the other type of association, and either type of association may influence self-reported liking under particular conditions.[2] Yet the two kinds of associations may have distinct antecedents, in that object-related associations stem from direct experiences with or communicated information about the object, whereas self-related associations are the product of self-perceptions of one's evaluative responses (see Gawronski et al., 2008). Even though the two kinds of associations may often show a high level of correspondence, there may be cases in which they dissociate, for example, when evaluative responses rooted in object-related associations are attributed to situational factors instead of internal attributes (e.g., Hofmann, Gschwendner, & Schmitt, 2009). In such cases, people's self-referential beliefs about whether they like or dislike a given attitude object may deviate from their actual evaluative response to that object. An illustrative example is the notion of aversive racism, in that aversive racists are assumed to experience negative feelings in response to racial outgroups, while being convinced that they have positive attitudes toward these groups (Dovidio & Gaertner, 2004).

Insight into the Effects of One's Mental Associations

A third question in the context of self-insight concerns the extent to which people are aware of the behavioral effects of their mental associations. In dual-process frameworks, awareness of the effects of mental associations is typically studied by means of behavioral control. A common assumption in dual-process theories is that people control for biasing influences on their behavior when three conditions are met. First, they have to be *motivated* to control their behavior for biasing influences. Second, they have to be *able* to engage in behavioral control. Third, they have to be *aware* of the biasing influence (e.g., Hall & Payne, 2010; Strack & Hannover, 1996; Wegener & Petty, 1997; Wilson & Brekke, 1994). To the extent that both the first and the second conditions are met, people are assumed to be unaware of the biasing influence if they fail to control their behavior despite their motivation and ability to do so. In such cases, lack of awareness may again involve one of three distinct components: (1) the mental associations themselves; (2) the relevant behavior; and (3) the causal relation between the two (see Figure 3.1). Thus, insight into the effects of mental associations can be limited if people are unaware of any of these components.

Unawareness of Mental Associations

To the extent that people can be unaware of momentarily activated associations and these associations nevertheless influence behavior, people may misattribute their behavior to other factors, which could lead to inaccurate self-beliefs. In line with this contention, Bar-Anan and colleagues (2010) showed that participants who were primed with a particular goal (e.g., affiliation) did not differ from control participants on a self-report measure of goal strength. Yet participants in the goal-priming condition were more likely to choose activities that were conducive to that goal. Importantly, when asked to explain their choices, participants misattributed their preferences to plausible reasons that were accessible and easy to communicate (e.g., stable dispositions) rather than their momentary goals, and the inaccurate self-beliefs resulting from these misattributions influenced subsequent choices in a manner that was consistent with their newly formed self-beliefs. These results are consistent with the proposition that awareness of the content of one's mental associations is an essential precondition for understanding their effects on one's behavior.

Unawareness of Behavior

A common implication of many dual-process theories is that implicit measures should be better predictors of spontaneous behavior, whereas explicit measures should show superior performance in the prediction of deliberate behavior (e.g., Fazio, 2007; Strack & Deutsch, 2004; Wilson, Lindsey, & Schooler, 2000). This prediction has been confirmed in a large number of studies that classified different kinds of behaviors on theoretical grounds as either spontaneous or deliberate (for reviews, see Friese, Hofmann, & Schmitt, 2008; Perugini, Richetin, & Zogmaister, 2010). The typical interpretation of these findings is that the spontaneous behaviors in these studies are difficult to control and therefore influenced by the automatically activated associations assessed by implicit measures. In other words, participants are assumed to be motivated to control their behavior, but they are unable to do so. Yet an alternative interpretation is that people are able to control at least some of the behaviors classified as spontaneous, but that they are unaware of how their mental associations affect these behaviors (see Gawronski et al., 2006). For example, speaking time (McConnell & Leibold, 2001) or spatial distance (Fazio et al., 1995) in social interactions with a black person seem relatively easy to control. However, people may be unaware of how these behaviors are affected by their evaluative associations regarding black people. As a result, they may not attempt to control these behaviors even if they have the motivation and the ability to do so (Strack & Hannover, 1996).

Unawareness of Causal Link

Even if people are consciously aware of their mental associations and the behaviors resulting from these associations, they may sometimes be unaware of the causal link between the two. One example in this regard is the impact of mental associations on the interpretation of ambiguous behavior. In a study by Gawronski, Geschke, and Banse (2003), for example, German participants were asked to form an impression of either a German or a Turkish individual on the basis of evaluatively ambiguous behavior. Consistent with previous research (e.g., Duncan, 1976; Sagar & Schofield, 1980), participants evaluated the behavior more negatively when the target was Turkish than when the target was German. However, this effect was moderated by participants' evaluative associations regarding Turks and Germans, such that the target's category membership influenced the interpretation of ambiguous behavior only for participants with a strong associative preference for Germans over Turks (see also Hugenberg & Bodenhausen, 2003). Importantly, the influence of evaluative associations was unaffected by participants' motivation to control prejudiced reactions. Instead, motivation to control prejudice moderated only the impact of evaluative associations on self-reported evaluations of Turkish people in general; that is, evaluative associations and self-reported evaluations showed a positive correlation only for participants low, but not for those high, in motivation to control prejudice (see Dunton & Fazio, 1997). Self-reported evaluations had no impact on the interpretation of ambiguous behavior. Thus, given that participants were generally able to control the influence of their evaluative associations on the interpretation of ambiguous behavior (i.e., participants were not under time pressure or otherwise cognitively depleted), these results suggest that participants were unaware of the impact of their evaluative associations on the interpretation of ambiguous behavior. In other words, evaluative associations influenced behavioral interpretations irrespective of participants' motivation and their ability to control for this influence (Strack & Hannover, 1996).

Another important factor in this context is the accuracy of people's naive theories about the causal impact of their mental associations on behavior (Strack, 1992; Wegener & Petty, 1997; Wilson & Brekke, 1994). Even if people are consciously aware of their thoughts and their behavior, causal relations between the two are not directly observable but have to be inferred from observed covariations. According to Wegner and Wheatley (1999), such inferences about mental causation are guided by three general principles. First, the thought should precede the behavior with a sufficiently short interval (*priority*). Second, the content of the thought should be compatible with the behavior (*consistency*). Third, the thought should be the only apparent cause of the behavior in that situation (*exclusivity*). Even though the presence of these conditions seems rather easy to establish in many situations, there can be conditions under which their assessment is hindered, thereby leading to inaccurate inferences of mental causation. Such distortions can go either way, in that they may lead to overestimations (e.g., Wegner, Sparrow, & Winerman, 2004) or underestimations (e.g., Wegner, Fuller, & Sparrow, 2003) of mental causation. For example, in a study by Wegner and colleagues (2003) participants were asked to give freely chosen, random answers to a set of yes–no questions. Even though participants were convinced that their responses were entirely random, they answered more questions correctly than would have been expected by chance, and this effect was more pronounced for easy compared with difficult questions. Interestingly, these effects generalized to situations when participants were asked to answer yes–no questions by sensing the inclinations of a confederate who did not even know the questions. Thus, one could argue that participants were aware of their thoughts of the correct answers, as well as their behavioral response to the question. Yet it seems that they were unaware of the causal link between the two.

To the extent that people draw inaccurate inferences about the causal links between their thoughts and their behaviors, the naive theories based on these inferences have the potential to further undermine people's attempts to control for biasing influences of their mental associations. Thus, extending the list of prerequisites for effective and contextually appropriate behavioral control, dual-process theorists argued that people need to have not only the necessary motivation, ability, and awareness but also an accurate theory of *how* their behavior is biased (Strack, 1992; Wegener & Petty, 1997; Wilson & Brekke, 1994). If their naive theories of mental causation are inaccurate, people may adjust their behavior in line with the implications of these theories even when their behavior is unbiased. More seriously, people may sometimes adjust their behavior in the wrong direction, thereby promoting rather than reducing bias (e.g., Petty & Wegener, 1993).

Relations between Different Components of Self-Insight

A final important question concerns the relation between the proposed components of self-insight. This issue has been a common source of confusion, in that the different components are often conflated in theoretical interpretations of empirical findings.

For example, in research on goal pursuit, effects of unconscious goal priming are often interpreted as evidence that people can pursue goals of which they are unaware (e.g., Bargh et al., 2001; Ferguson, 2008). However, as we have argued in this chapter, the fact that people can be unaware of the cause of a momentary goal does not mean that they are unaware of the goal itself. Similar confusion has been caused by different interpretations of Greenwald and Banaji's (1995) definition of *implicit attitudes* as "introspectively unidentified (or inaccurately unidentified) traces of past experience that mediate favorable or unfavorable feeling, thought, or action toward social objects" (p. 8). Whereas some researchers have interpreted this definition as implying unawareness of the causes of an attitude, others have referred to this definition in claiming unawareness of the attitude itself. Again, as we have outlined in this chapter, the two aspects of self-insight are conceptually distinct, and the former type of unawareness does not necessarily imply the latter.

In the preceding sections, we have argued that awareness of the contents of one's mental associations represents an important precondition for people's insight into both the causes and the effects of their mental associations (see Figure 3.1). As for the causes of one's mental associations, accurate knowledge presupposes (1) awareness of the relevant stimuli, (2) awareness of the mental associations themselves, and (3) awareness of the causal link between the two. Correspondingly, accurate knowledge about the effects of one's mental associations presupposes (1) awareness of the mental associations themselves, (2) awareness of the relevant behavior, and (3) awareness of the causal link between the two. Thus, accurate knowledge of the contents of one's mental associations represents a *necessary* precondition for insight into the causes and the effects of one's mental associations. Yet knowing the contents of one's mental associations is *insufficient* for accurate knowledge about the causes and the effects of these associations. For example, people may well be aware of their personal preferences, but they may be unaware of where these preferences come from or how these preferences influence their behavior (Nisbett & Wilson, 1997). From this perspective, comprehensive insight into one's mind includes all three components discussed in this chapter: the causes, the contents, and the effects of one's mental associations.

Conclusion

Our main goal in this chapter was to provide a conceptual analysis of self-insight from the perspective of dual-process theories. Even though dual-process theories differ in many regards (Gawronski & Creighton, in press), their shared distinction between automatic and controlled processes offers a valuable framework for understanding the mental underpinnings of self-insight. Toward this end, we have distinguished between insight into the causes, the contents, and the effects of one's mental associations, all of which are required for a comprehensive understanding of the working of one's mind. The implications of our analysis are applicable to any kind of mental association, including attitudes (i.e., object-evaluation associations), prejudice (i.e., group-evaluation associations), self-esteem (i.e., self-evaluation association), stereotypes (i.e., group-attribute association), self-concepts (i.e., self-attribute associations), and goals (i.e., means–ends-evaluation associations). Thus, we hope that our analysis will be useful for all researchers interested in self-knowledge, irrespective of their content area.

ACKNOWLEDGMENTS

Preparation of this chapter has been supported by the Canada Research Chairs Program (Grant No. 202555) and the Social Sciences and Humanities Research Council of Canada (Grant No. 410-2008-2247).

NOTES

1. Note that our analysis focuses on associations between mentally represented concepts, and therefore does not include self-knowledge of emotions or mood states. It also does not capture the role of cognitive feelings, such as processing fluency. Self-knowledge of emotions and mood states is discussed in more detail by Clore and Robinson (Chapter 12, this volume); cognitive feelings are discussed by Hofree and Winkielman (Chapter 13, this volume).

2. The distinction between actual evaluative responses and the self-concept of one's attitude may also explain differences between the standard IAT (Greenwald et al., 1998) and the personalized IAT (Olson & Fazio, 2004), in that the standard IAT assesses object-evaluation associations, whereas the personalized IAT assesses associations between the self and the attribute of liking or disliking a given object (for a discussion, see Gawronski, Peters, & LeBel, 2008).

REFERENCES

Baeyens, F., Eelen, P., & Van den Bergh, O. (1990). Contingency awareness in evaluative conditioning: A case for unaware affective-evaluative learning. *Cognition and Emotion, 4*, 3–18.

Baeyens, F., Eelen, P., Van den Bergh, O., & Crombez, G. (1992). The content of learning in human evaluative conditioning: Acquired valence is sensitive to US revaluation. *Learning and Motivation, 23*, 200–224.

Banaji, M. R. (2001). Implicit attitudes can be measured. In H. L. Roediger, J. S. Nairne, I. Neath, & A. Surprenant (Eds.), *The nature of remembering: Essays in remembering Robert G. Crowder* (pp. 117–150). Washington, DC: American Psychological Association.

Banse, R., Seise, J., & Zerbes, N. (2001). Implicit attitudes towards homosexuality: Reliability, validity, and controllability of the IAT. *Zeitschrift für Experimentelle Psychologie, 48*, 145–160.

Bar-Anan, Y., Wilson, T. D., & Hassin, R. R. (2010). Inaccurate self-knowledge formation as a result of automatic behavior. *Journal of Experimental Social Psychology, 46*, 884–894.

Bargh, J. A. (1994). The four horsemen of automaticity: Awareness, intention, efficiency, and control in social cognition. In R. S. Wyer & T. K. Srull (Eds.), *Handbook of social cognition* (pp. 1–40). Hillsdale, NJ: Erlbaum.

Bargh, J. A., Chen, M., & Burrows, L. (1996). Automaticity of social behavior: Direct effects of trait construct and stereotype activation on action. *Journal of Personality and Social Psychology, 71*, 230–244.

Bargh, J. A., Gollwitzer, P. M., Lee-Chai, A., Barndollar, K., & Trötschel, R. (2001). The automated will: Nonconscious activation and pursuit of behavioral goals. *Journal of Personality and Social Psychology, 81*, 1014–1027.

Bargh, J. A., & Pietromonaco, P. (1982). Automatic information processing and social perception: The influence of trait information presented outside of conscious awareness on impression formation. *Journal of Personality and Social Psychology, 43*, 437–449.

Bem, D. J. (1972). Self-perception theory. *Advances in Experimental Social Psychology, 6*, 1–62.

Blanton, H., & Jaccard, J. (2008). Unconscious racism: A concept in pursuit of a measure. *Annual Review of Sociology, 34*, 277–297.

Buhrmester, M. D., Blanton, H., & Swann, W. B. (2011). Implicit self-esteem: Nature, measurement, and a new way forward. *Journal of Personality and Social Psychology, 100*, 365–385.

Carver, C., & Scheier, M. F. (1981). *Attention and self-regulation: A control-theory approach to human behavior.* New York: Springer.

Custers, R., & Aarts, H. (2005). Positive affect as implicit motivator: On the nonconscious operation of behavioral goals. *Journal of Personality and Social Psychology, 89*, 129–142.

De Houwer, J., Hendrickx, H., & Baeyens, F. (1997). Evaluative learning with subliminally presented stimuli. *Consciousness and Cognition, 6*, 87–107.

De Houwer, J., Teige-Mocigemba, S., Spruyt, A., & Moors, A. (2009). Implicit measures: A normative analysis and review. *Psychological Bulletin, 135*, 347–368.

Devine, P. G. (1989). Stereotypes and prejudice: Their automatic and controlled components. *Journal of Personality and Social Psychology, 56*, 5–18.

Dijksterhuis, A. (2004). I like myself but I don't know why: Enhancing implicit self-esteem by subliminal evaluative conditioning. *Journal of Personality and Social Psychology, 86*, 345–355.

Dovidio, J. F., & Gaertner, S. L. (2004). Aversive racism. *Advances in Experimental Social Psychology, 36*, 1–52.

Duncan, B. L. (1976). Differential perception and attribution of intergroup violence: Testing the lower limits of stereotyping of Blacks. *Journal of Personality and Social Psychology, 34*, 590–598.

Dunton, B. C., & Fazio, R. H. (1997). An individual difference measure of motivation to control prejudiced reactions. *Personality and Social Psychology Bulletin, 23*, 316–326.

Epstein, S. (1994). Integration of the cognitive and the psychodynamic unconscious. *American Psychologist, 49*, 709–724.

Fazio, R. H. (1995). Attitudes as object–evaluation associations: Determinants, consequences, and correlates of attitude accessibility. In R. E. Petty & J. A. Krosnick (Eds.), *Attitude strength* (pp. 247–282). Mahwah, NJ: Erlbaum.

Fazio, R. H. (2007). Attitudes as object–evaluation associations of varying strength. *Social Cognition, 25*, 603–637.

Fazio, R. H., Jackson, J. R., Dunton, B. C., & Williams, C. J. (1995). Variability in automatic activation as an unobtrusive measure of racial attitudes: A bona fide pipeline? *Journal of Personality and Social Psychology, 69*, 1013–1027.

Ferguson, M. J. (2008). On becoming ready to pursue a goal you don't know you have: Effects of nonconscious goals on evaluative readiness. *Journal of Personality and Social Psychology, 95*, 1268–1294.

Friese, M., Hofmann, W., & Schmitt, M. (2008). When and why do implicit measures predict behaviour?: Empirical evidence for the moderating role of opportunity, motivation, and process reliance. *European Review of Social Psychology, 19*, 285–338.

Gawronski, B., & Bodenhausen, G. V. (2006). Associative and propositional processes in evaluation: An integrative review of implicit and explicit attitude change. *Psychological Bulletin, 132*, 692–731.

Gawronski, B., & Bodenhausen, G. V. (2011). The associative-propositional evaluation model: Theory, evidence, and open questions. *Advances in Experimental Social Psychology, 44*, 59–127.

Gawronski, B., & Creighton, L. A. (in press). Dual-process theories. In D. E. Carlston (Ed.), *The Oxford handbook of social cognition*. New York: Oxford University Press.

Gawronski, B., Geschke, D., & Banse, R. (2003). Implicit bias in impression formation: Associations influence the construal of individuating information. *European Journal of Social Psychology, 33*, 573–589.

Gawronski, B., Hofmann, W., & Wilbur, C. J. (2006). Are "implicit" attitudes unconscious? *Consciousness and Cognition, 15*, 485–499.

Gawronski, B., & LeBel, E. P. (2008). Understanding patterns of attitude change: When implicit measures show change, but explicit measures do not. *Journal of Experimental Social Psychology, 44*, 1355–1361.

Gawronski, B., Peters, K. R., & LeBel, E. P. (2008). What makes mental associations personal or extra-personal?: Conceptual issues in the methodological debate about implicit attitude measures. *Social and Personality Psychology Compass, 2*, 1002–1023.

Greenwald, A. G., & Banaji, M. R. (1995). Implicit social cognition: Attitudes, self-esteem, and stereotypes. *Psychological Review, 102*, 4–27.

Greenwald, A. G., Banaji, M. R., Rudman, L. A., Farnham, S. D., Nosek, B. A., & Mellott, D. S. (2002). A unified theory of implicit attitudes, stereotypes, self-esteem, and self-concept. *Psychological Review, 109*, 3–25.

Greenwald, A. G., McGhee, D. E., & Schwartz, J. L. K. (1998). Measuring individual differences in implicit cognition: The Implicit Association Test. *Journal of Personality and Social Psychology, 74*, 1464–1480.

Greenwald, A. G., & Nosek, B. A. (2009). Attitudinal dissociation: What does it mean? In R. E. Petty, R. H. Fazio, & P. Brinol (Eds.), *Attitudes: Insights from the new implicit measures* (pp. 65–82). Hillsdale, NJ: Erlbaum.

Hall, D. L., & Payne, B. K. (2010). Unconscious influences of attitudes and challenges to self-control. In R. R. Hassin, K. N. Ochsner, & Y. Trope (Eds.), *Self-control in society, mind, and brain* (pp. 221–242). New York: Oxford University Press.

Hofmann, W., De Houwer, J., Perugini, M., Baeyens, F., & Crombez, G. (2010). Evaluative conditioning in humans: A meta-analysis. *Psychological Bulletin, 136*, 390–421.

Hofmann, W., Gawronski, B., Gschwendner, T., Le, H., & Schmitt, M. (2005). A meta-analysis on the correlation between the Implicit Association Test and explicit self-report measures. *Personality and Social Psychology Bulletin, 31*, 1369–1385.

Hofmann, W., Gschwendner, T., Nosek, B. A., & Schmitt, M. (2005). What moderates implicit–explicit consistency? *European Review of Social Psychology, 16*, 335–390.

Hofmann, W., Gschwendner, T., & Schmitt, M. (2009). The road to the unconscious self not taken: Discrepancies between self- and observer-inferences about implicit dispositions from nonverbal behavioral cues. *European Journal of Personality, 23*, 343–366.

Hofmann, W., & Wilson, T. D. (2010). Consciousness, introspection, and the adaptive unconscious. In B. Gawronski & B. K. Payne (Eds.), *Handbook of implicit social cognition: Measurement, theory, and applications* (pp. 197–215). New York: Guilford Press.

Hugenberg, K., & Bodenhausen, G. V. (2003). Facing prejudice: Implicit prejudice and the perception of facial threat. *Psychological Science, 14*, 640–643.

Jones, E. E., & Nisbett, R. E. (1972). The actor and the observer: Divergent perceptions of the causes of behavior. In E. E. Jones, D. E. Kanouse, H. H. Kelley, R. E. Nisbett, S. Valins, & B. Weiner (Eds.), *Attribution: Perceiving the causes of behavior* (pp. 79–94). Morristown, NJ: General Learning Press.

Knight, D. C., Nguyen, H. T., & Bandettini, P. A. (2003). Expression of conditional fear with and without awareness. *Proceedings of the National Academy of Sciences USA, 100*, 15280–15283.

Krosnick, J. A., Betz, A. L., Jussim, L. J., & Lynn, A. R. (1992). Subliminal conditioning of attitudes. *Personality and Social Psychology Bulletin, 18*, 152–162.

Kruglanski, A. W., Shah, J. Y., Fishbach, A., Friedman, R., Chun, W. Y., & Sleeth-Keppler, D. (2002). A theory of goal-systems. *Advances in Experimental Social Psychology, 34,* 331–378.

McConnell, A. R., & Leibold, J. M. (2001). Relations among the Implicit Association Test, discriminatory behavior, and explicit measures of racial attitudes. *Journal of Experimental Social Psychology, 37,* 435–442.

Moors, A., & De Houwer, J. (2006). Automaticity: A conceptual and theoretical analysis. *Psychological Bulletin, 132,* 297–326.

Nisbett, R. E., & Wilson, T. D. (1977). Telling more than we can know: Verbal reports on mental processes. *Psychological Review, 84,* 231–259.

Olson, M. A., & Fazio, R. H. (2001). Implicit attitude formation through classical conditioning. *Psychological Science, 12,* 413–147.

Olson, M. A., & Fazio, R. H. (2004). Reducing the influence of extra-personal associations on the Implicit Association Test: Personalizing the IAT. *Journal of Personality and Social Psychology, 86,* 653–667.

Payne, B. K., Cheng, S. M., Govorun, O., & Stewart, B. D. (2005). An inkblot for attitudes: Affect misattribution as implicit measurement. *Journal of Personality and Social Psychology, 89,* 277–293.

Payne, B. K., & Gawronski, B. (2010). A history of implicit social cognition: Where is it coming from? Where is it now? Where is it going? In B. Gawronski & B. K. Payne (Eds.), *Handbook of implicit social cognition: Measurement, theory, and applications* (pp. 1–15). New York: Guilford Press.

Perugini, M., Richetin, J., & Zogmaister, C. (2010). Prediction of behavior. In B. Gawronski & B. K. Payne (Eds.), *Handbook of implicit social cognition: Measurement, theory, and applications* (pp. 255–277). New York: Guilford Press.

Petty, R. E., & Wegener, D. T. (1993). Flexible correction processes in social judgment: Correcting for context-induced contrast. *Journal of Experimental Social Psychology, 29,* 137–165.

Ranganath, K. A., Smith, C. T., & Nosek, B. A. (2008). Distinguishing automatic and controlled components of attitudes from direct and indirect measurement methods. *Journal of Experimental Social Psychology, 44,* 386–396.

Rydell, R. J., & McConnell, A. R. (2006). Understanding implicit and explicit attitude change: A systems of reasoning analysis. *Journal of Personality and Social Psychology, 91,* 995–1008.

Rydell, R. J., McConnell, A. R., Mackie, D. M., & Strain, L. M. (2006). Of two minds: Forming and changing valence-inconsistent implicit and explicit attitudes. *Psychological Science, 17,* 954–958.

Sagar, H. A., & Schofield, J. W. (1980). Racial and behavioral cues in black and white children's perceptions of ambiguously aggressive acts. *Journal of Personality and Social Psychology, 39,* 590–598.

Scarabis, M., Florack, A., & Gosejohann, S. (2006). When consumers follow their feelings: The impact of affective or cognitive focus on the basis of consumer choice. *Psychology and Marketing, 23,* 1015–1034.

Smith, C. T., & Nosek, B. A. (2011). Affective focus increases the concordance between implicit and explicit attitudes. *Social Psychology, 42,* 300–313.

Strack, F. (1992). The different routes to social judgments: Experiential versus informational strategies. In L. L. Martin & A. Tesser (Eds.), *The construction of social judgments* (pp. 249–275). Hillsdale, NJ: Erlbaum.

Strack, F., & Deutsch, R. (2004). Reflective and impulsive determinants of social behavior. *Personality and Social Psychology Review, 8,* 220–247.

Strack, F., & Hannover, B. (1996). Awareness of influence as a precondition for implementing correctional goals. In P. M. Gollwitzer & J. A. Bargh (Eds.), *The psychology of action: Linking cognition and motivation to behavior* (pp. 579–596). New York: Guilford Press.

Sweldens, S., Van Osselaer, S., & Janiszewski, C. (2010). Evaluative conditioning procedures and the resilience of conditioned brand attitudes. *Journal of Consumer Research, 37*, 473–489.

Walther, E., Gawronski, B., Blank, H., & Langer, T. (2009). Changing likes and dislikes through the backdoor: The US-revaluation effect. *Cognition and Emotion, 23*, 889–917.

Walther, E., & Nagengast, B. (2006). Evaluative conditioning and the awareness issue: Assessing contingency awareness with the four picture recognition test. *Journal of Experimental Psychology: Animal Behavior Processes, 32*, 454–459.

Wegener, D. T., & Petty, R. E. (1997). The flexible correction model: The role of naive theories of bias in bias correction. *Advances in Experimental Social Psychology, 29*, 141–208.

Wegner, D. M., Fuller, V. A., & Sparrow, B. (2003). Clever hands: Uncontrolled intelligence in facilitated communication. *Journal of Personality and Social Psychology, 85*, 5–19.

Wegner, D. M., Sparrow, B., & Winerman, L. (2004). Vicarious agency: Experiencing control over the movements of others. *Journal of Personality and Social Psychology, 86*, 838–848.

Wegner, D. M., & Wheatley, T. (1999). Apparent mental causation: Sources of the experience of will. *American Psychologist, 54*, 480–492.

Wicklund, R. A. (1975). Objective self-awareness. *Advances in Experimental Social Psychology, 8*, 233–275.

Wilson, T. D., & Brekke, N. (1994). Mental contamination and mental correction: Unwanted influences on judgments and evaluations. *Psychological Bulletin, 116*, 117–142.

Wilson, T. D., & Dunn, E. W. (2004). Self-knowledge: Its limits, value, and potential for improvement. *Annual Review of Psychology, 55*, 493–518.

Wilson, T. D., Dunn, D. S., Kraft, D., & Lisle, D. J. (1989). Introspection, attitude change, and attitude-behavior consistency: The disruptive effects of explaining why we feel the way we do. *Advances in Experimental Social Psychology, 22*, 287–343.

Wilson, T. D., Lindsey, S., & Schooler, T. Y. (2000). A model of dual attitudes. *Psychological Review, 107*, 101–126.

Wilson, T. D., Lisle, D. J., Schooler, J. W., Hodges, S. D., Klaaren, K. J., & LaFleur, S. J. (1993). Introspection can reduce post-choice satisfaction. *Personality and Social Psychology, 19*, 331–339.

Wilson, T. D., & Schooler, J. W. (1991). Thinking too much: Introspection can reduce the quality of preferences and decisions. *Journal of Personality and Social Psychology, 60*, 181–192.

Wittenbrink, B., Judd, C. M., & Park, B. (1997). Evidence for racial prejudice at the implicit level and its relationships with questionnaire measures. *Journal of Personality and Social Psychology, 72*, 262–274.

CHAPTER 4

Referential Processing and Competence as Determinants of Congruence between Implicit and Explicit Motives

OLIVER C. SCHULTHEISS
ALEXANDRA STRASSER

In this chapter, we approach the issue of self-knowledge from an information-processing perspective on the dissociation between implicit and explicit forms of motivation. We argue that the dissociation between these types of motivation is due to differences in the way that implicit and explicit motivational systems process information, namely, as nonverbal and verbal-symbolic codes, respectively. Therefore, congruence between both systems can be achieved through referential processing, that is, the translation of verbal codes into nonverbal codes and vice versa. This can happen as the result of the strategic translation of verbally represented goals into the imagined experience of goal pursuit and attainment, or as the result of individual differences in referential processing ability (referential competence). We review various measures of referential competence, their development, convergent and discriminant validity, and their ability to account for individual differences in motivational congruence. In closing, we discuss the role of referential processing in the coherence of personality and in affective disorders.

Conceptual Overview: Two-Systems Model of Motivation

From the perspective of motivation psychology, the issue of self-knowledge can be framed as an issue of *motivational congruence*, that is, the accurate explicit (i.e., conscious) representation of one's implicit (i.e., nonconscious) motives. For more than 50 years, researchers have examined this issue by devising a large variety of self-report instruments to measure explicit beliefs about one's motives, and correlating these with content-coding measures of implicit motivational needs, such as the Thematic Apperception Test (TAT; Morgan & Murray, 1935) or its descendant, the Picture Story Exercise (PSE; McClelland, Koestner, & Weinberger, 1989; Schultheiss & Pang, 2007; Smith, 1992). The self-report instruments were originally devised to measure the same motives assessed by the TAT and PSE, namely, people's needs for power, achievement, or affiliation (e.g., the Personality Research Form, or PRF; Jackson, 1984). Other self-report instruments were developed to assess personal goals in these domains of motivation (e.g., Brunstein, Schultheiss, & Grässmann, 1998; Pöhlmann & Brunstein, 1997) or the motivational themes of people's wishes (e.g., King, 1995).

However, when these explicit measures were correlated with the implicit measures of motives—the TAT or PSE—the variance overlap was usually in the minuscule positive range, despite the fact that, as we see shortly, both types of measures are valid predictors of various types of goal-directed behavior. Low correlations between implicit and explicit motive measures indicate that while some people hold explicit views of their motivational needs that are congruent with their implicit motives, roughly as many people's explicit views do not fit their implicit motives. Thus, whereas the former have valid beliefs about their implicit motives, the latter do not. A growing body of literature shows that lacking congruence between implicit and explicit levels of motivation is associated with impaired life satisfaction and emotional well-being, increased psychosomatic complaints and medication use, and clinically relevant levels of depressive symptoms (e.g., Baumann, Kaschel, & Kuhl, 2005; Brunstein et al., 1998; Hofer, Chasiotis, & Campos, 2006; Pueschel, Schulte, & Michalak, 2011; Schüler, Job, Fröhlich, & Brandstätter, 2008; Schultheiss, Jones, Davis, & Kley, 2008). Therefore, an emerging key question in the field is why implicit and explicit motive measures show so little overlap with each other and why some individuals have better insight into their implicit motives than others.

Building on earlier work by McClelland and colleagues (1989; Weinberger & McClelland, 1990) and others (Cantor & Blanton, 1996; LeDoux, 1996, 2002; Rolls, 1999), as well as on current concepts in the cognitive sciences and biopsychology (see Berridge & Robinson, 2003; Rolls, 2005; Schultheiss, 2007; Squire, 2004), Schultheiss (2001, 2008; see Figure 4.1) has described the properties of the implicit and explicit motivation systems as follows: The implicit system comprises a limited number of biologically based motives, of which the needs for power, affiliation, and achievement (often abbreviated as *n* Power, *n* Affiliation, *n* Achievement) have been most thoroughly studied in humans over the past 50 years. Each implicit motive represents a relatively stable capacity to experience a particular class of incentives as pleasurable. Thus, individuals high in *n* Power delight in having impact on other people; individuals high in *n* Affiliation cherish close, friendly contact with others; and individuals high in *n* Achievement get a kick out of mastering challenging tasks. Implicit motives preferentially respond to nonverbal stimuli, such as facial expressions, gestures, and so forth (e.g., Klinger, 1967; Schultheiss & Hale, 2007), and influence nondeclarative (i.e., procedural or autonomic) measures of motivation, such as hormone changes, cardiovascular responses, response speed on performance tasks, instrumental conditioning, nonverbal communication, and intuition-guided behavior (e.g., Brunstein & Maier, 2005; McClelland, 1979; Schultheiss & Brunstein, 2002; Schultheiss et al., 2005; Stanton & Schultheiss, 2009). Thus, the implicit system is geared toward processing nonverbal information and generating automatic, incentive-driven behavior aimed at maximizing pleasure.

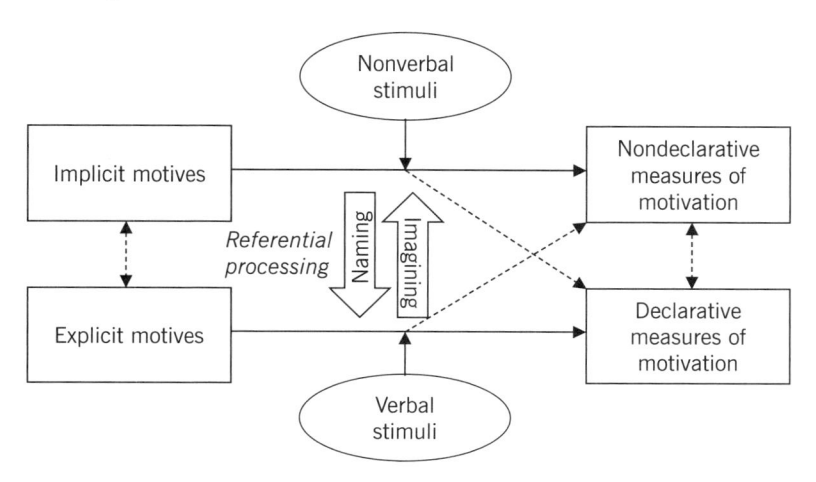

FIGURE 4.1. Information-processing model of implicit and explicit motivation (solid lines: significant correlation/influence; dashed lines: no significant correlation/influence). From Schultheiss (2008). Copyright 2008 by The Guilford Press. Adapted by permission.

The explicit system, in contrast, contains individuals' stable, language-based beliefs about themselves, that is, the motivational needs and values that people endorse and ascribe to themselves on questionnaire scales related to power, affiliation, or achievement. It also houses the long- and short-term goals people pursue in their daily lives, represented as verbal codes (e.g., "I want to become a doctor," "I want to practice my piano skills daily," "I want to spend more time with my partner"), and whose content and importance reflects the structure of peoples' explicit motivational values (Weinberger & McClelland, 1990). Owing to the demands and affordances of the sociocultural context individuals live in, the number of different values and goals in the explicit system can be quite large and is not inherently limited. The explicit system responds most readily to verbal incentives (e.g., demands, requests, suggestions) and influences declarative criterion measures of motivation, such as people's decisions, judgments, goal choices, and controlled forms of behavior. In summary, the explicit system is geared toward representing and processing verbal information in the service of effortful behavioral regulation.

The validity of this two-systems model of motivation is supported by research documenting that implicit and explicit motive measures are statistically distinct and predict different kinds of outcomes in response to different kinds of incentives (e.g., Biernat, 1989; Brunstein & Hoyer, 2002; Brunstein & Schmitt, 2004; Brunstein & Maier, 2005; Craig, Koestner, & Zuroff, 1994). A meta-analysis on achievement motivation by Spangler (1992) summarizes the main findings of a large body of research as follows: (1) Implicit and explicit motive measures have only marginal variance overlap (correlations typically settle in the low positive range of $r \sim .10$; see also Köllner & Schultheiss, 2011); (2) implicit motive measures are good predictors of spontaneous, intuition-guided forms of behavior (e.g., making inventions or showing leadership behavior), particularly in the presence of nonverbal incentives; and (3) explicit motive measures are good predictors of controlled and declarative forms of behavior (e.g., judgments, attitudes, grades), particularly in the presence of verbally transmitted social incentives.

Role of Strategic Referential Processing in Motivational Congruence: Evidence from Studies on Goal Imagery

According to the information-processing model proposed by Schultheiss (2001, 2008), the degree to which the implicit and the explicit motivational system can operate in tandem or independently depends on the degree of *referential processing* between the systems (see Figure 4.1; see also Weinberger & McClelland, 1990). *Referential processing* is a descriptive term for the translation of nonverbal representations into verbal ones through verbal labeling ("naming") and verbal representations into nonverbal ones through mental imagery ("imagining"). It was introduced by Paivio (1986), who argued that referential processing allows information exchange between verbal and nonverbal processing systems, but that it always requires additional processing time and effort relative to processing within verbal and nonverbal systems in which the representational format remains constant. For instance, reading a word only requires its perception and its transformation into a motor speech pattern, whereas naming an object requires its perception, the retrieval of an appropriate verbal label, then the transformation of the label into speech (see Figure 4.2 and Bucci & Freedman, 1978, for related arguments). The retrieval of the proper label represents the extra step necessary for referential processing from the nonverbal to the verbal system (or RP_{naming}). In the reverse case—$RP_{imagining}$—the retrieval of a nonverbal representation in response to a word (e.g., *flower*) also requires an additional processing step, namely, the formation of the appropriate mental image for the word. Research by Paivio and others (reviewed in Paivio, 1986, 2007) consistently shows that tasks that require processing only within the nonverbal system or within the verbal system are more efficiently accomplished than tasks that require referential processing between systems. In our view, the fact that the brain processes information in separate, parallel systems with different representational formats and that between-systems exchange

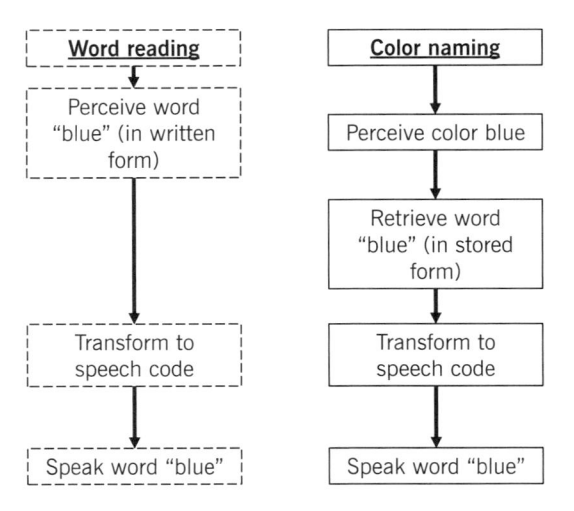

FIGURE 4.2. Process analysis of word-reading and color-naming tasks. Relative to reading words, naming things requires an additional processing step: retrieval of the proper word referent for a nonverbal entity. From Bucci and Freedman (1978). Copyright 1978 by John Wiley & Sons, Inc. Adapted by permission.

entails a cost provides the key to understanding why motivational systems are not necessarily and automatically marching in lockstep. If this view is correct, then strategic use of and stable individual differences in referential processing should be associated with variations in the congruence between implicit (i.e., nonverbal) and explicit (i.e., verbally mediated) motivational systems.

To address the question of whether strategic use of referential processing increases motivational congruence, Schultheiss and Brunstein (1999, 2002; see Schultheiss, 2001, for a more extensive portrayal and discussion of these and related studies) conducted three experimental studies in which one-half of participants vividly imagined the pursuit and attainment of an experimenter-assigned verbal goal ($RP_{imagining}$) and attend to their affective response to the experience (RP_{naming}), whereas the other half engaged in control tasks that did not require translation of the same goal into mental imagery. Across all studies, goal-imagery participants' commitment to the assigned goal and their behavioral efforts aimed at attaining it were significantly predicted by their implicit motives. In other words, they chose and behaved in a motivationally congruent manner. In contrast, among control group participants, goal commitment and implementation were not predicted by their implicit motives, reflecting a higher risk for motivational incongruence. These findings, replicated by Job and Brandstätter (2009), suggest that situationally induced referential processing can transiently increase between-systems congruence and tie the commitment to and execution of explicit goals to implicit motives. We speculate that individuals who have learned to employ referential processing strategically (e.g., who frequently and deliberately engage in mental simulations of future goal-related activities and pursuits) will also show higher levels of motivational congruence in their everyday lives. However, this conjecture still needs to be validated in future studies.

Note that in our view, referential processing does not allow individuals to gain direct access to the nonconscious processes involved in implicit motivation or those that aid the formation and maintenance of explicit self-views and goal hierarchies. Rather, referential processing aids motivational congruence by making the experiential reality of verbally encapsulated goals and values (= output of the explicit system) available to implicit motives ($RP_{imagining}$), and by labeling and representing in a person's verbal consciousness his or her motive-dependent affective response (= output of the implicit system) to the simulated experience (RP_{naming}). And it is precisely the process of binding "gut feelings" and their valid trigger stimuli in the mind that often goes awry because people may not pay attention to their affective responses or may misattribute them to the wrong triggers (see Schwarz & Clore's, 2007, distinction between incidental and integral feelings).

Individual Differences in Referential Processing: The Case for Referential Competence

But what if referential processing is not strategically employed or induced by an experimenter as in the Schultheiss and Brunstein (1999, 2002) studies? Can people still choose goals and endorse values that fit their implicit motives? As suggested by the low positive correlations between implicit and explicit measures of motivation observed in meta-analyses (Spangler, 1992), some people are able to achieve motivational congruence to some extent, but almost as many others fail to a similar extent. In our recent research, we have explored the possibility that individual differences in automatic engagement of referential processing—that is, *referential competence* (RC)—are responsible for the degree to which individuals' implicit motives and explicit values and goals are well matched or mismatched in the absence of strategically employed referential processing.

In the following section we first provide a brief history of the RC concept and its measurement. We then describe recent work suggesting that high RC is associated with motivational congruence and report additional validation data for various measures of RC.

Brief History of the RC Concept

Naming Things Takes Longer Than Reading Words

The observation that it takes longer to name things than to read their word referents is an old one in psychology. For instance, Ligon (1932) reported that the longer latency for naming things over reading words emerges as soon as children learn to read, well before they are practiced readers. A well-known example for the phenomenon is the Stroop test in which participants either have to read color names or name a series of colored areas corresponding to the color names. In the classic study (Stroop, 1935), participants took 41 seconds to read 100 color names printed in black (Card A), but 63 seconds to name the colors of 100 rectangular patches (Card B)—a difference of 22 seconds. Longer reaction times for reading versus naming is not specific to the color domain but has also been found for other stimuli, including objects, drawings, and geometric forms (Fraisse, 1969).

But the substantial sample-level difference between naming things and reading words is just half of the story here, albeit one that is very consistent with Paivio's (1986) proposition of a referential process that needs to be engaged for translating back and forth between verbal and nonverbal codes. The other half is in the substantial speed variations *between individuals* on each task (i.e., naming or reading). Probably the first researcher to make use of this variation as an individual-difference variable was Broverman (1960a, 1960b). Broverman used cards A and B from the Stroop task to measure participants' reading and naming abilities, respectively, then created adjusted difference scores (regression residuals) to classify individuals as conceptually dominant (better reading than naming) or perceptual–motor dominant (better naming than reading). Broverman used these scores to predict participants' performance on other cognitive tasks. Consistent with Paivio's (1986) dual-coding theory, conceptually dominant individuals performed particularly well on a task that required finding the appropriate word meaning (verbal system processing), whereas individuals with perceptual–motor dominance performed particularly well on a task requiring spatial–figural comparisons and transformations (nonverbal system processing). However, because dual-coding theory was not around at the time, Broverman made no attempt to relate the adjusted difference scores from the Stroop task to indicators of referential between-systems processing.

The first study to explore explicitly the concept of RC was conducted by Bucci and Freedman (1978). Like Broverman, they used cards A and B from Stroop's task to assess word-reading and color-naming times, respectively, then created a naming–reading difference score based on regression residuals. Participants were split into a high-RC group (color naming faster than predicted by word reading) and a low-RC group (color naming slower than predicted by word reading). The difference between the groups was solely due to differences in color-naming latencies, as groups did not significantly differ in their word-reading times. Unlike Broverman, however, Bucci and Freedman were not as much interested in how these groups differed in traditional cognitive tasks (verbal intelligence tests were included, too, but scores were not substantially related to RC) as in how well they were able to tell stories in response to the instruction to talk about a dramatic or interesting personal experience. High-RC individuals used specific, concrete language in their narrations, even if they talked about something as mundane as traveling to another city. They also used direct quotes and third-person singular pronouns frequently, but first-person pronouns relatively sparsely. In contrast, low-RC individuals used unspecific, abstract language, avoided quotes, and frequently used first-person pronouns (*I*). In other words, the high-RC group used language in a manner similar to that of an author of fiction, whereas the low-RC group did not.

In a replication study, Bucci (1984) again used the color-naming task to divide a sample into low- and high-RC individuals and to study how these groups differ when describing different color shades and providing short narratives of everyday experiences. Compared to the low-RC group, the high-RC group produced more metaphorical color terms (e.g., maroon, mauve, sienna, "like dried mud") and used more specific, concrete, and focused language in their narratives. They also made less use of the first-person pronoun. Together with the earlier study by Bucci and Freedman (1978), these findings suggest that high-RC individuals (i.e., who are quick at naming things), relative to those with low-RC ability, are habitually better at moving back and forth between verbal and nonverbal representations and at capturing nonverbal experience efficiently and accurately with words.

Content Analysis of Text: Ratings versus Word Counts

From these studies, Bucci and her collaborators advanced RC research by developing two new measures of referential processing. One was the derivation of scales for rating the quality of narrative language based on the findings for high-RC individuals in the Bucci (1984) and Bucci and Freedman (1978) studies. The referential activity (RA) scales assess the degree to which a speaker or writer is able to translate experience into words in a way that will evoke corresponding experiences for the listener or reader (Bucci & Kabasakalian-McKay, 1992). In other words, they measure how well narrators are able to capture and communicate nonverbal experience, including emotions and other "inner" events, in language that easily evokes vivid images in the reader's mind.

The four RA scales are Concreteness, Specificity, Clarity, and Imagery. The Concreteness and Imagery scales measure the sensory characteristics of language; the Specificity and Clarity scales reflect its degree of articulation, focus, and communicative quality. Moreover, Concreteness and Specificity indicate how *frequently* these dimensions are expressed in speech or writing; Clarity and Imagery are indicators of the *effectiveness* of the expressions. All dimensions are coded on a 10-point scale, ranging from 1 (*low level*) to 10 (*high level*). Because the four scales are substantially intercorrelated, an overall RA mean score can also be computed. The RA measure can be applied to different types of materials such as psychotherapy session protocols and PSE stories, and has been validated in studies on therapeutic progress (Bucci, 1995).

In our own research, we have found higher scores on the overall RA measure to be related to better RC, as reflected in smaller differences on the Stroop color-naming/word-reading task. In one unpublished study with 75 U.S. student participants, the correlation between RA, as assessed in six PSE stories and partialed for word count, and RC was $r = -.24$, $p < .05$. In another study, we obtained a similar, although slightly smaller correlation (see Table 4.1; note that the correlation is negative because higher RA ratings are associated with *smaller* differences between color-naming and word-reading latencies, signifying higher RC). While this result should not be surprising given the history of the development of the RA scales, it is, in our opinion, still remarkable that response latencies on a simple naming task consistently converge with judgments of the vividness and literary quality of imaginative stories. Our results also support the notion that a basic process of information exchange between nonverbal and verbal systems as assessed through the color-naming task determines to what extent nonverbal experience is accurately represented in narrative language and thus available for conscious reflection.

The other advance resulting from the color-naming task studies by Bucci and Freedman (1978) and Bucci (1984) was the development of a computerized RA (CRA) measure by Mergenthaler and Bucci (1999). The development of the system had its roots in the observed differences in word use between high-RC and low-RC individuals (e.g., use of first-person and third-person pronouns). Mergenthaler and Bucci's CRA measure consists of two dictionaries: One is a list of 63 words identified as characteristic for high RA (e.g., third-person singular pronouns, all articles, references to speaking). The other is a word list of 118 entries representing low RA (e.g., nonspecific quantifiers such as *any, more*; nonspecific actions in the present tense such as *make, try*; words representing negation and uncertainty). Bucci and Mergenthaler reported a correlation of around $r = .50$ between the CRA measure and the RA scales. Moreover, the high- and low-RA words cover about 50% of a text. A caveat provided by the authors is that the CRA measures may miss out on descriptions of bodily, sensory, and emotional states that are better captured by the RA scales. The CRA measure has not been validated with the color-naming task originally devised for the assessment of RC.

TABLE 4.1. Correlations between Referential Activity as Assessed in the PSE, RC as Assessed in Color-Naming and Clock Tasks, and Hedonic Tone Judgments and Response Latencies in 93 U.S. College Students

	1	2	3	4
1. Referential activity	—			
2. RC$_{color\ naming}$	–.16	—		
3. RC$_{clock\ task}$	–.22*	.18†	—	
4. Hedonic tone	–.06	.12	.18†	—
5. Hedonic tone$_{latency}$	–.22*	.13	.33**	–.04

Note. Unpublished data from Schultheiss et al. (2008, Study 1).
†$p < .10$; *$p < .05$; **$p < .005$.

The RA scales and the CRA measure can be used to assess not only situation- or stimulus-specific RP by examining individuals' RA fluctuations in response, for instance, to a therapist's suggestions (e.g., Bucci & Maskit, 2007) or one's child (e.g., Christian, Hoffman, Bucci, Crimmins, & Worth, 2010) but also stable individual differences in RC, as suggested by the overall consistency of a person's RA level from one situation to the next. For instance, in one study ($N = 83$) in which we used the RA rating scales to assess RC from PSE protocols, we found that individuals' RA levels were highly stable from one story to the next, as indicated by an internal consistency coefficient of .86. In another study, CRA analyses of individuals' personal-goal descriptions showed internal consistencies of .80 (high CRA lexicon) and .87 (low CRA lexicon).

Exploring the Reliability and Validity of RC: Schultheiss, Patalakh, Rawolle, Liening, and MacInnes (2011)

To test the hypothesis that RC is a predictor of the degree to which the implicit and the explicit motivational systems are in congruence with each other, Schultheiss and colleagues (2011) conducted a series of studies in which they examined the reliability and validity of Bucci's (1984) color-naming measure of RC. Across four studies, they assessed RC with a computer task requiring participants to name color patches (red, green, blue, and yellow) or to read color words ("red," "green," "blue," and "yellow") presented in random order on the screen (see Figure 4.3, Panel A, for a schematic overview). Responses were recorded via voice-key activation. Stimulus presentations were organized into eight blocks with 12 color-naming and 12 word-reading trials each. To obtain a pure measure of color-naming ability, net of effects of general mental speed or speech generation effects, Schultheiss and colleagues subtracted average word-naming latencies from average color-naming latencies and divided the difference by the average of both latencies. On average and across studies, participants were about 100 ms (milliseconds) slower at naming colors than they were at reading words. Participants' difference scores were moderately to highly consistent across blocks, with coefficients alpha ranging from .74 to .90 across studies. Moreover, overall RC scores showed high retest stability over a 2-week interval, $r = .80$. These findings suggest that the color-naming task captures stable and consistent individual differences in RC.

In three studies, Schultheiss and colleagues (2011) then examined to what extent the RC measure was associated with, or predicted, the degree to which individuals' explicit goal commitments and motivational values were aligned with their implicit motives in the domains of power, achievement, and affiliation at the between-subjects (Studies 2 through 4) and within-subjects level (Study 3). Motivational congruence was assessed (1) at the between-subjects level as the absolute difference between standardized implicit motives scores assessed per PSE and standardized explicit goal commitment (motive–goal congruence) or value (motive–value congruence) scores assessed per questionnaire and (2) at the within-subjects level as the degree to which the profile of story writing responses to PSE pictures correlated with questionnaire item responses to the same pictures (as assessed with the PSE questionnaire; Schultheiss, Yankova, Dirlikov, & Schad, 2009). The results can be summarized as follows.

First, higher RC was associated with higher motive–goal congruence, that is, better alignment between individuals' implicit motives and their explicit goal

Cognitive RC

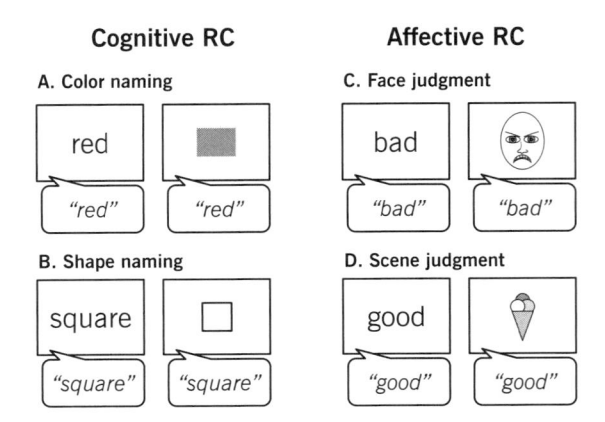

A. Color naming

red	[gray square]
"red"	"red"

B. Shape naming

square	[square outline]
"square"	"square"

Affective RC

C. Face judgment

bad	[angry face]
"bad"	"bad"

D. Scene judgment

good	[ice cream cone]
"good"	"good"

FIGURE 4.3. Schematic overview of tasks used to assess nonverbal-to-verbal RC (i.e., "naming").

commitments, across all three studies in which the effect was tested. This was true of both studies with cross-sectional design (Studies 2 and 3) and a study in which participants could indicate their preferences on a goal choice task (Study 4). Across studies, Schultheiss and colleagues (2011) report an average r of .275 for the association between the RC color-naming task and motive–goal congruence.

Second, RC was associated only marginally with motive–value congruence, that is, better alignment between individuals' implicit motives and the value they explicitly placed on specific types of motivation (power, achievement, affiliation), assessed at the between-subjects level in Study 2 and not significantly in Study 3. Schultheiss and colleagues (2011) explained this with the more enduring and passive nature of self-attributed motivational values relative to personal goals, which are more frequently formed and actively pursued and thus open more opportunities for RC to influence their selection in a motive-congruent way.

Third, RC was also associated with better motivational congruence at the within-subjects level (Study 3). The faster participants named colors, the stronger and more positive the correlations between the motive profiles of their PSE story writing responses and the profiles of their questionnaire responses to the same PSE picture cues. Within-subjects motivational congruence had no significant variance overlap with between-subjects motivational congruence, which indicates that whether individuals accurately judge their motivational needs vis-à-vis others is not directly linked to how much insight they have into variations of their motivational responses to different situational cues. It is therefore particularly impressive that RC predicts both types of motivational congruence in similar ways.

Fourth and finally, gender emerged as a moderator of the association between RC and motivational congruence. In Study 2, the association between RC and motive–goal congruence was stronger in women ($r = .48$) than in men ($r = .10$), and the previously mentioned association between RC and within-subjects congruence in Study 3 emerged only in women ($r = .38$), not in men ($r = -.08$). Given the absence of direct gender differences in RC or motivational congruence measures, these findings are intriguing and merit further research.

In summary, the Schultheiss and colleagues (2011) studies provide replicable evidence that RC, as assessed with a simple color-naming task, is a stable individual-difference variable that taps into individuals' ability to translate efficiently between verbal and nonverbal representations, and that predicts, as hypothesized by Schultheiss's (2008) information-processing model of motivation, the degree to which implicit and explicit motivational systems are in alignment.

Broadening the Measurement Basis of RC: Shape Naming, Valence Judgments, and Imaging to Words

In two studies, one conducted in the United States, the other in Germany (unpublished data from the Schultheiss and colleagues [2011] Studies 2 and 3), we have also explored to what extent other naming tasks converge with the color-naming task we have used as our cardinal measure of RC. Specifically, we have devised tasks that require participants to (1) name simple shapes and read their names (square, circle, triangle; *shape-naming task*); (2) judge happy ("good") and angry faces ("bad"), as well as read the words *good* and *bad* (*face-judgment task*); and (3) judge complex scenes from the International Affective Picture System (Lang, Bradley, & Cuthbert, 2008) preselected for having strong positive valence (e.g., *bunnies, ice cream*; "good") or negative valence (e.g., *plane crash, attacking dog*; "bad") and read the words *good* and *bad* (*scene-judgment task*). See Figure 4.3 for an overview of these tasks.

The structure of the three new tasks was similar to that of the color-naming task; that is, there was an equal number of randomly presented naming and reading trials in each block, responses were assessed per voice key, and response latency differences for naming and reading trials were aggregated across several blocks. Like color naming, the shape-naming task was assumed to tap a cognitive component of RC but had the advantage of circumventing problems with color vision, which are present in a small percentage of the population. In contrast, the face-judgment and scene-judgment tasks were assumed to tap into a more affective component of RC because they required participants to retrieve the proper label for the affect generated by a hedonically charged nonverbal cue.

Table 4.2 shows that all four tasks had substantial convergent validity, although the two cognitive RC tasks tended to correlate more strongly with each other than with the two affective RC tasks, and vice versa. Moreover, on the two cognitive tasks, object naming required about 100 ms more time than word reading. In contrast, valence judgments of faces and scenes on the two affective RC tasks required substantially more processing time, with a difference of about 180 ms relative to word reading. Somewhat counterintuitively, the cognitive RC tasks turned out to be better predictors of motivational congruence (both for the motive–goal and the motive–value indices) in U.S. and German samples than the affective RC tasks. When we combined the color-naming and shape-naming measures into a measure of cognitive RC, it was significantly correlated with motive–goal congruence ($r = .23$) and total congruence (i.e., the average of motive–goal, motive–value, and value–goal congruence; $r = .22$) in the U.S. sample, p's < .05, whereas a combined measure of the two affective RC tasks was not (motive–goal congruence, $r = .05$; total congruence, $r = .12$, p's > .10). Similarly, in the German sample, cognitive RC was associated with motive–goal congruence ($r = .18$, $p < .10$) and total congruence ($r = .16$, $p = .12$) but affective

TABLE 4.2. Descriptive Statistics and Correlations for Four Measures of RC and Four Motivational Congruence Indices in U.S. and German Students

	M	SD	1	2	3	4	5	6	7	8
1. Color naming										
U.S.	125	45	—							
Germany	96	39	—							
2. Shape naming										
U.S.	102	46	.50***	—						
Germany	104	36	.45***	—						
3. Face judgment										
U.S.	181	63	.24*	.49***	—					
Germany	173	41	.32***	.36***	—					
4. Scene judgment										
U.S.	193	55	.36***	.36***	.53***	—				
Germany	175	31	.21*	.26**	.40***	—				
5. Motive–value congruence										
U.S.	0.322	0.293	.18†	.06	.14	.02	—			
Germany	0.309	0.339	.08	.08	-.03	.04	—			
6. Motive–goal congruence										
U.S.	0.370	0.309	.34***	.05	-.00	.09	.26*	—		
Germany	0.341	0.297	.20*	.09	-.03	-.04	.22*	—		
7. Value–goal congruence										
U.S.	0.245	0.309	.13	.02	.12	-.00	.08	.10	—	
Germany	0.337	0.348	-.08	.18†	-.11	-.18†	.13	.16	—	
8. Total congruence										
U.S.	0.317	0.205	.30***	.07	.15	.08	.67***	.71***	.61***	—
Germany	0.329	0.219	.09	.18†	-.09	-.10	.68***	.65***	.67***	—

Note. Unpublished data from Schultheiss et al. (2011, Studies 2 and 3). Motive–value congruence scores represent log-transformed absolute difference scores between PSE motive and PRF scale z-scores, averaged across motivational domains (power, achievement, affiliation). Motive–goal congruence scores represent log-transformed absolute difference scores between PSE motive and idiographic goal commitment z-scores, averaged across motivational domains. Value–goal congruence scores represent log-transformed absolute difference scores between PRF scale and idiographic goal commitment z-scores, averaged across motivational domains. Total congruence scores represent the average of these three congruence scores. Higher values on all scores represent lower congruence. For measures of RC, raw difference scores in milliseconds; larger difference = less RC. For motivational congruence indices, larger index = less congruence. *N*'s 86 to 93 for U.S. students and 99 for German students.
†*p*<.10; **p*<.05; ***p*<.01; ****p*<.005.

RC was not (motive–goal congruence, $r=-.05$; total congruence, $r=-.11$, p's > .20). The correlation between cognitive and affective RC was .48 in the U.S. sample and .41 in the German sample. Future studies need to address whether the difference in the association between cognitive and affective RC on the one hand and motivational congruence measures on the other is robust and, if it is, why cognitive RC is a better predictor of motivational congruence than affective RC.

While all of these studies have used measures that assess RC_{naming} through a variety of labeling tasks, we have also explored $RC_{imagining}$, that is, the ease with which people can translate verbal experience into a nonverbal format (unpublished data from Schultheiss et al., 2008, Study 1). We based our research on earlier work by Paivio (1978), who assessed $RP_{imagining}$ by measuring how long participants took to figure out for which of two digital clock times (= symbolic information) the arms of a corresponding analog clock were closer together. To provide the correct answer, the digital clock information first needs to be translated into mental imagery of analog clock faces (= referential processing). Then, the clocks can be compared in the mind's eye and a decision can be made about the proximity of the two arms on each clock (see Figure 4.4 for an illustration). Our $RC_{imagining}$ measure consisted of 20 such comparisons, presented in two blocks of 10 trials. Participants' key-press response latencies were the dependent variable. To control for performance aspects that are inherent in the clock task but do not reflect referential translations per se (see Paivio, 1978, Experiment 3), we also measured participants' performance on 20 trials in which they had to judge which of two analog clock faces the hands were closer together

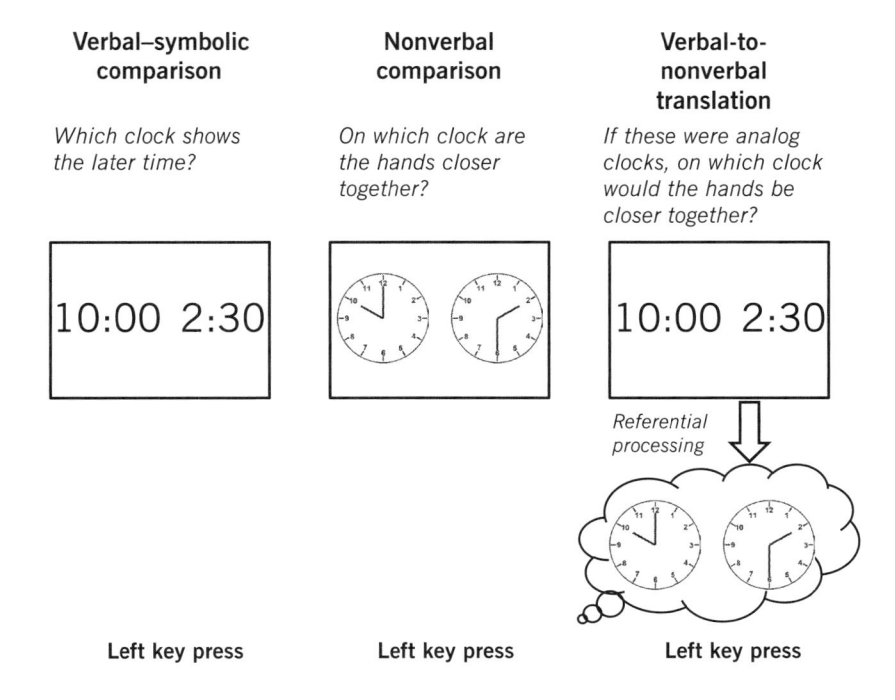

FIGURE 4.4. Schematic overview of clock task used to assess verbal-to-nonverbal RC (i.e., "imagining").

(nonverbal comparison) and another 20 trials on which they had to judge which of two digital times represented the later time (verbal–symbolic comparison).

Although all three performance measures were positively and significantly correlated with each other, regression analysis indicated that only the nonverbal–comparison control task was a significant unique predictor of variance in the $RC_{imagining}$ task, but not the verbal–symbolic comparison task. We therefore subtracted response latencies of the nonverbal–comparison task from latencies on the $RC_{imagining}$ task to obtain a net estimate of participants' ability for imaging to words. This yielded a normally distributed, corrected $RC_{imagining}$ measure with a mean of 3.16 seconds ($SD = 1.57$). Thus, on average participants took about 3 seconds to create a mental image in response to verbal–symbolic information, above and beyond the time they needed to make a comparison based on nonverbal information.

Does the clock task measure valid individual differences in RC? To provide an answer to this question, we used a two-pronged approach. First, we examined its convergent validity with the color-naming measure of RC, as well as with Bucci and Kabasakalian-McKay's (1992) text-coding measure of RA. To obtain a measure of the latter, we had a coder, who had achieved an 86% agreement overall with practice excerpts scored by experts in the instruction manual, code six PSE stories collected from each participant and used in our analyses the average RA sum score per participant, residualized for protocol length to control for differences in verbal fluency (longer stories tended to have higher RA ratings). Second, we tested the clock task's criterion validity by examining how well it predicted the speed with which participants could make judgments about their mood on a standard hedonic tone scale, as assessed via PC and key-press responses. Based on research on alexithymia (e.g., Sifneos, 1975) and dual attitudes (for a review, see Wilson, Lindsey, & Schooler, 2000), we reasoned that people who make mood judgments quickly are better at reading out nonverbal gut feelings and are also less likely to construct them through indirect, inferential means than people who take a long time to make such judgments.

Table 4.1 shows that RC as assessed by the clock task converged with the color-naming and the RA-coding measures of RC in the predicted manner: Longer net response times on the clock task were associated with longer net color-naming times and with less vivid and imagery-laden language in PSE stories. Of the three RC measures tested, the clock task was also the one most strongly associated with how quickly participants judged their mood. Those who took a long time translating digital clock information into an analog representation also took longer indicating how happy, satisfied, sad, or depressed they were. Notably, higher RA, as rated in PSE stories, was also associated with faster responses on the hedonic tone rating task. Note that the association between the color-naming task and the clock task does not simply reflect differences in overall response speed (an effect that may account for the comparatively large overlap of $r = .71$ between $RC_{imagining}$ and RC_{naming} measures reported by Paivio, Clark, Digdon, & Bons, 1989, p. 172), as this effect has been removed from the clock task RC measure by subtracting the effect of analog clock comparisons and from the color-naming RC measure by subtracting the effect of word-reading times. None of the RC measures was associated with mood per se, suggesting that individual differences in RC are not influenced by mood.

Overall, our explorations into the measurement of RC suggest that stable individual differences in referential processing can be obtained through a variety of measures that show meaningful patterns of variance overlap with each other, that predict valid criteria, and that provide a rich arsenal for further exploration of RC's role in personality and motivational congruence.

Further Explorations into the Convergent and Discriminant Validity of RC

So far we have focused on relationships between RC measures and their ability to predict congruence between motivational systems and other criteria. Over the course of several studies in which we have included the color-naming task as our RC measure, we have also examined its relationships with other measures that (1) assess phenomena that tap into similar cognitive abilities as RC (e.g., verbal fluency and verbal intelligence), or (2) assess constructs that are also related to the translation of affective–emotional information into a verbal format (i.e., alexithymia), or (3) have been shown to predict motivational congruence specifically. Here is what we found.

RC and Verbal Ability

Schultheiss and colleagues (2011) examined the overlap between the RC color-naming task and various measures of verbal fluency and verbal intelligence. Shorter color-naming latency differences were related to higher verbal fluency as assessed by the total word count on the PSE in one study (Study 2: $r=-.22$) but not in another (Study 3: $r=.06$). We explored this issue further by examining the overlap between color-naming RC and PSE word count in other, unpublished datasets, but without much evidence for a consistent association between RC and verbal fluency. Schultheiss and colleagues also examined correlations between RC and two measures of verbal intelligence. One test required participants to generate words with an assigned prefix or suffix; the other, to assign words to the most appropriate of four pictures (e.g., the word *frenetic* to the picture of a soccer game). RC was not reliably associated with participants' performance on either task (generating words: $r=-.02$; assigning the proper word: $r=-.17$). Replicating earlier findings by Bucci and Freedman (1978), who also failed to observe convergence between the color-naming RC task and verbal intelligence tests, these observations suggest that the color-naming RC task measures an ability that is not captured by traditional tests of verbal fluency or intelligence. They also suggest that traditional intelligence tests, which typically measure verbal and nonverbal abilities separately, but usually not their interplay, may miss out on a fundamental domain of human cognitive ability (see Paivio, 2007, for a thorough analysis and discussion of this issue).

RC and Alexithymia

The construct of *alexithymia*—literally the inability to read and verbalize one's emotions—has been used in clinical studies to explain why some patients have problems benefiting from psychotherapy and are restricted in their emotional lives (e.g., Sifneos, 1975; Taylor & Bagby, 2004). Schultheiss and colleagues (2011) used a standard measure of alexithymia, the Toronto Alexithymia Scale (TAS; Bagby, Parker, & Taylor, 1994), in two of their studies to examine the overlap of this measure with

RC (findings involving the TAS in Study 3 are reported here only and were not included in the original paper by Schultheiss et al., 2011). Color-naming RC scores were not significantly associated with TAS scores (Study 2: $r=.04$; Study 3: $r=-.15$, p's > .10). Neither was there any evidence that higher TAS scores were associated with less motivational congruence as indexed by higher motive-goal (Study 2: $r=.01$, n's; Study 3: $r=-.22$, $p<.05$) or motive–value difference scores (Study 2: $r=-.08$; Study 3: $r=.02$, p's > .10).

These findings stand in marked contrast to Bucci's observation that increases in referential processing are associated with episodes of emotional insight during psychotherapy, that is, with a transient reduction of alexithymia (e.g., Bucci, 1995). However, Bucci's research typically examines alexithymia as a process, not as a trait, and relies on actually measuring emotional insight procedurally rather than asking participants about whether they ascribe emotional insight to themselves. These two factors may account for the differences between the findings of Schultheiss and colleagues (2011), who also measured RC procedurally and assessed the criterion of motivational insight in a sophisticated manner, and typical work on alexithymia, which somewhat paradoxically relies on self-report methods such as the TAS to assess individuals' conscious insight into the limits of their emotional insight and relates the outcome of this assessment to other declarative measures of emotional processing. Schultheiss and colleagues therefore argued that the *construct* of alexithymia has considerable conceptual overlap with referential processing because both constructs deal with the verbalization of nonverbal experience, and that lacking overlap of the TAS *measure* of alexithymia with the measure of RC should not be viewed as conclusive evidence against such a link. Corroborating this line of thought, recent research sheds doubt on the validity of the TAS as a valid and specific measure of the alexithymia construct (e.g., Leising, Grande, & Faber, 2009; Parling, Mortazavi, & Ghaderi, 2010).

RC and Other Correlates of Motivational Congruence

Recent years have seen rising interest in the predictors and correlates of motivational congruence, and a number of moderators of the fit between a person's implicit and explicit motives have been identified. In several studies, we have started to explore the degree to which these moderators show variance overlap with RC.

Action orientation after failure (AOF), the ability to downregulate negative affect and thus to regain self-access (e.g., Kuhl, 2000), has been shown to predict the degree to which individuals choose goals that are congruent with their implicit motives (Baumann et al., 2005; Brunstein, 2001). However, in two studies in which we assessed AOF with a questionnaire measure (Kuhl, 1981), correlation coefficients between AOF and RC measures were low and nonsignificant. In the study in which we had measured RC_{naming} (color naming), $RC_{imagining}$ (clock task), and RA (ratings of PSE stories), none of the three measures was substantially associated with AOF (r's = .09, .00, and .05, respectively; $N=93$). In another study, RC_{naming} (color naming) and RA also failed to converge with AOF, r's(75) = .12 and –.15, respectively, p's > .20.

Another variable that has been implicated in motivational congruence is self-determination, that is, the ability to choose goals in a self-congruent manner and to be aware of one's feelings and preferences (Deci & Ryan, 1985). Thrash and Elliot

(2002) found that individuals with high scores on the Self-Determination Scale (SDS), a self-report measure of this ability, were better able to choose goals that were congruent with their implicit achievement motive than individuals with low scores on this scale. However, as in the case of AOF, we found SDS scores to be unrelated to RC (color naming) and RA (PSE story ratings), r's(75) = –.09 and .13, respectively, p's > .20.

Other moderators of motivational congruence, such as public and private self-consciousness (Thrash, Elliot, & Schultheiss, 2007) or identity status (Hofer, Busch, Chasiotis, & Kiessling, 2006), remain to be examined for their overlap with measures of RC. However, given the substantial differences between the assessment of these variables (declarative measures) and RC (procedural measures), we expect correlations to be generally low and to reflect a fundamental divide between self-ascribed and process-measured abilities.

Beyond Motivational Congruence: Referential Processing and the Functional Coherence of Personality

As the research we have reviewed here so far suggests, referential processing between verbal and nonverbal codes, both through the strategic use of goal imagery and through stable individual differences in RC, is a necessary prerequisite for motivational congruence, as assessed through measures of implicit motives and explicit goal pursuits. But does the congruence-enhancing effect of RP extend to other elements of personality, too?

Our answer to this question can only be speculative at this point because to our knowledge no research has explored the role of RP in other implicit–explicit dissociations. But we would venture this prediction: RP, either as a state or as a trait (i.e., RC), should play a critical role whenever nonverbally manifested dispositions (e.g., attachment styles, implicit attitudes) need to be represented accurately in language to become consciously available (e.g., as explicit representations of one's attachment style or social attitudes). If RP is high, conscious beliefs about oneself are more likely to represent a direct translation of nonverbal experience; if it is low, they are more likely to be the result of the ever-busy left-hemispheric interpreter's propensity for making inferences about the causes of one's behavior even when direct insight into the causes of this behavior is lacking (Gazzaniga, 1985; Nisbett & Wilson, 1977; Roser & Gazzaniga, 2004; Wilson, 2002). For instance, we would expect individual differences in RC to predict to what extent individuals' enduring self-attributed attachment styles, as assessed per questionnaire or other forms of self-report, converge with their habitual automatic emotional and behavioral responses to an attachment figure (see Crowell, Fraley, & Shaver, 2008). Likewise, we would expect the degree to which nonverbal indicators of transient emotions (e.g., behavioral and autonomic changes) converge with self-reported emotional states to depend on an individual's current RP, which in turn may depend on dispositional RC (see Mauss, Levenson, McCarter, Wilhelm, & Gross, 2005).

In contrast, we do not expect RP to be involved in within-systems congruence of the verbal system or the nonverbal system because the ease with which verbal concepts can be related to each other or with which nonverbal representations can be connected to other nonverbal representations represents processes that are distinct from RP as defined by Paivio (1986). Consistent with this conjecture, we have failed to find evidence for an effect of RC on the congruence between explicit goals and values (see Table 4.2). Both types of constructs are represented verbally, although at different levels of abstraction, and typically show a substantial degree of convergence in all individuals (e.g., Emmons & McAdams, 1991; King, 1995). For the same reason, we would not expect RP (or RC) to moderate the degree to which explicit attitudes converge with implicit attitudes that represent the strength of automatic associations between verbal concepts, such as Me and Happy (i.e., Implicit Association Test [IAT] and similar measures; e.g., Greenwald & Farnham, 2000). And indeed, a recent meta-analysis suggests that the term *implicit* should be used with caution in this context because attitudes assessed with the IAT correlate at .24 on average with questionnaire measures of attitudes (Hofmann, Gawronski, Gschwendner, Le, & Schmitt, 2005). The size of this overlap is similar to the overlap between explicit value and goal measures (e.g., King, 1995; Rawolle, Patalakh, & Schultheiss, 2011) and considerably larger than the correlation between implicit and explicit motive measures (see the first section of this chapter).

Insight into the role of RP in normal personality coherence can also be gained from studies on clinically relevant phenomena such as anxiety disorders, posttraumatic stress disorder (PTSD), and depression (see also Paivio, 2007, for a discussion of this issue). Borkovec and Inz (1990) have argued that generalized anxiety disorder (GAD) is characterized by an avoidance of mental imagery and a preponderance of verbal processing during worry. This suggests that anxiety predisposes individuals for enhanced processing of information within the verbal system and decreased referential processing between verbal and nonverbal systems. In support of this view, Baumann and colleagues (2005) found that individuals who reported a high rate of threats in their daily lives and who had difficulties regulating negative emotions resulting from perceived threats experienced reduced congruence between implicit and explicit levels of achievement motivation. Although RP was not assessed in this study, we speculate that the anxiety-inducing effects of threat reduced RP in these individuals, which in turn facilitated motive-incongruent goal choices.

A disorder in which the ties between different information-processing systems appear to be severely compromised is PTSD. Individuals suffering from PTSD have typically experienced trauma that later leads to unbidden flashbacks, intrusive memories, hypervigilance, and cognitive avoidance, among other symptoms (DSM-IV-TR; American Psychiatric Association, 2000). From a therapeutic perspective, one of the most problematic aspects of PTSD is the unpredictability and dissociation of the symptoms. It is as if the symptoms lead a life of their own, come and go unbidden, and are independent of a person's conscious recall of the trauma. In their dual-representation theory of PTSD, Brewin, Dalgleish, and Joseph (1996) have argued that the dissociative aspects of PTSD are due to the representation of the trauma and its situational context in two different types of memory: verbally accessible memories and situationally accessible memories, that is, memories triggered by situational cues that elicit emotional and behavioral responses. Dissociation of symptoms occurs because people suffering from PTSD are characterized by a lack of coherence between these two types of memories. It does not take much to recognize in the two different types of memories instantiations of Paivio's (1986) verbal and nonverbal processing systems or, in the parlance of modern cognitive approaches to learning and memory, declarative and nondeclarative systems (Squire, 2004). Brewin and colleagues' (1996) theory of dissociation in PTSD therefore indentifies low RP as a core problem in PTSD.

Low RP may be an outcome of trauma and threat, which can hinder the translation of anxiety-laden nonverbal experiences into verbal representations. But there is also evidence that low RP may represent a precursor for the development of PTSD. Gilbertson and colleagues (2006) compared soldiers with combat exposure with their monozygotic twin brothers who had not been exposed to combat. The brothers not exposed to combat thus served as a proxy measurement for precombat mental abilities in their exposed twins, as these abilities have a substantial amount of heritability. Soldiers who developed PTSD and their twins were characterized by low verbal ability, whereas soldiers who had not developed PTSD and their brothers scored in the normal range on measures of verbal ability. Although Gilbertson and colleagues did not directly assess individual differences in RC, their findings are consistent with the idea that low RC may increase the risk for developing PTSD after trauma. Gilbertson and colleagues endorse a similar conclusion when they state that "verbal mediation and intellectual sophistication may be critical to effective forms of coping with exposure to severely traumatic experiences, and the capacity to place such events into meaningful verbal concepts may reduce negative emotional impact" (p. 493).

Finally, Bucci and Freedman (1981) found lower RC, as assessed through a colornaming task, to be associated with more severe symptoms of depression in a small sample of female inpatients at a clinic. Due to the cross-sectional nature of the study and the small sample size, it is difficult to ascertain whether RP is generally involved in depression and, if so, whether it is a precursor, correlate, or consequence of depression. We venture the speculation, though, that low levels of RP, either as a disposition or as a strategy for achieving congruence, predispose individuals for the development of depression. As we outlined in the previous section, RP, both as a state and as a trait, is associated with motivationally congruent goal choices, and successful realization of motive-congruent goals is in turn related to heightened emotional well-being (Brunstein et al., 1998; Schultheiss et al., 2008) as well as low levels of depressive symptoms (Pueschel et al., 2011; Schultheiss et al., 2008).

Thus, the view we take here of the potential role of RP in clinical disorders is that RP facilitates between-systems coherence, and that this coherence is essential for effective and adaptive personality functioning. However short and necessarily incomplete our review of RP-related clinical phenomena may be, the perspective we present is consistent with other modern accounts of personality that emphasize the importance of fluid between-systems exchange for personality functioning (e.g., Kuhl, 2000, 2001) and with meta-theoretical approaches to psychotherapy and mental health that assign a pivotal role to self-congruence, that is, the coherence between different functional systems in the person (e.g., Bucci, 1997; Grawe, 2004).

Summary and Conclusion

According to the approach we have presented in this chapter, self-knowledge is preconditioned upon the accurate and efficient exchange of information between functionally separate verbal and nonverbal information-processing systems. Once the contents of the verbal system have been translated into a nonverbal format, systems that operate at the nonverbal level can process this information, and their output (e.g., affective responses) can be translated back into a verbal format to become available for conscious reflection. Integrity of the referential process is thus a necessary requirement for accurate self-beliefs that cut across different processing systems. Self-knowledge can be strategically enhanced through the deliberate translation of verbal codes into nonverbal ones and vice versa. Research on goal imagery (Schultheiss & Brunstein, 1999, 2002) represents only one example of the strategic use of referential processing to gain self-insight. Expressive writing that aims to capture everyday or special experiences in specific and concrete narrative language may represent another such strategy (see Pennebaker, 1997). Self-knowledge can also be better in some individuals than in others due to differences in RC, that is, the habitual ease and efficiency with which the referential process works, and future studies need to explore whether this ability can be increased through training. At this point, we simply hope that the tools for inducing and measuring referential processing we have presented in this chapter will provide researchers and practitioners with the necessary methods for understanding the origins of personality coherence and helping individuals to increase congruence between implicit and explicit levels of motivation.

ACKNOWLEDGMENT

We thank the editors and Allan Paivio for their helpful and constructive feedback on an earlier version of this chapter.

REFERENCES

American Psychiatric Association. (2000). *Diagnostic and statistical manual of mental disorders* (4th ed., text rev.). Washington, DC: Author.

Bagby, R. M., Parker, J. D., & Taylor, G. J. (1994). The twenty-item Toronto Alexithymia Scale—I: Item selection and cross-validation of the factor structure. *Journal of Psychosomatic Research, 38*(1), 23–32.

Baumann, N., Kaschel, R., & Kuhl, J. (2005). Striving for unwanted goals: Stress-dependent discrepancies between explicit and implicit achievement motives reduce subjective well-being and increase psychosomatic symptoms. *Journal of Personality and Social Psychology, 89*, 781–799.

Berridge, K. C., & Robinson, T. E. (2003). Parsing reward. *Trends in Neuroscience, 26*(9), 507–513.

Biernat, M. (1989). Motives and values to achieve: Different constructs with different effects. *Journal of Personality, 57*, 69–95.

Borkovec, T. D., & Inz, J. (1990). The nature of worry in generalized anxiety disorder: A predominance of thought activity. *Behaviour Research and Therapy, 28*, 153–158.

Brewin, C. R., Dalgleish, T., & Joseph, S. (1996). A dual representation theory of posttraumatic stress disorder. *Psychological Review, 103*, 670–686.

Broverman, D. M. (1960a). Cognitive style and intra-individual variation in abilities. *Journal of Personality, 28*, 240–256.

Broverman, D. M. (1960b). Dimensions of cognitive style. *Journal of Personality, 28*, 167–185.

Brunstein, J. C. (2001). Persönliche Ziele und Handlungs- versus Lageorientierung: Wer bindet sich an realistische und bedürfniskongruente Ziele? [Personal goals and action versus state orientation: Who builds a commitment to realistic and need-congruent goals?]. *Zeitschrift für Differentielle und Diagnostische Psychologie, 22*, 1–12.

Brunstein, J. C., & Hoyer, S. (2002). Implizites und explizites Leistungsstreben: Befunde zur Unabhängigkeit zweier Motivationssysteme [Implicit versus explicit achievement strivings: Empirical evidence of the independence of two motivational systems]. *Zeitschrift fur Pädagogische Psychologie, 16*, 51–62.

Brunstein, J. C., & Maier, G. W. (2005). Implicit and self-attributed motives to achieve: Two separate but interacting needs. *Journal of Personality and Social Psychology, 89*(2), 205–222.

Brunstein, J. C., & Schmitt, C. H. (2004). Assessing individual differences in achievement motivation with the Implicit Association Test. *Journal of Research in Personality, 38*(6), 536–555.

Brunstein, J. C., Schultheiss, O. C., & Grässmann, R. (1998). Personal goals and emotional well-being: The moderating role of motive dispositions. *Journal of Personality and Social Psychology, 75*(2), 494–508.

Bucci, W. (1984). Linking words and things: Basic processes and individual variation. *Cognition, 17*, 137–153.

Bucci, W. (1995). The power of the narrative: A multiple code account. In J. W. Pennebaker (Ed.), *Emotion, disclosure, and health* (pp. 93–122). Washington, DC: American Psychological Association.

Bucci, W. (1997). *Psychoanalysis and cognitive science: A multiple code theory.* New York: Guilford Press.

Bucci, W., & Freedman, N. (1978). Language and hand: The dimension of referential competence. *Journal of Personality, 46*, 594–622.

Bucci, W., & Freedman, N. (1981). The language of depression. *Bulletin of the Menninger Clinic, 45*, 334–358.

Bucci, W., & Kabasakalian-McKay, R. (1992). *Scoring referential activity: Instructions for use with transcripts of spoken narrative texts.* Ulm, Germany: Ulmer Textbank.

Bucci, W., & Maskit, B. (2007). Beneath the surface of the therapeutic interaction: The psychoanalytic method in modern dress. *Journal of the American Psychoanalytic Association, 55*, 1355–1397.

Cantor, N., & Blanton, H. (1996). Effortful pursuit of personal goals in daily life. In P. M. Gollwitzer & J. A. Bargh (Eds.), *The psychology of action: Linking cognition and motivation to behavior* (pp. 338–359). New York: Guilford Press.

Christian, C., Hoffmann, L., Bucci, W., Crimins, M., & Worth, M. (2010). Symbolization and emotional engagement in mothers' reports of child care activities. *International Journal of Applied Psychoanalytic Studies, 7*, 22–39.

Craig, J. A., Koestner, R., & Zuroff, D. C. (1994). Implicit and self-attributed intimacy motivation. *Journal of Social and Personal Relationships, 11*, 491–507.

Crowell, J. A., Fraley, R. C., & Shaver, P. R. (2008). Measurement of individual differences in adolescent and adult attachment. In J. Cassidy & P. R. Shaver (Eds.), *Handbook of attachment: Theory, research, and clinical applications* (2nd ed., pp. 599–634). New York: Guilford Press.

Deci, E. L., & Ryan, R. M. (1985). *Intrinsic motivation and self-determination in human behavior.* New York: Plenum Press.

Emmons, R. A., & McAdams, D. P. (1991). Personal strivings and motive dispositions: Exploring the links. *Personality and Social Psychology Bulletin, 17*, 648–654.

Fraisse, P. (1969). Why is naming longer than reading? *Acta Psychologica, 30*, 96–103.

Gazzaniga, M. S. (1985). *The social brain: Discovering the networks of the mind.* New York: Basic Books.

Gilbertson, M. W., Paulus, L. A., Williston, S. K., Gurvits, T. V., Lasko, N. B., Pitman, R. K., et al. (2006). Neurocognitive function in monozygotic twins discordant for combat exposure: Relationship to posttraumatic stress disorder. *Journal of Abnormal Psychology, 115*(3), 484–495.

Grawe, K. (2004). *Psychological therapy.* Ashland, OH: Hogrefe & Huber.

Greenwald, A. G., & Farnham, S. D. (2000). Using the Implicit Association Test to measure self-esteem and self-concept. *Journal of Personality and Social Psychology, 79*(6), 1022–1038.

Hofer, J., Busch, H., Chasiotis, A., & Kiessling, F. (2006). Motive congruence and interpersonal identity status. *Journal of Personality, 74*(2), 511–542.

Hofer, J., Chasiotis, A., & Campos, D. (2006). Congruence between social values and implicit motives: Effects on life satisfaction across three cultures. *European Journal of Personality, 20*(4), 305–324.

Hofmann, W., Gawronski, B., Gschwendner, T., Le, H., & Schmitt, M. (2005). A meta-analysis on the correlation between the implicit association test and explicit self-report measures. *Personality and Social Psychology Bulletin, 31*(10), 1369–1385.

Jackson, D. N. (1984). *Personality Research Form* (3rd ed.). Port Huron, MI: Sigma Assessment Systems, Inc.

Job, V., & Brandstätter, V. (2009). Get a taste of your goals: Promoting motive–goal congruence through affect-focus goal fantasy. *Journal of Personality, 77,* 1527–1560.

King, L. A. (1995). Wishes, motives, goals, and personal memories: Relations of measures of human motivation. *Journal of Personality, 63,* 985–1007.

Klinger, E. (1967). Modeling effects on achievement imagery. *Journal of Personality and Social Psychology, 7,* 49–62.

Köllner, M., & Schultheiss, O. C. (2011). *A meta-analysis of the correlation between implicit and explicit measures of motivational needs for achievement, affiliation, and power.* Manuscript in preparation.

Kuhl, J. (1981). Motivational and functional helplessness: The moderating effect of state versus action orientation. *Journal of Personality and Social Psychology, 40,* 155–170.

Kuhl, J. (2000). A functional-design approach to motivation and self-regulation: The dynamics of personality systems interactions. In M. Boekaerts, P. P. Pintrich, & M. Zeidner (Eds.), *Handbook of self-regulation* (pp. 111–169). New York: Academic Press.

Kuhl, J. (2001). *Motivation und Persönlichkeit: Interaktionen psychischer Systeme* [Motivation and personality: Interactions of mental systems]. Göttingen, Germany: Hogrefe.

Lang, P. J., Bradley, M. M., & Cuthbert, B. N. (2008). *International affective picture system (IAPS): Affective ratings of pictures and instruction manual* (Technical Report A-8). Gainesville: University of Florida.

LeDoux, J. E. (1996). *The emotional brain.* New York: Simon & Schuster.

LeDoux, J. E. (2002). *The synaptic self.* New York: Viking.

Leising, D., Grande, T., & Faber, R. (2009). The Toronto Alexithymia Scale (TAS-20): A measure of general psychological distress. *Journal of Research in Personality, 43,* 707–710.

Ligon, E. M. (1932). A genetic study of color naming and word reading. *American Journal of Psychology, 44,* 103–122.

Mauss, I. B., Levenson, R. W., McCarter, L., Wilhelm, F. H., & Gross, J. J. (2005). The tie that binds?: Coherence among emotion experience, behavior, and physiology. *Emotion, 5*(2), 175–190.

McClelland, D. C. (1979). Inhibited power motivation and high blood pressure in men. *Journal of Abnormal Psychology, 88,* 182–190.

McClelland, D. C., Koestner, R., & Weinberger, J. (1989). How do self-attributed and implicit motives differ? *Psychological Review, 96*, 690–702.

Mergenthaler, E., & Bucci, W. (1999). Linking verbal and non-verbal representations: Computer analysis of referential activity. *British Journal of Medical Psychology, 72*, 339–354.

Morgan, C., & Murray, H. A. (1935). A method for investigating fantasies: The Thematic Apperception Test. *Archives of Neurology and Psychiatry, 34*, 289–306.

Nisbett, R. E., & Wilson, T. D. (1977). Telling more than we can know: Verbal reports on mental processes. *Psychological Review, 84*, 231–259.

Paivio, A. (1978). Comparisons of mental clocks. *Journal of Experimental Psychology: Human Perception and Performance, 4*(1), 61–71.

Paivio, A. (1986). *Mental representations: A dual coding approach.* New York: Oxford University Press.

Paivio, A. (2007). *Mind and its evolution: A dual coding theoretical approach.* Mahwah, NJ: Erlbaum.

Paivio, A., Clark, J. M., Digdon, N., & Bons, T. (1989). Referential processing: Reciprocity and correlates of naming and imaging. *Memory and Cognition, 17*(2), 163–174.

Parling, T., Mortazavi, M., & Ghaderi, A. (2010). Alexithymia and emotional awareness in anorexia nervosa: Time for a shift in the measurement of the concept? *Eating Behaviors, 11*, 205–210.

Pennebaker, J. W. (1997). Writing about emotional experiences as a therapeutic process. *Psychological Science, 8*, 162–166.

Pöhlmann, K., & Brunstein, J. C. (1997). GOALS: Ein Fragebogen zur Messung von Lebenszielen [GOALS: A questionnaire for the assessment of life goals]. *Diagnostica, 43*, 63–79.

Pueschel, O., Schulte, D., & Michalak, J. (2011). Be careful what you strive for: The significance of motive–goal congruence for depressivity. *Clinical Psychology and Psychotherapy, 18*, 23–33.

Rawolle, M., Patalakh, M., & Schultheiss, O. C. (2011). *Clarifying the relationships between implicit motives, self-attributed needs, and personal goal commitments.* Manuscript submitted for publication.

Rolls, E. T. (1999). *The brain and emotion.* Oxford, UK: Oxford University Press.

Rolls, E. T. (2005). *Emotion explained.* Oxford, UK: Oxford University Press.

Roser, M., & Gazzaniga, M. S. (2004). Automatic brains—interpretive minds. *Current Directions in Psychological Science, 13*, 56–59.

Schüler, J., Job, V., Fröhlich, S. M., & Brandstätter, V. (2008). A high implicit affiliation motive does not always make you happy: A corresponding explicit motive and corresponding behavior are further needed. *Motivation and Emotion, 32*, 231–242.

Schultheiss, O. C. (2001). An information processing account of implicit motive arousal. In M. L. Maehr & P. Pintrich (Eds.), *Advances in motivation and achievement: Vol. 12. New directions in measures and methods* (pp. 1–41). Greenwich, CT: JAI Press.

Schultheiss, O. C. (2007). A memory-systems approach to the classification of personality tests: Comment on Meyer and Kurtz (2006). *Journal of Personality Assessment, 89*(2), 197–201.

Schultheiss, O. C. (2008). Implicit motives. In O. P. John, R. W. Robins, & L. A. Pervin (Eds.), *Handbook of personality: Theory and research* (3rd ed., pp. 603–633). New York: Guilford Press.

Schultheiss, O. C., & Brunstein, J. C. (1999). Goal imagery: Bridging the gap between implicit motives and explicit goals. *Journal of Personality, 67*, 1–38.

Schultheiss, O. C., & Brunstein, J. C. (2002). Inhibited power motivation and persuasive communication: A lens model analysis. *Journal of Personality, 70*, 553–582.

Schultheiss, O. C., & Hale, J. A. (2007). Implicit motives modulate attentional orienting to perceived facial expressions of emotion. *Motivation and Emotion, 31*(1), 13–24.

Schultheiss, O. C., Jones, N. M., Davis, A. Q., & Kley, C. (2008). The role of implicit motivation in hot and cold goal pursuit: Effects on goal progress, goal rumination, and depressive symptoms. *Journal of Research in Personality, 42*, 971–987.

Schultheiss, O. C., & Pang, J. S. (2007). Measuring implicit motives. In R. W. Robins, R. C. Fraley, & R. Krueger (Eds.), *Handbook of research methods in personality psychology* (pp. 322–344). New York: Guilford Press.

Schultheiss, O. C., Patalakh, M., Rawolle, M., Liening, S., & MacInnes, J. J. (2011). Referential competence is associated with motivational congruence. *Journal of Research in Personality, 45*, 59–70.

Schultheiss, O. C., Wirth, M. M., Torges, C. M., Pang, J. S., Villacorta, M. A., & Welsh, K. M. (2005). Effects of implicit power motivation on men's and women's implicit learning and testosterone changes after social victory or defeat. *Journal of Personality and Social Psychology, 88*(1), 174–188.

Schultheiss, O. C., Yankova, D., Dirlikov, B., & Schad, D. J. (2009). Are implicit and explicit motive measures statistically independent?: A fair and balanced test using the Picture Story Exercise and a cue- and response-matched questionnaire measure. *Journal of Personality Assessment, 91*, 72–81.

Schwarz, N., & Clore, G. L. (2007). Feelings and phenomenal experiences. In A. Kruglanski & E. T. Higgins (Eds.), *Social psychology: Handbook of basic principles* (2nd ed., pp. 385–407). New York: Guilford Press.

Sifneos, P. E. (1975). Problems of psychotherapy of patients with alexithymic characteristics and physical disease. *Psychotherapy and Psychosomatics, 26*, 65–70.

Smith, C. P. (Ed.). (1992). *Motivation and personality: Handbook of thematic content analysis.* New York: Cambridge University Press.

Spangler, W. D. (1992). Validity of questionnaire and TAT measures of need for achievement: Two meta-analyses. *Psychological Bulletin, 112*, 140–154.

Squire, L. R. (2004). Memory systems of the brain: A brief history and current perspective. *Neurobiology of Learning and Memory, 82*(3), 171–177.

Stanton, S. J., & Schultheiss, O. C. (2009). The hormonal correlates of implicit power motivation. *Journal of Research in Personality, 43*, 942–949.

Stroop, J. R. (1935). Studies of interference in serial verbal reactions. *Journal of Experimental Psychology, 18*, 643–662.

Taylor, G. J., & Bagby, R. M. (2004). New trends in alexithymia research. *Psychotherapy and Psychosomatics, 73*(2), 68–77.

Thrash, T., & Elliot, A. J. (2002). Implicit and self-attributed achievement motives: Concordance and predictive validity. *Journal of Personality, 70*, 729–756.

Thrash, T. M., Elliot, A. J., & Schultheiss, O. C. (2007). Methodological and dispositional predictors of congruence between implicit and explicit need for achievement. *Personality and Social Psychology Bulletin, 33*(7), 961–974.

Weinberger, J., & McClelland, D. C. (1990). Cognitive versus traditional motivational models: Irreconcilable or complementary? In E. T. Higgins & R. M. Sorrentino (Eds.), *Handbook of motivation and cognition: Vol. 2. Foundations of social behavior* (pp. 562–597). New York: Guilford Press.

Wilson, T. D. (2002). *Strangers to ourselves: Discovering the adaptive unconscious.* Cambridge, MA: Belknap Press.

Wilson, T. D., Lindsey, S., & Schooler, T. Y. (2000). A model of dual attitudes. *Psychological Review, 107*, 101–126.

CHAPTER 5

Self-Knowledge
From Philosophy to Neuroscience to Psychology

MATTHEW D. LIEBERMAN

The contemplation of self-knowledge has a long history within philosophy, a comparatively short history within psychology, and a vanishingly short history within neuroscience. Thus, if we wish to see whether neuroscience has something useful to tell us about the self, we would do well to situate it in the context of the 2,000-year dialogue that philosophers have had about the nature of the self and the paths by which we can know something about it.

This chapter is divided into two parts. In the first part, I consider various pronouncements by philosophers about the nature of self-knowledge and see what neuroscientists have had to say that supports or conflicts with those claims. In the second part, I start from the brain region, medial prefrontal cortex (MPFC), that has mostly commonly been associated with self-knowledge and self-related processes more generally, and examine the other psychological processes that invoke this region in order to try to make some progress in identifying the kinds of processes that are invoked when we think about the self or retrieve self-knowledge.

To avoid turning this into a mystery novel, here's the punchline. First, the MPFC may be more commonly activated by self-processing than anything else that has been studied; however, self-processing may just be a very prominent example of a broader class of processes. This is not to suggest that knowing the self is just like knowing *anything* else we know well (Greenwald & Banaji, 1989) because this is clearly not the case (Macrae, Moran, Heatherton, Banfield, & Kelley, 2004).

From Philosophy to Neuroscience

Ancient Greece Invokes the Challenge

The Ancient Greeks had profound influence over the course that Western civilization has taken over the past two millennia. Who would have guessed that the inscription "know thyself" above the Oracle at Delphi or Socrates' warning that the "unexamined life is not worth living" would have led to such an onslaught of interest, leading ultimately to countless self-help aisles in second-rate mall bookstores full of advice on how to understand oneself and how to use those insights to hack into one's own operating system and make changes for the better?

In 2002, Kelley and colleagues published the first neuroimaging paper on self-knowledge that identified the key region, MPFC, that has been the center of virtually every self-related functional magnetic resonance imaging (fMRI) study since (see Craik et al., 1999, for an earlier attempt). The paradigm was simple and straightforward. Participants were presented with a trait word such as *dependable* or *polite* on each of a series of trials. Additionally, on the same screen was an instruction cue that indicated the task to be performed for that trial. On some trials, participants indicated whether the trait word was self-descriptive. On other trials, participants indicated with whether the trait word described George Bush, a well-known public figure, and on still other trials, participants determined whether the trait word was presented in uppercase or lowercase letters (a task originally developed by Markus [1977] and Rogers, Kuiper, & Kirker [1977]).

Two regions were more active during self-reference trials compared to those that required referencing knowledge about another person: MPFC and an overlapping region of precuneus and posterior cingulate cortex (i.e., precuneus$_{PCC}$).

In the last decade, about three dozen neuroimaging studies of self-knowledge (or self-reference, as it is typically described in the neuroimaging literature) have been conducted. In a review of 32 of these studies (Lieberman, 2010; see also van Overwalle, 2009), MPFC was observed in 94% of the studies, with precuneus$_{PCC}$ appearing in 63% of the studies. The only other region appearing in more than half of the studies, at 53%, was dorsomedial prefrontal cortex (DMPFC), a region commonly associated with thinking about the mental states of others.

If we are to heed the instruction to "know thyself" from a neuroscience perspective, this first study provided the bedrock, the foundation upon which to build. But the studies using variants of this paradigm have also led to as many questions as answers. It is also important to note a terminological difference between self-knowledge research within neuroscience and social psychology. Within social-cognitive neuroscience, encoding new information about the self (coming to know the self), making judgments about the self, or retrieving self-related information are all considered self-knowledge processes. In contrast, within social psychology, self-knowledge more frequently refers to the accuracy of people's beliefs about themselves. Neuroscientists would probably refer to this as self-insight or the accuracy of self-beliefs, rather than self-knowledge per se. Regardless of the terminology, there is precious little research on the neural bases of self-knowledge accuracy, but what little there is, is quite consistent with self-reference findings, implicating MPFC in this as well (Beer, John, Scabini, & Knight, 2006; Schmitz, Rowley, Kawahara, & Johnson, 2006; Schnyer,

Nicholls, & Verfaelli, 2005). For the remainder of this chapter, however, I use *self-knowledge* to refer more broadly to all aspects of knowledge about the self, including the processes involved in accessing this information.

Enlightenment and Temporality of the Self

In 1689, John Locke, a British empiricist and one of the intellectual giants of the early Enlightenment period, included a chapter in *An Essay Concerning Human Understanding* titled "Identity and Diversity." Here, he wrote about memory as the basis on which identity stands, concluding that "as far as consciousness can extend backwards in time to any past action or thought, so far reaches the identity of that person" (1689/1975, p. 335). He immediately appreciated the neuropsychological implication of his claim:

> But yet possibly it will still be objected: Suppose I wholly lose the memory of some parts of my life, beyond a possibility of retrieving them, so that perhaps I shall never be conscious of them again; yet am I not the same person that did those actions, had those thoughts that I once was conscious of, though I have now forgot them? To which I answer, that we must here take notice what the word "I" is applied to; which, in this case, is the man only. And the same man being presumed to be the same person, "I" is easily here supposed to stand also for the same person. (p. 342)

He then went on to suggest that this final supposition is incorrect; while an amnesic is literally the same man, Locke contends he is no longer the same person, no longer in possession of the same identity, because he cannot recall the information that was the basis of his former identity. He was not suggesting that the man is not the same because he has changed in some minor fashion. Rather, he claimed that these are two distinct individuals because there is no overlap in their memories.

Klein, Loftus and Kihlstrom (1996) were able to examine Locke's claim directly in one of the first social cognitive neuroscience experiments ever conducted. They studied a patient who was temporarily amnesic due to head injury. They found that this patient possessed trait self-knowledge that was largely equivalent to that observed outside of the amnesic state. She made trait ratings of herself during her amnesic state and afterward, and these two sets of ratings correlated .74, almost identical to the test–retest correlation of control subjects ($r = .78$). In other words, even though this patient could not remember the episodes in her life that would have led her to believe she was, say, generous, she still knew she was a generous person.

In separate behavioral research, Klein, Loftus, Trafton, and Fuhrman (1992) observed that remembering specific episodes of past behavior was only relevant to making self-judgments in domains where one had relatively little experience. Specifically, subjects were asked to remember trait-specific memories immediately prior to making trait self-judgments, and this only facilitated the speed of self-judgments in low-experience domains. Lieberman, Jarcho, and Satpute (2004) followed up this work with an fMRI study comparing self-knowledge (i.e., self-reference) in high- and low-experience domains. Consistent with Klein and colleagues, this study revealed that the medial temporal lobe, central to the storage of episodic memories, was only involved in self-knowledge for low-experience domains. In contrast, high-experience domain self-knowledge was associated with MPFC and precuneus$_{PCC}$ along with other regions associated with more automatic or implicit processes. Together, these studies suggest that, on the whole, as brilliant as he was, Locke had it wrong about the relationship of memory to identity. Except perhaps in new domains of experience, our sense of self outlives the memories that may have given rise to the original self-insights (see also Hastie & Park, 1986).

John Butler, a lesser known philosopher from the Enlightenment period, who wrote the chapter "Of Personal Identity" in his book *The Analogy of Religion* (1736/1819 [reprinted in *Works*, 1896]), goes in quite the opposite direction from Locke, suggesting that memory is not enough to forge together the identities of the same man at two different points in time. Butler takes the "ever-changing river" approach to the self, suggesting that states of consciousness are what define the self, and just as a river is never the same at two different points in time, neither is consciousness, and thus neither is the self. He wrote:

> No one can any more remain one and the same person two moments together than two successive moments can be one and the same moment.... And from hence it must follow that it is a fallacy upon ourselves to charge our present selves with anything we did... or that our present self will be interested in what will befall us tomorrow. (p. 213)

On the one hand, this statement comes across as semantic hairsplitting, but from a psychological perspective there does seem to be some truth to the fact that, at times, we do treat our future and past selves as distinct from the current self (Libby & Eibach, 2002). Oftentimes an apology amounts to being distant enough from the actions of a past self that one can promise such actions will never happen again. It is as if someone else was responsible for those actions, and we promise not to bring that irresponsible person around again. On the flip side, *temporal discounting* is the study of the fact that we are much less motivated by the pleasures and pains of our future self compared to those we can receive today (Loewenstein & Elster, 1992).

fMRI research on past and future selves backs up Butler's account, at least from a psychological, if not an ontological, perspective. Simply put, MPFC is more active when one reflects on the current self rather than either the past or future self. D'Argembeau, Xue, Lu, Van der Linden, and Bechara (2008) asked individuals to indicate whether traits were self-descriptive or other-descriptive, and varied whether participants were answering about the target now or from a prior period of time. The only three regions that were more active when thinking about the current self than any of the other combinations were MPFC, DMPFC, and precuneus$_{PCC}$. A follow-up study that included past, present, and future perspectives on the self (D'Argembeau et al., 2010) observed greater MPFC activity for the present compared to the past and future perspectives (see also Ersner-Hershfield, Wimmer, & Knutson, 2009). Similarly, work on mindfulness meditation has found that prior to mindfulness training, individuals who are very caught up in the self of the moment show much greater MPFC activity than after being trained in mindfulness to take a more detached view of the self (Farb et al., 2007; see also Way, Creswell, Eisenberger, & Lieberman, 2010). In contrast, lateral parietal regions were more active when considering the self in other time periods, consistent with another recent study on imagining the self taking a walk in past, present, or future periods (Nyberg, Kim, Habib, Levine, & Tulving, 2010).

Sources and Components of Self in Modern Philosophy

The modern period of philosophy is commonly dated to middle of the 19th century. There are countless philosophers from this period who have weighed in on the nature of the self and our knowledge of it, but unfortunately social cognitive neuroscience research has yet to yield studies relevant to most of them. I am going to cheat a little here by turning to William James, who is often considered the founder of modern experimental psychology in America but was first and foremost a philosopher. In his work, *Psychology*, an abbreviated version of his massive two-volume opus *Principles of Psychology*, James posited a key division between components of the self:

> The consciousness of Self involves a stream of thought, each part of which as "I" can remember those which went before, know the things they knew, and care paramountly for certain ones among them as "Me." ... This Me is an empirical aggregate of things objectively known. The I which knows them cannot itself be an aggregate. (1892, p. 215)

Similarly, in *Principles* he discussed the two elements of the self as "an objective person, known by a passing subjective thought and recognized as continuing in time. Hereafter, let us use the words ME and I for the empirical person and the judging Thought" (1890, p. 371).

According to this account, an active part of the self is involved in experiencing the world, one's phenomenological point of view, and reflecting on the passive part of the self that represents our repository of self-knowledge. There is a special file cabinet of self-knowledge called the ME, and the I is what fills the file cabinet and can later peruse its contents. Given how computationally distinct these two components of the self would have to be, one might naturally expect to see different brain regions involved in each.

Very few of the fMRI studies on self-knowledge can address this question because most confound the act of self-reference (i.e., the I reflecting on the self) with activating self-knowledge (i.e., the ME that is reflected upon). A few studies have made some attempt to separate these, but they yield somewhat different conclusions. One study took a developmental approach, comparing adults and 10-year-old children as they made self-referential judgments (Pfeifer, Lieberman, & Dapretto, 2007). Here, the assumption was that to the extent the I and ME are separable, the I's act of retrieving self-knowledge might be more automatic in adults than in children but the ME, the repository of self-knowledge, would be much more developed and consolidated (see also Wang, Lee, Sigman, & Dapretto, 2006). Thus, we hypothesized that regions more active during self-reference in children would correspond more to the I, and regions that were more active in adults might correspond more to the ME. MPFC and precuneus$_{PCC}$ were two of the only regions that were more active in the children than in the adults. In contrast, the lateral temporal cortex and angular gyrus were the only regions more active in adults than in children. Similarly, Blakemore, den Ouden, Choudhury, and Frith (2007) asked people to imagine their intentions in various situations and found that adolescents activated MPFC more than adults, whereas adults activated superior temporal sulcus to a greater degree.

From these two studies alone, one might conclude that MPFC is more associated with the act of self-reflection than with the contents of self-knowledge. This would be consistent with the view that the prefrontal cortex is generally more involved in orchestrating information and behavioral responses elsewhere in the brain than in storing that content directly. Unfortunately, the other two relevant studies suggest the opposite conclusion. Both of these studies (Moran, Heatherton, & Kelley, 2009; Rameson, Satpute, & Lieberman, 2010) compared explicit self-knowledge, during which individuals explicitly reflected on the self, to implicit self-knowledge, during which self-relevant images were presented without any instruction to consider their self-relevance. To the extent that the I and the ME, in James's formulation, are separable, one would expect I-specific activations to be absent in the implicit conditions. Instead, both studies found significant overlap in the MPFC region recruited by both explicit and implicit tasks. Rameson and colleagues (2010) also found overlap in precuneus$_{PCC}$ across the two tasks. In other words, these two studies suggest that MPFC is involved in the representation of self-knowledge, not just the manipulation of self-knowledge through self-reflection processes. Combined with the previous two studies, the only thing we can conclude is that the jury is still out and more research is needed.

Gilbert Ryle, a 20th-century British philosopher, was described as both a behaviorist and a phenomenologist, sometimes in reference to the same work. In his most famous work, *The Concept of Mind*, he devoted an entire chapter to self-knowledge, in which he concluded:

> The sorts of things I can find out about myself are the same as the sorts of things I can find out about other people, and the methods of finding them out are much the same.... John Doe's ways of finding out about John Doe are the same as John Doe's ways of finding out about Richard Roe. (1949, pp. 155–156)

These words led to Bem's (1972) influential self-perception approach to self-knowledge. Bem opened his chapter on self-perception theory with the following:

> Individuals come to "know" their own attitudes, emotions, and other internal states partially by inferring them from observations of their own overt behavior and/or the circumstances in which this behavior occurs. Thus, to the extent that internal cues are weak, ambiguous, or uninterpretable, the individual is functionally in the same position as an outside observer. (1972, p. 2)

I quote Bem at length here to point out an important distinction between Bem and Ryle. It is commonly assumed that Bem held the same position as Ryle, when in fact Bem was always careful to suggest that self-observation is only necessary when internal cues are insufficient to form a judgment. Ryle, on the other hand, implied that all self-knowledge is generated through external sources.

Although no neuroscience research to date has examined the generation of self-knowledge through observing one's own behavior, there is strong evidence that processing the self through internal and external sources of information rely on independent neural networks. When people view external manifestations of themselves, whether it is images of their own faces or a video feed showing their own arm movements in real time, a network of lateral frontal and parietal regions, particularly on the right side of the brain, is recruited (Lieberman, 2007). In contrast, when people focus on internal characteristics such as their feelings, preferences, dispositions, and goals for the future, the characteristic MPFC and precuneus$_{PCC}$ activations are found.

This dissociation between internally focused and externally focused self-processes (Lieberman, 2007, 2010) has a number of implications for how we understand the self. First, it casts doubt on the unity of self-awareness and self-knowledge processes. By extension, it casts doubt on whether the "mirror test" of self-awareness (Gallup, 1970) is a test of generic self-awareness or is instead merely a test of physical self-recognition. Second, it may help explain why in the face of overwhelming evidence to the contrary, nearly all people behave as if mind–body dualism is true. The fact that the brain evolved separate systems for consideration of our own minds and bodies may render us incapable of experiencing them as one thing.

From Neuroscience to Psychology

As can be seen, neuroscience has been able to weigh in on at least a few of the claims made over the millennia by those who have opined most famously about the nature of self-knowledge. What else can we learn from neuroscience about the self? If we know the regions that tend to be involved in self-knowledge, what good does that do psychologists?

What Else Do We Know about MPFC?

Across the three dozen or so fMRI studies of self-knowledge (i.e., self-reference), MPFC is unequivocally the touchstone region. Publishing a paper on the neural bases of self-knowledge without activations in MPFC is likely to be difficult. Even though rostral anterior cingulate cortex (rACC) is adjacent to MPFC and self-knowledge tasks often produce activations overlapping the two regions, as an editor I have witnessed harsh reviews of papers that have rACC but not MPFC activations during self-reference. It must be pointed out that although self-reference tasks almost uniformly activate MPFC, this does not imply that MPFC is a "self" region or that activation there necessarily implies that self-referential processes are occurring.

I do think it is safe to say that the MPFC plays a uniquely human role in self and social cognition. MPFC is the only region of the prefrontal cortex that is verifiably larger in humans than in other primates after researchers control for brain and body size (Semendeferi et al., 2001). Moreover, this region has disproportionately greater spacing between neurons than in other primates, thought to allow for more complex connectivity (Semendeferi et al., 2011). Thus there is something distinctive about this region in humans compared with other species.

A variety of studies provide the link from MPFC to social cognition, rather than to self-processes only. For instance, Mitchell and colleagues (Mitchell, Banaji, & Macrae, 2005; Mitchell, Macrae, & Banaji, 2006) have found in a number of studies that when individuals judge the psychological characteristics of those similar to themselves they recruit MPFC rather than the DMPFC usually observed during social cognition (Frith & Frith, 2003). Mitchell has suggested that this occurs because when people try to make sense of similar others, they use the self as a template and project their understanding of themselves onto the similar others.

A self-based explanation cannot account for the MPFC activations typically seen when people make judgments about close others who are not necessarily similar to themselves (van Overwalle, 2009). A recent set of studies by Krienen, Tu, and Buckner (2010) pitted closeness and similarity against one another and found that MPFC activity was more sensitive to closeness than to similarity. When making judgments of a friend whom one acknowledges is not very similar to oneself, robust MPFC activity cannot easily be attributed to a self-projection process.

MPFC has increasingly been associated with empathy processes as well. MPFC activity has been associated with the accuracy of empathic judgments (Zaki, Weber, Bolger, & Ochsner, 2009). Additionally, MPFC activity during an empathy task predicts helping in everyday life (Rameson, Morelli, & Lieberman, 2012). Given that one of the hallmarks of adult empathy is a focus on the needs and experience of the other person rather than on oneself, these findings are hard to reconcile with a "self"-focused account of MPFC.

Finally, MPFC is emerging as a key player in the neural bases of persuasion. Multiple laboratories have now observed MPFC to be more active in response to persuasive messages (Chua, Liberzon, Welsh, & Strecher, 2009; Falk, Berkman, & Lieberman, 2011, in press; Falk, Berkman, Mann, Harrison, & Lieberman, 2010) and in predicting whether people will change their behavior.

Two Theories of MPFC and DMPFC Function

So what does this all mean? What does MPFC really do? In truth, we really don't know yet. Whatever it does will have implications for our understanding of self-processes, including self-knowledge. I have a theory that I think is more than half-baked, but certainly not fully baked. A key fact driving my own theorizing is the asymmetry in MPFC and DMPFC involvement in thinking about the self and thinking about others. As mentioned earlier, when thinking about the self, MPFC is activated in nearly every study, and DMPFC is activated about half the time. In contrast, when thinking about others, DMPFC is activated in nearly every study (91%), and MPFC is reported in one-third (33%) of studies. Thus, it seems that MPFC and DMPFC are not clearly identified as self and social cognition regions per se. It is more plausible to suppose that MPFC is responsible for a mental process that *tends* to be recruited more often when thinking about the self than about others (but it can be involved in either), and that DMPFC is responsible for a mental process that *tends* to be recruited more often when thinking about others than about the self (but it also can be involved in either). So this is our starting point. Any account of the functions of these two regions needs to accommodate that asymmetry.

Generic and Idiosyncratic Theories of People

At least two processing distinctions fit this bill reasonably well. They are related distinctions but are positioned at different levels of analysis. The first and more straightforward of these is a cognitive distinction between generic and idiosyncratic representations of people. We have a representation of the generic individual, his or her goals and preferences, and how the generic individual is likely to respond in various situations. This is precisely what more than half a century of studies on attribution processes has focused on (Jones et al., 1971). For instance, we would probably all represent the generic person in such a way that we would expect that with a gun pointed to his or her head, the person would feel fear, think about ways to survive or escape this ordeal, and be willing to engage in various low-cost behaviors such as shouting that teen heartthrob "Justin Bieber is my favorite singer of all time," if it would secure freedom. I do not need to know about the person's unique characteristics to make this assessment. It is exactly this sort of generic assessment that theory of mind tasks use repeatedly to measure one person's ability to consider the mental states of another person.

Two important things should be noted about the use of these generic theories of people. First, as social psychologists well know, the fact that people have these theories, use them endlessly, and believe in their utility in no way guarantees that the theories are correct. Second, and more importantly for our current purposes, these same generic theories can be applied to ourselves as well as to others. That is, when I consider what I would do if a gun were held to my head, I might draw on the same generic theory that I use to forecast the reactions of people in general (Karniol, 2003). While we can use this generic theory of people when thinking about others or ourselves, we are probably likely to draw on it more frequently for thinking about others rather than ourselves. For judging others, this generic theory is all we have to go on, but for ourselves we have other kinds of information (Pronin, 2009).

In addition to a generic theory of people, we also have idiosyncratic theories of particular individuals. Idiosyncratic theories no doubt come into play when imagining whether one's father or one's 14-year-old niece would yell "I love Justin Bieber" based solely on a verbal request (without a gun or other threat). Of course, our most idiosyncratic theory of any individual is reserved for ourselves. We have deeply idiosyncratic theories of ourselves. Thus, idiosyncratic theories probably are recruited more often when thinking about the self than about others. At a first approximation, the differential application of generic and idiosyncratic knowledge when thinking about self and others comports well with the ratio of MPFC and DMPFC activations for each target, self and other. This account also accommodates the finding of greater MPFC when thinking about similar others (Mitchell et al., 2005) because this could reflect the projection of one's idiosyncratic self-theory and also accommodate the finding of greater MPFC when thinking about close others (Krienen et al., 2010) who are not similar, as we are likely to have idiosyncratic theories of them as well.

Why would the brain be set up to separate these functions, and what are the implications for our understanding of self-knowledge? One possibility is that generic and idiosyncratic social knowledge functions evolved at different points in our history. A second and more interesting possibility is that there are different computational requirements for each, and that the requirements are sufficiently at odds with one another that it is too computationally costly to try to represent both functions in the same brain region. McClelland, McNaughton, and O'Reilly (1995) gave an elegant demonstration of something analogous in the domain of memory. They were addressing why semantic and episodic memory (i.e., memory for generalities and memory for specific instances) are represented separately in the brain. They created computational simulations that repeatedly produced "catastrophic interference" when episodic and semantic memories were represented in a single system.

This latter account is exciting because it would suggest that there are likely computational differences involved in idiosyncratic and generic bases of self-knowledge. Given that these two kinds of self-knowledge do not feel phenomenologically different on first pass, this is a case where neuroimaging might help us draw psychological distinctions and suggest avenues of psychological research we might otherwise overlook.

This account would also suggest the possibility that self-knowledge and self-representation more generally might have been an accidental side effect of needing to represent others in one's group idiosyncratically. Evolutionarily, this might have been the greater press. If this is the case, we should expect that in human children and in other species, the development of idiosyncratic, more so than generic, theories of others would be linked to the development of self-knowledge.

Immersive and Transactional Social Experience

The second possible distinction is phenomenological rather than computational in nature (see Buber [1937] for a similar distinction described from a philosophical perspective and Clark & Mills [1979] on exchange and communal processing which has much in common with the current distinction). Many of our social interactions and the social cognition that supports them are transactional in nature. We are focused on a particular transaction, and other individuals, who happen to have minds that we must take into account, are a means to an end rather than an end in themselves. During these interactions, other people only vaguely rise above the level of other objects or perhaps complex machines that are represented in terms of input–output patterns. At a restaurant, I am aware that if I motion my hand in a certain way the waiter will bring the check over. The waiter is simply a means to an end and this is a two-way street. Many of the canned compliments from people in the service industries do not represent a genuine interest in the customer but rather an understanding of reciprocity and ingratiation that are likely to increase sales and tips. Driving on the road with other cars is probably an ideal example of transactional social cognition. I know that the other cars are being operated by people with minds, and my theory of those minds is integral to how I behave in relation to those other cars, but I am not the least bit interested in those people as ends in themselves.

Transactional social experience is closely aligned with generic theories of people, but here I am focusing on the distinctly diminished sense of human interaction that often parallels the use of this generic theory. Transactional social experience is also not the same as dehumanization (Harris & Fiske, 2006), in that we can and do have transactional experiences with all the people we are closest with in life. Though, to be sure, dehumanization likely increases the tendency to treat others in transactional terms.

While we do not typically treat ourselves transactionally, we certainly can, and our memories of what we did or felt in the past are certainly influenced at times by our generic theories of how the average person would react in that situation. Thus, if DMPFC supports social cognition framed in a transactional way, it would follow that we would see it often in the kinds of abstract theory of mind tasks typically used in fMRI research and only occasionally when people think about themselves.

Naturally, we do not always treat other people in a transactional manner. Sometimes another person's humanity jumps out at us, and the full appreciation that the person is a sentient being full of hopes, desires, fears, and all the rest captures us. There are times when we really *connect* with another person in a way that has strong emotional and physiological components. This occurs when we empathize or sympathize with what someone else is going through. It probably also happens when actors using the Stanislavski method are fully immersed in the experience of the characters they are playing. And finally, it also happens when we relive, rather than simply recall, our own past experiences. Put another way, we treat ourselves in a far more immersive than transactional way compared with how we treat others, and our degree of connectedness with the other is likely to mediate this variable. Thus, if MPFC supports social cognition that is more immersive in nature, it would follow that we would see it most often when we think about ourselves, a target whose experience we can really dive into, and also in some situations when we think about others.

While the transactional and generic theory of mind accounts line up with one another quite nicely, the immersive and idiosyncratic accounts have an important difference. Certainly it is the case that the more idiosyncratic the knowledge we have of a person, the more easily we can find ourselves in an immersive encounter with that individual. However, it is also the case that we can have an immersive experience with someone about whom we have no idiosyncratic knowledge whatsoever. When we see a starving child on late-night television our understanding is immediate, emotional, and immersive—we are brought into the world of that child—but not based on specialized knowledge we have of the individual. At this point, it is unclear exactly how to reconcile the two accounts, but each focuses on ways of knowing and encountering people (including ourselves) rather than on the distinction between self and other processing per se.

Conclusions?

It is largely out of convention rather than necessity that there is a conclusions section here. The truth is that there are still far more questions than answers about the manner by which the brain supports self-knowledge, and what it has to tell us that is of psychological interest. We know that thinking about oneself, whether about one's autobiographical past, one's trait self-knowledge, or one's current preferences, all activate MPFC extremely reliably, and precuneus$_{PCC}$ and DMPFC somewhat reliably. We know that these are our primary targets for connecting the study of self-knowledge to the brain, that these are the regions where we would expect to see dissociations based on key psychological distinctions within self-knowledge processes and contents. However, what is mostly known is that these are the targets. The further utility of this brain mapping largely awaits further studies from psychologists who find the benefit to using dissociations and convergences at the level of the brain to complement the use of techniques such as self-report, reaction times, and memory clustering.

I have suggested two possible accounts of what MPFC (and DMPFC) may do in a larger, functional sense and how this might relate to how we think about self-knowledge. Neither of these accounts is fully fleshed out, but they at least suggest a method by which neuroscience may genuinely contribute to the psychological study of self-knowledge. If we can identify the functions of these regions that self-knowledge clearly relies upon, then we may be able to derive additional insights about what is involved in the formation, representation, and retrieval of self-knowledge.

REFERENCES

Beer, J. S., John, O. P., Scabini, D., & Knight, R. T. (2006). Orbitofrontal cortex and social behavior: Integrating self-monitoring and emotion–cognition interactions. *Journal of Cognitive Neuroscience, 18*, 871–879.

Bem, D. J. (1972). Self-perception theory. In L. Berkowitz (Ed.), *Advances in experimental social psychology* (pp. 1–62). New York: Academic Press.

Blakemore, S.-J., den Ouden, H., Choudhury, S., & Frith, C. (2007). Adolescent development of the neural circuitry for thinking about intentions. *Social Cognitive and Affective Neuroscience, 2*, 130–139.

Buber, M. (1937). *I and thou.* New York: Scribners & Sons.

Butler, J. (1819). *The analogy of religion.* Hartford, CT: Samuel T. Goodrich. (Original work published 1736)

Butler, J. (1896). *The works of John Butler.* Oxford, UK: Clarendon Press.

Chua, H. F., Liberzon, I., Welsh, R. C., & Strecher, V. J. (2009). Neural correlates of message tailoring and self-relatedness in smoking cessation programming. *Biological Psychiatry, 65*, 165–168.

Clark, M. S., & Mills, J. (1979). Interpersonal attraction in exchange and communal relationships. *Journal of Personality and Social Psychology, 37*, 12–24.

Craik, F. I. M., Moroz, T. M., Moscovitch, M., Stuss, D. T., Winocur, G., Tulving, E., et al. (1999). In search of the self: A positron emission tomography study. *Psychological Science, 10*, 26–34.

D'Argembeau, A., Stawarczyk, D., Majerus, S., Collette, F., Van der Linden, M., & Salmon, E. (2010). Modulation of medial prefrontal and inferior parietal cortices when thinking about past, present, and future selves. *Social Neuroscience, 5*, 187–200.

D'Argembeau, A., Xue, G., Lu, Z.-L., Van der Linden, M., & Bechara, A. (2008). Neural correlates of envisioning emotional events in the near and far future. *NeuroImage, 40*, 398–407.

Ersner-Hershfield, H., Wimmer, G. E., & Knutson, B. (2009). Saving for the future self: Neural measures of future self-continuity predict temporal discounting. *Social Cognitive and Affective Neuroscience, 4*, 85–92.

Falk, E. B., Berkman, E. T., & Lieberman, M. D. (2011). Neural activity during health messaging predicts reductions in smoking above and beyond self-report. *Health Psychology, 30*, 177–185.

Falk, E. B., Berkman, E. T., & Lieberman, M. D. (in press). From neural responses to population behavior: Neural focus group predicts population level media effects. *Psychological Science.*

Falk, E. B., Berkman, E. T., Mann, T., Harrison, B., & Lieberman, M. D. (2010). Predicting persuasion-induced behavior change from the brain. *Journal of Neuroscience, 30*, 8421–8424.

Farb, N. A. S., Segal, Z. V., Mayberg, H., Bean, J., McKeon, D., Fatima, Z., et al. (2007). Attending to the present: Mindfulness meditation reveals distinct neural modes of self-reference. *Social Cognitive and Affective Neuroscience, 2*, 313–322.

Frith, U., & Frith, C. D. (2003). Development and neurophysiology of mentalizing. *Philosophical Transactions of the Royal Society B: Biological Sciences, 358*, 459–473.

Gallup, G. G., Jr. (1970). Chimpanzees: Self-recognition. *Science, 167*, 86–87.

Greenwald, A. G., & Banaji, M. R. (1989). The self as a memory system: Powerful, but ordinary. *Journal of Personality and Social Psychology, 57*, 41–54.

Harris, L. T., & Fiske, S. T. (2006). Dehumanizing the lowest of the low: Neuroimaging responses to extreme outgroups. *Psychological Science, 17*, 847–853.

Hastie, R., & Park, B. (1986). The relationship between memory and judgment depends on whether the judgment task is memory-based or on-line. *Psychological Review, 93*, 258–268.

James, W. (1890) *Principles of psychology* (Vol. 1). New York: Holt.

James, W. (1892). *Psychology*. New York: Holt.

Jones, E. E., Kanouse, D. E., Kelley, H. H., Nisbett, R. E., Valins, S., & Weiner, B. (1971). *Attribution: Perceiving the causes of behavior*. Morristown, NJ: General Learning Press.

Karniol, R. (2003). Egocentrism versus protocentrism: The status of self in social prediction. *Psychological Review, 110*, 563–580.

Kelley, W. M. C., Macrae, C. N., Wyland, C. L., Caglar, S., Inati, S., & Heatherton, T. F. (2002). Finding the self?: An event-related fMRI study. *Journal of Cognitive Neuroscience, 14*, 785–794.

Klein, S. B., Loftus, J., & Kihlstrom, J. F. (1996). Self-knowledge of an amnesic patient: Toward a neuropsychology of personality and social psychology. *Journal of Experimental Psychology, 125*, 250–260.

Klein, S. B., Loftus, J., Trafton, J. G., & Fuhrman, R. W. (1992). Use of exemplars and abstractions in trait judgments: A model of trait knowledge about the self and others. *Journal of Personality and Social Psychology, 63*, 739–753.

Krienen, F. M., Tu, P. C., & Buckner, R. L. (2010). Clan mentality: Evidence that the medial prefrontal cortex responds to close others. *Journal of Neuroscience, 30*, 13906–13915.

Libby, L. K., & Eibach, R. P. (2002). Looking back in time: self-concept change affects visual perspective in autobiographical memory. *Journal of Personality and Social Psychology, 82*, 167–179.

Lieberman, M. D. (2007). Social cognitive neuroscience: A review of core processes. *Annual Review of Psychology, 58*, 259–289.

Lieberman, M. D. (2010). Social cognitive neuroscience. In S. T. Fiske, D. T. Gilbert, & G. Lindzey (Eds.). *Handbook of social psychology* (5th ed., pp. 143–193). New York: McGraw-Hill.

Lieberman, M. D., Jarcho, J. M., & Satpute, A. B. (2004). Evidence-based and intuition-based self-knowledge: An fMRI study. *Journal of Personality and Social Psychology, 87*, 421–435.

Locke, J. (1689/1975). *An essay concerning human understanding*. Oxford, UK: Oxford University Press.

Loewenstein, G., & Elster, J. (1992) *Choice over time*. New York: Russell Sage Foundation.

Macrae, C. N., Moran, J. M., Heatherton, T. F., Banfield, J. F., & Kelley, W. M. (2004). Medial prefrontal activity predicts memory for self. *Cerebral Cortex, 14*, 647–654.

Markus, H. (1977). Self-schemata and processing information about the self. *Journal of Personality and Social Psychology, 35*, 63–78.

McClelland, J. L., McNaughton, B. L., & O'Reilly, R. C. (1995). Why are there complimentary learning systems in the hippocampus and neocortex: Insights from the successes and failures of connectionist models of learning and memory. *Psychological Review, 102*, 419–457.

Mitchell, J. P., Banaji, M. R., & Macrae, C. N. (2005). The link between social cognition and self-referential thought in the medial prefrontal cortex. *Journal of Cognitive Neuroscience, 17,* 1306–1315.

Mitchell, J. P., Macrae, C. N., & Banaji, M. R. (2006). Dissociable medial prefrontal contributions to judgments of similar and dissimilar others. *Neuron, 50,* 655–663.

Moran, J. M., Heatherton, T. F., & Kelley, W. M. (2009). Modulation of cortical midline structures by implicit and explicit self-relevance evaluation. *Social Neuroscience, 4,* 197–211.

Nyberg, L., Kim, A. S. N., Habib, R., Levine, B., & Tulving, E. (2010). Consciousness of subjective time in the brain. *Proceedings of the National Academy of Sciences USA, 107,* 22356–22359.

Pfeifer, J. H., Lieberman, M. D., & Dapretto, M. (2007). "I know you are but what am I?!": An fMRI study of self-knowledge retrieval during childhood. *Journal of Cognitive Neuroscience, 19,* 1323–1337.

Pronin, E. (2009). The introspection illusion. *Advances in Experimental Social Psychology, 41,* 1–67.

Rameson, L. T., Morelli, S. A., & Lieberman, M. D. (2012). The neural correlates of empathy: Experience, automaticity, and prosocial behavior. *Journal of Cognitive Neuroscience, 24,* 235–245.

Rameson, L. T., Satpute, A. B., & Lieberman, M. D. (2010). The neural correlates of implicit and explicit self-relevant processing. *NeuroImage, 50,* 701–708.

Rogers, T. B., Kuiper, N. A., & Kirker, W. S. (1977). Self-reference and the encoding of personal information. *Journal of Personality and Social Psychology, 35,* 677–688.

Ryle, G. (1949). *The concept of mind.* New York: Barnes & Noble.

Schmitz, T. W., Rowley, H. A., Kawahara, T. N., & Johnson, S. C. (2006). Neural correlates of self-evaluative accuracy after traumatic brain injury. *Neuropsychologia, 44,* 762–773.

Schnyer, D. M., Nicholls, L., & Verfaellie, M. (2005). The role of VMPC in metamemorial judgments of content retrievability. *Journal of Cognitive Neuroscience, 17,* 832–846.

Semendeferi, K., Schleicher, A., Zilles, K., Armstrong, E., & Van Hoesen, G. W. (2001). Evolution of the hominoid prefrontal cortex: Imaging and quantitative analysis of area 10. *American Journal of Physical Anthropology, 114,* 224–241.

Semendeferi, K., Teffer, K., Buxhoeveden, D. P., Park, M. S., Bludau, S., Amunts, K., et al. (2011). Spatial organization of neurons in the frontal pole sets humans apart from great apes. *Cerebral Cortex, 21,* 1485–1497.

van Overwalle, F. (2009). Social cognition and the brain: A meta-analysis. *Human Brain Mapping, 30,* 829–858.

Wang, A. T., Lee, S. S., Sigman, M., & Dapretto, M. (2006). Developmental changes in the neural basis of interpreting communicative intent. *Social Cognitive and Affective Neuroscience, 1,* 107–121.

Way, B. M., Creswell, J. D., Eisenberger, N. I., & Lieberman, M. D. (2010). Dispositional mindfulness and depressive symptomatology: Correlations with limbic and self-referential neural activity during rest. *Emotion, 10,* 12–24.

Zaki, J., Weber, J., Bolger, N., & Ochsner, K. (2009). The neural bases of empathic accuracy. *Proceedings of the National Academy of Sciences, USA, 106,* 11382–11387.

CHAPTER 6

Blind Spots to the Self
Limits in Knowledge of Mental Contents and Personal Predispositions

JASON CHIN
MICHAEL MRAZEK
JONATHAN SCHOOLER

In a world filled with mysteries, one might hope to take solace in there being at least one thing we can know with certainty, namely, ourselves. Indeed, Descartes' famous declaration "I think therefore I am" is fundamentally grounded in the observation that knowledge of the occurrence of our own thoughts is the only thing we can know with utmost assurance. While the privileged knowledge of the existence of our own experience may well represent a critical foundation for constructing an understanding of reality (e.g., Schooler, Hunt, & Schooler, 2011), alas, even this apparent epistemological stronghold has its weaknesses. In particular, while our knowledge of the existence of our experience may be unassailable, we can nevertheless be victims to major blind spots[1] with respect to both the contents of our thoughts and the nature of our personal dispositions.

The example of mind wandering while reading nicely illustrates the limitations of our knowledge of the current contents of thought. In many situations there can be some genuine practical advantage to mind wandering. Examples such as a long drive, a tedious lecture, or a shower all represent situations in which it may be possible to reflect on one's experiences or to plan one's day without unduly compromising performance on the primary activity. But reading is a special case, in that there is arguably no circumstance in which it is possible to read successfully while simultaneously thinking about topics entirely unrelated to what is being read. In such cases, one is simply getting further and further away from the place in the text that will have to be returned to once one's engagement in mindless reading is finally noticed. Nevertheless, despite its evident futility, most of us are all too familiar with the experience of suddenly realizing that while our eyes have been dutifully moving across the page, our minds have been fundamentally elsewhere. While the regular practice of such futile musings might initially seem paradoxical, their occurrence gains greater clarity when understood in terms of the notion that we can temporarily lose track of the current contents of thought (Schooler, 2002). Accordingly, as we discuss in greater detail shortly, the reason why people's minds wander during reading, even though this is an entirely self-defeating activity, is simply that they have temporarily lost track of the fact that their minds have strayed from the text.

While our awareness of the current contents of thought is one domain in which our self-knowledge can be sorely lacking, it is not the only area. Given that we are constant witnesses to our every experience, it might seem as if we should have a reasonably firm understanding of our basic traits and predispositions. And indeed, such a view has some merit. The predictive success of personality measures stems to a significant degree from the fact that individuals are in many cases able to provide reasonably accurate reports of their general predispositions. Nevertheless, recent research suggests that there are times when individuals can be notably uncertain about important personal predispositions, and in particular, their capacity for generous behavior. As will be argued, not only do people maintain significant uncertainty about such traits, but this uncertainty can also serve as motivation for prosocial behavior. Accordingly, when uncertainty about their capacity for prosocial behavior is made salient, people become motivated to resolve the ambiguity by engaging in prosocial behaviors so as to persuade themselves that they do in fact possess this trait.

In this chapter we review evidence for blind spots both in our awareness of the current contents of thought (in particular, the occurrence of mind wandering), and in our certainty regarding personal predispositions (in particular, the capacity for generosity). As will be seen, an understanding of blind spots in mental contents and personal traits is markedly enhanced by a consideration of the role of motivation. Under some circumstances individuals may be motivated to turn a blind eye to genuine self-knowledge, whereas in other contexts, self-knowledge can be an important motivating factor driving people to engage in behaviors that may (accurately or inaccurately) inform their self-understanding.

Limitations in Awareness of the Contents of Thought

Consideration of evidence in support of the claim that one can lose track of the contents of one's own mind may be clarified by first introducing a distinction between two ways in which individuals can be conscious of an experience. In one sense, individuals are always conscious of any experience they are having. If an individual is experiencing a daydream, then, by definition, that daydream is conscious. In this sense, the person can be said to be experientially conscious of the daydream. At the same time, if we do not explicitly realize that we are daydreaming, then we may be said to lack "meta-awareness" of the fact that we were daydreaming. The example of mind wandering while reading thereby illustrates a distinction between experience and meta-awareness (Schooler, 2002). Accordingly, experience or experiential consciousness corresponds to the contents of consciousness, in this case, whatever it is that the person is daydreaming about. In contrast, *meta-awareness*, also known as meta-consciousness or metacognitive awareness, can be defined as one's explicit knowledge about the current contents of thought. The sudden noticing that one's mind has wandered represents a canonical example of a state of experiential consciousness reaching meta-awareness. Other examples include explicitly identifying one's emotional state (Schooler & Mauss, 2009), recognizing the occurrence of an unwanted thought (Wenzlaff & Wegner, 2000; Winkielman & Schooler, 2009), and appreciating that one is employing a particular mental strategy (Schooler & Smallwood, 2009). In short, whereas experiential consciousness is a continuous process that carries on throughout waking hours, meta-awareness is an intermittent process whereby individuals only periodically take stock of what they are thinking about (for recent reviews, see Chin & Schooler, 2010; Winkielman & Schooler, 2011).

In recent years, a growing body of research has supported the contention that individuals are only intermittently meta-aware of the experience of mind wandering (i.e., of the fact that their attention has drifted away from a task to unrelated concerns). This claim is supported by two strands of evidence, both revealing the frequency and consequences of mind wandering without meta-awareness: the self-caught/probe-caught paradigm and the zone-out/tune-out paradigm (Schooler, Smallwood, et al., 2011). We review each in turn.

Self-Caught/Probe-Caught Mind Wandering

One approach for documenting mind wandering in the absence of meta-awareness is combining self-catching and experience-sampling measures into a single paradigm. The self-catching measure asks participants to press a response key every time they notice for themselves that they have engaged in mind wandering. This measure provides a straightforward assessment of the mind-wandering episodes that have reached meta-awareness. By contrast, the experience-sampling measure probes participants at unpredictable intervals to ask whether they were mind wandering. When used in conjunction with the self-caught measure, experience sampling can catch people mind wandering before they notice it themselves.

A number of studies have effectively used the self-caught/probe-caught methodology to illuminate the relationship between mind wandering and meta-awareness. This approach was initially used to examine mind wandering while reading (Schooler, Reichle, & Halpern, 2004). Whereas participants regularly self-caught themselves mind wandering (approximately four times in a 45-minute period), they nevertheless were regularly caught mind wandering (about 15% of experience-sampling probes). Strikingly, and in support of the fundamental difference between mind-wandering episodes that are accompanied versus not accompanied by meta-awareness, there was a strong correlation between probe-caught mind wandering and comprehension performance, but no such relationship occurred with self-caught mind wandering. It may be that when individuals self-catch mind-wandering episodes, they are able to engage in the self-regulation process necessary to avoid comprehension failures.

Further evidence that meta-awareness of mind-wandering episodes allows self-regulation comes from comparison of gaze behavior prior to self-caught and probe-caught mind wandering. In an eye-tracking experiment, the eye movements of readers became especially erratic, with fewer words being fixated and more off-text fixations, in the 2.5 seconds immediately before the subjects' self-caught mind wandering (Reichle, Reineberg, & Schooler, 2010). This finding suggests that either an increasing meta-awareness of mind wandering leads readers to more completely disengage from the text, or that the especially erratic movement of the eyes causes readers to become meta-aware of their own mind wandering. Future research will be necessary to disentangle these two accounts and to better understand the relationship among mind wandering, meta-awareness of such lapses, and eye movements during reading.

Additional studies have examined the impact of two mind-altering experiences hypothesized to undermine individuals' meta-awareness: alcohol intoxication and cigarette craving. In one study, 54 male social drinkers consumed a moderate dose of alcohol (0.82 g/kg) or a placebo beverage, then performed a task assessing mind wandering during reading (Sayette, Reichle, & Schooler, 2009). Compared with those who drank the placebo, participants who drank alcohol were more likely to report that they were mind wandering when probed. After accounting for this increase in mind wandering, alcohol also lowered the probability of catching oneself mind wandering. These data suggest that alcohol increases mind wandering while simultaneously reducing the likelihood of noticing one's mind wandering.

In another study, 44 smokers, who were either nicotine-deprived (crave condition) or nondeprived (low-crave condition), performed the same mind-wandering task used in the previously described alcohol study (Sayette, Schooler, & Reichle, 2010). Smokers in the cigarette-crave condition were significantly more likely than the low-craving smokers to acknowledge that their mind was wandering when they were probed. When this more than threefold increase in zoning out was accounted for, craving also lowered the probability of self-catching mind wandering. As with the alcohol findings discussed earlier, it appears that cigarette craving simultaneously increases mind wandering while reducing the metacognitive capacity to notice it. The findings derived from the self-caught/probe-caught paradigm therefore suggest that the failures of self-regulation associated with both alcohol consumption and cigarette craving may result from a compromised ability to notice one's distracted state and therefore regulate it accordingly.

Experience Sampling of Aware versus Unaware Mind Wandering

A second methodology that has been used to examine fluctuations in meta-awareness of mind wandering entails combining the experience-sampling methodology with a judgment of participants' immediately prior state of meta-awareness. In this procedure, participants are intermittently queried regarding whether or not they were mind wandering, and if mind wandering, are asked to indicate whether they had been aware of this fact. In response to such queries, participants routinely indicated that they had been unaware of their mind wandering up until the time of the probe. Moreover, when participants classify mind-wandering episodes as unaware, their performance and neurocognitive activity systematically differ from when they report having been aware that they were mind wandering.

Consistent with findings using the self-caught/probe-caught methodology, retrospective classifications of unaware mind-wandering episodes (termed *zoning out*) and aware episodes (termed *tuning out*) indicate that zoning out is more strongly associated with comprehension failures than tuning out (Smallwood, McSpadden, & Schooler, 2008). Similarly, reports of zoning out seem to be most closely linked to failures in response inhibition (Smallwood, Beach, Schooler, & Handy, 2008; Smallwood, McSpadden, Luus, & Schooler, 2008) and in understanding the narrative structure of a novel (Smallwood, McSpadden, & Schooler, 2008). Together these results suggest that mind wandering in the absence of awareness is especially damaging to task performance.

Neurocognitive measures also reveal differences in the degree of activation between mind-wandering episodes that have been classified as aware versus unaware. In a combined experience sampling/functional magnetic resonance imaging study, mind wandering with awareness activated similar brain regions to those observed during mind wandering without awareness (Christoff, Gordon, Smallwood, Smith, & Schooler, 2009). These brain regions, however, were more strongly activated when mind wandering occurred without awareness. This greater activation is consistent with the results of behavioral studies indicating a more severe performance detriment associated with zoning out. The anterior prefrontal cortex (Brodmann's area) was one brain region that was significantly more strongly recruited during unaware episodes of mind wandering. Notably, anterior prefrontal cortex recruitment has been directly linked to engagement of cognitive meta-awareness (Gallagher & Frith, 2003). The observation that this same brain region became specifically more recruited during unaware episodes of mind wandering may seem surprising at first. However, the anterior prefrontal cortex may be involved in mind wandering through its role in the maintenance of thought. Its recruitment during mind wandering in the absence of awareness may make it more difficult for meta-awareness to be implemented.

The Relationship between Motivation and Self-Knowledge of Fleeting Mental States

The evidence reviewed so far suggests that fluctuations of meta-awareness of mind wandering may be a natural consequence of inherent limitations in cognitive capacity. Being meta-aware of one's mental states is necessarily a resource-demanding task, so it is not always feasible to dedicate resources both to the task at hand and to meta-awareness of ongoing mental processes. Evidence consistent with this view comes from the finding that manipulations that compromise cognitive resources (e.g., alcohol, craving) specifically undermine individuals' capacity to notice that they are mind wandering.

While simple limits in cognitive resources are certainly one compelling source of variations in meta-awareness of mental states, they are not the only source. In particular, it seems likely that motivation may also play a role. Indeed, the relationship between motivation and meta-awareness may well go both ways. On the one hand, it seems likely that someone who is highly motivated to pay attention to what he or she is doing will be more motivated to check in regularly to make sure that his or her mind is where it is supposed to be. On the other hand, there may be times when, for a variety of possible reasons, individuals may be disinclined to acknowledge what they are thinking about to themselves. In such cases, the frequency of meta-awareness might be curtailed. We consider in turn these two sides of the relationship between motivation and meta-awareness.

One context in which motivation for meta-awareness of mental states might be enhanced is following deliberate self-reflection. A recent study examined this possibility by fostering a self-reflective state of mind in participants and subsequently measuring meta-awareness of mind wandering (Mrazek, Smallwood, & Schooler, 2012). Participants in one group rated whether adjectives were descriptive of themselves, while a control condition rated whether the adjectives described the President of the United States. Following this manipulation, the self-caught/probe-caught methodology was employed to assess meta-awareness of mind wandering while participants completed a short global/local detection task. Relative to the control condition, members of the self-reflective condition reported comparable amounts of mind wandering at the experience-sampling probes but self-caught their mind wandering significantly more often. This result suggests that the motivation to reflect on one's personality, which was cultivated during the adjective-rating task, led to an increased likelihood of becoming meta-aware of one's mind wandering.

A second line of research provides evidence for situations in which motivation may dampen individuals' motivation to notice the contents of their thought. In this study (Baird, Smallwood, Fishman, Mrazek, & Schooler, 2012), the contents of mind-wandering episodes were systematically biased using a thought suppression paradigm originally employed by Wegner and Gold (1995). Participants first were asked to think about a previous relationship that had ended. Then, they were instructed to try not to think about the relationship while simultaneously engaging in a resource-demanding task (i.e., reading). Based on Wegner and Gold's findings, we hypothesized that this would cause individuals to mind-wander regularly about the former relationship while reading. We also anticipated that the frequency of such intrusions would depend on whether individuals had terminated the relationship themselves (what Wegner and Gold referred to as "cold flames") or whether the partner had ended the relationship ("hot flames"). Using a self-catching procedure, Wegner and Gold found that hot flames reported fewer intrusive thoughts about their former relationship than did cold flames. However, we reasoned that this might not be because hot flames actually had fewer thoughts about their former partners, but rather because they were motivated not to acknowledge those thoughts when they occurred. In other words, individuals who have been "dumped" by their partner may prefer not to acknowledge that they are thinking about the individuals who spurned them. To test this hypothesis, we included both the self-caught and probe-caught measures. Consistent with the findings of Wegner and Gold, we found that hot flames were less likely spontaneously to self-catch thoughts about their former partner than were cold flames. However, in striking contrast, we found that hot flames were significantly more likely than cold flames to be caught thinking about their partners by the probes. Apparently, in this paradigm, individuals who have been spurned think about their partners at least as much as those who have not—they simply are less willing to acknowledge this fact to themselves.

The Baird and colleagues (2012) study suggests that motivation may play an important role in mediating the frequency with which individuals take stock of their mental states. If an individual is disinclined to want to think about someone, as is likely the case for partners who have been spurned, then he or she may be relatively less willing to acknowledge such thoughts to him- or herself when they occur. This view offers another way to think about the mental processes sometimes attributed to Freudian repression. Accordingly, rather than keeping thoughts from entering consciousness, motivational processes may instead prevent individuals from acknowledging the occurrence of those thoughts when they happen. Indeed, such an account is consistent with case studies of corroborated recovered memories of sexual abuse[2] (Schooler, 2001). In a number of these cases, conversations with partners of abuse victims revealed that victims had talked about the allegedly repressed memory during a period in which they subsequently claimed the memory had been unavailable. One interpretation of these unacknowledged episodes of retrieval is that the victims recalled the abuse but lacked meta-awareness of the fact that they were recalling it. In other words, like the hot flames in Schooler and colleagues' study, they may have been motivated not to let the unwanted thought reach the level of meta-awareness. According to this view, when memories of genuine abuse are characterized as recovered, the recovery may not be of the memory itself. Rather, it may entail a newfound willingness to acknowledge the memory when it comes to mind.

In summary, consideration of variations in individuals' awareness of their fleeting mental states and, in particular, of their tendency to mind-wander, suggests that individuals routinely lose track of the current contents of thought. Such failure of self-knowledge about one's current mental contents appear to be driven by multiple sources. On some occasions it may simply reflect limited cognitive resources. Meta-awareness is resource-demanding and so it is simply infeasible to maintain continuous explicit monitoring of the contents of thought. On other occasions, failures of meta-awareness may be more frequent as individuals become, for various reasons, disinclined to acknowledge to themselves what they are thinking about. While motivations may sometimes lead to attenuated self-knowledge, in other cases, such as when people are put into a self-reflective state of mind, motivation for meta-awareness may be increased, and individuals may become increasingly inclined to take stock of their mental states. As will be seen, this motivation for enhanced self-knowledge becomes increasingly important when we consider the case of knowledge for personal traits, the domain we turn to next.

Self-Signaling and Uncertainty about Personal Traits

Under many circumstances individuals possess a relatively robust appreciation of their personal traits and dispositions. Under such circumstances, individuals are often motivated to procure personal information that accords with their preconceived beliefs about their self-concept (Swann, Rentfrow, & Guinn, 2003). However, in other situations, people can be uncertain about their personal traits and predispositions. In these latter circumstances, people are motivated to resolve this lack of self-insight, even if they might uncover something unsavory.

Trope and Brickman (1975) were among the first to document the impact of inducing trait uncertainty on people's motivation to gain self-knowledge. These researchers primed participants to feel uncertain about whether they possessed a novel ability. They then presented participants with the chance to construct a self-diagnostic test for which they could select alternatives of varying diagnosticity and difficulty. Their results demonstrated that participants primed with uncertainty showed a stronger preference for diagnostic items, even if these items represented a greater chance of failure. Research performed in applied settings has found parallel results. For example, Ashneel and Lievens (2007) found that in workplace settings, workers who were more uncertain about themselves were more likely to seek out performance feedback from supervisors.

These studies reveal that uncertainty about performance can motivate individuals to seek information about their abilities. But what about more core predispositions? Does uncertainty similarly motivate information-seeking behaviors about enduring personality traits? Recent theorizing on what is known as *self-signaling theory* posits that individuals are often uncertain about their core traits and consequently engage in various behaviors to put themselves in a favorable light with respect to traits about which they are uncertain. Self-signaling (Bodner & Prelec, 2003) proposes that when people are uncertain about traits, they will be motivated to engage in behaviors that signal positive trait information about themselves to themselves because it feels good to gain such information. This type of positive affect is referred to as *diagnostic utility*. Acts of self-signaling can include any type of behavior that reveals information about the self (for a related perspective, see self-perception theory; Bem, 1972), such as resisting the temptation to break a diet, which demonstrates self-control.

In its original conception, self-signaling was presented as a useful theoretical model for understanding previous psychological findings (Bodner & Prelec, 2003). Notably, self-signaling theorists described Quattrone and Tversky's (1984) study, which found that people are willing to endure greater pain when told that a high pain tolerance is associated with longevity. This finding is perplexing under traditional models of utility, which expect that people would prefer to avoid such a seemingly unnecessary source of pain. Under self-signaling, however, this pain seeking is interpreted as resulting from a motivation to infer possessing the trait of good health.

Critically, the motivation to self-signal assumes some level of self-uncertainty about the trait in question (Bodner & Prelec, 2003). With regard to the pain example (Quattrone & Tversky, 1984), a person who somehow knows exactly when he or she will die would have no reason to endure the frigid waters of longevity. This trial would tell nothing that is not already known. In the realm of self-control, a person who is completely certain that he or she possesses self-control would gain no diagnostic utility from resisting a temptation—there is nothing left to learn about the self in this regard. Self-signaling theory would therefore suggest that, independent of one's current self-evaluation, increased uncertainty surrounding a self-evaluation should promote self-signaling. This prediction was the focus of a recent set of studies in our laboratory and represents the first test of this key assumption of self-signaling theory.

In a recent set of studies, Smallwood and Schooler (2011) examined the relationship between uncertainty about prosocial tendencies and individuals' likelihood of engaging in such behaviors. The goal of this research was (1) to document the specific role that trait uncertainty plays in modulating self-signaling behavior, and (2) to demonstrate that people are routinely uncertain about their proclivity for prosocial

Blind Spots to the Self

behavior. The basic logic of this series of studies was that individuals who are especially uncertain about how prosocial they are should be particularly motivated to behave in ways that signal to themselves that they are indeed kind and generous.

Study 1 of this series took a correlational route, measuring the relationship between uncertainty about one's generosity and volunteer behavior. In this study, participants completed a questionnaire that asked them to indicate (1) how generous they viewed themselves to be, (2) how certain they were of their generosity, and (3) how many hours they tended to volunteer in a typical month. As predicted, this study found that participants who were more uncertain about their generosity reported volunteering more often than those who were more confident about their level of generosity.

Given Study 1's limitation as a correlational investigation, Study 2's main purpose was to provide causal evidence linking uncertainty about moral characteristics and helping behavior. To create uncertainty, participants took a computer-based test that included bogus self-report and implicit measures of personality. Participants were then randomly assigned to receive feedback about their personality, with this feedback varying in the amount of certainty the computer supposedly ascribed to it. After the experimental manipulations, participants were given the chance to agree to perform a small helping task in the future. Finally, Study 2 also included a response inhibition task designed to examine whether uncertain participants experienced increased enduring activation of helping concepts. The results of Study 2 revealed that participants receiving uncertain feedback were more likely to agree to help the experimenter by filling out additional questionnaires in the future. Furthermore, uncertain participants had more difficulty ignoring words related to helping during a subsequent color-naming task.

Study 3 was designed to test the effect of negative subjective uncertainty on helping. In particular, this study experimentally manipulated certainty and uncertainty about lacking compassion, using a sham physiological test that was alleged to reveal individuals' propensity for compassion. To broaden the generality of the research, Study 3 also featured a new measure of prosocial behavior, namely, the number of pens participants picked up after a clumsy confederate dropped several of them. The results of this study demonstrated that negative uncertainty had an effect on helping similar to that of positive uncertainty. Participants made to feel uncertain about being noncompassionate were most helpful (i.e., picked up the most pens), while certain participants helped less than controls who received no feedback.

Finally, Study 4 included both positive and negative compassion feedback in order to compare their relative effects and to explore a potential interaction between uncertainty and the valence of feedback. Helping, in Study 4 required a more tangible sacrifice because participants were asked to donate cash to a fire relief fund. Importantly, this request was solicited from participants as they walked across the campus after they believed they had finished the experiment. Since the experimenter was not in any way involved with the prosocial request, this study addressed the possibility that the results from previous studies were due to participants' possible concern that the experimenter was not appreciating their prosociality. This study revealed that uncertainty increased donations, independent of the valence of feedback, and even when the experimenter was seemingly unaware of the prosocial behavior. There was also a separate effect for feedback valence, as participants made to feel noncompassionate helped more, a finding that supports previous research regarding prosociality's self-enhancing function (Sachdeva, Iliev, & Medin, 2009).

Collectively, these studies on the impact of inducing trait uncertainty on prosocial behavior lead to two important conclusions regarding people's self-knowledge of their basic predispositions. First the fact that participants were powerfully influenced by being given ambiguous information about their prosocial proclivities suggests that this is a predisposition about which people can be genuinely uncertain. Second, the finding that priming people's uncertainty about their compassion enhances prosocial behavior illustrates the motivating power of self-signaling. When individuals are uncertain about their personal traits, they can become highly motivated to engage in behaviors that will help to prove that their predispositions are as they would desire them to be.

One final observation about self-signaling in the context of self-knowledge is also warranted. In order for self-signaling to operate, individuals cannot realize that they are engaging in it. If people behave in a prosocial manner simply to prove that they are prosocial, then this no longer provides any information about whether or not they are genuinely prosocial. Thus, an ironic aspect of self-signaling is that in order to gain self-knowledge from it, one must suspend self-knowledge about its usage.

Conclusions

This review reveals that people can possess serious blind spots in their self-knowledge of both their current thought processes and their general predispositions. Our thoughts routinely lapse into topics entirely unrelated to the situation at hand, yet often manage to do so below the radar of awareness. We are capable of significant degrees of uncertainty about personal predispositions as central as our capacity for generosity, yet we primarily respond to this deficit only when it is brought to our attention. Strikingly, and in keeping with referring to these deficits in self-knowledge as "blind spots," these pockets of ignorance frequently go unnoticed. A notable aspect of blind spots in vision is that they exist without our realizing it. Although the gaps in self-knowledge revealed in this analysis are certainly not as hidden as those associated with visual blind spots, the parallels are nevertheless notable. In the case of mind wandering, not only do we frequently experience major lapses in our mental processes but more often than not such lapses also occur without our realizing it. This fact is evidenced by (1) the frequency with which people are caught in mind wandering by experience-sampling probes before they catch the episodes themselves, and (2) the substantial proportion of times after being caught by such probes that people report they previously had failed to notice the lapse. Similarly, in the case of our own generosity, we seem to be lacking in knowledge about both the full extent of our capacity for prosocial behavior (as evidenced by the fact that priming uncertainty about this trait has such robust effects), and the efforts we go to in order to remedy this uncertainty (as noted, self-signaling is only effective if people don't realize they are doing it).

As the alleged inscription at the Oracle at Delphi "Know Thyself" famously reveals, the goal of self-knowledge is an old and venerable one. However, our success in this regard is most clearly variable. Not only do we routinely lack self-knowledge about important mental contents and personal predispositions but we are also routinely unaware of this deficit. While such blind spots in self-knowledge may abound, unlike visual blind spots, they may prove far more remediable. Recent evidence suggests for example, that meditation practices that enhance "mindfulness" (Wallace & Shapiro, 2006) can reduce people's tendency to experience mental lapses (Mrazek, Smallwood, & Schooler, 2011) and may enhance their awareness of experiential states (Schooler & Mauss, 2009; Sze, Gyurak, Yuan, & Levenson, 2010). While such practices may well prove to be particularly helpful in ameliorating the negative consequences of certain deficits in self-knowledge, this analysis also raises the possibility that there may be other circumstances in which self-knowledge can be counterproductive. Indeed, a relatively straightforward implication of the self-signaling data discussed here is that gaining self-knowledge about one's level of prosociality can reduce the motivation for self-signaling and thereby dampen one's inclination to engage in prosocial acts. Moreover, as suggested, the very process of self-signaling may be undermined if attention is drawn to the fact that one is engaging in a behavior for that purpose (Chin & Schooler, 2012). Thus, while there are certainly many situations in which knowing oneself is an admirable goal, it seems there are at least some cases where blind spots in self-knowledge may be quite functional.

NOTES

1. Our use of the term *blind spot* is in keeping with Pronin, Lin, and Ross's (2002) discussion of bias blind spots (see also Hansen & Pronin, Chapter 21, this volume). Like Pronin and colleagues, we use the metaphor of the visual blind spot to illustrate salient gaps in individuals' self-knowledge. However, here we suggest that such blind spots extend beyond perceptions of bias to awareness of current mental states (e.g., mind wandering) and enduring personal traits (e.g., generosity).

2. Importantly, we are not claiming that all memories characterized as recovered necessarily correspond to actual episodes of abuse. Indeed there are good reasons to believe that many so-called "recovered" memories are actually the product of therapists' suggestions. However, in these cases there was compelling corroborative evidence indicating that the memories actually corresponded to genuine episodes of abuse. Corroboration of the forgetting, however, was less clear. Indeed, as discussed in a number of cases, it appeared that individuals' claims of amnesia had been distorted quite possibly as a consequence of failures in their metacognitive capacity to acknowledge the memories when they came to mind.

ACKNOWLEDGMENTS

The writing of this chapter was supported through United States Department of Education Grant No. R3OJA110277 to Jonathan Schooler. We thank Sierra Yates Robart for comments on an earlier draft.

REFERENCES

Asneel, F., & Lievens, F. (2007). The relationship between uncertainty and desire for feedback: A test of competing hypotheses. *Journal of Applied Social Psychology, 37*, 1–34.

Baird, B., Smallwood, J., Fishman, D., Mrazek, M. D., & Schooler, J. W. (2012). *Unnoticed unwanted thoughts: Suppressed conscious thoughts evade detection and undermine control*. Manuscript in preparation.

Bem, D. J. (1972). Self-percepton theory. In L. Berkowitz (Ed.), *Advances in social psychology* (Vol. 6, pp. 1–62). New York: Academic Press.

Bodner, R., & Prelec, D. (2003). Self-signaling and diagnostic utility in everyday decision making. In I. Brocas & J. D. Carillo (Eds.), *The psychology of economic decisions, volume 1: Rationality and well-being* (pp. 105–123). Oxford, UK: Oxford University Press.

Chin, J., & Schooler, J. W. (2010). Meta-awareness. In W. Banks (Ed.), *Encyclopedia of consciousness* (pp. 33–41). Oxford, UK: Elsevier.

Chin, J. M., & Schooler, J. W. (2012). *Doing good to feel good: The value of pure intentions*. Unpublished Working Paper, University of British Columbia, Vancouver.

Christoff, K., Gordon, A. M., Smallwood, J., Smith, R., & Schooler, J. W. (2009). Experience sampling during fMRI reveals default network and executive system contributions to mind-wandering. *Proceedings of the National Academy of Sciences USA, 106,* 8719–8724.

Gallagher, H. L., & Frith, C. D. (2003). Functional imaging of "theory of mind." *Trends in Cognitive Science, 7,* 77–83.

Mrazek, M. D., Smallwood, J., & Schooler, J. W. (2011). *Mindfulness and mind-wandering: Finding convergence through opposing constructs*. Manuscript under review.

Mrazek, M. D., Smallwood, J., & Schooler, J. W. (2012). *Self-reflection increases meta-awareness of mind-wandering*. Manuscript in preparation.

Pronin, E., Lin, D. Y., & Ross, L. (2002) The bias blind spot: Perceptions of bias in self versus others. *Personality and Social Psychological Bulletin, 28,* 369–381.

Quattrone, G. A., & Tversky, A. (1984). Causal versus diagnostic contingencies: On self-deception and on the voter's illusion. *Journal of Personality and Social Psychology, 46,* 237–248.

Reichle, E. D., Reineberg, A. E., & Schooler, J. W. (2010). Eye movements during mindless reading. *Psychological Science, 21*(9), 1300–1310.

Sachdeva, S., Iliev, R., & Medin, D. L. (2009). Sinning saints and saintly sinners: The paradox of moral self regulation. *Psychological Science, 20,* 523–528.

Sayette, M. A., Reichle, E. D., & Schooler, J. W. (2009). Lost in the sauce: The effects of alcohol on mind-wandering. *Psychological Science, 20,* 747–752.

Sayette, M. A., Schooler, J. W., & Reichle, E. D. (2010). Out for a smoke: The impact of cigarette craving on zoning-out during reading. *Psychological Science, 21,* 26–30.

Schooler, J. W. (2001). Discovering memories in the light of meta-awareness. *Journal of Aggression, Maltreatment and Trauma, 4,* 105–136.

Schooler, J. W. (2002). Re-representing consciousness: Dissociations between consciousness and meta-consciousness. *Trends in Cognitive Science, 6,* 339–344.

Schooler, J. W., Hunt, T., & Schooler, J. N. (2011). Reconsidering the metaphysics of science from the inside out. In S. Schmidt & H. Wallach (Eds.), *Neuroscience consciousness and spirituality* (pp. 157–194). New York: Springer.

Schooler, J. W., & Mauss, I. B. (2009). To be happy and to know it: The experience and meta-awareness of pleasure. In K. Berridge & M. Kringlebach (Eds.), *Pleasures of the brain* (pp. 244–254). New York: Oxford University Press.

Schooler, J. W., Reichle, E. D., & Halpern, D. V. (2004). Zoning-out during reading: Evidence for dissociations between experience and meta-consciousness. In D. T. Levin (Ed.), *Thinking and seeing: Visual metacognition in adults and children* (pp. 204–226). Cambridge, MA: MIT Press.

Schooler, J. W., & Smallwood, J. (2009). Meta-cognition. In A. Cleermans, T. Bayne, & P.

Wilken (Eds.) *Oxford handbook of consciousness* (pp. 443–445). Oxford, UK: Oxford University Press.

Schooler, J. W., Smallwood, J., Christoff, K., Handy, T. C., Reichle, E. D., & Sayette, M. A. (2011). Meta-awareness, perceptual decoupling and the wandering mind. *Trends in Cognitive Science, 15*, 319–326.

Smallwood, J., Beach, E., Schooler, J. W., & Handy, T. C. (2008). Going AWOL in the brain: Mind-wandering reduces cortical analysis of external events. *Journal of Cognitive Neuroscience, 20*, 458–469.

Smallwood, J., McSpadden, M. C., Luus, B., & Schooler, J. W. (2008). Segmenting the stream of consciousness: The psychological correlates of temporal structures in the time series data of a continuous performance task. *Brain and Cognition, 66*(1), 50–56.

Smallwood, J., McSpadden, M. C., & Schooler, J. W. (2008). When attention matters: The curious incident of the wandering mind. *Memory and Cognition, 36*(6), 1144–1150.

Swann, W. B., Jr., Rentfrow, P. J., & Guinn, J. S. (2003). Self-verification: The search for coherence. In M. R. Leary & J. P. Tangney (Eds.), *Handbook of self and identity* (pp. 367–383). New York: Guilford Press.

Smallwood, J., & Schooler, J. W. (2011). [Moral uncertainty promotes moral behavior]. Unpublished raw data, University of California, Santa Barbara.

Sze, J. A., Gyurak, A., Yuan, J. W., & Levenson, R. W. (2010). Coherence between emotional experience and physiology: Does body awareness training have an impact? *Emotion, 10*, 803–814.

Trope, Y., & Brickman, P. (1975). Difficulty and diagnosticity as determinants of choice among tasks. *Journal of Personality and Social Psychology, 31*, 918–925.

Wallace, A. B., & Shapiro, S. L. (2006). Mental balance and well-being: Building bridges between Buddhism and Western psychology. *American Psychologist, 61*(7), 690–701.

Wegner, D. M., & Gold, D. B. (1995). Fanning old flames: Emotional and cognitive effects of suppressing thoughts of a past relationship. *Journal of Personality and Social Psychology, 68*, 782–792.

Wenzlaff, R. M., & Wegner, D. M. (2000). Thought suppression. *Annual Review of Psychology, 51*, 59–91.

Wilson, T. D., Dunn, D. S., Bybee, J. A., Hyman, D. B., & Rotondo, J. A. (1984). Effects of analyzing reasons on attitude–behavior consistency. *Journal of Personality and Social Psychology, 47*, 5–16.

Winkielman, P. W., & Schooler, J. W. (2009). Unconscious, conscious, and metaconscious in social cognition. In F. Strack & J. Förster (Eds.), *Social cognition: The basis of human interaction* (pp. 49–69). New York: Psychology Press.

Winkielman, P., & Schooler, J. W. (2011). Splitting consciousness: Unconscious, conscious, and metaconscious processes in social cognition. *European Review of Social Psychology, 22*, 1–35.

CHAPTER 7
Other People as a Source of Self-Knowledge

SANJAY SRIVASTAVA

I have a friend—let's call her Felicia—who has said a number of times over the years that she does not photograph well. Recently Felicia was stopped on the street by a professional fashion photographer who wanted to take her picture for a fashion and style blog. Felicia assented—reluctantly, I think—and a few weeks later the photographs appeared online. One of Felicia's friends (OK, it was me) came across the blog post and put up a link on Facebook, and within minutes, Felicia responded—rather predictably—that she thought she looked terrible in the pictures. But after compliments and "likes" from friends started accumulating, Felicia modified her stance a little bit, allowing that she was coming around to liking, or at least accepting, the photos.

This chapter explores whether other people's perceptions might be a source of self-knowledge. My anecdote about Felicia is meant to illustrate a major tension in trying to make sense of whether and how feedback from others might be incorporated into the self. On the one hand, a typical adult's self-concept is pretty stable: Most people have a strong sense of who they are. And it is arguably a good thing if someone's sense of self does not rise and fall with every offhanded comment that someone else has made because a stable sense of self provides a sense of stability and order to one's place in the world. On the other hand, the self-concept may not be entirely impervious to social feedback. Many people are interested in learning about themselves. Moreover, it is probably pretty difficult to remain completely unaffected by what others are saying.

Many psychologists, from William James onward, have been interested in "the social self." The self is intimately, and perhaps inextricably, entwined with the social world. We compare ourselves to others (Festinger, 1954); we look for our place within some groups and apart from others (Tajfel & Turner, 1979) and as members of a larger society (Erikson, 1950); we try to learn about the self by imagining the impressions we make on others (Mead, 1934). It hardly makes sense to imagine a self-concept without incorporating the social world.

Many "social" theories of the self are primarily about what and how the self thinks about the social world: The social world is important because it is something that the individual mentally represents, and those mental representations are involved in the process of building a self-concept. Such social-cognitive processes are clearly important in understanding the bases of self-knowledge, but they may not be the only way that other people are involved. Other people may matter not just as mental representations, but in a more truly "social" way.

My goal in this chapter is to try to look beyond these individual-centered social-cognitive approaches and ask to what extent other people—not just mental representations of the social world but actual human beings—might affect self-knowledge. I consider some of the ways that other people's impressions of an individual could affect that individual's self-knowledge. More specifically, I focus on the perhaps counterintuitive notion that other people could potentially contribute to *accurate* self-views. To set a manageable scope for this chapter, I focus on an admittedly narrow subset of social knowledge—knowledge of one's social roles and personal attributes (e.g., personality traits). I acknowledge up front that "self-knowledge" is a much broader domain that includes many other things: knowledge of one's preferences and goals, of one's physical body, and much more (cf. Markus, 1983; Neisser, 1988).

An Early Perspective: Reflected Appraisals

Reflected appraisals—perceptions of how others perceive the self (i.e., "What do other people think of me?")—are a particularly interesting species of metaperception (perceptions of perceptions), and are probably the most widely studied form of metaperception (see Carlson & Kenny, Chapter 15, this volume). Reflected appraisals were central to symbolic interactionist theories of how the self develops (Cooley, 1902; Mead, 1934). The symbolic interactionists proposed that people form a sense of self by first learning or inferring how others perceive them (i.e., by forming reflected appraisals). Over time, reflected appraisals become internalized into a self-concept (components of which are often called *direct self-appraisal* in the context of symbolic interactionism).[1]

Kinch (1963) proposed a series of postulates that formalized the symbolic interactionist theory. If two of these postulates hold true, then actual social others will affect the self by way of reflected appraisals. The first postulate is that reflected appraisals must be based on the actual behaviors of other people. The second postulate is that direct self-appraisals must be based on reflected appraisals. With regard to accuracy, we can add that in order for a person to acquire accurate self-views from others, others must be able to accurately perceive the individual's roles and attributes, and the person must behave in ways that are based on those perceptions.

On the last point, there is substantial evidence that people are able to perceive one another with at least some degree of accuracy (e.g., Funder, 1987, 1995; Kenny & Albright, 1987), and sometimes with greater accuracy than individuals have in perceiving themselves (Vazire, 2010). Attributes that are reputational in nature, such as *social status* (defined as one's prominence in the eyes of others), are another area where others might have better information than the self (Srivastava & Anderson, 2011). There is also evidence that perceptions guide interpersonal behavior (e.g., Bargh, Chen, & Burrows, 1996; Jussim, 1991; Snyder & Swann, 1978). Thus, it is reasonable to suppose that if reflected appraisals affect direct self-appraisals, then they may promote accuracy. But what does contemporary research say about Kinch's original postulates? Do people use others' behavior to form reflected appraisals; and do people then use those reflected appraisals as a basis for forming direct self-appraisals?

In research on adults, reflected appraisals as a route to self-knowledge have had a rocky history. Reflected appraisals correlate with direct self-appraisals and others' perceptions, but causation and underlying mechanisms have been difficult to establish (e.g., Kenny & DePaulo, 1993; Shrauger & Schoeneman, 1979; Tice & Wallace, 2005). By contrast, stronger evidence has been found among adolescents (e.g., Cole, 1991; Felson, 1985, 1993; Harter, 1999; Pfeifer et al., 2009). For example, in a longitudinal study, Felson (1985) found that reflected appraisals prospectively predicted adolescents' self-appraisals of physical attractiveness. And in a neuroimaging study, Pfeifer and her colleagues (2009) found that during a self-reflection task, there was greater overlap between regions used for self-perception and other-perception among adolescents than among adults, suggesting that adolescents may be more heavily drawing upon representations of other people's minds when directly appraising the self. One plausible interpretation of these and other findings is that an adolescent's still-forming self-concept is more open to influences of all kinds, including input from the social world; by contrast, adults have more stored self-appraisals and therefore have less need to look outward to fill in the gaps. Another proposed explanation is that adults are more likely to refer to internal guideposts, such as possible selves, and less likely to make social comparisons when drawing inferences about the self (Harter, 1999).

Reflected appraisals are an important part of the history of research on self-knowledge, and they continue to be of great interest, particularly in research on development of the self during childhood and adolescence (Pfeifer et al., 2009). They present one possible pathway for others to affect self-knowledge; but reflected appraisals are not necessarily the only way. It is possible for others to affect the self-concept without a mental representation of others' perceptions being formed along the way (Srivastava & Beer, 2005). In the remainder of this chapter I consider a variety of ways, not just reflected appraisals, that other people could affect the self-concept.

The Loyal Resistance: Motivated Self-Perception

Before further considering whether and how other people might influence self-knowledge, it is important to weigh the evidence for why such influences may be limited. Several prominent theories of the self have suggested that the self-perception process is guided by motives that would make it resistant to social influences. The *self-enhancement* perspective argues that people are motivated to form and maintain positive self-views. The *self-verification* perspective proposes that people are motivated to maintain consistency and coherence in their self-views. These motives are reviewed in detail in other chapters in this volume (Schriber & Robins, Chapter 8;

Helzer & Dunning, Chapter 23; Strube, Chapter 24)—here I focus on the potential these motives have for derailing social influences on accurate self-views.

Self-Enhancement

Perhaps the most widely studied motivation in self-perception is self-enhancement. The *self-enhancement motive* is the desire to have an evaluatively positive self-concept. (Sometimes self-enhancement is also described as a motive to maintain high self-esteem.) Researchers have discovered a number of different psychological processes that have the effect of increasing or maintaining the positivity of the self-concept. Many of these processes can make people resistant to information from others that might otherwise be used to update the self-concept.

One such process is the *self-serving attributional bias*: a tendency to attribute the causes of positive events to one's own personality, while attributing negative events to factors outside of one's own control (e.g., Bradley, 1978). Two meta-analyses have found that the self-serving bias is present in many different kinds of samples (Campbell & Sedikides, 1999; Mezulis, Abramson, Hyde, & Hankin, 2004). The magnitude of the self-serving bias is typically quite substantial, but it is moderated by a number of factors, including culture, age, and self-esteem. For example, the self-serving bias is larger in Western samples than in Asian samples, though it is still present in the latter (Mezulis et al., 2004). It is also larger among individuals with higher self-esteem.

A self-serving attributional bias would lead individuals to dismiss social information or feedback that is evaluatively negative. Instead of being seen as potentially diagnostic of the self, negative information from others would be attributed to other causes, such as transient factors ("I'm just having a bad day") or others' inaccurate perceptions ("He doesn't know the real me"). Self-serving biases do not operate as strongly on positive social information; but because most people see themselves positively already (e.g., Alicke & Govorun, 2005), such information does not have much potential to change the existing self-concept.

Even when feedback temporarily overcomes self-serving biases, over time such biases might creep back in to erase openness to personal growth. For example, in a study of reactions to "360 feedback" given to managers, in the form of leadership ratings made by their coworkers, managers who initially believed they were good leaders but who received low leadership ratings from others—in other words, managers who demonstrably self-enhanced and were directly confronted with others' perceptions of them—described themselves as highly motivated to improve their performance after hearing the feedback. However, when the researchers followed up 6 months later, the motivation had not resulted in managers' taking any concrete steps to improve performance (Atwater & Brett, 2005).

For some individuals, the self-enhancement motive can go beyond cognitive biases and spill into overt behavioral resistance as well. Individuals who are highly narcissistic typically have high but unstable self-esteem, meaning that their very positive self-concepts can be easily perturbed by external events (Jordan, Spencer, Zanna, Hoshino-Browne, & Correll, 2003; Raskin, Novacek, & Hogan, 1991). In an effort to preserve their high self-esteem, narcissists who are insulted by another person are prone to lash out aggressively (Bushman & Baumeister, 1998). It is not entirely clear why narcissists do not just use cognitive strategies like everybody else.

However, one possibility is that it may be due to poor impulse control (Vazire & Funder, 2006). Poor impulse control would make it relatively difficult for narcissists to use complex cognitive strategies; it would also make it difficult for them to conform to social norms against aggression when under a perceived threat. The end result is that although narcissists respond behaviorally to negative social information about themselves—indicating that at some level the information is registering with them—they are willing to go to extraordinary lengths to prevent that information from affecting their self-concepts.

Self-Verification

Self-verification theory proposes that humans have a fundamental motive to confirm their existing self-views (Swann, 2011). An assumption of self-verification theory is that people use self-views "in making predictions about their worlds, guiding behavior, and maintaining a sense of coherence, place, and continuity" (p. 5). In order for people to reap these benefits their long-standing self-views must remain stable. Otherwise, predictions and behavioral plans would be in constant flux, and the personal and social world would be experienced as chaotic and incoherent.

To fulfill these pragmatic and epistemic needs for a stable self, people engage in a variety of intrapsychic and interpersonal processes that make them resistant to social information that might otherwise change their self-concept. Caspi and Roberts (2001) discussed three categories of person–environment transactions—selection, evocation, and reaction—that can be a basis for either continuity or change in personality. Research on self-verification theory has shown that these three kinds of transactions contribute to continuity in the self-concept. First, people select social environments that provide them feedback that is consistent with their existing self-concepts (Swann, Pelham, & Krull, 1989). Second, people try to evoke feedback from others that verifies their existing self-views (e.g., Swann, Wenzlaff, Krull, & Pelham, 1992). Third, people react to social information in ways that let them keep their existing self-views intact—for example, people selectively attend more to self-consistent information than to self-inconsistent information (Swann & Read, 1981).

In contrast to the self-enhancement motive, the self-verification motive can make people resistant to both positive and negative social information; all that is necessary is that the new information conflict with an already-existing self-view. A recent meta-analysis found evidence for both self-enhancement and self-verification motives (Kwang & Swann, 2010). In critical tests where the two motives might conflict (i.e., when an individual has a well-established negative self-view, such as Felicia's long-standing belief that she looks bad in photographs), self-verification was typically somewhat stronger, but the relative effect sizes were moderated by a number of factors. In particular, the threat of social rejection appears to weaken the self-verification motive. Rejection is powerful enough to affect self-views directly, in the form of lower self-esteem (Leary, Tambor, Terdal, & Downs, 1995; Srivastava & Beer, 2005). This suggests that in a hierarchy of motives, the need to belong may take priority over the need to maintain a stable and coherent sense of self. This tradeoff suggests a possible avenue for lowering resistance to potential social sources of self-knowledge, a point to which I return later.

Benefits of Resistance to Change

Motives to self-enhance and to self-verify can make the self resistant to the influences of social information. Such resistance may have benefits: Theories that have examined the social and psychological functions served by the self suggest that it may be maladaptive for the self-concept to be overly malleable. A stable sense of self helps organize goal-directed behavior. Goals are organized hierarchically and must be mentally represented and managed in some coherent way (Carver & Scheier, 1999). McAdams (1985) proposed that at the highest level of organization, the self is represented in a narrative structure—a life story—that integrates different parts of the self into a coherent whole. The life story, in turn, is created through smaller stories that define situated components of the self; and much of this development occurs during adolescence (Habermas & Bluck, 2000; McLean, Pasupathi, & Pals, 2007). It is thus not possible to change self-views that are tied into the life story without reverberations for the entire narrative. In the case of major, life-changing events, a new and coherent resolution—not easily achieved—is important for preserving healthy psychological functioning (Pals, 2006). Another function of a stable sense of self is *prediction*—anticipating or simulating how one might behave in novel situations in the future. For example, Bowlby (1979) proposed that people have working models that they use to predict how the self and others will behave in close relationships, and they plan behavior accordingly. Furthermore, insofar as self-views guide behavior, a stable sense of self makes an individual more predictable by others, which has advantages in relationships and social groups (Swann, 2011).

Conversely, a too-unstable self-concept would undermine functions such as goal pursuit and predictability. At the outside limits, a self-concept that is very easily perturbed by social input can create a risk for poor social adjustment and psychopathology (e.g., Crocker & Wolfe, 2001; Jordan et al., 2003; Kernis, Grannemann, & Mathis, 1991; Lieb, Zanarini, Schmahl, Linehan, & Bohus, 2004). In light of these considerations, it is reasonable to be skeptical about whether a functioning self-concept could nevertheless be open to influence by social others under some circumstances.

Under What Conditions Might Others Contribute to Self-Knowledge?

In spite of the evidence reviewed earlier, self-enhancement and self-verification motives—and the variety of associated psychological mechanisms that may inoculate the self against social input—are not necessarily all-determining. The theories and research on these motives, as well as a variety of other theoretical perspectives, suggest that at least under some conditions people might be open to acquiring self-knowledge through input from other people.

Younger Age

One factor that may make the self more open to social influence is age. Development of a consolidated self-concept begins in childhood and continues through adolescence (e.g., Harter, 1990; Measelle, Ablow, Cowan, & Cowan, 1998). But many of the processes that make the self resistant to social influence depend on already having a well-established and stable self-concept (Swann, 2011). As a result, the self-concepts of younger people may be more open to social input. Some developmental studies support this idea, indicating that reflected appraisals may be more influential on direct self-appraisals during childhood and adolescence than they are during adulthood (Felson, 1985; Pfeifer et al., 2009).

Expert Others

People may be more open to receiving social feedback about the self when they believe that others have special expertise. For example, in a study of clinical feedback, college students were more likely to accept negative personality feedback when it came from a PhD clinical psychologist than when it came from a fellow undergraduate (Halperin, Snyder, Shenkel, & Houston, 1976; see also Albright & Levy, 1995). Such expertise is probably important for a classic experimental method for manipulating self-esteem—providing false feedback from personality tests (e.g., Aronson & Mettee, 1968). The appearance of authority of these tests, and of the experimenter who delivers the feedback, are likely an important part of the stagecraft of such experiments.

Attributes That Are Defined by Others' Perceptions

Some attributes might be considered by folk perceivers to have an objective existence apart from human perception. This folk belief has been dubbed "naive realism" by Ross and Ward (1996). Research on naive realism has demonstrated that people often believe that their own perceptions are less biased than other people's perceptions (Pronin, Gilovich, & Ross, 2004). Naive realism may help sustain self-enhancement or self-verification processes by allowing individuals to dismiss others' perceptions when they conflict with self-perceptions (see Hansen & Pronin, Chapter 21, this volume).

However, some attributes depend more heavily on others' perceptions. For example, reputational attributes such as social status, likeability, and attractiveness are defined primarily by how one is seen by others (e.g., Srivastava & Anderson, 2010). Reputational attributes might be more changeable by social feedback than attributes that people believe have an objective existence outside of others' perceptions (Felson, 1985).

Novel Components of the Self

Although a great deal of development of self and identity occurs in adolescence, change can continue throughout the lifespan (Helson & Srivastava, 2001; McAdams et al., 2006). Ongoing identity development in middle adulthood is associated with psychological maturity and resilience (Pals, 2006). However, a wholesale remaking of the self-concept is exceedingly rare in healthy adults; rather, healthy adult development, particularly during early and middle adulthood, is characterized by increasing complexity and differentiation in the self (Labouvie-Vief, 2003).

One way that the self can become more complex is through the development of more circumscribed, context-dependent self-views. For example, theories and research on the relational self have demonstrated that people form distinct mental representations of themselves with specific other people (Andersen & Chen, 2002; Chen, Boucher, & Tapias, 2006). Such relational selves can be thought of as a set of if–then propositions (e.g., "IF I am with my son, THEN I am goofy"). Although relational selves are somewhat influenced by prior experiences in close relationships, they can vary considerably within one person across different relationships (Baldwin, Keelan, Fehr, Enns, & Koh-Rangarajoo, 1996). New relationships may thus be a context for ongoing development of the self during adulthood that is not constrained by an existing self-concept, and therefore may be open to social input.

Incentives to Change

As discussed earlier, one argument for why the adult self-concept may be resistant to change is based in an analysis of the functions of the self. The self-concept is used to predict and guide behavior and to understand the world, and a stable self-concept is thought to be important for these functions (Swann, 2011). However, careful consideration of a functional approach leaves open the possibility that the self-concept may become more malleable when other important functions would be served by changing.

One situation where research has shown that self-verification processes are weaker, and therefore the self might be open to change, is when the individual faces the threat of social rejection. For example, members of dating couples seek self-verifying negative feedback less than members of married couples; this effect may be because losing one's partner is less of a concern in marriage (Swann, De La Ronde, & Hixon, 1994). A recent meta-analysis found that when rejection risk was higher, self-verification motives were weaker (Kwang & Swann, 2010). Instead, people were more likely to try to impress their partners in an effort to keep the relationship intact. This suggests that the self-verification motive (and perhaps other self-perception motives) is malleable when faced with competing goals.

When Should People Trust Social Input?

The factors listed in this section may make people more open to social input about the self. Are these the right sources and situations? Many of these are arguably times or situations when openness to social input could be rational or adaptive (or both), which implies a certain amount of pragmatism. Younger people and people in novel situations or roles have less prior information to go on; when that is the case, the views of older or more experienced others may compare favorably to a nascent or uncertain self-view. Experts are more likely to have valid information than nonexperts.

A variety of factors can make others' social perceptions a more accurate, potential source for valid self-knowledge (Funder, 1995). Accuracy is higher among perceivers who are extraverted (Akert & Panter, 1988), intelligent (Havenstein & Alexander, 1991), and highly motivated (Smith, Ickes, Hall, & Hodges, 2010). Others are more accurate in perceiving traits that are highly evaluative and that have more observable behavioral manifestations (Vazire, 2010). Perceivers are more accurate when their attentional resources are not divided (Biesanz, Neuberg, Smith, Asher, & Judice, 2001). All of these findings suggest that people could benefit from seeking input from particular other people, under particular circumstances, and about particular traits. However, it remains to be tested whether people are more sensitive to these differences—for example, whether people are more willing to incorporate social feedback into their self-views when it comes from smart extraverts.

How Would Others Affect the Self?: Some Possible Mechanisms

What psychological and interpersonal mechanisms might make it possible for others' perceptions to feed into self-knowledge? Research on behavioral confirmation has shown that after perceivers form an impression of someone, the perceivers often act in ways that elicit behavior that is consistent with their initial perception. Some of the earliest research on behavioral confirmation involved observations of teachers bringing their students' behavior in line with teachers' initial impressions (e.g., Rosenthal & Jacobson, 1968). Subsequent laboratory experiments expanded on this framework, for example, by showing that perceivers elicited socially engaged behavior from targets they believed to be attractive (Snyder, Tanke, & Berscheid, 1977). In over four decades of work, researchers have demonstrated that behavioral confirmation can occur across a wide range of situations and attributes (see Snyder & Stukas, 1999, for a review).

A variety of psychological and social mechanisms appear to be involved in mediating behavioral confirmation effects. For example, Chen and Bargh (1997) showed that when social stereotypes are implicitly activated in perceivers, the perceivers can unintentionally and automatically act out those stereotypes and elicit reciprocal behavior (e.g., behaving with hostility toward an interaction partner after a black stereotype is implicitly activated). At a more fine-grained level, a meta-analysis by Harris and Rosenthal (1985) identified a variety of nonverbal behaviors, including smiling, eye contact, and speech rate, that appear to mediate the link between perceivers' expectations and targets' behavior. Such behaviors can function as reinforcers: When the target behaves as expected, the perceiver responds in ways that the target finds rewarding. Such low-level reinforcement processes do not need to involve formation of a metaperception. That could explain why, for example, Srivastava and Beer (2005) found that being liked by others made people evaluate themselves positively, but the effect was not mediated by reflected appraisals.

After perceivers have elicited confirmatory behavior, the self-concept can subsequently be updated through a variety of mechanisms. When elicited behavior clashes with what were previously well-established (though not necessarily accurate) components of the self-concept, cognitive dissonance can be reduced by revising the self-concept (Festinger, 1957). Alternatively, when behavior is elicited in a domain where the individual was not already committed to a particular self-view, self-perception of the behavior might lead an individual to infer a new self-view as a result (Bem, 1967; Chaiken & Baldwin, 1981).

Behavioral confirmation is not the only mechanism by which others may influence self-views. In social situations, people often need to share certain beliefs and perceptions in order to feel connected to others and to accomplish collective goals

(Hardin & Higgins, 1996). According to the *affiliative social tuning hypothesis*, one of the ways that a person can try to build a shared reality is by adjusting his or her beliefs to be more in "tune" with what that person thinks others think (Sinclair, Huntsinger, Skorinko, & Hardin, 2005). In a series of experiments, Sinclair, Hardin, and Lowery (2006) found that when people were motivated to affiliate with another person, they adjusted their self-views to be more consistent with their metaperceptions—in this case, with others' ostensible gender- and race-based stereotypes. In contrast to behavioral confirmation processes, the perceivers in these experiments did not have to behave in any way that elicited stereotype-consistent behavior (other than expressing their endorsement of the stereotypes).

The study by Sinclair and her colleagues (2006) focused on how believing that others hold inaccurate stereotypes can distort self-views. But the same social tuning mechanism would increase accuracy (rather than decreasing it) when metaperceptions are accurate. Thus, in circumstances when metaperceptions are derived from others' accurate perceptions, social tuning would be another mechanism by which others can promote accurate self-knowledge.

An Example: Social Influences on Self-Knowledge of Status

One area in which other people may exert a substantial influence on self-knowledge is in the domain of status perceptions. *Status*, as I am using the term here, is defined as respect and influence in the eyes of other people (Srivastava & Anderson, 2011). In a variety of studies of naturalistic group interactions, status self-perceptions have been found to depend on social input in some interesting ways.

Status has several of the characteristics discussed earlier that make it a prime candidate for being open to influences through social input. It is a reputational attribute—that is, it is defined by what other people think. Status is also context-specific: A person can have high status in one group and low status in another. And people often encounter new contexts where they must figure out their new, context-specific status, such as through changes in the workplace. The novelty of the associated situation-specific self-views may make them malleable.

A less obvious but crucial characteristic of status is that it is connected to social rejection. Specifically, a number of studies have found that overestimation of one's own status incurs social costs in the form of rejection by the group (Anderson, Ames, & Gosling, 2008; Anderson, Srivastava, Beer, Spataro, & Chatman, 2006). This probably happens for a number of reasons. Status is typically organized in hierarchies, so when individuals act as though they have high status, they are implying that others have lower status (Tiedens & Fragale, 2003). And individuals with high status also can claim a number of privileges, such as speaking whenever they please and telling others what to do (Anderson & Berdahl, 2002; Galinsky, Gruenfeld, & Magee, 2003). Because groups reject individuals who overestimate their status, the threat of rejection seems to dampen self-enhancement and self-verification biases. Overestimation of one's own status can also come with more tangible sanctions, such as being denied resources and rewards by other group members (Anderson et al., 2008).

As a result of these incentives and sanctions, people are typically quite accurate in perceiving their own status—more so than in perceiving other attributes, such as the Big Five personality characteristics (Srivastava & Anderson, 2011). Indeed, individuals who have an especially strong need to belong to social groups are especially likely to be accurate in perceiving their own status (Anderson et al., 2006). Their motivation probably makes them especially responsive to the prospect of rejection, and willing to revise their self-views as a result. By contrast, narcissists tend to persist in overestimating their status, even in the face of group sanctions (Anderson et al., 2008). Narcissists' difficulties with impulse control, combined with their need to maintain high self-esteem, probably make it difficult for them to defer to other people's directives or even to acknowledge that they ought to do so.

Conclusions

People may be able to learn about themselves from other people—but in healthy adults, there are significant limitations to this potential. A mostly stable sense of self helps in predicting and planning future behavior, and provides a sense of epistemic stability. But a completely calcified sense of self would not be adaptive either. Nevertheless, people may be open to using social feedback to acquire self-knowledge when they think that others are in a position to offer valuable information, when the resulting changes to the self-concept would be circumscribed, and when updating their self-knowledge would serve some important goal or function.

Having made a case for social input contributing to accurate self-views, I want to conclude by acknowledging some shortcomings of this case. The process I have discussed here is an almost-complete loop—from actual attributes of an individual to others' perceptions and back to the individual's self-knowledge, with many intermediate steps along the way. Most of the studies and theories I have cited are piecemeal, addressing just one or another bit of this proposed cycle. A valuable direction for future research would be to complete the loop—that is, to coherently demonstrate the entire cycle in action at once. Doing so would help illuminate a social self that is truly social—not just in mentally representing the social world, but in a deeper sense of being interconnected with other people.

NOTE

1. These influences of others on the self were part of a larger cycle in which the self also affected others; such reciprocal interactions are an important part of the larger theoretical model.

REFERENCES

Akert, R. M., & Panter, A. T. (1988). Extraversion and the ability to decode nonverbal communication. *Personality and Individual Difference, 9,* 965–972.

Albright, M. D., & Levy, P. E. (1995). The effects of source credibility and performance rating discrepancy on reactions to multiple raters. *Journal of Applied Social Psychology, 25,* 577–600.

Alicke, M. D., & Govorun, O. (2005). The better-than-average effect. In M. D. Alicke, D. A.

Dunning , & J. I. Krueger (Eds.), *The self in social judgment* (pp. 85–106). New York: Psychology Press.

Andersen, S. M., & Chen, S. (2002). The relational self: An interpersonal social-cognitive theory. *Psychological Review, 109*, 619–645.

Anderson, C. P., Ames, D. R., & Gosling, S. D. (2008). Punishing hubris: The perils of status self-enhancement in teams and organizations. *Personality and Social Psychology Bulletin, 34*, 90–101.

Anderson, C., & Berdahl, J. L. (2002). The experience of power: Examining the effects of power on approach and inhibition tendencies. *Journal of Personality and Social Psychology, 83*, 1362–1377.

Anderson, C., Srivastava, S., Beer, J. S., Spataro, S. E., & Chatman, J. A. (2006). Knowing your place: Self-perceptions of status in social groups. *Journal of Personality and Social Psychology, 91*, 1094–1110.

Aronson, E., & Mettee, D. R. (1968). Dishonest behaviour as a function of differential levels of induced self-esteem. *Journal of Personality, 9*, 121–127.

Atwater, L. E., & Brett, J. F. (2005). Antecedents and consequences of reactions to developmental 360° feedback. *Journal of Vocational Behavior, 66*, 532–548.

Baldwin, M. W., Keelan, J. P. R., Fehr, B., Enns, V., & Koh-Rangarajoo, E. (1996). Social-cognitive conceptualization of attachment working models: Availability and accessibility effects. *Journal of Personality and Social Psychology, 71*, 94–109.

Bargh, J. A., Chen, M., & Burrows, L. (1996). Automaticity of social behavior: Direct effects of trait construct and stereotype activation on action. *Journal of Personality and Social Psychology, 71*, 230–244.

Bem, D. (1967). Self-perception: An alternative interpretation of cognitive dissonance phenomena. *Psychological Review, 74*, 183–200.

Biesanz, J. C., Neuberg, S. L., Smith, D. M., Asher, T., & Judice, T. N. (2001). When accuracy-motivated perceivers fail: Limited attentional resources and the reemerging self-fulfilling prophecy. *Personality and Social Psychology Bulletin, 27*, 621–629.

Bowlby, J. (1979). *The making and breaking of affectional bonds*. London: Tavistock.

Bradley, G. W. (1978). Self-serving biases in the attribution process: A reexamination of the fact or fiction question. *Journal of Personality and Social Psychology, 36*, 56–71.

Bushman, B. J., & Baumeister, R. F. (1998). Threatened egotism, narcissism, self-esteem, and direct and displaced aggression: Does self-love or self-hate lead to violence? *Journal of Personality and Social Psychology, 75*, 219–229.

Campbell, W. K., & Sedikides, C. (1999). Self-threat magnifies the self-serving bias: A meta-analytic integration. *Review of General Psychology, 3*, 23–43.

Carver, C. S., & Scheier, M. F. (1999). Stress, coping, and self-regulatory processes. In L. A. Pervin & O. P. John (Eds.), *Handbook of personality: Theory and research* (2nd ed., pp. 553–575). New York: Guilford Press.

Caspi, A., & Roberts, B. W. (2001). Personality development across the life span: The argument for change and continuity. *Psychological Inquiry, 12*, 49–66.

Chaiken, S., & Baldwin, M. W. (1981). Affective–cognitive consistency and the effect of salient behavioral information on the self-perception of attitudes. *Journal of Personality and Social Psychology, 41*, 1–12.

Chen, M., & Bargh, J. A. (1997). Nonconscious behavioral confirmation processes: The self-fulfilling nature of automatically-activated stereotypes. *Journal of Experimental Social Psychology, 33*, 541–560.

Chen, S., Boucher, H. C., & Tapias, M. P. (2006). The relational self revealed: Integrative conceptualization and implications for interpersonal life. *Psychological Bulletin, 132*, 151–179.

Cole, D. A. (1991). Change in self-perceived competence as a function of peer and teacher evaluation. *Developmental Psychology, 27*, 682–688.

Cooley, C. H. (1902). *Human nature and the social order.* New York: Scribner.

Crocker, J., & Wolfe, C. T. (2001). Contingencies of self-worth. *Psychological Review, 108*, 593–623.

Erikson, E. (1950). *Childhood and society.* New York: Norton.

Felson, R. (1985). Reflected appraisal and the development of self. *Social Psychology Quarterly, 48*, 71–78.

Felson, R. (1993). The (somewhat) social self: How others affect self-appraisals. In J. Suls (Ed.), *The self in social perspective* (Vol. 4, pp. 1–26). Hillsdale, NJ: Erlbaum.

Festinger, L. (1954). A theory of social comparison processes. *Human Relations, 7*, 117–140.

Festinger, L. (1957). *A theory of cognitive dissonance.* Stanford, CA: Stanford University Press.

Funder, D. C. (1987). Errors and mistakes: Evaluating the accuracy of social judgment. *Psychological Bulletin, 101*, 75–90.

Funder, D. C. (1995). On the accuracy of personality judgment: A realistic approach. *Psychological Review, 102*, 652–670.

Galinsky, A. D., Gruenfeld, D. H., & Magee, J. C. (2003). From power to action. *Journal of Personality and Social Psychology, 85*, 453–466.

Habermas, T., & Bluck, S. (2000). Getting a life: The emergence of the life story in adolescence. *Psychological Bulletin, 126*, 748–769.

Halperin, K., Snyder, C. R., Shenkel, R. J., & Houston, B. K. (1976). Effects of source status and message favorability on acceptance of personality feedback. *Journal of Applied Psychology, 61*, 85–88.

Hardin, C. D., & Higgins, E. T. (1996). Shared reality: How social verification makes the subjective objective. In R. M. Sorrentino & E. T. Higgins (Eds.), *Handbook of motivation and cognition: Vol. 3. The interpersonal context* (pp. 28–84). New York: Guilford Press.

Harris, M. J., & Rosenthal, R. (1985). Mediation of interpersonal expectancy effects: 31 meta-analyses. *Psychological Bulletin, 97*, 363–386.

Harter, S. (1990). Self and identity development. In S. Shirley & G. R. Elliott (Eds.), *At the threshold: The developing adolescent* (pp. 352–387). Cambridge, MA: Harvard University Press.

Harter, S. (1999). *The construction of the self: A developmental perspective.* New York: Guilford Press.

Havenstein, N. M., & Alexander, R. A. (1991). Rating ability in performance judgments: The joint influence of implicit theories and intelligence. *Organizational Behavior and Human Decision Processes, 50*, 300–323.

Helson, R., & Srivastava, S. (2001). Three paths of adult development: Conservers, seekers, and achievers. *Journal of Personality and Social Psychology, 80*, 995–1010.

Jordan, C. H., Spencer, S. J., Zanna, M. P., Hoshino-Browne, E., & Correll, J. (2003). Secure and defensive high self-esteem. *Journal of Personality and Social Psychology, 85*, 969–978.

Jussim, L. (1991). Social perception and social reality: A reflection–construction model. *Psychological Review, 98*, 54–73.

Kenny, D. A., & Albright, L. (1987). Accuracy in interpersonal perception: A social relations analysis. *Psychological Bulletin, 102*, 390–402.

Kenny, D. A., & DePaulo, B. M. (1993). Do people know how others view them?: An empirical and theoretical account. *Psychological Bulletin, 114*, 145–161.

Kernis, M. H., Grannemann, B. D., & Mathis, L. C. (1991). Stability of self-esteem as a moderator of the relation between level of self-esteem and depression. *Journal of Personality and Social Psychology, 61,* 80–84.

Kinch, J. W. (1963). A formalized theory of the self-concept. *American Journal of Sociology, 68,* 481–486.

Kwang, T. & Swann, W. B., Jr. (2010). Do people embrace praise even when they feel unworthy?: A review of critical tests of self-enhancement versus self-verification. *Personality and Social Psychology Review, 15,* 263–280.

Labouvie-Vief, G. (2003). Dynamic integration: Affect, cognition, and the self in adulthood. *Current Directions in Psychological Science, 12,* 201–206.

Leary, M. R., Tambor, E. S., Terdal, S. K., & Downs, D. L. (1995). Self-esteem as an interpersonal monitor: The sociometer hypothesis. *Journal of Personality and Social Psychology, 68,* 518–530.

Lieb, K., Zanarini, M. C., Schmahl, C., Linehan, M. M., & Bohus, M. (2004). Borderline personality disorder. *Lancet, 364,* 453–461.

Markus, H. (1983). Self-knowledge: An expanded view. *Journal of Personality, 51,* 543–565.

McAdams, D. P. (1985). *Power, intimacy, and the life story: Personological inquiries into identity.* New York: Guilford Press.

McAdams, D. P., Bauer, J. J., Sakaeda, A., Anyidoho, N. A., Machado, M. A., Magrino, K., et al. (2006). Continuity and change in the life story: A longitudinal study of autobiographical memories in emerging adulthood. *Journal of Personality, 74,* 1371–1400.

McLean, K. C., Pasupathi, M., & Pals, J. L. (2007). Selves creating stories creating selves: A process model of self-development. *Personality and Social Psychology Review, 11,* 262–278.

Mead, G. H. (1934). *Mind, self, and society.* Chicago: University of Chicago Press.

Measelle, J. R., Ablow, J. C., Cowan, P. A., & Cowan, C. P. (1998). Assessing young children's self-perceptions of their academic, social and emotional lives: An evaluation of the Berkeley Puppet Interview. *Child Development, 69,* 1556–1576.

Mezulis, A., Abramson, L., Hyde, J. S., & Hankin, B. L. (2004). Is there a universal positivity bias in attributions?: A meta-analytic review of individual, developmental, and cultural differences in the self-serving attributional bias. *Psychological Bulletin, 130,* 711–746.

Neisser, U. (1988). Five kinds of self-knowledge. *Philosophical Psychology, 1,* 35–59.

Pals, J. L. (2006). Narrative identity processing of difficult life experiences: Pathways of personality development and positive self-transformation in adulthood. *Journal of Personality, 74,* 1079–1110.

Pfeifer, J. H., Masten, C. L., Borofsky, L. A., Dapretto, M., Fuligni, A. J., & Lieberman, M. D. (2009). Neural correlates of direct and reflected self-appraisals in adolescents and adults: When social perspective-taking informs self-perception. *Child Development, 80,* 1016–1038.

Pronin, E., Gilovich, T. D., & Ross, L. (2004). Objectivity in the eye of the beholder: Divergent perceptions of bias in self versus others. *Psychological Review, 111,* 781–799.

Raskin, R. N., Novacek, J., & Hogan, R. (1991). Narcissistic self esteem management. *Journal of Personality and Social Psychology, 60,* 911–918.

Rosenthal, R., & Jacobson, L. (1968). *Pygmalion in the classroom.* New York: Holt, Rinehart & Winston.

Ross, L., & Ward, A. (1996). Naive realism in everyday life: Implications for social conflict and misunderstanding. In T. Brown, E. S. Reed, & E. Turiel (Eds.), *Values and knowledge. The Jean Piaget Symposium Series* (pp. 103–135). Hillsdale, NJ: Erlbaum.

Shrauger, J. S., & Schoeneman, T. J. (1979). Symbolic interactionist view of self-concept: Through the looking glass darkly. *Psychological Bulletin, 86,* 549–573.

Sinclair, S., Hardin, C., & Lowery, B. (2006). Self-stereotyping in the context of multiple social identities. *Journal of Personality and Social Psychology, 90,* 529–542.

Sinclair, S., Huntsinger, J., Skorinko, J. L., & Hardin, C. (2005). Social tuning of the self: consequences for the self-evaluations of stereotype targets. *Journal of Personality and Social Psychology, 89,* 160–175.

Smith, J. L., Ickes, W., Hall, J., & Hodges, S. D. (Eds.). (2010). *Managing interpersonal sensitivity: Knowing when—and when not—to understand others.* New York: Nova Science.

Snyder, M., & Stukas, A. A. (1999). Interpersonal processes: The interplay of cognitive, motivational, and behavioral activities in social interaction. *Annual Review of Psychology, 50,* 273–303.

Snyder, M., & Swann, W. B., Jr. (1978). Hypothesis testing processes in social interaction. *Journal of Personality and Social Psychology, 36,* 1202–1212.

Snyder, M., Tanke, E. D., & Berscheid, E. (1977). Social perception and interpersonal behavior: On the self-fulfilling nature of social stereotypes. *Journal of Experimental Social Psychology, 35,* 656–666.

Srivastava, S., & Anderson, C. (2011). Accurate when it counts: Perceiving power and status in social groups. In J. L. Smith, W. Ickes, J. A. Hall, & S. D. Hodges (Eds.), *Managing interpersonal sensitivity: Knowing when—and when not—to understand others* (pp. 41–58). New York: Nova Science.

Srivastava, S., & Beer, J. S. (2005). How self-evaluations relate to being liked by others: Integrating sociometer and attachment perspectives. *Journal of Personality and Social Psychology, 89,* 966–977.

Swann, W. B., Jr. (2011). Self-verification theory. In P. A. M. Van Lange, A. W. Kruglanski, & E. T. Higgins (Eds.), *Handbook of theories of social psychology* (Vol. 2, pp. 23–42). London: Sage.

Swann, W. B., Jr., De La Ronde, C., & Hixon, J. G. (1994). Authenticity and positivity strivings in marriage and courtship. *Journal of Personality and Social Psychology, 66,* 857–869.

Swann, W. B., Jr., Pelham, B. W., & Krull, D. S. (1989). Agreeable fancy or disagreeable truth?: How people reconcile their self-enhancement and self-verification needs. *Journal of Personality and Social Psychology, 57,* 782–791.

Swann, W. B., Jr., & Read, S. J. (1981). Acquiring self-knowledge: The search for feedback that fits. *Journal of Personality and Social Psychology, 41,* 1119–1128.

Swann, W. B., Jr., Wenzlaff, R. M., Krull, D. S., & Pelham, B. W. (1992). The allure of negative feedback: Self-verification strivings among depressed persons. *Journal of Abnormal Psychology, 101,* 293–306.

Tajfel, H., & Turner, J. C. (1979). An integrative theory of intergroup conflict. In W. G. Austin & S. Worchel (Eds.), *The social psychology of intergroup relations* (pp. 33–48). Monterey, CA: Brooks-Cole.

Tice, D. M., & Wallace, H. M. (2005). The reflected self: Creating yourself as (you think) others see you. In M. R. Leary & J. P. Tangney (Eds.), *Handbook of self and identity* (pp. 91–105). New York: Guilford Press.

Tiedens, L. Z., & Fragale, A. R. (2003). Power moves: Complementarity in dominant and submissive nonverbal behavior. *Journal of Personality and Social Psychology, 84,* 558–568.

Vazire, S. (2010). Who knows what about a person?: The Self–Other Knowledge Asymmetry (SOKA) model. *Journal of Personality and Social Psychology, 98,* 281–300.

Vazire, S., & Funder, D. C. (2006). Impulsivity and the self-defeating behavior of narcissists. *Personality and Social Psychology Review, 10,* 154–165.

CHAPTER 8
Self-Knowledge
An Individual-Differences Perspective

ROBERTA A. SCHRIBER
RICHARD W. ROBINS

Socrates, the celebrated philosopher who lived by the adage "Know Thyself," was in his time declared the wisest man in the world. After the pronouncement came from the Oracle of Delphi, Socrates was dubious and set out to test the claim's veracity. He traveled around Greece speaking to every poet and politician, artisan, and academic who might constitute proof to the contrary. He found none. In fact, time and time again, Socrates was surprised to find that there was little remarkable about the most reputable; that underlings often outshone their superiors; and that the majority of individuals, from the most exalted to the common, tended to make exaggerated claims about their knowledge and ability. Socrates finally conceded to being the wisest man in the world, noting that at least "I do not think I know what I do not know." Why did Socrates have such self-insight? And, why did those around him perceive themselves as wiser than they truly were?

In this chapter, we discuss theory and research on *individual differences* in the degree to which people have insight into their personal characteristics, including their talents, abilities, and traits. In most cases, we are concerned with directional biases in self-perception, that is, with variability in the extent to which people over- versus underestimate their strengths and weaknesses. Whether our biases are positive or negative (they are typically quite flattering), an individual-differences approach can help us understand the mechanisms underlying these biases and their consequences for psychological and social functioning.

First, we briefly discuss self-enhancement as a general phenomenon that is by no means observed in everyone, and then review the most prominent explanatory accounts of self-enhancement. Specifically, we ask: What are the psychological mechanisms that contribute to self-enhancing (vs. self-diminishing) tendencies? Next, we describe the various methods that have been used to operationalize individual differences in self-enhancement, with an emphasis on procedures that use an explicit criterion for gauging the accuracy of people's beliefs about themselves. Last, we address the contentious question of whether self-enhancement is adaptive. Is self-insight the path to truth, beauty, and happiness, as Socrates argued, or are people better off maintaining positive illusions about themselves? The answer, as we discuss below, may hinge on the way in which these illusions are conceptualized and assessed. Throughout this chapter, narcissism is used as a vivid example of, and explanatory framework for, how and why individuals tend to bend the truth about themselves—to themselves.

Explaining Individual Differences in Self-Enhancement

Self-Enhancement as the Norm but not the Rule

The notion that individuals strive to protect their self-worth by maintaining self-enhancing illusions has long been considered a truism in psychology (Allport, 1937; Greenwald, 1980; Taylor & Brown, 1988). As Sedikides, Horton, and Gregg (2007) aptly put it, "Most people, most of the time, see themselves through rose-colored glasses" (p. 783). Yet this quote also highlights the complementary view—not everyone self-enhances, and not all the time. Indeed, most studies that have compared self-evaluations to an external criterion have found a relatively weak self-enhancement effect, typically around one-third of a standard deviation (e.g., John & Robins, 1994; Robins & John, 1997a). One explanation for the weak effect is that most people self-enhance, but few individuals have severely distorted views of themselves. Another possibility involves the presence of substantial individual differences in both the magnitude and direction of the effect; that is, some people have extremely inflated self-views, others have only mild positive illusions, and still others have accurate or even overly negative views. This possibility is difficult to evaluate because most studies of self-enhancement report only aggregate statistics (i.e., main effects) about the general tendency in the sample.

In one of the first studies to report individual-level statistics, John and Robins (1994) used a simulated managerial task in which participants competed for a fixed pool of money that was allocated by group consensus. At the end of the task, participants ranked their own performance as well as that of the other group members, and were also ranked by a panel of expert observers (11 psychologists trained to evaluate performance in the task). On average, participants ranked themselves more positively than they were ranked by their peers or by the observers. However, substantial individual differences also emerged. Although 60% of participants evaluated themselves overly positively, 36% evaluated themselves overly negatively, and more than 50% were accurate within one rank of the peer and observer consensus rankings. Similar percentages were reported by Robins and John (1997a) and by Paulhus (1998). In organizational studies, the proportion of self-enhancers is even smaller and may not exceed the proportion of self-diminishers (Atwater & Yammarino, 1992), presumably because employees expect that their self-evaluations will be compared with supervisor ratings. Thus, many individuals do not exhibit self-enhancement biases, and a nontrivial number actually see themselves more negatively than others see them.

Do these self-enhancing versus self-diminishing tendencies reflect transient fluctuations around a general effect or the operation of a chronic and deep-seated facet of personality? Consistent with the latter possibility, a number of studies have demonstrated that the broad and stable trait of narcissism is strongly associated with individual differences in self-enhancement (e.g., John & Robins [1994] reported correlations in the .40s). The link generalizes across a wide range of contexts, operationalizations of self-enhancement, and self- and observer-based measures of narcissism (Campbell, Rudich, & Sedikides, 2002; Colvin, Block, & Funder, 1995; Kernis & Sun, 1994; Kwan, John, Robins, & Kuang, 2008; Paulhus, 1998; Robins & Beer, 2001; Robins & John, 1997a). The relation between self-enhancement and narcissism is critical, as it demonstrates that individual differences in self-enhancement are not due to measurement error and other sources of random variability but, rather, are systematic and psychologically meaningful. That is, they function more like a trait than a state.[1]

What accounts for these systematic biases in self-perception? Two classes of explanations have been advanced: (1) *cognitive–informational accounts*, which focus on the information available to the self, prior beliefs and expectancies, and processes of attention, encoding, and retrieval of self-relevant information, and (2) *motivational–affective accounts*, which focus on the motive to maintain and enhance self-esteem, self-presentational concerns such as the need for social approval, and the desire to reduce negative affect—especially shame—and increase positive affect—especially pride (see also Helzer & Dunning, Chapter 23, this volume, for an account of cognitive and motivational factors underlying accurate and biased self-perception).

Cognitive–Informational Accounts

Early accounts of self-enhancement, or "self-serving biases" as they were sometimes referred to in the 1970s, emphasized the role of cognitive processes. Reflecting the dominant paradigm of the time, individuals were assumed to function like idealized scientists, dispassionately forming opinions about themselves based on the available data, without considering the favorability of the information. From this perspective, biases in self-perception arise because people are not very good scientists and reach conclusions based on faulty data and information-processing deficits, rather than because they want to feel good about themselves. For example, the well-documented *self-serving attribution bias*—the tendency to take credit for success but blame others or the situation for failure—was assumed to reflect a cognitive self-system that was oriented toward maintaining consistency and biased by prior beliefs and expectancies (Miller & Ross, 1975).

If we think about self-perception using the computer analogical terms that reflect a "cold" cognition (i.e., not motivational) view of the mind, consideration of the neural "hardware"—its development and defects—can be telling with regard to the processes that subserve an accurate versus biased view of the self. For example, cognitive development greatly fosters accuracy in self-knowledge (Trzesniewski, Kinal, & Donnellan, 2011). Children's self-views tend to be overly positive early in childhood but become progressively more accurate as children develop the capacity to self-reflect, to understand and integrate positive and negative information, as well as to make and use comparative judgments (e.g., "I am worse than my peers at math") (Jacobs, Bleeker, & Constantino, 2003; Lagattuta & Thompson, 2007; Trzesniewski et al., 2011). Moreover, from an information-processing standpoint, these cognitive changes are complemented by the increasing availability of relevant information due to a greater focus on grades and other forms of social comparison as children enter middle school. Consistent with these developmental changes, the self-serving attribution bias tends to decline from childhood to adolescence and adulthood (Mezulis, Abramson, Hyde, & Hankin, 2004).

Aside from these normative cognitive changes, biases in self-perception may derive from breakdowns or malfunctions in the neural hardware—biases that, as such, do not reflect motivated processes. For example, although self-serving attribution biases decline as children show increasing levels of cognitive maturity, they tend to increase again in old age, returning to the same level of distortion as in childhood. The spike in self-serving attributions in old age may reflect the increasing prevalence of dementias and other forms of neural pathology that impair accurate self-knowledge. Loss of self-insight is a core symptom of frontotemporal dementia (FTD). Rankin, Baldwin, Pace-Savitsky, Kramer, and Miller (2005) found that patients with FTD overestimated their positive traits (e.g., extraversion) and underestimated their negative traits (e.g., coldheartedness) relative to informant reports. The bias appeared to come from patients with FTD having based their self-reports on their premorbid personality, as if they had failed to update their self-knowledge. Similarly, patients with damage to the orbitofrontal cortex evidence positive distortions, as well as deficits in the capacity to experience and "use" self-conscious emotions, such as embarrassment, to effectively regulate their social behavior (Beer, 2007; Beer, John, Scabini, & Knight, 2006). Further implicating frontal regions, Kwan and colleagues (2007) showed that transcranial magnetic stimulation (which serves to suppress activity) of the medial prefrontal cortex reduced the degree to which participants engaged in self-enhancement, defined as perceiving themselves more positively than they perceived others.

Other types of neural pathology do not seem to impair self-knowledge dramatically, raising the question of which processes, specifically, allow for accurate self-views. For example, individuals with autism spectrum disorders (ASDs) exhibit pervasive deficits in social functioning that presumably stem from neurocognitive impairments in self-awareness and awareness of others' mental and emotional states. To the extent that individuals with ASDs lack the interest or ability to self-reflect and to make sense of others' reactions toward them, they should have inaccurate self-views. However, in a recent study, we found that children and adolescents with ASDs did not exhibit particularly pronounced self-perceptual biases and showed the same level of self–parent agreement on the Big Five traits as typically developing individuals, suggesting a comparable level of self-knowledge (Schriber & Robins, 2011). Also, Klein, Loftus, and Kihlstrom (1996) found that a patient with amnesia was able to report accurately on her changed personality despite not being able to recall specific memories of the behaviors, reactions, and experiences that constituted that change. Although studies such as these do not necessarily speak to individual differences in self-enhancement in typically functioning individuals, they do raise provocative questions about the cognitive mechanisms that underlie self-knowledge, and point to the possibility that individuals may be differentially wired to process, store, and retrieve self-relevant information that promotes or inhibits self-knowledge.[2]

Another line of research addressing cognitive mechanisms involves studies that compare first- versus third-person perspective on the self (Sutin & Robins, 2008). At the time of encoding, all self-perceivers have incomplete data by virtue of being confined to a first-person perspective—we cannot, as the poet Robert Burns noted, "see oursels as ithers see us." Using Funder's (1999) terminology, cues about one's personality may not be observable or detectable to the self, so perhaps it is inevitable that individuals fill in the blanks with what they think or expect to be the case, however misguided. Does closing this informational gap diminish self-enhancing biases?

Apparently not. Using the same group discussion task from John and Robins (1994), Robins and John (1997a) had half their participants evaluate themselves immediately after the task and the other half after watching a video recording of their performance taken from the potentially more reality-disclosing viewpoint of an observer (i.e., with the camera angled directly at them). Contrary to an information-processing account, reversing visual perspective (and thus becoming one's own observer) did not reduce the magnitude of the self-enhancement effect. Moreover, the observer-perspective condition *accentuated* the effect of narcissism, with the self-evaluations of high narcissists becoming more positively distorted and the self-evaluations of low narcissists becoming more realistic. Similarly, the self-serving attribution bias persists even after researchers controlled for imperfect information-processing strategies such as selective attention, differential information accessibility, or memory differences (Sedikides, Campbell, Reeder, & Elliot, 1998). When biases persist in the absence of informational differences, motivational factors are likely to be at play.

There is little doubt that individuals show biases in the way they process information about themselves. The question is whether these biases stem exclusively, or even primarily, from the basic cognitive machinery involved in the formation of self-evaluations, or from motivational and affective processes. Research accumulating over the past few decades suggests that we often lack not only the cognitive capacity to perceive ourselves accurately but also the motivational will to do so, as exposing the truth about ourselves can lead to painful feelings of shame and burst the bubble of inflated pride.

Motivational–Affective Accounts

Motivational theories generally assume that self-enhancement comes from a fundamental need to gain, protect, and otherwise maintain feelings of self-worth; that is, perceiving oneself through rose-colored glasses is an important way to regulate self-esteem (Taylor & Brown, 1988). From a motivational perspective, individual differences in self-enhancement reflect variability in the strength of the motivation to enhance and protect one's self-worth. This view has been supported by studies that measure or manipulate variables (e.g., ego involvement, ego threat) that activate or increase the intensity of the self-enhancement motive and studies that document an association between self-enhancement and stable individual-difference variables, such as narcissism, that are believed to reflect an excessive and chronic need to enhance self-worth.

Individual differences in self-enhancement arise, in part, from individual differences in the degree to which, and domains in which, individuals are ego-involved (Crocker & Wolfe, 2001). For example, Robins and Beer (2001, Study 1) found that individuals who reported that it was highly important to perform well in a group discussion task overestimated their performance to a greater extent than did individuals who found it less important. By extension, self-enhancement occurs primarily in domains that matter to individuals (e.g., Sedikides, Gaertner, & Toguchi, 2003). Paulhus and John (1998) discussed the existence of two types of self-enhancement biases, egoistic and moralistic, that derive from the extent to which individuals are concerned about excelling in the agentic versus communal domains. Individuals exhibiting an egoistic bias have an inflated sense of self-worth that is founded on positive distortions for agentic traits such as extraversion, achievement, intelligence, and talent. In contrast, individuals with a moralistic bias have an inflated view of their moral character that is founded on positive distortions for communal traits such as agreeableness, conscientiousness, moral uprightness, and likeability (Paulhus & Buckels, Chapter 22, this volume).[3]

Moreover, self-enhancement is not only "offensive," such as when one takes a gratuitous opportunity to self-aggrandize, but also "defensive," particularly in the face of ego threat. Individuals often act in ways that counter and minimize any potential damage from those times "when favorable views about oneself are questioned, contradicted, impugned, mocked, challenged, or otherwise put in jeopardy" (Baumeister, Smart, & Boden, 1996, p. 8). Ego threat can be operationalized in a variety of ways, such as negative information about one's performance, one's personality, or the quality of one's social interactions, and its regulation can be observed in a variety of responses, such as emotional reactions, attributions, and evaluations of feedback source. Regarding this emphasis on "protecting" the self, Campbell and Sedikides (1999) point out that ego threat—and, hence, self-enhancement—can vary across both persons and situations with those same variables that are linked to ego involvement: self-esteem, high task importance, achievement motivation, self-focused attention, competitiveness, and success expectancy.

Regarding more chronic and deeply rooted dispositions that anchor tendencies to distort self-views in the service of self-esteem regulation, research points to the centrality of narcissism as an all-encompassing theoretical framework. For example, research on the underlying cognitive processes, such as ego involvement, and concomitant emotional states, such as pride and shame, suggests that self-enhancement stems from the kind of dysregulated self-esteem system that characterizes highly narcissistic individuals (Tracy, Cheng, Martens, & Robins, 2011). After all, if self-enhancement is fostered by ego involvement, then imagine its propensity in narcissists, who are generally and chronically ego-involved. Moreover, if self-enhancement subserves self-esteem regulation (especially in the face of threat), then imagine its function for narcissists, who jealously and vigilantly guard their penchant to feel good about themselves.

Narcissism, both as a clinical disorder and as a normal dimension of personality functioning, involves having a grandiose sense of self-importance—a conviction of being special and superior—that is bolstered by unrealistically exaggerated beliefs about one's achievements and talents. As such, distortions in self-knowledge are part and parcel of being narcissistic. Moreover, narcissists need others to buy into and feed these distortions. They have a strong desire to be revered and, lacking empathy, use others not only as an audience but also as a means to an end, being interpersonally competitive, exploitative, and aggressive (Morf & Rhodewalt, 2001; Rosenthal

& Hooley, 2010; Sedikides, Campbell, Reeder, Elliot, & Gregg, 2002). Ultimately, narcissists care more about being admired than liked and seem to lack the social graces that place at least a thin veneer of constraint on egotism and hostility (Robins, Tracy, & Shaver, 2001).[4]

Despite narcissists' loud proclamations of self-love, theoretical accounts of narcissism suggest that narcissists' incessant attempts to self-promote come more from a deficit rather than a surplus of positive self-regard. Boyd (2000) observes that narcissists are not unlike Humpty Dumpty from Lewis Carroll's *Through the Looking Glass*: Humpty Dumpty is condescending, aloof, and arrogant toward Alice as he sits atop a high wall alone, occasionally dropping the King's name; however, his outside manner defends his inner fragility, his fear of falling down, of becoming undone. According to Kernberg (1975), this paradoxical personality pattern develops when a child with cold, rejecting parents protects him- or herself from their indifference and/or aggression by inflating his or her sense of self-worth. Kohut (1977) also places blame on cold, rejecting parents; their failure to "mirror" their children's grandiosity prevents them from internalizing the views by which they can esteem themselves in the absence of external validation; nor do they learn to trust in the good of others. In contrast to Kernberg and Kohut, Millon (1981) considered parental indulgence and excessive admiration as root causes of narcissism.

Otway and Vignoles (2006) provided empirical support for a blend of the preceding views, suggesting that a combination of parental devaluation and parental overvaluation predict adult narcissism. They conclude: "The future narcissist receives constant praise from his or her caregiver, but this is accompanied by implicit messages of coldness and rejection rather than warmth and acceptance and, thus . . . the praise—which is also indiscriminate—may come to seem unreal" (p. 113). A prospective, 20-year longitudinal study (Cramer, 2011) finds a stronger effect for the harsher brand of parenting—authoritarian and indifferent parenting behaviors—particularly toward children already evidencing in preschool indicators of narcissism (e.g., the desire to be the center of attention, low impulse control, interpersonal antagonism).

Work on the developmental determinants of narcissism thus converges on a picture in which a child who is made to feel that he or she is or should be perfect is shown that he or she falls short of perfection. This brings about the central feature of narcissism: a dissociation between conscious feelings of superiority and an unconscious sense of inadequacy. From this perspective, self-enhancement is not simply a mechanism to reinforce high explicit self-esteem, but, rather, is an attempt to regulate an unconscious, or only partially conscious, sense of inadequacy and vulnerability that is countered by strong conscious feelings of superiority. By adulthood, the narcissist's positive and negative self-representations may become so highly dissociated that the positive self is the only operative representation within the individual's explicit self-knowledge. As a result, narcissists endorse explicitly self-aggrandizing items, such as "If I ruled the world it would be a much better place," yet score low on measures of implicit self-esteem (Jordan, Spencer, Zanna, Hoshino-Browne, & Correll, 2003; Sakellaropoulo & Baldwin, 2007; Zeigler-Hill, 2006). This structural split in the self-representational system—explicit feelings of grandiosity coexisting with implicit feelings of inadequacy—may make the entire self vulnerable to threats to self-worth, promoting a defensive self-regulatory style characterized by a denial of the bad and an exaggerated emphasis on the good.

That the postulated fragile core of narcissism drives self-aggrandizement has received empirical support. For example, Bosson, Brown, Zeigler-Hill, and Swann (2003) found evidence for self-enhancement only among those high self-esteem individuals who also had low implicit self-esteem. Gregg and Sedikides (2010) even propose that low implicit self-esteem alone, regardless of level of explicit self-esteem, may undergird narcissism. They found that narcissism was related to lower levels of two implicit self-esteem measures (go/no-go association task, name-letter task), and that these associations persisted and even increased when explicit self-esteem was partialed out.

Such studies provide important insights into the nature of narcissism and its links to self-esteem and self-enhancement. However, in our view, this account of narcissism is incomplete without consideration of shame and pride, which we believe fuel the sense of inadequacy and grandiosity. Shame has been identified as the "keystone" affect in narcissism (Wright, O'Leary, & Balkin, 1989), with narcissism considered a mechanism to cope with excessive shame. Although narcissists are not liable to experience consciously, let alone report, shame, at least one study (Edelstein, Yim, & Quas, 2010) has observed physiological indicators of shame in narcissistic individuals (specifically, heightened cortisol reactivity in narcissistic males confronted with a stressful evaluative task). Our previous work suggests that narcissists avoid painful feelings of shame by inflating their feelings of self-worth via "hubristic"—as opposed to "authentic"—pride. Hubristic pride (i.e., feelings of arrogance and conceit) is related to a wide range of maladaptive outcomes, including aggression, low implicit self-esteem, problematic relationships, and depression; "authentic" pride, which is rooted in experiences of mastery and achievement, is related to genuine feelings of self-worth and other indicators of well-being and adjustment (Tracy, Cheng, Robins, & Trzesniewski, 2009; Tracy et al., 2011; Tracy & Robins, 2007).

Ultimately, nondefensive, genuine self-esteem is quite different from the defensive, illusory self-esteem that characterizes narcissistic self-aggrandizement, and their solid versus fragile cores lead to important differences in the steps individuals take to regulate their self-views. For example, Hepper, Gramzow, and Sedikides (2010) found that high self-esteem (controlling for narcissism) and narcissism (controlling for self-esteem) were both associated with the tendency to see self-relevant events in a favorable light. However, high self-esteem individuals also reported using self-affirmation, whereas narcissists reported defensiveness and soliciting/playing up positive feedback. Other research suggests that narcissists regulate implicit shame by seeking external indicators of their self-worth (e.g., others' approval, good grades, a compliment from a stranger), which they take as proof of the veracity of their positive self-representations to allow for the maintenance of hubristic pride. Still, these contingencies make self-esteem labile (Kernis, 2001). Consistent with this focus on positivity embracement, Horvath and Morf (2010) found that narcissists are more oriented toward using grandiosity, as opposed to the denial of worthlessness, to self-define and self-promote, whereas high self-esteem individuals, being more mindful of social acceptability, only moderately self-aggrandize and take the safer route of denying their negative characteristics. Finally, impulsivity fuels the narcissist's shortcuts toward securing self-worth (Vazire & Funder, 2006), as narcissists seek immediate means by which to enhance their self-concept, such as suppressing limitations and exaggerating strengths, rather than use of more deliberate approaches, such as developing their skills and capabilities.

Taken together, we believe the research to date supports the idea that individual differences in self-enhancement stem largely from a set of motivational and affective processes that are well captured by narcissistic tendencies toward aggrandizement and dysfunctional self-esteem regulation. Note that we are not equating narcissism with self-enhancement. Although all narcissists, by definition, are self-enhancers (either covertly or overtly), we do not believe that all self-enhancers are narcissists. Many individuals who exhibit self-enhancement tendencies do not possess the complex panoply of other attributes that characterize the narcissistic personality, including exhibitionism, exploitativeness, entitlement, and lack of empathy. However, we believe that most forms of self-enhancement, whether exhibited by narcissistic or non-narcissistic individuals, derive from the same underlying process—a defensive form of self-esteem regulation, where the desire to protect one's self-worth from threat, and accompanying feelings of shame, leads to positive, self-serving distortions. At the same time, we do not rule out the possibility that some instances of self-enhancement, particularly measured, circumscribed, and situated illusions that provide a rosy tint on reality rather than a wholesale distortion, primarily reflect the operation of cognitive–informational biases, such as selective encoding of schema-consistent information, rather than the kind of molten, top-down motivational–affective processes that characterize narcissistic self-esteem regulation.[5]

Assessing Individual Differences in Self-Enhancement

Finding an Accuracy Criterion

What is the best way to determine whether a person has self-knowledge? At first, the answer seems simple: To assess self-knowledge, one need only compare a person's self-view with what that person is truly like. But therein lies the problem. Assessing biases in self-perception requires some measure of reality or the "truth" about a person, to separate those individuals who are truly biased from those who have positive (or negative) but *accurate* self-views. Such "accuracy criteria" have proven difficult to find, as there is no "gold standard" for measuring a person's traits, capabilities, needs, and so on. For most attributes, we have only indirect measures from which the constructs must be inferred. Researchers interested in biases in self-knowledge typically rely on three types of accuracy criteria: social consensus, pragmatic criteria, and objective criteria (see also Back & Vazire, Chapter 9, this volume).

Many early researchers operationalized self-insight as the extent to which people's perceptions of themselves concur with how they are seen by others, that is, the *social consensus*. As Allport (1937) noted, "Proof positive of what a man *is* in the biophysical sense is difficult to obtain; ultimately, therefore, the most practical index of a man's insight . . . [is] the relation of what a man thinks he is to what others (especially psychologists) think he is" (p. 321, original emphasis). Social consensus is operationalized as the aggregate judgment of multiple observers, such as friends, spouses, coworkers, bosses, expert clinicians, and fellow participants in laboratory tasks (e.g., Funder, 1999; Robins & John, 1997b; Vazire, 2006; 2010). This criterion is especially helpful for assessing attributes that elude objective measurement, such as most global personality traits.

One problem with social consensus criteria is that different types of informants have different and circumscribed perspectives, which may limit their validity. For this reason, Kenny (2004) suggests conceptualizing the social consensus as the judgment that arises out of all possible perceivers observing all possible behaviors that a target emits. This conceptualization can remain only an ideal for obvious reasons. Furthermore, it is important to consider that the suitability of using others' views as a comparison point might vary with the attribute judged. Work by Vazire and colleagues (Vazire & Mehl, 2008; Vazire, 2010) suggests that informant reports may be less valid for difficult-to-observe traits such as neuroticism.

Another form of accuracy is *pragmatic accuracy*, or whether a judgment is predictive of behavior and/or functionally suited to a perceiver's needs (Swann, 1984). For example, an employer might perceive a prospective employee as being diligent and competent during an interview and hire him, hoping that his judgment is accurate in that it predicts good job performance. In self-perception, a judgment is similarly "accurate" if it is useful to the individual and related to successful task accomplishment, goal attainment, and other desirable outcomes. For example, Oltmanns and colleagues (e.g., Fiedler, Oltmanns, & Turkheimer, 2004; Oltmanns, Gleason, Klonsky, & Turkheimer, 2005) examined self- versus other-ratings of personality disorders for predicting success in military training and found that, in general, other-ratings are incrementally more predictive than self-ratings for outcomes such as early discharge from the military.

Finally, in some contexts, relatively *objective criteria* are available. For example, self-perceptions of intelligence or academic ability can be compared to standardized test scores (Borkenau & Liebler, 1993; Robins & Beer, 2001; Wright, 2000). Objective criteria can also be collected in everyday life, such as with experience-sampling devices (e.g., Vazire & Mehl, 2008), or in the laboratory, by obtaining direct measures of task performance (e.g., Robins & John, 1997b) or by recording and coding relevant behaviors (e.g., Gosling, John, Craik, & Robins, 1998). For example, a measure of talkativeness, itself useful as an indicator of extraversion, can be comprised of the amount of time and number of times that a participant speaks in a group interaction (Vazire, 2010). Indeed, to the extent that behavioral acts are building blocks of personality (Buss & Craik, 1983), counts of trait-relevant behaviors can be especially apt for measuring a person's attributes. However, not all attributes (e.g., neuroticism) are indexable by concrete, observable behaviors. Moreover, an objective external criterion should ideally capture a representative sample of behavior, which is difficult to accomplish in the laboratory (Vazire & Mehl, 2008).

Given the difficulty of obtaining external measures of what a person is like, many studies of self-enhancement have tried to circumvent the problem by inferring bias from seeming inconsistencies in people's judgments. For example, research on the "better-than-average effect" demonstrated that people's self-ratings are, on average, more positive than their ratings of a hypothetical "average other" (e.g., Brown, 1986). This finding has been widely interpreted as evidence of self-enhancement because, according to the researchers, it is logically impossible for the majority of people to be better than average. Aside from the flawed reasoning (the majority of people *can* be legitimately above the statistical mean if the distribution is skewed), research on the better-than-average effect does not provide information about the degree to which any particular *individual* is self-enhancing, accurate, or self-diminishing because many individuals who rate themselves above average may, in fact, be above average. Furthermore, such a measure could reflect misconceptions concerning the meaning of *average* and be influenced by nonmotivated cognitive tendencies such as heuristics and anchoring (Chambers & Windschitl, 2004). Although approaches like this are assumed to tap distorted self-views, they cannot be direct operationalizations of individual differences in those distortions because they have no external indicator of reality (Colvin et al., 1995; John & Robins, 1994).

Operationalizing Bias

Once a relevant criterion has been identified and measured, another thorny methodological issue remains—how to measure the discrepancy between the criterion and the self-evaluation. In many studies, the correlation between the criterion and the self-evaluation has been used as an indicator of accuracy. However, this method, while intuitive, is actually uninformative regarding self-enhancement bias. A perfect correlation can exist even when the entire sample's self-ratings are substantially higher (or lower) than the criterion. Moreover, self-criterion correlations cannot be used to measure individual differences in bias because they can be computed only at the sample level, and no individual score can be derived.[6]

Instead, assessing individual differences in bias requires a measure of directional deviations between self-perceptions and the criterion. The easiest procedure for doing this is to compute a *simple difference score*; that is, to subtract the criterion measure from the self-evaluation. This procedure requires that both measures be on the same metric. Another common procedure involves computing a *residualized difference score* (e.g., Colvin et al., 1995; Paulhus, 1998; Paulhus, Harms, Bruce, & Lysy, 2003; Robins & Beer, 2001). Here, the criterion measure is used to predict the self-evaluation via multiple regression, and the residuals are retained. Because all shared variance with the criterion has been removed (in effect, partialing out reality), residual scores reflect the magnitude and direction of bias relative to the criterion, with positive residuals indicating self-enhancement and negative residuals, self-diminishment.

Kim, Chiu, and Zou (2010) raised concerns about both simple and residualized difference scores. They noted that correlations with these measures are generally interpreted as reflecting an association between the variable of interest (e.g., narcissism) and the full range of individual differences in self-enhancement, from self-diminishment to self-aggrandizement. However, depending on the actual range of observed difference/residual scores, such correlations may reflect the difference between self-enhancers and accurate individuals (if the difference scores cover only positive values) or the difference between self-diminishers and accurate individuals (if the difference scores cover only negative values). To address this problem, Kim and his colleagues recommend using individuals' self-evaluations, the criterion measure, and the interaction between the two to gauge the actual correlates of self-enhancement (or self-diminishment). The interaction reflects the relation between positive or negative (mis)perceptions and the outcome variable when actual trait level is high or low according to the criterion measure.

Kwan, John, Kenny, Bond, and Robins (2004; Kwan, John, Robins, & Kuang, 2008) also critiqued difference and residual scores, but for different reasons than Kim and his colleagues. They argued that research comparing self-ratings to ratings *of* others (e.g., the average college student) does not take into account that self-perceivers may be justified in seeing themselves positively (e.g., they might actually perform better or be higher on the trait than everyone else), whereas research comparing self-ratings to ratings *by* others (i.e., social consensus) does not take into account that self-perceivers may tend to see everyone, not just themselves, more positively. To address these problems, Kwan and her colleagues developed a measure of self-enhancement that identifies the unique variance in self-evaluation that is independent of how one is generally perceived by others and how one general rates others (e.g., the tendency to see everyone, including the self, positively).[7]

Ultimately, in selecting a method for gauging individual differences in self-enhancement bias, we recommend that researchers follow a few simple guidelines. First, researchers should present conceptual and empirical arguments for why the criterion they used is appropriate. For example, social consensus is a better criterion for physical attractiveness than for subjective well-being. Second, the criterion should be measured reliably and validly, following the same measurement principles (e.g., aggregation across independent observations) that are used in scale construction. Third, researchers should specify precisely how they are computing the discrepancy between self-evaluations and the criterion, which assumptions are entailed in that choice, and which potential confounds might influence the findings. Fourth, whichever method one chooses, any conclusions about the nature of self-enhancement—its causes and consequences—should make specific reference to the criterion, as divergence from one type of criterion may not have the same psychological implications as divergence from another type. Indeed, an important next step in research on self-enhancement is to examine convergences across different operationalizations of bias and to identify their distinct psychological implications.

Finally, given the limitations of any one criterion, researchers should use multiple criteria to assess bias. For example, Robins and John (1997a) used three criteria to examine self-enhancement in evaluations of performance in a group discussion task—two social consensus criteria (aggregated judgments of peers and psychologists) and one objective outcome (amount of bonus money obtained from the group); the convergence of findings across all three criteria provided more powerful evidence about individual differences in self-perception bias than any single criterion.

Adaptive and Maladaptive Consequences of Positive Illusions

Xenophon (370 B.C./1864) related that Socrates "had been admired beyond all men for the cheerfulness and tranquillity with which he lived" (p. 505); he further quoted Socrates as having said, "I would not admit to any man that he has lived either better or with more pleasure than myself" (p. 506). Indeed, it is generally agreed that Socrates had extraordinary health and constitutional strength, and that at the time of his death, though 70 years old, both his body and mind were as vital as ever. Can it be that the most insightful man is also the happiest and healthiest? Does accuracy in self-knowledge yield more benefits than bias? That is, given that individuals can vary from self-enhancement to self-insight to self-effacement, who is most likely to flourish?

The case of Socrates flies in the face of the widespread contention that positively skewing the truth about oneself is adaptive. This position emerged in the late 1970s (e.g., Alloy & Abramson, 1988) and rose to prominence when Taylor and Brown (1988) published a provocative article on the widespread benefits of a *triad* of positive illusions: having an overly positive view about oneself, exaggerating one's level of control over events, and being overly optimistic about one's future. Researchers who align with this position have associated positive illusions with better emotional health (Taylor & Armor, 1996), better intellectual striving (e.g., higher motivation, persistence, and performance; Felson, 1984; Willard & Gramzow, 2009), more fulfilling interpersonal relationships, and faster recovery from trauma and illness (Bonanno, Rennicke, & Dekel, 2005; Gupta & Bonanno, 2010; Taylor, Lerner, Sherman, Sage, & McDowell, 2003).

Alternatively, self-enhancement has been linked to substantial costs. For example, not knowing one's limits appears to lead to imprudent risk taking (Baumeister, Heatherton, & Tice, 1993), ineffective action planning (Oettingen & Gollwitzer, 2001), disengagement from academic endeavors (Robins & Beer, 2001), and worse grades (Kwan, John, et al., 2008). Also, adverse emotional and physical health consequences may come from the repressive and/or defensive coping linked with self-enhancement (Rutledge, Linden, & Davies, 2000; Shedler, Mayman, & Manis, 1993). And interpersonally, self-enhancers may be judged harshly and rejected by others because of their pompous, self-centered, and narcissistic tendencies (Colvin et al., 1995; Kwan, John, Kenny, Bond, & Robins, 2004; Robins & John, 1997a).

Based on the checkered evidence, any global characterization of self-enhancement as either good or bad seems unjustified. Self-enhancement may be adaptive, maladaptive, or both—a "mixed blessing," according to Paulhus (1998). Thus, it is important to understand the factors that underlie the divergent findings. The consequences of self-enhancement may depend on (1) the type of outcome assessed, (2) the domain in which the self-enhancement occurs, (3) the time frame of the outcome, and (4) how self-enhancement is operationalized and assessed.

Type of Outcome

Kurt and Paulhus (2008) argued that self-enhancement leads to adaptive *intrapsychic* outcomes, such as self-esteem and optimism, but maladaptive *interpersonal* outcomes, such as hostility, defensiveness, and arrogance. Consistent with this, self-enhancers appear to be self-confident and happy (Taylor & Armor, 1996), and their positive outlooks may set the stage for positive attitudes and ambitions in the future (Robinson & Ryff, 1999). They also appear to fare better emotionally in the aftermath of negative events: In a prospective study on the impact of self-enhancement on posttraumatic resilience, self-enhancement was linked to less distress, less appraisal of threat, and better coping (Gupta & Bonanno, 2010).

However, if the outcome is defined in terms of interpersonal functioning, then self-enhancement is more likely to be maladaptive (Colvin et al., 1995; Paulhus, 1998). Self-enhancers are prone to social derision (Schlenker & Leary, 1982), and narcissistic individuals have problems maintaining long-term romantic relationships (Campbell, 1999; Wink, 1991). These interpersonal problems are no doubt fostered by the greater priority narcissistic individuals place on agentic versus communal goals (Roberts & Robins, 2000). Indeed, even in their relationships, narcissistic individuals are primarily hoping to enhance their self-worth rather than experience intimacy, warmth, or honesty (Campbell, 1999; Campbell, Brunell, & Finkel, 2006). Given that much of life is interpersonally mediated (e.g., whether one "plays well with others" can affect whether one seems like a suitable relationship partner, a candidate for a promotion, or a deserving recipient of aid), the negative effects of self-enhancement on interpersonal relations can create a widespread constellation of collateral problems.

Domain of Self-Enhancement

Whereas the most adverse consequences of self-enhancement seem to occur for interpersonal outcomes, it is self-enhancement on agentic, not communal, dimensions that seems to be the most deleterious. A prime example is status self-enhancement. Functionalist accounts of status imply that individuals who have an inflated perception of their status will act in ways that violate the status hierarchy and hinder cooperation, leading them to be ostracized from the group. Consistent with this account, individuals who overestimate their status in a group tend to be less accepted, liked, and trusted by other group members, less desired as future work partners, and less well compensated for their work; in contrast, overestimating one's acceptance in the group does not have these adverse outcomes, presumably because those who overestimate their acceptance have an overarching goal of getting along with others (Anderson, Ames, & Gosling, 2004; Anderson, Srivastava, Beer, Spataro, & Chatman, 2006). Because only status self-enhancement is punished, people take much more care to perceive their status accurately compared to their level of acceptance, even erring on the side of underestimating their status (Anderson et al., 2006).

However, status needs an audience, and Willard and Gramzow (2009, Study 4) reasoned that it is important to consider whether self-enhancement is *intrapsychic* (i.e., striving to convince oneself of one's worth) or *interpersonal* (i.e., striving to convince others of one's worth). To tap into these different processes, Willard and Gramzow manipulated the context—private versus public—in which self-reports of grade point average (GPA) were obtained. In a private context, self-reporting should be more indicative of a person's true self-views, as the expectations and demands of others are less salient and the impetus to engage in impression management is weaker. Interestingly, they found that self-enhancement borne from public self-focus, which was manipulated by the presence of a video camera, occurred to the same degree as private self-enhancement, but it did not have the same correlates. Specifically, public self-enhancers did *not* reap the benefits of private self-enhancers—increased positive affect and improved grades.

Time-Course Matters

Several studies suggest that self-enhancement yields short-term benefits but long-term costs. Robins and Beer (2001) found that overestimation of performance in a group discussion task predicted immediate rises in positive affect, but exaggerated beliefs about academic ability (relative to SAT scores and high school GPA) were associated with declines in self-esteem and well-being over the course of college. Moreover, self-enhancement did not predict superior academic performance—as proponents of the benefits of positive illusions would have expected—and self-enhancers were even slightly less likely to graduate. In the social arena, Paulhus (1998) found that among group members meeting for the first time, self-enhancers were better liked and perceived more favorably on a variety of attributes (e.g., Big Five traits, performance, adjustment). However, over the course of several weeks, self-enhancers came to be actively disliked, ultimately being regarded as conceited, defensive, and hostile. Consistent with this finding, several studies have demonstrated that narcissistic individuals are initially seen in a dazzling light, managing to charm others on the basis of brief glimpses into their personalities, such as short self-introductions (Back, Schmukle, & Egloff, 2010); 30-second audio recordings of their answers to the question "What do you enjoy doing?" (Friedman, Oltmanns, Gleason, & Turkheimer, 2006); and mere photographs (Back et al., 2010; Vazire, Naumann, Rentfrow, & Gosling, 2008). Interestingly, Back and his colleagues (2010) found that the exploitativeness/entitlement component of narcissism, which is the component most associated with toxic interpersonal outcomes, was largely responsible for narcissists' initial charm, even judged solely from photographs.

Measurement of Self-Enhancement

Finally, the consequences of self-enhancement may depend on how self-enhancement is operationalized. If self-enhancement is defined by the tendency to view oneself more positively than one views others, then the outcomes are often favorable. However, if self-enhancement is defined by the tendency to view oneself more positively than one is viewed by others, then outcomes are often unfavorable (Kurt & Paulhus, 2008). As previously discussed, however, neither of these operationalizations produces a "pure" measure of self-enhancement because self-perceivers may be justified in seeing themselves positively (in the case of the former index) or may tend to see *everyone* positively (in the case of the latter index). Kwan and colleagues (2008) found that when controlling for how participants were rated *by* others, all positive correlations between self-enhancement relative to perceptions *of* others and task performance disappeared, whereas significant correlations with narcissism, hypersensitivity, and defensiveness emerged. When using their unconfounded measure of self-enhancement, Kwan and colleagues found that self-enhancement was associated with lower levels of resilience, worse grades, poorer social skills, and higher levels of defensiveness and narcissism.

Taken together, the studies reviewed here argue against facile conclusions about the adaptive or maladaptive consequences of individual differences in self-enhancement. Instead, a comprehensive evaluation of this issue requires consideration of how the consequences vary across contexts, domains of self-enhancement, time frames, and operationalizations of self-enhancement. In our view, the field direly needs a meta-analysis to integrate the large and diverse literature on this issue and better understand the various moderators.

Concluding Remarks

So, why did Socrates have such self-insight? And why did the people around him perceive themselves as wiser than they truly were? In this chapter, we have focused on several factors, both situational and especially dispositional, that might account for individual differences in self-insight, which subsumes the self-enhancement biases exhibited by the targets of Socrates' sweeping survey of Greece. Because it is unlikely that these individuals were simply "wired" differently than Socrates, we can postulate that they were characterized by different motivations, in line with motivational accounts of self-enhancement. For example, it could be that they were particularly invested in seeming wise and were even threatened by such a sharply questioning man, leading them to self-enhance, whereas Socrates was driven by his strong motivation to seek the truth, and his corresponding ideal that "the unexamined life is not worth living." Many of these individuals might have even been narcissists, and we have emphasized throughout this chapter how narcissism constitutes a conceptual framework for understanding the psychological mechanisms that underlie self-enhancement.

Our review of theory and research on self-enhancement also reveals a number of methods that might have facilitated Socrates' attempt to determine which of the self-anointed wise men he met in his travels around Greece truly merited that designation and which were self-aggrandizing frauds. Ideally, Socrates would have had all the purported wise men rate each other using a round-robin design and would have proceeded to identify the unique variance in their self-evaluations that reflected overestimation relative to the social consensus. He might also have developed objective and pragmatic criteria for wisdom, and then gauged the degree to which each wise man's self-evaluations corresponded to those criteria. Finally, Socrates might have compared the life outcomes experienced by each wise man to better understand the consequences of individual differences in self-knowledge. Although the individuals who thought they were wiser than they truly were may have experienced "mixed blessings," the fact that Socrates teemed with life and joy until his death lends weight to the edict that one should "Know Thyself."

Ultimately, to the extent that self-enhancement comes from threat, insecurity, fragility, inner loathing, or a fear of how one appears to others, it may behoove one to consider the possibility that the capacity to confront all parts of yourself and "wrestle with your demons" will, in the words of playwright August Wilson, "cause your angels to sing."

NOTES

1. To say that self enhancement is trait-like does not imply that it manifests itself independently of the situational context. Indeed, self-enhancement biases are particularly pronounced in some contexts and virtually absent in others. The question is not whether the general tendency varies across contexts, but whether individual differences in the tendency are systematic and linked to psychologically meaningful constructs and outcomes. We might see self-enhancers responding to an evaluative context by further self-promotion or by an expression of hostility toward the evaluator. Those without the trait might respond with anxiety and

disengagement, or by working harder to maximize the chances of success. Clearly these different ways of responding to the same situation have important implications for interpersonal behavior and real-world outcomes.

2. We are assuming here that evidence linking neural pathology to self-enhancement implicates information-processing mechanisms. However, it is possible, albeit less likely, that the relevant brain regions subserve top-down motivational processes, such as self-esteem regulation. Separating cognitive and motivational accounts has long been a complex issue (Tetlock & Levi, 1980). This is even more evident as our understanding of the brain deepens and cognition, motivation, and emotion are increasingly seen as interdependent, perhaps even indistinguishable, processes (Barrett, 2009). For example, as a result of damage to, among other regions, the orbitofrontal cortex—one area that has been related to self-enhancement—Phineas Gage exhibited profound changes in his personality, becoming more erratic, irreverent, impatient, and disagreeable. It seems more plausible that these changes reflected a disruption of the capacity for cognitive control, valence judgments, and other low-level cognitive functions rather than a diminished motivation to please others. Of course, these low-level cognitive changes might cascade up and produce disruptions of higher-level processes such as impression management (or in the case of self-enhancement, self-esteem regulation) that reinforce and perhaps even accentuate the personality changes, but this would still implicate basic cognitive processes as the critical factor.

3. Motivational differences in these domains have been invoked to explain cultural differences in self-enhancement. Although some researchers (e.g., Heine & Hamamura, 2007) have argued that individuals in collectivistic cultures do not show a general self-enhancement motive, it may be that these individuals self-enhance on communal traits, whereas individuals from individualistic cultures self-enhance on agentic traits (Sedikides, Gaertner, & Vevea, 2005). Thus, cultural differences may be another source of individual differences in self-enhancing tendencies, and may partially align with Paulhus and John's (1998) distinction between egoistic and moralistic self-enhancement.

4. Despite their general lack of self-insight, narcissistic individuals do recognize that they possess narcissistic traits (e.g., arrogance), that they see themselves more positively than they are seen by others, and that they make a good first impression but become less well liked after others get to know them better (Carlson, Vazire, & Oltmanns, 2011).

5. Most theory and research concerning self-perception biases has focused on self-enhancement and neglected the question of why people self-diminish. Whether and why some individuals hold unrealistically negative self-views, be it on occasion or as a general tendency, is a fertile avenue for future research. Indeed, narcissism may provide insights into self-diminishment biases to the extent that narcissists, particularly covert/vulnerable narcissists (Dickinson & Pincus, 2003), are believed to fluctuate between highly self-enhancing and highly self-critical perceptions of themselves. Moreover, a narcissism perspective might help explain why, for example, both self-enhancers and self-diminishers are prone to depression (Kim & Chiu, 2011).

6. One exception is that within-person profile correlations can be computed between multiple self-ratings (e.g., of the Big Five) and multiple criterion measures. However, these correlations reflect the degree to which an individual accurately perceives his or her overall trait configuration (e.g., that he or she is more extraverted than conscientious), not the degree to which he or she exhibits a positivity bias.

7. Kwan and colleagues' self-enhancement index requires the use of a round-robin design, where every participant rates every other participant. An alternative is to use a ranking format, which eliminates differences in scale usage (e.g., in five-person groups, rankings of self and other group members must have a mean of 3). A self-enhancement index derived from ranking data is nearly perfectly correlated with the Kwan index (Kwan et al., 2008).

REFERENCES

Alloy, L. B., & Abramson, L. Y. (1988). Depressive realism: Four theoretical perspectives. In L. B. Alloy (Ed.), *Cognitive processes in depression* (pp. 223–265). New York: Guilford Press.

Allport, G. W. (1937). *Personality: A psychological interpretation.* New York: Holt.

Anderson, C., Ames, D. R., & Gosling, S. D. (2008). Punishing hubris: The perils of overestimating one's status in a group. *Personality and Social Psychology Bulletin, 34,* 90–101.

Anderson, C., Srivastava, S., Beer, J. S., Spataro, S. E., & Chatman, J. A. (2006). Knowing your place: Self-perceptions of status in face-to-face groups. *Journal of Personality and Social Psychology, 91,* 1094–1110.

Atwater, L. E., & Yammarino, F. J. (1992). Does self-other agreement on leadership perceptions moderate the validity of leadership and performance predictions? *Personnel Psychology, 45,* 141–164.

Back, M. D., Schmukle, S. C., & Egloff, B. (2010). Why are narcissists so charming at first sight?: Decoding the narcissism–popularity link at zero acquaintance. *Journal of Personality and Social Psychology, 98,* 132–145.

Baumeister, R. F., Heatherton, T. F., & Tice, D. M. (1993). When ego threats lead to self-regulation failure: Negative consequences of high self-esteem. *Journal of Personality and Social Psychology, 64,* 141–156.

Baumeister, R. F., Smart, L., & Boden, J. M. (1996). Relation of threatened egotism to violence and aggression: The dark side of high self-esteem. *Psychological Review, 103,* 5–33.

Beer, J. S. (2007). Neural systems of self-conscious emotions and their underlying appraisals. In J. L. Tracy, R. W. Robins, & J. P. Tangney (Eds.), *The self-conscious emotions: Theory and research* (pp. 53–67). New York: Guilford Press.

Beer, J. S., John, O. P., Scabini, D., & Knight, R. T. (2006). Orbitofrontal cortex and social behavior: Integrating self-monitoring and emotion-cognition interactions. *Journal of Cognitive Neuroscience, 18,* 871–879.

Bonanno, G. A., Rennicke, C., & Dekel, S. (2005). Self-enhancement among high exposure survivors of the September 11th terrorist attack: Resilience or social maladjustment? *Journal of Personality and Social Psychology, 88,* 984–998.

Borkenau, P. & Liebler, A. (1993). Convergence of stranger ratings of personality and intelligence with self-ratings, partner-ratings, and measured intelligence. *Journal of Personality and Social Psychology, 65,* 546–553.

Bosson, J. K., Brown, R. P., Zeigler-Hill, V., & Swann, W. B., Jr. (2003). Self-enhancement tendencies among people with high explicit self-esteem: The moderating role of implicit self-esteem. *Self and Identity, 2,* 167–187.

Boyd, J. H. (2000). The "soul" of the psalms compared to the "self" of Kohut. *Journal of Psychology and Christianity, 19,* 219–231.

Brown, J. D. (1986). Evaluations of self and others: Self-enhancement biases in social judgments. *Social Cognition, 4,* 353–376.

Buss, D. M., & Craik, K. H. (1983). The act frequency approach to personality. *Psychological Review, 90,* 105–126.

Campbell, W. K. (1999). Narcissism and romantic attraction. *Journal of Personality and Social Psychology, 77,* 1254–1270.

Campbell, W. K., Brunell, A. B., & Finkel, E. J. (2006). Narcissism, interpersonal self-regulation, and romantic relationships: An agency model approach. In K. D. Vohs & E. J. Finkel (Eds.), *Self and relationships: Connecting intrapersonal and interpersonal processes* (pp. 57–83). New York: Guilford Press.

Campbell, W. K., Rudich, E., & Sedikides, C. (2002). Narcissism, self-esteem, and the positivity of self-views: Two portraits of self-love. *Personality and Social Psychology Bulletin, 28*, 358–368.

Campbell, W. K., & Sedikides, C. (1999). Self-threat magnifies the self-serving bias: A meta-analytic integration. *Review of General Psychology, 3*, 23–43.

Carlson, E. N., Vazire, S., & Oltmanns, T. F. (2011). You probably think this paper's about you: Narcissists' perceptions of their personality and reputation. *Journal of Personality and Social Psychology, 101*, 185–201.

Chambers, J. R., & Windschitl, P. D. (2004). Biases in social comparative judgments: The role of nonmotivated factors in above-average and comparative-optimism effects. *Psychological Bulletin, 130*, 813–838.

Colvin, C. R., Block, J., & Funder, D. C. (1995). Overly positive self-evaluations and personality: Negative implications for mental health. *Journal of Personality and Social Psychology, 68*, 1152–1162.

Cramer, P. (2011). Young adult narcissism: A 20 year longitudinal study of the contribution of parenting styles, preschool precursors of narcissism, and denial. *Journal of Research in Personality, 45*, 19–28.

Crocker, J., & Wolfe, C. T. (2001). Contingencies of self-worth. *Psychological Review, 108*, 593–623.

Dickinson, K. A., & Pincus, A. L. (2003). Interpersonal analysis of grandiose and vulnerable narcissism. *Journal of Personality Disorders, 17*, 188–207.

Edelstein, R. S., Yim, I. S., & Quas, J. A. (2010). Narcissism predicts heightened cortisol reactivity to a psychosocial stressor in men. *Journal of Research in Personality, 44*, 565–572.

Feldman Barrett, L. (2009). The future of psychology: Connecting mind to brain. *Perspectives in Psychological Science, 4*, 326–339.

Felson, R. B. (1984). The effect of self-appraisals of ability on academic performance. *Journal of Personality and Social Psychology, 47*, 944–952.

Fiedler, E. R., Oltmanns, T. F., & Turkheimer, E. (2004). Traits associated with personality disorders and adjustment to military life: Predictive validity of self and peer reports. *Military Medicine, 169*, 207–211.

Friedman, J. N. W., Oltmanns, T. F., Gleason, M. E. J., & Turkheimer, E. (2006). Mixed impressions: Reactions of strangers to people with pathological personality traits. *Journal of Research in Personality, 40*, 395–410.

Funder, D. C. (1999). *Personality judgment: A realistic approach to person perception.* San Diego, CA: Academic Press.

Gosling, S., John, O. P., Craik, K. H., & Robins, R. W. (1998). Do people know how they behave?: Self-reported act frequencies compared with on-line codings by observers. *Journal of Personality and Social Psychology, 74*, 1337–1349.

Greenwald, A. G. (1980). The totalitarian ego: Fabrication and revision of personal history. *American Psychologist, 35*, 603–618.

Gregg, A. P., & Sedikides, C. (2010). Narcissistic fragility: Rethinking its links to explicit and implicit self-esteem, *Self and Identity, 9*, 142–161.

Gupta, S., & Bonanno, G. A. (2010). Trait self-enhancement as a buffer against potentially traumatic events: A prospective study. *Psychological Trauma: Theory, Research, Practice, and Policy, 2*, 83–92.

Heine, S. J., & Hamamura, T. (2007). In search of East Asian self-enhancement. *Personality and Social Psychology Review, 11*, 4–27.

Hepper, E. G., Gramzow, R. H., & Sedikides, C. (2010). Individual differences in self-enhancement and self-protection strategies: An integrative analysis. *Journal of Personality, 78*, 781–814.

Horvath, S., & Morf, C. C. (2010). To be grandiose or not to be worthless: Different routes to self-enhancement for narcissism and self-esteem. *Journal of Research in Personality, 44*, 585–592.

Jacobs, J. E., Bleeker, M. M., & Constantino, M. J. (2003). The self-system during childhood and adolescence: Development, influences, and implications. *Journal of Psychotherapy Integration, 13*, 33–65.

John, O. P., & Robins, R. W. (1994). Accuracy and bias in self-perception: Individual differences in self-enhancement and the role of narcissism. *Journal of Personality and Social Psychology, 66*, 206–219.

Jordan, C. H., Spencer, S. J., Zanna, M. P., Hoshino-Browne, E., & Correll, J. (2003). Secure and defensive high self-esteem. *Journal of Personality and Social Psychology, 85*, 969–978.

Kenny, D. A. (2004). PERSON: A general model of interpersonal perception. *Personality and Social Psychology Review, 8*, 265–280.

Kernberg, O. (1975). *Borderline conditions and pathological narcissism*. New York: Aronson.

Kernis, M. H. (2001). Following the trail from narcissism to fragile self-esteem. *Psychological Inquiry, 12*, 223–225.

Kernis, M. H., & Sun, C. R. (1994). Narcissism and reactions to interpersonal feedback. *Journal of Research in Personality, 28*, 4–13.

Kim, Y.-H., & Chiu, C.-Y. (2011). Emotional costs of inaccurate self-assessments: Both self-effacement and self-enhancement can lead to dejection. *Emotion, 11*, 1096–1104.

Kim, Y.-H., Chiu, C.-Y., & Zou, Z. (2010). Know thyself: Misperceptions of actual performance undermine achievement motivation, future performance, and subjective well-being. *Journal of Personality and Social Psychology, 99*, 395–409.

Klein, S. B., Loftus, J., & Kihlstrom, J. F. (1996). Self-knowledge of an amnesic patient: Toward a neuropsychology of personality and social psychology. *Journal of Experimental Psychology: General, 125*, 250–260.

Kohut, H. (1977). *The restoration of the self*. Madison, CT: International Universities Press.

Kurt, A., & Paulhus, D. L. (2008). Moderators of the adaptive value of self-enhancement: Operationalization, domain, and adjustment criterion. *Journal of Research in Personality, 42*, 839–853.

Kwan, V. S. Y., Barrios, V., Ganis, G., Gorman, J., Lange, C., Kumar, M., et al. (2007). Assessing the neural correlates of self-enhancement bias: A transcranial magnetic stimulation study. *Experimental Brain Research, 182*, 379–385.

Kwan, V. S. Y., John, O. P., Kenny, D. A., Bond, M. H., & Robins, R. W. (2004). Reconceptualizing individual differences in self-enhancement bias: An interpersonal approach. *Psychological Review, 111*, 94–110.

Kwan, V. S. Y., John, O. P., Robins, R. W., & Kuang, L. L. (2008). Conceptualizing and assessing self-enhancement bias: A componential approach. *Journal of Personality and Social Psychology, 94*, 1062–1077.

Lagattuta, K. H., & Thompson, R. A. (2007). The development of self-conscious emotions: Cognitive processes and social influences. In J. L. Tracy, R. W. Robins, & J. P. Tangney (Eds.), *The self-conscious emotions: Theory and research* (pp. 91–113). New York: Guilford Press.

Mezulis, A. H., Abramson, L. Y., Hyde, J. S., & Hankin, B. L. (2004). Is there a universal positivity bias in attributions?: A meta-analytic review of individual, developmental, and cultural differences in the self-serving attributional bias. *Psychological Bulletin, 130*, 711–747.

Miller, D. T., & Ross, M. (1975). Self-serving biases in the attribution of causality: Fact or fiction? *Psychological Bulletin, 82*, 213–225.

Millon, T. (1981). *Disorders of personality: DSM III: Axis II*. Chichester, UK: Wiley.

Morf, C. C., & Rhodewalt, F. (2001). Unraveling the paradoxes of narcissism: A dynamic self-regulatory processing model. *Psychological Inquiry, 12*, 177–196.

Oettingen, G., & Gollwitzer, P. M. (2001). Goal setting and goal striving. In A. Tesser & N. Schwarz (Eds.), *Intraindividual processes: Blackwell handbook of psychology* (pp. 329–347). Malden, MA: Blackwell.

Oltmanns, T. F., Gleason, M. E. J., Klonsky, E. D., & Turkheimer, E. (2005). Meta-perception for pathological personality traits: Do we know when others think that we are difficult? *Consciousness and Cognition: An International Journal, 14*, 739–751.

Otway, L. J., & Vignoles, V. L. (2006). Narcissism and childhood recollections: A quantitative test of psychoanalytic predictions. *Personality and Social Psychology Bulletin, 32*, 104–116.

Paulhus, D. L. (1998). Interpersonal and intrapsychic adaptiveness of trait self-enhancement: A mixed blessing? *Journal of Personality and Social Psychology, 74*, 1197–1208.

Paulhus, D. L., Harms, P. D., Bruce, M. N., & Lysy, D. C. (2003). The over-claiming technique: Measuring self-enhancement independent of ability. *Journal of Personality and Social Psychology, 84*, 890–904.

Paulhus, D. L., & John, O. P. (1998). Egoistic and moralistic biases in self-perception: The interplay of self-deceptive styles with basic traits and motives. *Journal of Personality, 66*, 1025–1060.

Rankin, K. P., Baldwin, E., Pace-Savitsky, C., Kramer, J. H., & Miller, B. L. (2005). Self awareness and personality change in dementia. *Journal of Neurology Neurosurgery and Psychiatry, 76*, 632–639.

Roberts, B. W., & Robins, R. W. (2000). Broad dispositions, broad aspirations: The intersection of personality traits and major life goals. *Personality and Social Psychology Bulletin, 26*, 1284–1296.

Robins, R. W., & Beer, J. S. (2001). Positive illusions about the self: Short-term benefits and long-term costs. *Journal of Personality and Social Psychology, 80*, 340–352.

Robins, R. W., & John, O. P. (1997a). Effects of visual perspective and narcissism on self-perception: Is seeing believing? *Psychological Science, 8*, 37–42.

Robins, R. W., & John, O. P. (1997b). The quest for self-insight: Theory and research on accuracy and bias in self-perception. In R. T. Hogan, J. A. Johnson, & S. R. Briggs (Eds.), *Handbook of personality psychology* (pp. 649–679). New York: Academic Press.

Robins, R. W., Tracy, J. L., & Shaver, P. R. (2001). Shamed into self-love: Dynamics, roots, and functions of narcissism. *Psychological Inquiry, 12*, 230–236.

Robinson, M. D., & Ryff, C. D. (1999). The role of self-deception in perceptions of past, present, and future happiness. *Personality and Social Psychology Bulletin, 25*, 596–608.

Rosenthal, S. A., & Hooley, J. M. (2010). Narcissism assessment in social–personality research: Does the association between narcissism and psychological health result from a confound with self-esteem? *Journal of Research in Personality, 44*, 453–465.

Rutledge, T., Linden, W., & Davies, R. F. (2000). Psychological response styles and cardiovascular health: Confound or independent risk factor? *Health Psychology, 19*, 441–451.

Sakellaropoulo, M., & Baldwin, M. W. (2007). The hidden sides of self-esteem: Two dimensions of implicit self-esteem and their relation to narcissistic reactions. *Journal of Experimental Social Psychology, 43*, 995–1001.

Schlenker, B. R., & Leary, M. (1982). Audiences reactions to self-enhancing, self-denigrating, and accurate self-presentations. *Journal of Experimental Social Psychology, 18*, 89–104.

Schriber, R. A., & Robins, R. W. (2011). *Self-insight in individuals with autism spectrum disorders*. Unpublished manuscript, University of California, Davis.

Sedikides, C., Campbell, W. K., Reeder, G., & Elliot, A. J. (1998). The self-serving bias in relational context. *Journal of Personality and Social Psychology, 74*, 378–386.

Sedikides, C., Campbell, W. K., Reeder, G., Elliot, A. J., & Gregg, A. P. (2002). Do others bring out the worst in narcissists?: The "others exist for me" illusion. In Y. Kashima, M. Foddy, & M. Platow (Eds.), *Self and identity: Personal, social, and symbolic* (pp. 103–123). Mahwah, NJ: Erlbaum.

Sedikides, C., Gaertner, L., & Toguchi, Y. (2003). Pancultural self-enhancement. *Journal of Personality and Social Psychology, 84*, 60–70.

Sedikides, C., Gaertner, L., & Vevea, J. L. (2005). Pancultural self-enhancement reloaded: A meta-analytic reply to Heine (2005). *Journal of Personality and Social Psychology, 89*, 539–551.

Sedikides, C., Horton, R. S., & Gregg, A. P. (2007). The why's the limit: Curtailing self-enhancement with explanatory introspection. *Journal of Personality, 75*, 783–824.

Shedler, J., Mayman, M., & Manis, M. (1993). The illusion of mental health. *American Psychologist, 48*, 1117–1131.

Sutin, A. R., & Robins, R. W. (2008). When the "I" looks at the "Me": Autobiographical memory, visual perspective, and the self. *Consciousness and Cognition, 17*, 1386–1397.

Swann, W. B., Jr. (1984). The quest for accuracy in person perception: A matter of pragmatics. *Psychological Review, 91*, 457–477.

Taylor, S. E., & Armor, D. A. (1996). Positive illusions and coping with adversity. *Journal of Personality, 64*, 873–898.

Taylor, S. E., & Brown, J. (1988). Illusion and well-being: A social psychological perspective on mental health. *Psychological Bulletin, 103*, 193–210.

Taylor, S. E., Lerner, J. S., Sherman, D. K., Sage, R. M., & McDowell, N. K. (2003). Portrait of the self-enhancer: Well adjusted and well liked or maladjusted and friendless? *Journal of Personality and Social Psychology, 84*, 605–615.

Tetlock, P. E. & Levi, A. (1980). Attribution bias: On the inconclusiveness of the cognition–motivation debate. *Journal of Experimental Social Psychology, 18*, 68–88.

Tracy, J. L., Cheng, J. T., Martens, J. P., & Robins, R. W. (2011). The emotional dynamics of narcissism: Inflated by pride, deflated by shame. In. W. K. Campbell, & J. D. Miller (Eds.), *Handbook of narcissism and narcissistic personality disorder: Theoretical approaches, empirical findings, and treatments* (pp. 330–343). New York: Wiley.

Tracy, J. L., Cheng, J. T., Robins, R. W., & Trzesniewski, K. (2009). Authentic and hubristic pride: The affective core of self-esteem and narcissism. *Self and Identity, 8*, 196–213.

Tracy, J. L., & Robins, R. W. (2007). The psychological structure of pride: A tale of two facets. *Journal of Personality and Social Psychology, 92*, 506–525.

Trzesniewski, K. H., Kinal, M. P.-A., & Donnellan, M. B. (2011). Self-enhancement and self-protection in developmental context. In M. Alicke, & C. Sedikides (Eds.), *Handbook of self-enhancement and self-protection* (pp. 341–357). New York: Guilford Press.

Vazire, S. (2006). Informant reports: A cheap, fast, and easy method for personality assessment. *Journal of Research in Personality, 40*, 472–481.

Vazire, S. (2010). Who knows what about a person?: The Self–Other Knowledge Asymmetry (SOKA) model. *Journal of Personality and Social Psychology, 98*, 281–300.

Vazire, S., & Funder, D. C. (2006). Impulsivity and the self-defeating behavior of narcissists. *Personality and Social Psychology Review, 10*, 154–165.

Vazire, S., & Mehl, M. R. (2008). Knowing me, knowing you: The accuracy and unique predictive validity of self-ratings and other-ratings of daily behavior. *Journal of Personality and Social Psychology, 95*, 1202–1216.

Vazire, S., Naumann, L. P., Rentfrow, P. J., & Gosling, S. D. (2008). Portrait of a narcissist:

Manifestations of narcissism in physical appearance. *Journal of Research in Personality, 42,* 1439–1447.

Willard, G., & Gramzow, R. H. (2009). Beyond oversights, lies, and pies in the sky: Exaggeration as goal projection. *Personality and Social Psychology Bulletin, 35,* 477–492.

Wink, P. M. (1991). Two faces of narcissism. *Journal of Personality and Social Psychology, 61,* 590–597.

Wright, F., O'Leary, J., & Balkin, J., (1989). Shame, guilt, narcissism, and depression: Correlates and sex differences. *Psychoanalytic Psychology, 6,* 217–230.

Wright, S. S. (2000). Looking at the self in a rose-colored mirror: Unrealistically positive self-views and academic performance. *Journal of Social and Clinical Psychology, 19,* 451–462.

Xenophon. (1864). *The Anabasis, or expedition of Cyrus, and the memorabilia of Socrates* (J. S. Watson, Trans.). New York: Harper & Bros. (Original work published 370 B.C.)

Zeigler-Hill, V. (2006). Discrepancies between implicit and explicit self-esteem: Implications for narcissism and self-esteem instability. *Journal of Personality, 74,* 119–143.

PART II
DOMAINS OF SELF-KNOWLEDGE

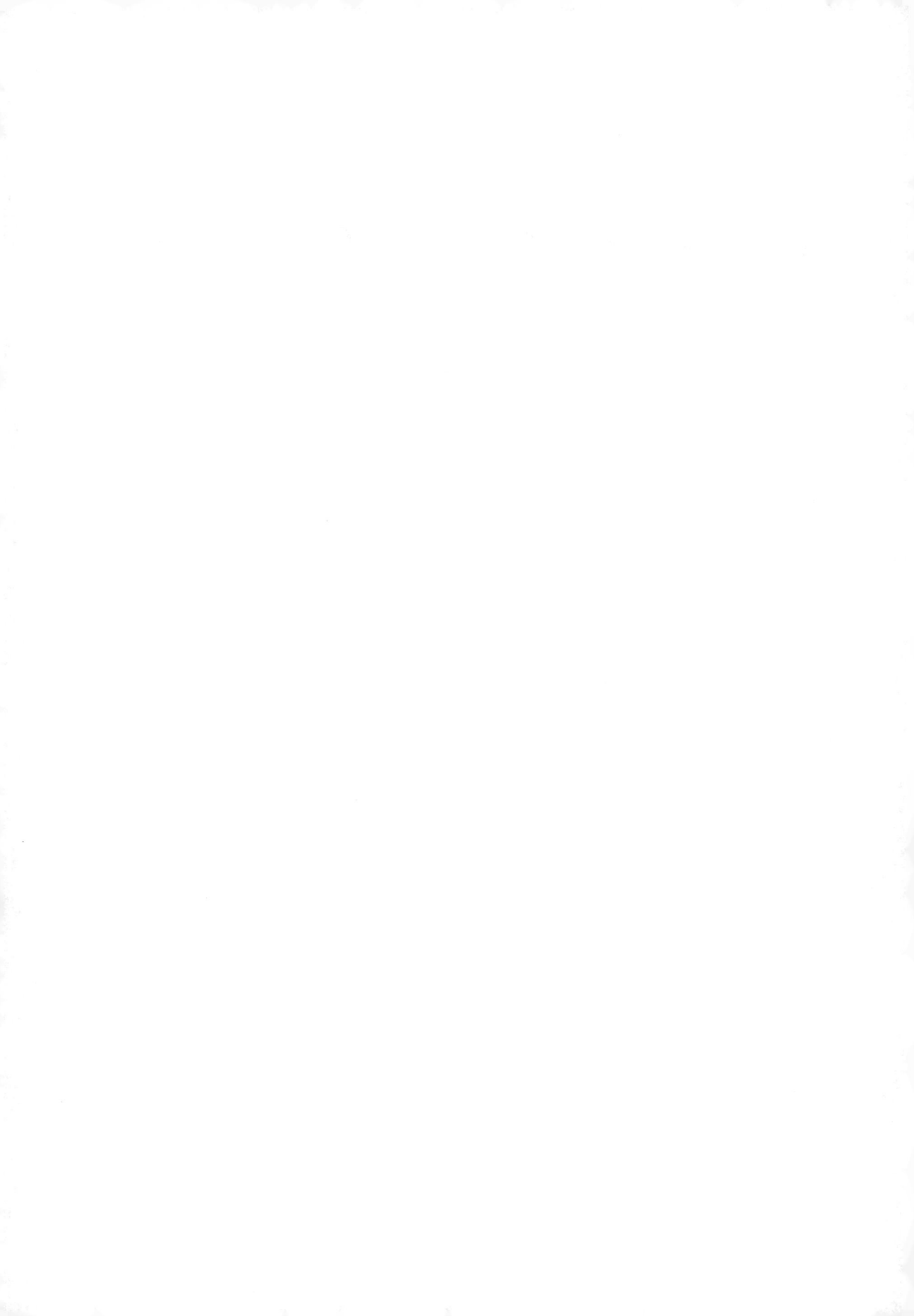

CHAPTER 9
Knowing Our Personality

MITJA D. BACK
SIMINE VAZIRE

Do we know our own personality? What are the blind spots in our self-views of our personality and why do they exist? Are some people more accurate in their self-descriptions than others? How can we improve our self-insight? And should we? The question of personality self-knowledge (PSK) has always fascinated the human mind. Philosophers have struggled with the quest for self-insight for centuries, many poets and songwriter have expressed the promises and pitfalls of knowing oneself, and tons of popular self-help books try to persuade individuals how to get a better sense of their "real" personality.

This preoccupation with PSK is mirrored by people's everyday thoughts and behaviors. People often think about and describe themselves in terms of their most important personality traits. Performing a Google search for the phrase "I am a person who" results in more than 300 million hits, most of which lead to straightforward trait self-descriptions. For example, Brigitte describes herself as a person "who is very outgoing and open minded," Sherry thinks that she is an individual "who is chronically worried," Fiona sees herself as someone "who is courteous and helpful," and Steve is convinced that he is a person "who has a God-given talent for organizing." Others describe themselves as a person "who gets scared easily"; "who is very lazy, carefree, laid back"; "who hates people"; "who makes many mistakes"; "who is ambitious, optimistic, playful"; "who is open-minded, introspective, confident"; "who is often swift to anger"; "who is chronically late"; "who is calm and relaxed"; "who takes a long time to warm up to others." These individuals all seem to have a clear sense of what kind of people they are. But are they indeed correct in their self-descriptions? Is Brigitte really more extraverted and open to experiences than others? Is it true that Sherry is relatively low in emotional stability?[1]

Unfortunately, despite the ubiquitous nature of personality self-descriptions and the value placed on correct self-views, there has been little empirical research on the accuracy of those views (for overviews, see Robins & John, 1997; Vazire & Carlson,

2010; Wilson, 2002, 2009; Wilson & Dunn, 2004). There exist optimistic and pessimistic opinions regarding the quality of people's PSK, both in lay and academic psychology. On the one hand, the privileged access of the self to one's personality seems to be obvious. No one but ourselves can better describe how we generally feel, what we admire and value in life—in short what kind of person we are. Consequently, the vast majority of contemporary personality psychologists use people's self-reports to measure personality traits (Funder, 2001; Gosling, Vazire, Srivastava, & John, 2004; Vazire, 2006). On the other hand, people often express skepticism about others' (usually not their own) exaggerated or distorted self-views. In fact, social-psychological research has pointed to many biases in people's explicit self-views, including introspective limits, self-enhancement, and socially desirable responding (Greenwald & Banaji, 1995; Nisbett & Wilson, 1977; Taylor & Brown, 1988; see also Hansen & Pronin, Chapter 21, and Helzer & Dunning, Chapter 23, this volume).

In summary, although we regularly rely on our own and others' personality self-descriptions, empirical knowledge about the general degree of PSK, its underlying processes, determinants and consequences, is still limited. In the following sections we first define PSK and distinguish different domains of PSK. For each domain, we then provide a short summary of the existing evidence for PSK. Afterward, we present a process model of PSK and use this model to explain existing blind spots in people's personality self-views. Finally, we discuss some future prospects, including the study of moderators and the adaptiveness of PSK.

Definitions and Measurement: What Is PSK?

From a naive point of view the definition of PSK is straightforward: PSK is the agreement between people's self-views of their personality and their real personality. However, things get complicated when we try to analyze PSK empirically. Whereas people's self-views are indeed relatively easy to define and measure, there is no simple definition of "real" personality and no direct way to measure it. As empirical research on PSK cannot be conducted without a criterion measure against which people's self-descriptions are evaluated, a working definition and measures of real personality are needed.

According to a realistic approach to personality, there is not a single, best measure but many reasonable measures of "real" personality (Funder, 1999). Besides people's explicit self-concept (as measured by self-reports) three sources of data capture meaningful individual differences: the implicit self-concept of personality (Asendorpf, Banse, & Mücke, 2002; Back, Schmukle, & Egloff, 2009; Wilson, Lindsey, & Schooler, 2000), actual behavior (Back & Egloff, 2009; Baumeister, Vohs, & Funder, 2007; Furr, 2009; Vazire & Mehl, 2008), and people's reputations (i.e., what others think of someone's personality; Hofstee, 1994; Hogan & Roberts, 2000; Vazire, 2010). The implicit self is typically measured by indirect tests of personality (e.g., implicit association tests [IATs] for the measurement of personality; Asendorpf et al., 2002; Back, Schmukle, et al., 2009; Egloff & Schmukle, 2002; Schmukle, Back, & Egloff, 2008). Actual behavior can best be assessed by direct behavioral observation in meaningful social situations (Back & Egloff, 2009; Back, Schmukle, et al., 2009; Back, Schmukle, & Egloff, 2010, 2011; Borkenau, Mauer, Riemann, Spinath,

& Angleitner, 2004; Funder, Furr, & Colvin, 2000; Mehl, Gosling, & Pennebaker, 2006; Vazire, 2010; Vazire & Mehl, 2008). Finally, people's reputations are usually measured by personality reports of knowledgeable informants such as friends or family members (Vazire, 2006). All of these measures represent reasonable criteria for people's "real" personality.

In line with this realistic approach to personality, we broadly define PSK as accurate explicit self-perceptions of how one regularly thinks, feels, and behaves, and awareness of how those patterns are interpreted by others (Vazire & Carlson, 2010). Following this definition, PSK can be measured as correlations of explicit self-reports of personality with criterion measures of people's "real" self-related cognitions and emotions (e.g., indirect personality measures), behaviors (e.g., observations of actual behavior), and reputations (e.g., personality reports from knowledgeable informants).

This definition allows us to distinguish at least four domains of PSK (see Figure 9.1). First, one can ask how well people's explicit personality self-views converge with their implicit self-concept of personality (*explicit–implicit consistency*). According to dual-process models, individuals process information about themselves and their environment in both an explicit (i.e., controlled or conscious) and an implicit (i.e., automatic or unconscious) mode (Bargh & Chartrand, 1999; Dijksterhuis & Nordgren, 2006; Epstein, 1994; Fazio, 1990; Greenwald et al., 2002; Strack & Deutsch, 2004; Wilson et al., 2000; see Evans, 2008, for a recent review; see also Gawronski & Bodenhausen, Chapter 3, this volume). With respect to personality, an explicit self-concept encompassing propositional representations of one's personality ("I am an extraverted person") can be distinguished from an implicit self-concept of personality consisting of associative and less consciously accessible representations of one's

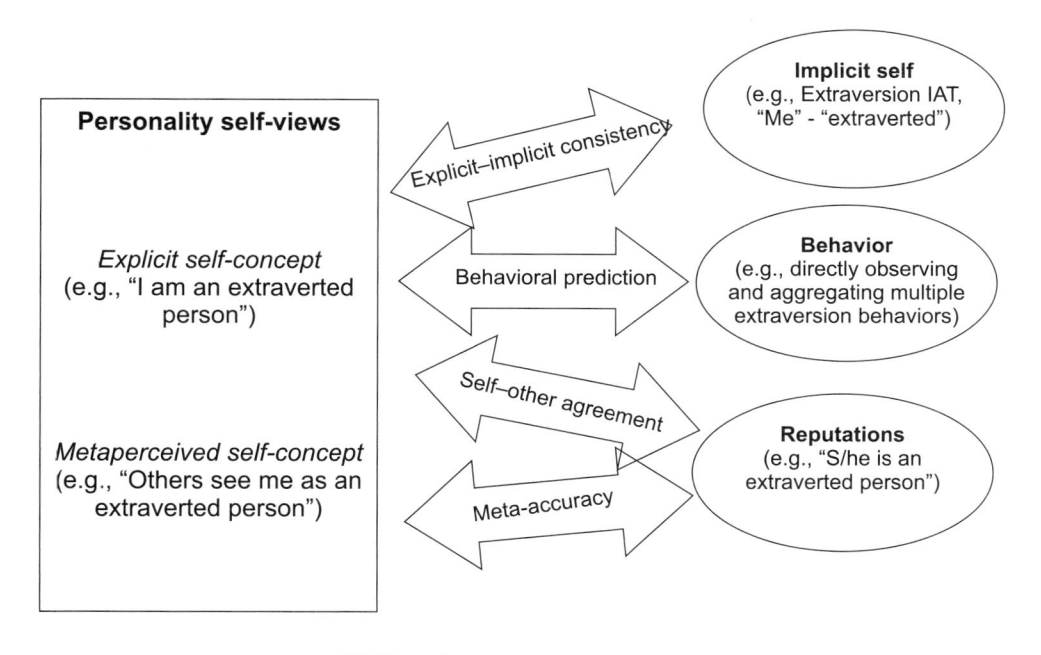

FIGURE 9.1. Four domains of PSK.

personality ("Me"—"extraverted") (Asendorpf et al., 2002; Back, Schmukle, et al., 2009). The amount of explicit–implicit consistency can be interpreted as the explicit access to one's inner self. It indicates how much people's conscious self-descriptions are in line with their implicit self-related representations (cf. Hofmann & Wilson, 2010).

Second, one can ask how well people's explicit personality self-views converge with their actual behavior (*behavioral prediction*). Predicting actual behavior is often regarded as the "gold standard" for the validation of any personality measure (Back, Schmukle, et al., 2009; Funder, 1999; Kenny, 1994): A personality measure is as good as its ability to predict relevant behavior. A measure of extraversion should, for example, predict how much people engage in extraverted behavior. The same logic can be applied to the study of PSK: PSK is high when people's self-reports are good predictors of how they actually behave. Behavioral prediction can be measured by correlating personality self-reports with corresponding behavioral measures. In doing so, it is important not to rely on behavioral self-reports, which are neither conceptually nor empirically identical to actual behaviors (e.g., Back & Egloff, 2009; Gosling, John, Craik, & Robins, 1998; Todd, Penke, Fasolo, & Lenton, 2007; Vazire & Mehl, 2008; West & Brown, 1975). Instead, one should use behavioral observation techniques to assess people's actual behaviors within meaningful social situations (cf. Back & Egloff, 2009). As social behaviors are multiply determined and single behavioral observations contain a lot of error variance, aggregation across behavioral observers, time points, and situational settings is generally recommended (Ahadi & Diener, 1989; Funder, 1999; Kenrick & Funder, 1988).

Third, PSK can be analyzed by asking how well people's explicit personality self-views converge with others' perceptions of their personality (*self–other agreement*). In this case, the criterion is others' opinions about one's personality (i.e., one's reputation), and high PSK would be indicated by a high consensus between the self's and others' judgments about one's personality. How others see us contains important information with respect to what we are like. This is particularly true for others who are well acquainted. Friends, spouses, and family members have the chance to observe us in multiple social situations. They notice what kinds of people, situations, and tasks we prefer, they know the life decisions we made, and they have very direct access to our everyday actual behavior—even more direct access than we ourselves have (Funder, 1999; Hofstee, 1994). This is particularly true for personality traits that are reputational in nature, such as being charming or funny. We can only be charming or funny if others find us so.

PSK as self–other agreement is usually measured by correlating personality self-reports with other-reports. To enhance the validity of other-reports—and thereby the validity of a PSK analysis based on self–other agreement—personality judgments are averaged across multiple informants. Choosing informants from different social contexts (e.g., friend, family, coworker) has the additional advantage that the aggregated other-reports are based on different aspect of a target's life, possibly resulting in a more complete reflection of the target's real personality. Usually, these informants are nominated by the target persons themselves. One potential problem with this self-nomination approach is that people who are nominated by a target usually also like the target. This might lead to distorted (and probably less accurate) personality judgments (Leising, Erbs, & Fritz, 2010). Therefore, it can be helpful (although more difficult) also to obtain ratings from informants independent of the target's preferences (i.e., people who are well acquainted with the target but do not particularly like him or her).

Fourth, PSK can be studied by asking how well people know how others view their personality (*meta-accuracy*). This approach is covered in depth by Carlson and Kenny (Chapter 15, this volume), so we do not define it in detail here.

Each of the four approaches to PSK has its benefits and shortcomings. Explicit–implicit consistency is a limited approach to PSK because the validity of indirect tests of personality is uncertain. Many indirect tests lack sufficient reliability (Bosson, Swann, & Pennebaker, 2000; Schmukle, 2005), and the indirect personality test with the best reliability estimates, the IAT (Egloff, Schwerdtfeger, & Schmukle, 2005; Nosek, Greenwald, & Banaji, 2007), has been criticized due to potential methodological confounds and because it is still not sufficiently clear what it really measures (Back, Schmukle, & Egloff, 2005; Buhrmester, Blanton, & Swann, 2011; Perugini & Banse, 2007). The IAT has, however, been shown to predict meaningful actual behaviors over and above personality self-reports (see Schnabel & Asendorpf, 2010, for an overview), at least for Neuroticism, Extraversion, and to a lesser degree Agreeableness (Back, Schmukle, et al., 2009).

On the one hand, behavioral prediction is arguably the most appropriate way to validate personality self-reports. On the other hand, it is also the most complex and difficult. Researchers need to choose appropriate situations that evoke meaningful behavioral differences, theoretically define a priori what kind of behaviors indicate each personality trait under investigation, and apply specified (and often tedious) behavioral observation techniques to assess a multitude of behavioral criteria (Vazire, Gosling, Dickey, & Schapiro, 2007). Perhaps it is too time-consuming or we do not have the chance to observe Brigitte's extraversion behavior in her everyday life. Or if we try, we might choose the wrong situation or the wrong (or too few) behavioral criteria.

Both the self–other agreement and the meta-accuracy approaches assume that observers' judgments are valid measures of an actor's personality. As others might be wrong about our personality, each outcome of a self–other agreement or meta-accuracy analysis is disputable. For the same reasons, self–other agreement and meta-accuracy analyses might also result in an inflated estimate of PSK. If Fiona's child, friend, and coworkers also think Fiona is agreeable (high self–other agreement) and Fiona thinks that others see her as agreeable (high meta-accuracy), one could still argue that Fiona and her acquaintances are all mistaken and Fiona is in fact not very agreeable. There are, however, good reasons to assume that this is an overly pessimistic view of the self–other agreement and meta-accuracy approaches. Although well-acquainted others are also prone to a number of biases (Leising et al., 2010; Vazire, 2010), their judgments do contain valid information about our personality (Funder, 1999). Specifically, other-reports can often predict actual behavior above and beyond self-reports of personality (e.g., Kolar, Funder, & Colvin, 1996; Vazire, 2010; Vazire & Mehl, 2008).

In summary, all four approaches to PSK give us some important information about how well people know their personality. Most people would agree that someone whose self-concept is mirrored by his or her implicit self, everyday behavior, and reputation, and who knows his or her reputation, has more self-knowledge than someone whose self-concept lacks these characteristics. In the following section, we summarize prior empirical findings for each approach to PSK.[2]

Empirical Findings: What Do People Know about Their Personality?

How well do people know their inner self? The correspondence between the explicit and implicit self-concept of personality (explicit–implicit consistency) has been an important topic of psychological research since the first attempts to assess the implicit self-concept of personality via projective measures such as the Thematic Apperception Test (TAT; Murray, 1943). Over the last few decades, renewed attention to implicit measures (Banse & Greenwald, 2007; Bosson et al., 2000; De Houwer, 2006; Nosek et al., 2007) has also led to a renewed interest in explicit–implicit consistency (cf. Hofmann & Wilson, 2010). One of the most prominent indirect measures is the Implicit Association Test (IAT; Greenwald, McGhee, & Schwartz, 1998). In contrast to other implicit measures of personality, personality IATs routinely demonstrate good reliability as well as incremental predictive validity (Back, Schmukle, et al., 2009; Schnabel & Asendorpf, 2010).[3]

Interestingly, IAT measures and self-report measures of the same construct tend to be only slightly associated. Two reviews have reported an average correlation between implicit and explicit measures of $r = .24$ (Hofmann, Gawronski, Gschwendner, Le, & Schmitt, 2005; Nosek, Banaji, & Greenwald, 2002). In a similar type of analysis, Nosek (2005) reported an average correlation of $r = .36$. There are, however, important differences in the strength of associations depending on the domain assessed, with correlations ranging between $r = .08$ (age attitude) and $r = .52$ (attitudes toward political candidates) (Nosek et al., 2002). Concerning personality dispositions, explicit–implicit consistency tends to be even lower than the average effects. Correlation coefficients of $r = .17$ for the association between implicit and explicit self-esteem (Nosek et al., 2002) and of $r = .21$ for the association between implicit and explicit self-concept (Hofmann, Gawronski, et al., 2005) have been reported. Similarly, weak positive correlations have been found for implicit and explicit anxiety measures, with a mean of $r = .14$ (Egloff & Schmukle, 2002). For studies that investigated the explicit and implicit self-concept for all of the Big Five dimensions, the average explicit–implicit consistency was $r = .11$ (Back, Schmukle, et al., 2009), $r = .18$ (Grumm & von Collani, 2007), $r = .15$ (Schmukle, Back, & Egloff, 2008, Study 1), $r = .13$ (Schmukle et al., 2008, Study 2), and $r = .08$ (Steffens & Schulze König, 2006), respectively (weighted mean $r = .13$). In summary, average correlations between the measures of the explicit and implicit self-concept of personality tend to be rather low, despite high reliabilities of the individual measures (Egloff et al., 2005).

Within the Big Five, the trait domain seems to moderate the explicit–implicit consistency. For the five studies that examined the explicit and implicit Big Five, mean consistency was strongest for Extraversion (weighted mean $r = .26$), weaker for Conscientiousness ($r = .18$) and Neuroticism ($r = .17$), and absent for Openness ($r = .01$) and Agreeableness ($r = -.02$). A variety of other dispositional and situational context moderators of the association between implicit and explicit measures have been discussed (Hofmann, Gawronski, et al., 2005; Hofmann, Gschwendner, & Schmitt, 2005;

Nosek, 2005). These moderators can be grouped into two classes: awareness and adjustment (Hofmann, Gschwendner, et al., 2005). *Awareness* refers to the degree to which individuals are able to form an accurate propositional representation of their underlying associative representation. Dispositions (e.g., private self-consciousness, self-focused attention; Hofmann, Gschwendner, et al., 2005) or situational contexts (e.g., cognitive elaboration, i.e., thinking about feelings and mental states; Egloff, Weck, & Schmukle, 2008; Karpinski, Steinman, & Hilton, 2005; Nosek, 2005) that foster translation processes between the explicit and implicit self-concept of personality should lead to a stronger explicit–implicit consistency (see Schultheiss & Strasser, this volume).

Adjustment, or bias, refers to the degree to which individuals change their explicit self-concept descriptions due to adaptation to social norms and self-presentation concerns. The more people adjust their personality self-descriptions because of their dispositions (e.g., self-monitoring, social desirability) or the situational context (e.g., private vs. public reporting) the less they should converge with implicit measures (Hofmann, Gschwendner, et al., 2005; Nosek, 2005). Thus, whereas the overall consistency between the explicit and implicit self-concept of personality is typically low, individuals' insight into the inner self may vary as a function of the self-perceiver's dispositions and the situational context.

Probably the most convincing argument for high PSK would be findings that indicate people's personality self-views converge with their actual behavior (behavioral prediction). If people behave in the same way they describe themselves, they probably know pretty well who they are. In fact, during the long-lasting debates around the stability, cross-situational consistency, and predictive validity of personality, weak or even absent correlations between personality self-reports and observable behaviors were the most important argument against the usefulness of broad personality self-descriptions (Mischel, 1968; Nisbett & Wilson, 1977). On the other hand, it was argued that personality measures can predict behavior when behavior is observed in adequate (i.e., personality-relevant) situations and behavioral indicators are sufficiently aggregated across behavioral observers, time points and situational settings (Epstein, 1983; Funder, 1999; Kenrick & Funder, 1988).

In recent years a few studies have examined the relationship between personality self-reports and actual behavior across a broad range of traits (e.g., Back, Schmukle, et al., 2009; Borkenau et al., 2004; Kolar et al., 1996; Mehl et al., 2006; Spain, Eaton, & Funder, 2000; Vazire, 2010). Confirming earlier research, these studies typically found a modest positive correlation between people's self-descriptions and their actual behaviors (between .20 and .35 averaged across the Big Five; see Vazire & Carlson, 2010). In the German Observational Study of Adult Twins (GOSAT), Peter Borkenau and colleagues (2004) videotaped targets in 15 social situations designed to provoke diverse personality-related behaviors and assessed Big Five and intelligence personality judgments based on these behaviors for each situation. The average correlation between the targets' personality self-reports and behavioral judgments aggregated across situations and traits was $r = .22$ for the Big Five. Additionally, some task- and trait-specific effects on the predictive validity of self-reports were revealed. For example, Openness self-reports were more strongly related to behavioral judgments based on a pantomime situation ($r = .29$) than on a situation where participants had to sing a song ($r = .06$).

The latter finding points to the possibility that behavioral prediction can be enhanced by aggregating across behavioral criteria specifically designed to match the trait dimension of interest. This approach was pursued in the Mainz Observation of Behavior Study (Back, Schmukle, et al., 2009). Based on a systematic investigation of theoretical and empirical approaches to personality and social behavior, behavioral aspects of the Big Five were defined and subsequently assigned to a multitude of concrete actual behaviors for each of the five dimensions. For the measurement of these behaviors, 130 participants were observed in a diverse set of relevant social situations, including speaking situations, interpersonal interactions, creativity tasks, helping situations, performance tasks, body-oriented tasks, and unstructured situations. Several trained expert raters objectively coded or rated more than 50 predefined behavioral criteria. A meaningful behavioral criterion was subsequently adopted for each of the Big Five dimensions by aggregating across rater and behavioral criteria. Personality self-reports were then used as predictors of these behavioral aggregates. Results underlie the predictive validity of personality self-reports: Explicit measures of Neuroticism ($r=.36$), Extraversion ($r=.38$), Openness ($r=.31$), Agreeableness ($r=.35$), and Conscientiousness ($r=.30$) each predicted corresponding behavioral aggregates.

Meaningful relations between people's personality self-descriptions and their actual behavior were also found in a naturalistic context. Mehl and colleagues (2006) examined people's everyday behaviors and choice of situations using the Electronically Activated Recorder (EAR; Mehl, Pennebaker, Crow, Dabbs, & Price, 2001), a device that captures auditory recordings during people's daily lives. Personality self-reports predicted a number of corresponding actual behaviors. People who described themselves as agreeable, for instance, swore less than more disagreeable individuals. Self-proclaimed extraverts talked more, whereas those who thought of themselves as introverted spent more time alone. The more participants described themselves as conscientious, the more time they spent in class. The mean effect size of the significant real-life behavioral correlates was .27 (see Vazire & Carlson, 2010).

Vazire and Mehl (2008) performed an even more direct test of people's knowledge of their behavior. Participants were asked how they typically behave (e.g., "Compared to the average person, how often do you talk to someone of the opposite sex?"), and these self-reports were then compared with their actual behaviors as measured by the EAR over a 4-day period (e.g., percentage of person's EAR recordings that were coded as talking with the opposite sex). PSK was again significant (e.g., $r=.31$ for the ability to judge how much one talks with the opposite sex) with a mean correlation of .26. Participants' PSK varied depending on the behavioral domain. For example, people were better at judging how much they watch TV ($r=.55$) and worse at judging how much they talk one-on-one ($r=-.06$). Although such trait domain-specific findings often differ depending on the situational context investigated and the level of behavioral aggregation, there also seem to be systematic moderator effects. In her self–other knowledge asymmetry (SOKA) model, for instance, Vazire (2010) suggests that people are better at judging their own internal traits (e.g., neuroticism) and not so good at judging their highly evaluative traits (e.g., intelligence).

In summary, self-reports of personality and self-reports of concrete behaviors do regularly predict socially relevant behaviors. These results clearly show that people's personality self-reports have some validity: They are related to what people actually do. On the other hand, because predictive validities were far from perfect, there are substantial blind spots in personality self-views when it comes to predicting actual behavior. Brigitte might be correct in assuming that she is relatively extraverted, but she might not recognize that there are still some others out there who are even more expressive and outgoing than herself.

Is our self-view mirrored by what others think of our personality? Research on the accuracy of personality judgments at zero acquaintance has shown that our self-perceptions converge even with personality impressions of complete strangers. This has been shown for judgments based on real-life encounters (e.g., Levesque & Kenny, 1993), thin slices of videotaped behavior (e.g., Borkenau & Liebler, 1992; Borkenau et al., 2004), streams of thought (Holleran & Mehl, 2008), written short stories (Küfner, Back, Nestler, & Egloff, 2010), offices and bedrooms (Gosling, Ko, Mannarelli, & Morris, 2002), music preferences (Rentfrow & Gosling, 2006), personal websites (Marcus, Machilek, & Schutz, 2006; Vazire & Gosling, 2004), online social networking profiles (Back, Stopfer, et al., 2010) and even physical appearance (e.g., Borkenau & Liebler, 1992; Naumann, Vazire, Rentfrow, & Gosling, 2009) and e-mail addresses (Back, Schmukle, & Egloff, 2008).

Self–other agreement, however, increases with level of acquaintance (Biesanz, West, & Millevoi, 2007; Funder & Colvin, 1988; Funder, Kolar, & Blackman, 1995; Watson, Hubbard, & Wiese, 2000), a well-established finding that is partly due to the increasing amount of distinct behavioral information available (e.g., Borkenau et al., 2004). Thus, self–other agreement in PSK is usually studied using personality judgments by well-acquainted others, such as spouses or friends, as criterion measures. And how well do our self-views correspond with our friends' or spouses' opinions of us? Pretty well. In the GOSAT study (Borkenau et al., 2004), for example, each participant described him- or herself and was described by two close acquaintances using the self- and third-person version of the NEO Five Factor Inventory (NEO-FFI; German version: Borkenau & Ostendorf, 1993). A mean self–other agreement of .45 was found, ranging from .39 for Conscientiousness to .54 for Extraversion.

Meta-analyses of self–other agreement for close others yielded very similar results of .49 (Kenny, 1994), and .44 (Connolly, Kavanagh, & Viswesvaran, 2007), respectively. In their summary of other exemplary single studies on the topic, Vazire and Carlson (2010) report a mean self–other agreement of .40. Interestingly, whereas self–other agreement is stronger for observable traits (e.g., Extraversion) and often absent for more internal traits (e.g., Neuroticism) in zero- or short-term acquaintance contexts, it is relatively consistent across observable and internal traits for long-term acquaintances (i.e., close others; Connolly et al., 2007, Table 3). Thus, when compared to others who know us well, our personality self-perceptions clearly contain some truth across all of the five broad trait domains, although there are still discrepancies.

Are people aware of these discrepancies? Do they know how others see them (even if others disagree with their self-views)? Empirically, results on meta-accuracy as a form of PSK are mixed (Carlson & Kenny, Chapter 15, this volume; Kenny, 1994; Kenny & DePaulo, 1993; Levesque, 1997). A recent summary of existing studies on generalized and dyadic meta-accuracy reports similar average findings (Vazire & Carlson, 2010): Whereas people seem to have at least some idea about their general reputations (*generalized meta-accuracy*; mean $r = .44$), their ability to judge who specifically views them in a certain way is rather limited (*dyadic meta-accuracy*; mean

$r = .14$ for new acquaintances and $r = .17$ for well-acquainted others). When people are asked how other social partners from different contexts view them (e.g., parents vs. friends), evidence for dyadic meta-accuracy is stronger (Carlson & Furr, 2009; see Carlson & Kenny, Chapter 15, this volume, for details).

So what have we learned from prior studies on PSK? Do people know their personality or are they hopelessly mistaken? The truth lies between these extreme positions. Personality self-views moderately predict actual behaviors and reputations; people have some idea about these reputations but little insight into their implicit dispositions and how they are viewed by particular other people. Thus, PSK does exist, but it is far from being perfect. Another way to look at the validity of explicit personality self-views is to compare it with the predictive validity of others or the implicit self. Studies that directly compare how well the explicit self and others predict actual behavior (e.g., Vazire, 2010) and studies comparing the predictive validity of the explicit and implicit self (e.g., Back, Schmukle, et al., 2009) show that our explicit self is often as good a predictor of our actual behavior as are others or our implicit self. Sometimes acquaintances are better, other times our self-views are better, and still other times our implicit self seems to be the best judge of who we really are. Moreover, in many cases, all of these approaches to personality have some validity and independently predict actual behavior. Thus, on the one hand, personality self-views are not mere illusions of the self—they are related to reality. On the other hand, we are clearly not the flawless and superior judges of ourselves we often assume ourselves to be. For all four domains of PSK, our self-views have important blind spots.

This has implications for individuals' daily social lives, the appropriate assessment of personality, and the theoretical understanding of PSK. For individual human beings, an appropriate reaction to these results would be to adjust the amount of faith they put in their own and others' personality self-descriptions. All too often in social interactions, we trust our own self-view but distrust other's self-views when they do not correspond to our own perceptions (Hansen & Pronin, Chapter 21, this volume; Pronin, Kruger, Savitsky, & Ross, 2001). In light of prior empirical findings on PSK, we should put more (but not too much) faith in the self-descriptions of others and a bit less faith in our own self-descriptions.

From a practical assessment perspective, findings underline the importance and utility of personality self-reports: They tell us a lot about true personality differences between people. On the other hand, results clearly show that personality self-reports are not the same as "real personality." They are subject to a number of biases and often deviate substantially from how people really are. Consequently, when measuring personality, self-reports should be complemented by other valid methodological approaches, such as other-reports and implicit tests. Combining different perspectives on personality and aggregating across multiple heterogeneous personality tests can probably enhance the validity of our personality measures substantially.

From a theoretical perspective, the existence of various blind spots can be used as a starting point to understand better the processes that determine whether PSK is achieved or not. What steps need to be taken for explicit personality self-reports to predict implicit personality, behavior, and reputation? What are the potential biases during these steps? In the following section, we describe processes that theoretically influence PSK and use these processes to explain the blind spots for each of the four PSK domains.

Knowing Our Personality 141

Processes: What Are the Reasons for the Blind Spots in PSK?

How can we understand PSK and the existing blind spots in personality self-views? We present a process model of PSK that summarizes and integrates existing models of explicit–implicit consistency (Hofmann, Gschwendner, et al., 2005; Hofmann & Wilson, 2010), behavior prediction (behavioral process model of personality: Back, Schmukle, et al., 2009; SOKA model: Vazire, 2010); self-perception and self–other agreement (Bem, 1967; Brunswik, 1956; Funder, 1999; Kenny, 1994, Chap. 9; Swann & Bosson, 2008), and meta-accuracy (Kenny, 1994, Chap. 8). The integrative model explains PSK by outlining the processes that influence and mediate among the distinct aspects of personality: the explicit self, implicit self, actual behavior, and reputations (see Figure 9.2).

At its core the model is a description of how personality is expressed and perceived in a social context. In accordance with identity negotiation theory (Swann & Bosson, 2008), it is assumed that our self both influences our reputations and is influenced by our reputations via social feedback (Srivastava & Beer, 2005). As described in process models of personality judgment (e.g., the lens model [Brunswik, 1956] or the realistic accuracy model [Funder, 1999]) reputations are based on the perception and utilization of observable behavioral cues that are more or less related to our personality. Additionally, as described in self-perception theory (Bem, 1967),

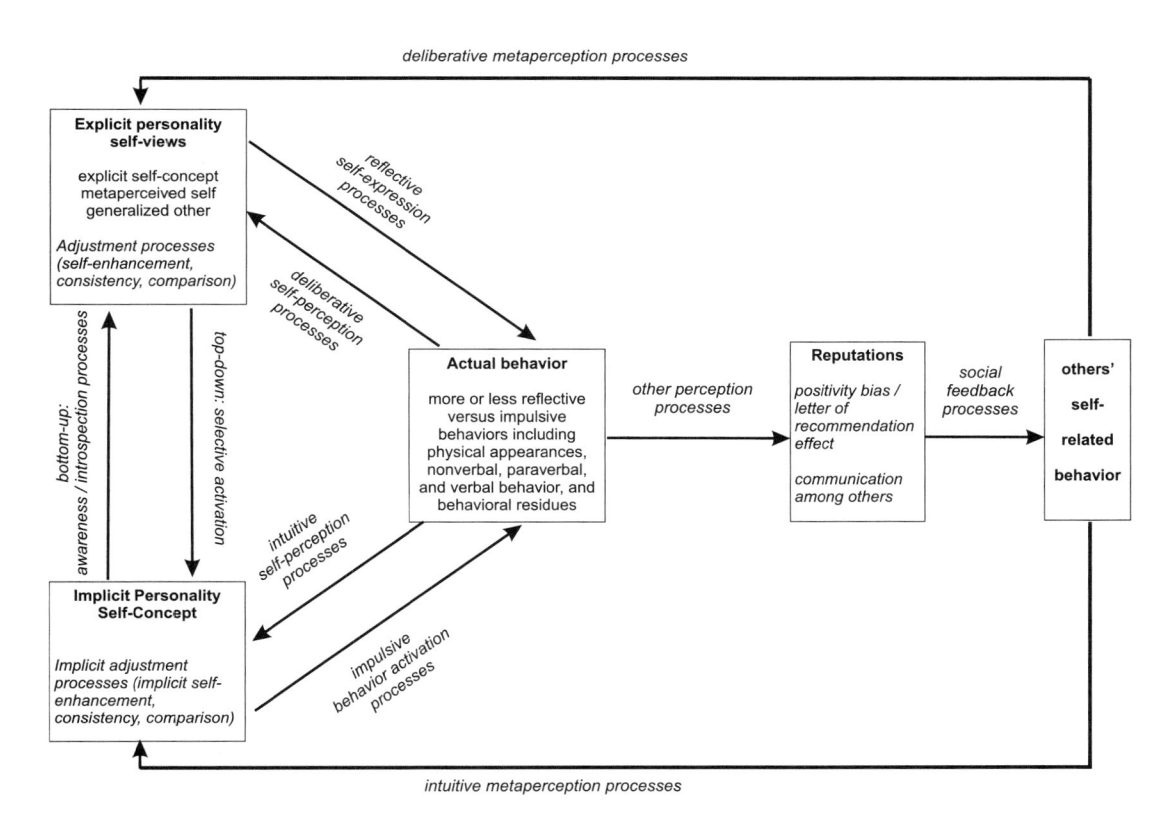

FIGURE 9.2. A process model of PSK.

behavioral cues can be perceived by the actor him- or herself and incorporated into his or her self-concept. Finally, in line with dual-process models (Back, Schmukle, et al., 2009; Fazio & Olson, 2003; Hofmann, Gschwendner, et al., 2005; Hofmann & Wilson, 2010; Strack & Deutsch, 2004), we assume that (at least some) aspects of the self-concept can be decomposed into structurally distinct, albeit related implicit and explicit components that jointly determine more or less controlled versus spontaneous actual behavior (see also Gawronski & Bodenhausen, Chapter 3, and Schultheiss & Strasser, Chapter 4, this volume).

Various specific intra- and interpersonal processes influence this dynamic chain of actions (see Figure 9.2 for details). We now briefly describe the most important processes and discuss how they might explain the bright spots (accurate self-perceptions) and blind spots (biased self-perception) in PSK.

Motivated Blind Spots in the Explicit Self

A number of important adjustment processes take place within the intrapersonal dynamics of explicit self-views (Hofmann, Gschwendner, et al., 2005; Hofmann & Wilson, 2010; Robins & John, 1997; Wilson & Dunn, 2004). We constantly adjust both our explicit self-concept and our interpersonal expectations (metaperceptions) by means of *self-enhancement processes* (John & Robins, 1994; Kwan, John, Kenny, Bond, & Robins, 2004; Robins & Beer, 2001; Taylor & Brown, 1988), as well as *consistency processes* (perceiving one's characteristics and one's reputations as a coherent unit across time and situations) and *comparison processes* (comparing one's own characteristics with those of others) (Festinger, 1954, 1957; Heider, 1958). For a discussion of how these motives influence self-views, we refer readers to other chapters in this volume (Schriber & Robins, Chapter 8; Helzer & Dunning, Chapter 23; Leary & Toner, Chapter 25).

Explaining the Blind Spots in Explicit–Implicit Consistency

Many of our mental states and behaviors are the result of automatic processes that are not directly accessible to our conscious selves (Bargh, 1997; Wilson, 2002). As summarized earlier, prior research on explicit–implicit consistency suggests that we are (on average) not very successful (although not completely wrong) in knowing our inner self. According to the behavioral process model of personality (Back, Schmukle, et al., 2009) the amount of *explicit–implicit consistency* in personality self-views can be interpreted as the correspondence among one's reflective and impulsive cognitive, emotional, and behavioral processes as they typically function. The typical operation of reflective processes (across time and multiple situations)—how people typically perceive and categorize situations, which behavioral options they prefer, and how they deliberately realize these preferences—condense into propositional representations of the self (the explicit self-concept). The typical functioning of impulsive processes—how situational cues are automatically processed and what kinds of actions are automatically performed—should lead to chronic associative links among associative network elements, including those between self- and trait concepts. The low average explicit–implicit consistency points to the possibility that these reflective and impulsive processes typically operate largely independently (although they jointly predict actual behavior).

What are potential pathways that could override these seemingly separated spheres? A direct link between the explicit and implicit self can be achieved via bottom-up or top-down processes (Peters & Gawronski, 2011): First, subtle experiential states of awareness (Strack & Deutsch, 2004) or activation of implicit self-associations might lead to an increased accessibility of newly activated self-knowledge that can then be integrated in one's propositional representations (i.e., explicit self-concept). This might be fostered by thinking about oneself (elaboration). Egloff and colleagues (2008), for instance, found that writing about anxiety-arousing situations substantially strengthened the relationship between implicit and explicit anxiety measures ($r = .55$ instead of $r = -.06$ in the control condition; see also Schultheiss and Strasser, Chapter 4, this volume, for a more detailed discussion). Second, intentional revision of explicit personality aspects of the self may result in selective activation of implicit self-associations, and thus in corresponding changes in the implicit self-concept of personality (Peters & Gawronski, 2011).

There is also a more indirect potential path to explicit–implicit consistency via the self-perception of behavior (Bem, 1967, 1972). Individuals may become aware of (implications of) their implicit self-concept via self-inference (e.g., by reconstructing their behaviors and behavioral outcomes; see "Explaining the Blind Spots in Behavior Prediction" below). For example, Fiona's view of herself as very agreeable might be somewhat altered when she perceives her own nonverbal signs of impatience (which primarily result from her implicit disagreeableness). One's own behavior can also be perceived more indirectly and automatically affect the implicit self-concept (Strack, Martin, & Stepper, 1988; Strack & Neumann, 2000). Thus, theoretically, explicit–implicit consistency could also result from the implicit perception of one's own reflective behaviors. Even more indirectly, the explicit and implicit self might converge because impulsive and reflective behaviors affect one's reputation, which in turn influences others' behavior toward us (see "Explaining the Blind Spots in Self–Other Agreement and Meta-Accuracy" below). These feedback behaviors might then lead to alterations in one's explicit and implicit self-concept via deliberative and intuitive metaperceptions, which should also enhance explicit–implicit consistency.

The disjunctions between explicit and implicit self-concepts are probably due to the fact that these direct and indirect processes often break down or are not even initiated. Most importantly, the explicit self often fails to integrate implicit aspects of the self. As a case in point, people seem to be not very willing to integrate (or capable of integrating) self-perceptions of their nonverbal behavior (most of which is impulsively activated) into their explicit self-concept. This was shown in a recent study by Hofmann, Gschwendner, and Schmitt (2009). Participants filled out an explicit measure of Extraversion and performed an Extraversion IAT. They were then videotaped while simulating a television commercial. Afterwards, participants watched their own video and were asked to judge their nonverbal behavior and again their degree of extraversion. The same video was also played to neutral observers who also rated the participants' behavior and extraversion. In contrast to neutral observers, self-perceivers didn't detect nonverbal behaviors related to implicit extraversion and didn't use them for their subsequent explicit extraversion judgments. This was shown even when participants were provided with motivation (monetary incentive) and a comparative context (videos of people high and low in Extraversion; Study 2). Similar results were found in the domain of speech anxiety (Study 3). People thus seem to "have a 'blind spot' with respect to the nonverbal behavioural manifestations of their unconscious selves, even though neutral observers may readily detect and utilize this information for dispositional inferences" (Hofmann et al., 2009, p. 343). In summary, although there are many potential ways to relate the explicit and implicit self, each of these potential relations is subject to a number of (very effective) biases resulting in substantial blind spots. For more on this topic, we refer readers to other chapters in this volume (Gawronski & Bodenhausen, Chapter 3; Schultheiss & Strasser, Chapter 4).

Explaining the Blind Spots in Behavior Prediction

Why aren't people more aware of how they behave? One of the most important obstacles to behavior prediction is that many behavioral processes relevant to personality operate outside conscious awareness on a rather automatic level. The explicit self-concept of personality only captures the reflective, controlled part of observable behaviors. This boundary condition of the explicit self is often referred to as a *lack of awareness* (see "Explaining the Blind Spots in Explicit–Implicit Consistency") or *introspective limits* (Greenwald & Banaji, 1995; Wilson, 2002). People have only limited access to certain aspects of the self, which nevertheless influence the everyday behaviors people show. Another important reason for the limited predictive validity of personality self-reports is the motivational processes outlined above. People may misperceive even controlled behaviors due to both self-deception and impression management processes (Paulhus, 1984; Paulhus, Bruce, & Trapnell, 1995; Paulhus & Reid, 1991; see also Paulhus & Buckels, Chapter 22, this volume).

Both factors—lack of awareness and motivated biases—undermine people's ability to act in line with how they describe themselves (*self-expression*) and thus undermine the convergence between the explicit self and actual behavior (behavioral prediction PSK). To behave in accordance with their personality self-views, people have to successfully engage in a variety of self-expression processes. They have to have a clear sense of what kind of behaviors fit their self-views; they have to possess the necessary abilities to perform these behaviors. These behaviors have to be controllable, and there has to be an appropriate situational context. The more people distort their self-views (bias) and the more the behavioral domain is influenced by impulsive processes that have not been integrated to people's explicit self (lack of awareness), the more difficult self-expression is and the lower will be the predictive validity of personality self-views.

Another route to behavioral prediction PSK is to observe one's behavior correctly and bring one's self-views in line with that behavior. According to self-perception theory (Bem, 1967, 1972), the perception of one's own overt behavior is crucial to understanding personality self-views. Some traits (e.g., anxiousness) are of a more internal nature and can thus provide strong internal cues (e.g., anxiety) that can be directly used to infer one's own personality (e.g., "I am a person who is easily scared"). Many other traits, however, provide weaker or more ambiguous internal cues. As a consequence, self-perceivers—much in the same way as outside observers—have to infer their inner self by relying on the observable external cues they themselves produce. Here again, motivated biases and implicit processes are obstacles to accurate self-perception.

Vazire's (2010) SOKA model summarizes the informational and motivational blind spots of the self in comparison to others as judges: People are not in a very good position to observe their own behavior objectively and even when put in this position (by video feedback or other information about their behavior) they are reluctant to integrate incongruent information into their explicit self-concept. Consistent with the SOKA model, it was shown that the self is a better judge of more internal and less observable traits, such as neuroticism, and others are better judges of highly evaluative traits, such as intellect (Vazire, 2010).

Another seldom-investigated potential pathway to behavioral prediction is via the reputations that result from one's behaviors. In principle, people could learn about their behavior (e.g., Fiona behaves aggressively) because their reputations (e.g., Fiona is aggressive) are based on their behaviors and might lead others to give (more or less explicit) behavioral feedback (e.g., telling Fiona not to be so aggressive; avoiding controversial discussions with Fiona) that can then be perceived (e.g., Fiona: "People seem to think I am aggressive") and integrated into one's explicit personality self-concept (e.g., Fiona: "I must be less agreeable than I thought"). There are, however, even more processes involved, each of which is again subject to multiple biases: Reputations are also based on behaviors not related to the explicit self; others might give no or ambiguous feedback; the self might incorrectly perceive others' feedback; perceived feedback might be distorted by motivated processes; and so forth (see the following section). The importance of accurate perceptions of other's behavior is not restricted to direct feedback behavior. As one's own personality score is relationally defined (more or less extraverted than others) people have to correctly estimate others' personality (by detecting and using others' behavior) for accurate comparison processes and self-views.

Explaining the Blind Spots in Self–Other Agreement and Meta-Accuracy

There are three ways to explain levels of self–other agreement (Kenny, 1994): self-verification, consensual behavior observation, and feedback integration. According to the *self-verification* view (Swann, 1987, 1990, 2012), people have a strong motivation to have their self-views confirmed by others (even when these self-views are negative) and try to convince others to agree with their self-views. Following this logic, self–other agreement can be seen as the result of successful self-presentation processes (Baumeister, 1982; DePaulo, 1992): People have to communicate their explicit self by means of behavioral expression, and others have to use these behavioral cues for their personality judgments. Of course, many things can go awry in this process, including the self failing to express its explicit personality (see the earlier discussion of self-expression), and others misperceiving the self's behavior or interpreting it in ways not anticipated by the self.

Another explanation is that the self and others (partially) use the same information to infer the self's personality: observable behavior. According to this *consensual behavior observation* approach, self–other agreement is limited by biases during both self- and other-perception (see earlier discussion). On the other hand, there can also be cases in which self–other agreement is strengthened because the self and others use the same biased information. According to the consensual behavior observation view, self–other agreement depends on (1) the existence of relevant behavioral information that is (2) available to both the self and the perceiver, (3) the detection of such information by both parties, and (4) a consensual utilization based on shared meaning systems (cf. Funder, 1999; Kenny, 1994).

A third way to explain self-other agreement (and lack thereof) is that we learn to see ourselves as others see us. What others think about us (reputation) is reflected in their behavior toward us, and we perceive this behavior and use it to evaluate ourselves. The process of *feedback integration* is described in symbolic interactionism (Cooley, 1902; Mead, 1934; Shrauger & Schoeneman, 1979) and more recently in sociometer theory (Back, Krause, et al., 2009; Denissen, Penke, Schmitt, & Van Aken, 2008; Kavanagh, Robins, & Ellis, 2010; Leary & Baumeister, 2000). According to feedback integration, the more we correctly detect and accept others' opinions about ourselves, the higher self–other agreement will be. Probably the most important obstacle to the integration of feedback is that others rarely give straightforward personality feedback (Blumberg, 1972; Felson, 1980), particularly if it is negative (Tesser & Rosen, 1975). Even if others try to give such feedback, it will probably be rather ambiguous and subtle. Moreover, even if valid behavioral feedback cues exist and are detected, people often refrain from accepting such feedback due to the motivational processes described earlier.

Analogous to the self–other agreement processes described, one can distinguish three ways to understand meta-accuracy: as self-perception, as behavior observation, or as the result of perceived feedback. For a discussion of these processes, see Carlson and Kenny (Chapter 15, this volume).

Only parts of the process model have been empirically tested. To our knowledge, no study has investigated more than two domains of PSK at once. It is therefore too early to summarize which of the processes is most important in explaining the bright and blind spots in PSK. When reviewing prior studies one can nevertheless identify some empirical trends. Motivational processes influencing the explicit self seem to be a general threat to PSK: People have a pronounced tendency to see themselves as they want to see themselves, making it hard to integrate any incongruent incoming information. Explicit–implicit consistency seems to be the domain of PSK where people know the least about themselves. Besides methodological issues, such as low stability of implicit measures, this seems to be due to limited cross talk between the explicit and implicit self (unless it is experimentally induced). Moreover, people seem to be reluctant to perceive and integrate their own automatic behaviors. Behavioral prediction is achieved by a mixture of partially successful self-expression and self-perception processes, and is limited because some behaviors are not initiated in a reflective manner. For self–other agreement and meta-accuracy, the perception and integration of feedback seems to be less influential than the use of observable behaviors by the self and others, and the reliance on one's self-views as a proxy for metaperceptions. Future research might broaden its scope and investigate PSK from all four perspectives, including as many of the discussed processes as possible.

On a more general level, the process model of PSK shows that the association between our explicit personality self-views and our implicit personality traits, behaviors, and reputations—PSK—relies on a complex variety of processes, each of which is prone to a number of potential biases. It is important to note that all of the processes described can and probably do operate simultaneously. Given the large number of potential biases it is understandable that our personality self-views are not as perfect as we usually assume they should be. Perhaps then the moderate amount of PSK can be viewed in a more optimistic way: PSK is very difficult to achieve, but people nevertheless know something about their personality. In the next sections, we very briefly discuss four topics that are important future prospects in the study of PSK: the structure of PSK, moderators of PSK, ways to improve PSK, and the adaptiveness of PSK.

Will the Real PSK Please Stand Up?: The Structure of PSK

We have discussed four different ways to define, measure, and analyze PSK. Although, behavioral prediction is probably the most convincing approach, each of the three other approaches captures important unique aspects of PSK. It is still an important open basic question in PSK research whether the four aspects of PSK should be seen as interchangeable measures of the same underlying ability or whether they represent independent PSK constructs. According to the process model outlined here, one would expect these PSK domains to be positively related. Many of the processes discussed affect more than one, or even all, of the PSK domains. Motivated self-perception and self-presentation, for instance, undermine PSK globally. Probably a hierarchical structure with a broad PSK factor and between two and four subordinate PSK facets will be most appropriate to describe the structure of PSK.[4]

Can We Identify Good Traits, Good Information, and Good Judges?: Moderators of PSK

Based on his realistic accuracy model, Funder (1999) has derived a number of main effects and interactive moderator effects on the accuracy of other-perceptions. Similarly, the outlined process model of PSK can be applied to identify potential moderators of the ability to know oneself. The processes described may each vary as a function of the trait being investigated, the person who judges him- or herself, and the information available in a given situation. Thus characteristics of the trait, the information, and the judge can be analyzed as moderators of PSK.

As a case in point, one can ask: Who is a good judge of his or her own personality? An important feature of PSK is that the judge and the target are the same person. Thus, a good judge of the self (who detects and uses a lot of valid information about the self in an unbiased fashion) automatically also needs to be a good target (who gives away much valid information about the self). The outlined process model can be used to derive and empirically test who should be good at PSK. For example, one could argue that a good judge of the self should have a high information-processing capacity (i.e., intelligence) because that person needs to carry out correctly various complex cognitive processes simultaneously. He or she should be open to new experiences particularly concerning one's own feelings and self-views, and have an emotionally stable personality because this should foster the integration of new information. Extraversion, particularly an expressive behavioral style, should be helpful because it fosters the expression of one's self-views by means of observable behavioral acts. Finally, an agreeable nature should be related to higher PSK because it helps one's acquaintances to accomplish the difficult task of giving honest personality feedback. Thus, in summary, one could expect intelligent, emotionally stable, extraverted, and agreeable people to be particularly good judges of themselves. Whether this is true, whether these traits affect PSK in an additive or interactive fashion, and whether moderator effects differ depending on PSK domain, are all exciting, open research questions.

Can We Shine a Light on the Blind Spots in Personality Self-Views?: Improving PSK

As PSK is far from perfect, there is much room for improvement. The outlined process model can be applied to create interventions for improving PSK. To change successfully people's self-insight into their personality, treatments would have to strengthen the processes that mediate the associations among the variables of interest (e.g., explicit and implicit self-views). This might include training sessions for reduced bias (training to perceive incoming information about oneself objectively), reflections about one's inner self (training to get a sense of one's gut feelings and automatic motivational tendencies), self-expression (training to show others how one feels and what one thinks), self-observation of behavior (training to get an observer's perspective on one's own behavior), and social feedback (training to allow for honest personality feedback).

Prior attempts to improve people's self-insight have been astonishingly unsuccessful. People are very resistant to changing their self-concept even when facing relatively clear-cut and contradictory information (e.g., Hofmann et al., 2009). In one study, people failed to change their self-perceptions even after listening to audio recordings of their own behavior, recorded over 4 days in their natural environment. Not only did people resist changing their perceptions of their own personality, they also failed to change their perceptions of how they come across to others and how they behave (Vazire, Mehl, & Carlson, 2010).

Perhaps to have a lasting effect on others' self-views, social feedback has to be more intense. To be successful, approaches to improving PSK will probably have to involve longitudinal treatments with various social partners in multiple social contexts. Moreover, people's ability to learn and unlearn self- and other-perception processes and behavioral expression processes by means of explicit instructions is limited. Thus, treatments for improving PSK might have to include social interactions that foster the implicit learning of these processes (Funder, 1999; Hammond, 1996). As Funder (1999) has put it, the best advice for improving one's self-knowledge is to "mix with many different people in a wide range of social settings. Travel. Meet the kind of people you do not ordinarily meet. Most important, *be sure to seek feedback*" (p. 205, original emphasis).

Do We Really Want to Know Ourselves?: Adaptiveness of PSK

Why should we improve our self-insight? What is so good about knowing how one really is? There is no clear-cut answer to these questions. There would probably be more consensus if PSK clearly had positive consequences on our lives and a lack of PSK was related to dissatisfaction, interpersonal problems, and a lack of success. This is an open empirical question, but we would indeed expect PSK to be related to positive intrapersonal, interpersonal, and institutional outcomes (Ozer & Benet-Martinez, 2006). People base many of their most important decisions in life on their self-views. The better they know themselves, the more their behaviors should be in line with their inner feelings, the better they should be able to understand others' reactions toward them, and the more informed their life decisions should be. Only limited empirical data speak to this issue, most of which stems from research on self-enhancement research, a subdomain of PSK research (see Leary & Toner, Chapter 25, and Schriber & Robins, Chapter 8, this volume). Clearly, more research on different aspects of PSK using multiple outcome measure is needed to find out how adaptive it is to know oneself.

PSK is an important and complex topic that psychologists have only started to investigate. Strangely enough, our own personality seems in fact to be one of our greatest mysteries. The good news is that this mystery can be studied empirically, which is an extremely fascinating endeavor.

NOTES

1. Throughout this chapter, we use the five-factor model of personality (Goldberg, 1990; John, Naumann, & Soto, 2008; McCrae & John, 1992) as a guiding framework and describe PSK for the broad Big Five personality dimensions Neuroticism (Emotional Stability), Extraversion, Openness to Experience, Agreeableness, and Conscientiousness. Of course PSK can be analyzed for other traits as well, including ability-related traits such as intelligence, evaluative traits such as "funny," facets of the Big Five such as self-esteem or sociability, and more contextualized individual differences such as values or coping styles.

2. See Vazire and Carlson (2010) for a more complete review of existing empirical studies on PSK.

3. The IAT measures the strength of associations between concepts by comparing response times in two combined discrimination tasks. Participants are required to sort stimuli representing four concepts using only two responses, each assigned to two of the four concepts. The underlying assumption of the IAT is that if two concepts are highly associated, the sorting task will be easier (i.e., faster) when the two associated concepts share the same response key than when they share different response keys. The IAT can be applied to assess aspects of the implicit self-concept of personality by combining the categorization of items into the categories "me" and "others," with the classification of items into two opposing personality trait categories. For example, the IAT has been used to measure the implicit self-concept of Extraversion (Mierke & Klauer, 2003; Schmukle & Egloff, 2005). Here, categorization into the categories "me" and "others" was combined with a classification of items into Extraversion and Introversion categories. By measuring the relative ease of categorizing "me" and Extraversion items versus "others" and Introversion items as compared to "me" and Introversion items versus "others" and Extraversion items, the IAT effect thus represents an indicator of the implicit self-concept of Extraversion.

4. Here, we conceptualized PSK as the ability to accurately judge one's present personality traits, operationally defined as the traitwise correlation between one's trait self-view and a reasonable criterion measure of the "true" trait standing. Future research might additionally analyze the ability to predict one's past and future personality (Wilson, 2009), and thereby

apply different concepts of self-criterion consistency (Fleeson & Noftle, 2008; Furr, 2008; Furr & Funder, 2004).

REFERENCES

Ahadi, S., & Diener, E. (1989). Multipe determinants and effect size. *Journal of Personality and Social Psychology, 56,* 398–406.

Asendorpf, J. B., Banse, R., & Mücke, D. (2002). Double dissociation between implicit and explicit personality self-concept: The case of shy behavior. *Journal of Personality and Social Psychology, 83,* 380–393.

Back, M. D., & Egloff, B. (2009). Yes we can!: A plea for direct behavioural observation in personality research. *European Journal of Personality, 23,* 403–405.

Back, M. D., Krause, S., Hirschmüller, S., Stopfer, J. M., Egloff, B., & Schmukle, S. C. (2009). Unraveling the three faces of self-esteem: A new information-processing sociometer perspective. *Journal of Research in Personality, 43,* 933–937.

Back, M. D., Schmukle, S. C., & Egloff, B. (2005). Measuring task-switching ability in the Implicit Association Test. *Experimental Psychology, 52,* 167–179.

Back, M. D., Schmukle, S. C., & Egloff, B. (2008). How extraverted is *honey.bunny77@hotmail.de*? Inferring personality from e-mail addresses. *Journal of Research in Personality, 42,* 1116–1122.

Back, M. D., Schmukle, S. C., & Egloff, B. (2009). Predicting actual behavior from the explicit and implicit self-concept of personality. *Journal of Personality and Social Psychology, 97,* 533–548.

Back, M. D., Schmukle, S. C., & Egloff, B. (2010). Why are narcissists so charming at first sight?: Decoding the narcissism–popularity link at zero acquaintance. *Journal of Personality and Social Psychology, 98,* 132–145.

Back, M. D., Schmukle, S. C., & Egloff, B. (2011). A closer look at first sight: Social relations lens model analysis of personality and interpersonal attraction at zero acquaintance. *European Journal of Personality, 25,* 225–238.

Back, M. D., Stopfer, J. M., Vazire, S., Gaddis, S., Schmukle, S. C., Egloff, B., et al. (2010). Facebook profiles reflect actual personality not self-idealization. *Psychological Science, 21,* 372–374.

Banse, R., & Greenwald, A. G. (2007). Personality and implicit social cognition research: Past, present and future. *European Journal of Personality, 21,* 371–382.

Bargh, J. A. (1997). The automacity of everyday life. In R. S. Wyer (Ed.), *Advances in social cognition* (Vol. 10, pp. 1–61). Mahwah, NJ: Erlbaum.

Bargh, J. A., & Chartrand, T. L. (1999). The unbearable automaticity of being. *American Psychologist, 54,* 462–479.

Baumeister, R. F. (1982). A self-presentational view of social phenomena. *Psychological Bulletin, 91,* 3–26.

Baumeister, R. F., Vohs, K. D., & Funder, D. C. (2007). Psychology as the science of self-reports and finger movements: Whatever happened to actual behavior? *Perspectives on Psychological Science, 2,* 396–403.

Bem, D. J. (1967). Self-perception: An alternative interpretation of cognitive dissonance phenomena. *Psychological Review, 74,* 183–200.

Bem, D. J. (1972). Self-perception theory. In L. Berkowitz (Ed.), *Advances in experimental social psychology* (Vol. 6, pp. 1–62). New York: Academic Press.

Biesanz, J. C., West, S. G., & Millevoi, A. (2007). What do you learn about someone over time?: The relationship between length of acquaintance and consensus and self-other agreement in judgments of personality. *Journal of Personality and Social Psychology, 92,* 119–135.

Blumberg, H. H. (1972). Communication of interpersonal evaluations. *Journal of Personality and Social Psychology, 23,* 157–162.

Borkenau, P., & Liebler, A. (1992). Trait inferences: Sources of validity at zero acquaintance. *Journal of Personality and Social Psychology, 62,* 645–657.

Borkenau, P., Mauer, N., Riemann, R., Spinath, F. M., & Angleitner, A. (2004). Thin slices of behavior as cues of personality and intelligence. *Journal of Personality and Social Psychology, 86,* 599–614.

Borkenau, P., & Ostendorf, F. (1993). *NEO-Fünf-Faktoren Inventar (NEO-FFI)* [NEO-Five-Factor Inventory]. Göttingen, Germany: Hogrefe.

Bosson, J. K., Swann, W. B., & Pennebaker, J. W. (2000). Stalking the perfect measure of implicit self-esteem: The blind men and the elephant revisited. *Journal of Personality and Social Psychology, 79,* 631–643.

Brunswik, E. (1956). *Perception and the representative design of experiments.* Berkeley: University of California Press.

Buhrmester, M. D., Blanton, H., & Swann, W. B. (2011). Implicit self-esteem: Nature, measurement, and a new way forward. *Journal of Personality and Social Psychology, 100,* 365–385.

Carlson, E. N., & Furr, R. M. (2009). Evidence of differential meta-accuracy: People understand the different impressions they make. *Psychological Science, 20,* 1033–1039.

Connolly, J. J., Kavanagh, E. J., & Viswesvaran, C. (2007). The convergent validity between self and observer ratings of personality: A meta-analytic review. *International Journal of Selection and Assessment, 15,* 110–117.

Cooley, C. H. (1902). *Human nature and the social order.* New York: Scribner.

De Houwer, J. (2006). What are implicit measures and why are we using them. In R. W. Wiers & A. W. Stacy (Eds.), *The handbook of implicit cognition and addiction* (pp. 11–28). Thousand Oaks, CA: Sage.

Denissen, J. J. A., Penke, L., Schmitt, D. P., & Van Aken, M. A. G. (2008). Self-esteem reactions to social interactions: Evidence for sociometer mechanisms across days, people, and nations. *Journal of Personality and Social Psychology, 95,* 181–196.

DePaulo, B. M. (1992). Nonverbal behavior and self-presentation. *Psychological Bulletin, 111,* 203–243.

Dijksterhuis, A., & Nordgren, L. F. (2006). A theory of unconscious thought. *Perspectives on Psychological Science, 1,* 95–109.

Egloff, B., & Schmukle, S. C. (2002). Predictive validity of an Implicit Association Test for assessing anxiety. *Journal of Personality and Social Psychology, 83,* 1441–1455.

Egloff, B., Schwerdtfeger, A., & Schmukle, S. C. (2005). Temporal stability of the Implicit Association Test–Anxiety. *Journal of Personality Assessment, 84,* 82–88.

Egloff, B., Weck, F., & Schmukle, S. C. (2008). Thinking about anxiety moderates the relationship between implicit and explicit anxiety measures. *Journal of Research in Personality, 42,* 771–778.

Epstein, S. (1983). The stability of confusion: A reply to Mischel and Peake. *Psychological Review, 90,* 179–184.

Epstein, S. (1994). Integration of the cognitive and the psychodynamic unconscious. *American Psychologist, 49,* 709–724.

Evans, J. S. B. T. (2008). Dual-processing accounts of reasoning, judgment, and social cognition. *Annual Review of Psychology, 59,* 255–278.

Fazio, R. H. (1990). Multiple processes by which attitudes guide behavior: The MODE model as an integrative network. In M. P. Zanna (Ed.), *Advances in experimental social psychology* (Vol. 23, pp. 75–109). San Diego, CA: Academic Press.

Fazio, R. H., & Olson, M. A. (2003). Implicit measures in social cognition research: Their meaning and use. *Annual Review of Psychology, 54*, 297–327.

Felson, R. B. (1980). Communication barriers and the reflected appraisal process. *Social Psychology Quarterly, 43*, 223–233.

Festinger, L. (1954). A theory of social comparison processes. *Human Relations, 7*, 117–140.

Festinger, L. (1957). *A theory of cognitive dissonance.* Evanston, IL: Row, Peterson.

Fleeson, W., & Noftle, E. E. (2008). Where does personality have its influence?: A supermatrix of consistency concepts. *Journal of Personality, 76*, 1355–1385.

Funder, D. C. (1999). *Personality judgement: A realistic approach to person perception.* San Diego, CA: Academic Press.

Funder, D. C. (2001). Personality. *Annual Review of Psychology, 52*, 197–221.

Funder, D. C., & Colvin, C. R. (1988). Friends and strangers: Acquaintanceship, agreement, and the accuracy of personality judgment. *Journal of Personality and Social Psychology, 55*, 149–158.

Funder, D. C., Furr, R. M., & Colvin, C. R. (2000). The Riverside Behavioral Q-Sort: A tool for the description of social behavior. *Journal of Personality, 68*, 451–489.

Funder, D. C., Kolar, D. C., & Blackman, M. C. (1995). Agreement among judges of personality: Interpersonal relations, similarity, and acquaintanceship. *Journal of Personality and Social Psychology, 69*, 656–672.

Furr, R. M. (2009). Personality psychology as a truly behavioural science. *European Journal of Personality, 23*, 369–401.

Furr, R. M. (2008). A framework for profile similarity: Integrating similarity, normativeness, and distinctiveness. *Journal of Personality, 76*, 1267–1316.

Furr, R. M., & Funder, D. C. (2004). Situational similarity and behavioral consistency: Subjective, objective, variable-centered, and person-centered approaches. *Journal of Research in Personality, 38*, 421–447.

Goldberg, L. R. (1990). An alternative "description of personality": The Big-Five factor structure. *Journal of Personality and Social Psychology, 59*, 1216–1229.

Gosling, S. D., John, O. P., Craik, K. H., & Robins, R. W. (1998). Do people know how they behave?: Self-reported act frequencies compared with on-line codings by observers. *Journal of Personality and Social Psychology, 74*, 1337–1349.

Gosling, S. D., Ko, S. J., Mannarelli, T., & Morris, M. E. (2002). A room with a cue: Personality judgments based on offices and bedrooms. *Journal of Personality and Social Psychology, 82*, 379–398.

Gosling, S. D., Vazire, S., Srivastava, S., & John, O. P. (2004). Should we trust web-based studies?: A comparative analysis of six preconceptions about Internet questionnaires. *American Psychologist, 59*, 93–104.

Greenwald, A. G., & Banaji, M. R. (1995). Implicit social cognition: Attitudes, self-esteem, and stereotypes. *Psychological Review, 102*, 4–27.

Greenwald, A. G., Banaji, M. R., Rudman, L. A., Farnham, S. D., Nosek, B. A., & Mellot, D. S. (2002). A unified theory of implicit attitudes, stereotypes, self-esteem, and self-concept. *Psychological Review, 109*, 3–25.

Greenwald, A. G., McGhee, D. E., & Schwartz, J. L. K. (1998). Measuring individual differences in implicit cognition: The Implicit Association Test. *Journal of Personality and Social Psychology, 74*, 1464–1480.

Grumm, M., & von Collani, G. (2007). Measuring Big-Five personality dimensions with the Implicit Association Test—Implicit personality traits or self-esteem? *Personality and Individual Differences, 43*, 2205–2217.

Hammond, S. (1996). *The thin book of appreciative inquiry.* Plano, TX: Thin Books.

Heider, F. (1958). *The psychology of interpersonal relations.* Hillsdale, NJ: Erlbaum.

Hofmann, W., Gawronski, B., Gschwendner, T., Le, H., & Schmitt, M. (2005). A meta-analysis on the correlation between the Implicit Association Test and explicit self-report measures. *Personality and Social Psychology Bulletin, 31*, 1369–1385.

Hofmann, W., Gschwendner, T., & Schmitt, M. (2005). On implicit–explicit consistency: The moderating role of individual differences in awareness and adjustment. *European Journal of Personality, 19*, 25–49.

Hofmann, W., Gschwendner, T., & Schmitt, M. (2009). The road to the unconscious self not taken: Discrepancies between self- and observer-inferences about implicit dispositions from nonverbal behavioural cues. *European Journal of Personality, 23*, 343–366.

Hofmann, W., & Wilson, T. D. (2010). Consciousness, introspection, and the adaptive unconscious. In B. Gawronski & B. K. Payne (Eds.), *Handbook of implicit social cognition: Measurement, theory, and applications* (pp. 197–215). New York: Guilford Press.

Hofstee, W. K. B. (1994). Who should own the definition of personality? *European Journal of Personality, 8*, 149–162.

Hogan, R., & Roberts, B. W. (2000). A socioanalytic perspective on person/environment interaction. In W. B. Walsh, K. H. Craik, & R. H. Price (Eds.), *New directions in person–environment psychology* (pp. 1–24). Hillsdale, NJ: Erlbaum.

Holleran, S. E., & Mehl, M. R. (2008). Let me read your mind: Personality judgments based on a person's natural stream of thought. *Journal of Research in Personality, 42*, 747–754.

John, O. P., Naumann, L. P., & Soto, C. J. (2008). Paradigm shift to the integrative Big Five trait taxonomy: History, measurement, and conceptual issues. In O. P. John, R. W. Robins, & L. A. Pervin (Eds.), *Handbook of personality: Theory and research* (3rd ed., pp. 114–158). New York: Guilford Press.

John, O. P., & Robins, R. W. (1994). Accuracy and bias in self-perception: Individual differences in self-enhancement and the role of narcissism. *Journal of Personality and Social Psychology, 66*, 206–219.

Karpinski, A., Steinman, R. B., & Hilton, J. L. (2005). Attitude importance as a moderator of the relationship between implicit and explicit attitude measures. *Personality and Social Psychology Bulletin, 31*, 949–962.

Kavanagh, P. S., Robins, S. C., & Ellis, B. J. (2010). The mating sociometer: A regulatory mechanism for mating aspirations. *Journal of Personality and Social Psychology, 99*, 120–132.

Kenny, D. A. (1994). *Interpersonal perception: A social relations analysis.* New York: Guilford Press.

Kenny, D. A., & DePaulo, B. M. (1993). Do people know how others view them?: An empirical and theoretical account. *Psychological Bulletin, 114*, 145–161.

Kenrick, D. T., & Funder, D. C. (1988). Profiting from controversy: Lessons from the person–situation debate. *American Psychologist, 43*, 23–34.

Kolar, D. W., Funder, D. C., & Colvin, C. (1996). Comparing the accuracy of personality judgments by the self and knowledgeable others. *Journal of Personality, 64*, 311–337.

Küfner, A. C. P., Back, M. D., Nestler, S., & Egloff, B. (2010). Tell me a story and I will tell you who you are!: Lens model analyses of personality and creative writing. *Journal of Research in Personality, 44*, 427–435.

Kwan, V. S. Y., John, O., P., Kenny, D. A., Bond, M. H., & Robins, R. W. (2004). Reconceptualizing individual differences in self-enhancement bias: An interpersonal approach. *Psychological Review, 111*, 94–110.

Leary, M. R., & Baumeister, R. F. (2000). The nature and function of self-esteem: Sociometer theory. *Advances in Experimental Social Psychology, 32*, 1–62.

Leising, D., Erbs, J., & Fritz, U. (2010). The letter of recommendation effect in informant ratings of personality. *Journal of Personality and Social Psychology, 98*, 668–682.

Levesque, M. J. (1997). Meta-accuracy among acquainted individuals: A social relations analysis of interpersonal perception and metaperception. *Journal of Personality and Social Psychology, 72,* 66–74.

Levesque, M. J., & Kenny, D. A. (1993). Accuracy of behavioral predictions at zero acquaintance: A social relations analysis. *Journal of Personality and Social Psychology, 65,* 1178–1187.

Marcus, B., Machilek, F., & Schutz, A. (2006). Personality in cyberspace: Personal Web sites as media for personality expressions and impressions. *Journal of Personality and Social Psychology, 90*(6), 1014–1031.

McCrae, R. R., & John, O. P. (1992). An introduction to the five-factor model and its applications. *Journal of Personality, 60,* 175–215.

Mead, G. H. (1934). *Mind, self, and society.* Chicago: University of Chicago Press.

Mehl, M. R., Gosling, S. D., & Pennebaker, J. W. (2006). Personality in its natural habitat: Manifestations and implicit folk theories of personality in daily life. *Journal of Personality and Social Psychology, 90,* 862–877.

Mehl, M. R., Pennebaker, J. W., Crow, D. M., Dabbs, J., & Price, J. H. (2001). The Electronically Activated Recorder (EAR): A device for sampling naturalistic daily activities and conversations. *Behavior Research Methods, Instruments, and Computers, 33,* 517–523.

Mierke, J., & Klauer, K. C. (2003). Method-specific variance in the Implicit Association Test. *Journal of Personality and Social Psychology, 85,* 1180–1192.

Mischel, W. (1968). *Personality and assessment.* New York: Wiley.

Murray, H. A. (1943). *Thematic Apperception Test manual.* Cambridge, MA: Harvard University Press.

Naumann, L. P., Vazire, S., Rentfrow, P. J., & Gosling, S. D. (2009). Personality judgments based on physical appearance. *Personality and Social Psychology Bulletin, 35,* 1661–1671.

Nisbett, R. E., & Wilson, T. D. (1977). Telling more than we can know: Verbal reports on mental processes. *Psychological Review, 84,* 231–259.

Nosek, B. A. (2005). Moderators of the relationship between implicit and explicit evaluation. *Journal of Experimental Psychology: General, 134,* 565–584.

Nosek, B. A., Banaji, M. R., & Greenwald, A. G. (2002). Harvesting implicit group attitudes and beliefs from a demonstration website. *Group Dynamics, 6,* 101–115.

Nosek, B. A., Greenwald, A. G., & Banaji, M. R. (2007). The Implicit Association Test at age 7: A methodological and conceptual review. In J. A. Bargh (Ed.), *Social psychology and the unconscious: The automaticity of higher mental processes* (pp. 265–292). New York: Psychology Press.

Ozer, D. J., & Benet-Martinez, V. (2006). Personality and the prediction of consequential outcomes. *Annual Review of Psychology, 57,* 401–421.

Paulhus, D. L. (1984). Two component models of socially desirable responding. *Journal of Personality and Social Psychology, 46,* 598–609.

Paulhus, D. L., Bruce, M. N., & Trapnell, P. D. (1995). Effects of self-presentation strategies on personality profiles and their structure. *Personality and Social Psychology Bulletin, 21,* 100–108.

Paulhus, D. L., & Reid, D. B. (1991). Enhancement and denial in socially desirable responding. *Journal of Personality and Social Psychology, 60,* 307–317.

Perugini, M., & Banse, R. (2007). Personality, implicit self-concept and automaticity. *European Journal of Personality, 21,* 257–261.

Peters, K. R., & Gawronski, B. (2011). Mutual influences between the implicit and explicit self-concepts: The role of memory activation and motivated reasoning. *Journal of Experimental Social Psychology, 47,* 436–442.

Pronin, E., Kruger, J., Savitsky, K., & Ross, L. (2001). You don't know me but I know you: The illusion of asymmetric insight. *Journal of Personality and Social Psychollogy, 81*, 639–656.

Rentfrow, P. J., & Gosling, S. D. (2006). Message in a ballad: The role of music preferences in interpersonal perception. *Psychological Science, 17*, 236–242.

Robins, R. W., & Beer, J. S. (2001). Positive ilusions about the self: Short-term benefits and long-term costs. *Journal of Personality and Social Psychology, 80*, 340–352.

Robins, R. W., & John, O. P. (1997). The quest for self-insight: Theory and research on accuracy in self-perception. In R. Hogan, J. Johnson, & S. Briggs (Eds.), *Handbook of personality psychology* (pp. 649–679). New York: Academic Press.

Schmukle, S. C. (2005). Unreliability of the Dot Probe Task. *European Journal of Personality, 19*, 595–605.

Schmukle, S. C., Back, M. D., & Egloff, B. (2008). Validity of the five-factor model for the implicit self-concept of personality. *European Journal of Psychological Assessment, 24*, 263–272.

Schmukle, S. C., & Egloff, B. (2005). A latent state–trait analysis of implicit and explicit personality measures. *European Journal of Psychological Assessment, 21*, 100–107.

Schnabel, K., & Asendorpf, J. B. (2010). The self-concept: New insights from implicit measurement procedures. In B. Gawronski & B. K. Payne (Eds.), *Handbook of implicit social cognition* (pp. 408–425). New York: Guilford Press.

Shrauger, J. S., & Schoeneman, T. J. (1979). Symbolic interactionist view of self-concept: Through the looking glass darkly. *Psychological Bulletin, 86*, 549–573.

Spain, J. S., Eaton, L. G., & Funder, D. C. (2000). Perspectives on personality: The relative accuracy of self versus others for the prediction of emotion and behavior. *Journal of Personality, 68*, 837–867.

Srivastava, S., & Beer, J. S. (2005). How self-evaluations relate to being liked by others: Integrating sociometer and attachment perspectives. *Journal of Personality and Social Psychology, 89*, 966–977.

Steffens, M. C., & Schulze König, S. (2006). Predicting spontaneous Big-Five behavior with Implicit Association Tests. *European Journal of Psychological Assessment, 22*, 13–20.

Strack, F., & Deutsch, R. (2004). Reflective and impulsive determinants of social behavior. *Personality and Social Psychology Review, 8*, 220–247.

Strack, F., Martin, L. L., & Stepper, S. (1988). Inhibiting and facilitating conditions of the human smile: A nonobtrusive test of the facial feedback hypothesis. *Journal of Personality and Social Psychology, 54*, 768–777.

Strack, F., & Neumann, R. (2000). Furrowing the brow may undermine perceived fame: The role of facial feedback in judgments of celebrity. *Personality and Social Psychology Bulletin, 26*, 762–768.

Swann, W. B., Jr. (1987). Identity negotiation: Where two roads meet. *Journal of Personality and Social Psychology, 53*, 1038–1051.

Swann, W. B., Jr. (1990). To be adored or to be known: The interplay of self-enhancement and self-verification. In E. T. Higgins & R. M. Sorrentino (Eds.), *Handbook of motivation and cognition: Vol. 2. Foundations of social behavior* (pp. 408–448). New York: Guilford Press.

Swann, W. B., Jr. (2012). Self-verification theory. In P. A. M. Van Lange, A. W. Kruglanski, & E. T. Higgins (Eds.), *Handbook of theories of social psychology* (pp. 23–42). London: Sage.

Swann, W. B., Jr., & Bosson, J. K. (2008). Identity negotiation: A theory of self and social interaction. In O. P. John, R. W. Robins, & L. A. Pervin (Eds.), *Handbook of personality: Theory and research* (pp. 448–471). New York: Guilford Press.

Taylor, S. E., & Brown, J. D. (1988). Illusion and well-being: A social psychological perspective on mental health. *Psychological Bulletin, 103*, 193–210.

Tesser, A., & Rosen, S. (1975). The reluctance to transmit bad news. In L. Berkowitz (Ed.), *Advances in experimental social psychology* (Vol. 8, pp. 194–232). San Diego, CA: Academic Press.

Todd, P. M., Penke, L., Fasolo, B., & Lenton, A. P. (2007). Different cognitive processes underlie human mate choices and mate preferences. *Proceedings of the National Academy of Sciences of the USA, 104,* 15011–15016.

Vazire, S. (2006). Informant reports: A cheap, fast, and easy method for personality assessment. *Journal of Research in Personality, 40,* 472–481.

Vazire, S. (2010). Who knows what about a person?: The self–other knowledge asymmetry (SOKA) model. *Journal of Personality and Social Psychology, 98*(2), 281–300.

Vazire, S., & Carlson, E. N. (2010). Self-knowledge of personality: Do people know themselves? *Social and Personality Psychology Compass, 4,* 605–620.

Vazire, S., & Gosling, S. D. (2004). E-perceptions: Personality impressions based on personal websites. *Journal of Personality and Social Psychology, 87,* 123–132.

Vazire, S., Gosling, S. D., Dickey, A. S., & Schapiro, S. J. (2007). Measuring personality in nonhuman animals. In R. W. Robins, R. C. Fraley, & R. F. Krueger (Eds.), *Handbook of research methods in personality psychology* (pp. 190–206). New York: Guilford Press.

Vazire, S., & Mehl, M. R. (2008). Knowing me, knowing you: The accuracy and unique predictive validity of self-ratings and other-ratings of daily behavior. *Journal of Personality and Social Psychology, 95,* 1202–1216.

Vazire, S., Mehl, M. R., & Carlson, E. N. (2010). *Shining a light on the blind spots in self-perception.* Paper presented at the 15th European Conference on Personality, Brno, Czech Republic.

Watson, D., Hubbard, B., & Wiese, D. (2000). General traits of personality and affectivity as predictors of satisfaction in intimate relationships: Evidence from self- and partner-ratings. *Journal of Personality, 68,* 413–449.

West, S. G., & Brown, T. J. (1975). Physical attractiveness, the severity of emergency and helping: A field experiment and interpersonal simulation. *Journal of Experimental Social Psychology, 11,* 531–538.

Wilson, T. D. (2002). *Strangers to ourselves: Discovering the adaptive unconscious.* Cambridge, MA: Belknap Press.

Wilson, T. D. (2009). Know thyself. *Perspectives on Psychological Science, 4,* 384–389.

Wilson, T. D., & Dunn, E. W. (2004). Self-knowledge: Its limits, value, and potential for improvement. *Annual Review of Psychology, 55,* 493–518.

Wilson, T. D., Lindsey, S., & Schooler, T. Y. (2000). A model of dual attitudes. *Psychological Review, 107,* 101–126.

CHAPTER 10

Knowing Our Attitudes and How to Change Them

PABLO BRIÑOL
RICHARD E. PETTY

People know many objective facts about themselves, such as their age and how tall they are. It might seem obvious that people also would know their more subjective likes and dislikes—what they value and what they disdain—and know why they feel this way. However, research suggests that this is more complicated than it may first appear. In this chapter we review social-psychological studies on what people know about their attitudes, where they come from, and how they can be changed. We will see that although people have various notions (naive theories) about different aspects of their attitudes, these theories may or may not be accurate. We address whether or not this matters. We argue that both what people actually know about their attitudes and what they *think* they know can have important implications for how they process information about the world and how likely they are to modify and act on their attitudes.

Attitudes refer to general evaluations individuals have regarding people (including themselves), places, objects, and issues (e.g., ice cream is good; chocolate-covered cockroaches are nasty). Although some people enjoy evaluation more than others and are thus more likely to form attitudes (Jarvis & Petty, 1996), virtually everyone has attitudes about a diversity of objects and issues (Bargh, Chaiken, Govender, & Pratto, 1992). Attitudes are important because of their influence on people's choices and actions; that is, all else being equal, people decide to buy the products they like the most, attend the university they evaluate most favorably, and vote for the Presidential candidate they approve of most strongly. People who do not know what their attitudes are, they might not know how to act ("Should I buy chocolate or vanilla ice cream?"). Yet, as we see shortly, people do not always know what their attitudes are. And, even if people know their attitudes, they may not know where these attitudes come from, on what they are based, and what they do. After tackling these issues, we turn to the question of whether people know how and when they can change their own attitudes and the attitudes of others.

Knowing about Attitudes, Their Bases and Consequences

Explicit versus Implicit Attitude Measures

Because researchers initially made the seemingly reasonable assumption that people have knowledge of their own attitudes, most attitude measurement procedures simply ask people to report their evaluations (e.g., "On a scale where −5 means *extremely bad* and +5 means *extremely good*, how would you rate your evaluation of ice cream?"). Indeed, much research suggests that attitudes often come to mind automatically upon merely encountering an attitude object and can be reported rather quickly (e.g., see Bargh, Chaiken, Raymond, & Hymes, 1996; Fazio, Sanbonmatsu, Powell, & Kardes, 1986). An interesting puzzle, however, is that sometimes when researchers use implicit measures of attitudes such as the evaluative priming procedure (Fazio, Jackson, Dunton, & Williams, 1995) or the Implicit Association Test (Greenwald, McGhee, & Schwartz, 1998) that assess evaluations that come to mind automatically, they find that the attitudes observed are different from the ones that people report on more deliberative self-assessments (e.g., Greenwald, Poehlman, Uhlmann, & Banaji, 2009). For example, when responding to an object such as the self or a member of a racial minority group, people might explicitly say that they like (or dislike) the object, but an implicit measure tapping into an automatic evaluation might show that the opposite evaluation comes to mind spontaneously.

Although much of the time implicit and explicit measures tell the same story about one's attitudes, what does it mean when these measures produce different outcomes? There are a number of possibilities (see Petty, Fazio, & Briñol, 2009). In what might be called a *single attitude* approach, some have argued that the automatic attitude that comes to mind spontaneously is the "real" attitude (e.g., Dijksterhuis, Albers, & Bongers, 2009), whereas the explicit measure represents an evaluation colored by "downstream" influences (e.g., see Gawronski & Bodenhausen, 2006; Olson & Fazio, 2009). Importantly, the fact that downstream influences modify what people explicitly report as their attitude does not mean that people are unaware of their automatic evaluative tendencies. For example, people might not report a gut feeling because of fear that it might not be approved of by society (Olson & Fazio, 2003). Or a person might know what evaluative reaction automatically comes to mind but choose not to report it because he or she is uncertain of its origin or has concerns that it is inappropriate to rely on gut feelings. In support of the latter possibility, in one study (Loersch, McCaslin, & Petty, 2011), college students received neutral verbal information about a target person, as well as positive or negative associative information (i.e., pleasant or unpleasant pictures) presented subliminally (i.e, outside of conscious awareness). Prior research had suggested that the former information affected explicit measures, whereas the latter did not. When the standard attitude instructions were given, the subliminal associative information did not affect explicit attitude reports as in past research (see Rydell & McConnell, 2006). However, when instructed that going with gut feelings was legitimate, explicit measures of attitudes were influenced by the subliminal affective stimuli.

Other research further indicates that when people are led to believe (or already believe) that relying on their intuitions is legitimate, explicit and implicit measures become more highly correlated (see Jordan, Whitfield, & Ziegler-Hill, 2007; Ranganath, Smith, & Nosek, 2008). In general, the available research suggests that people sometimes have insight into their automatic evaluative reactions but choose not to rely upon these feelings when making explicit attitude reports because of social desirability fears or concerns that this information is not diagnostic or valid. It is also possible that people might not even notice these quick reactions unless they are motivated (or prompted) to search for them. In such cases, the explicit attitudes reported would presumably be based on a search for information people have about the object in memory or by factors in the immediate context. For example, a negative reaction might come to mind immediately upon presentation of an attitude object (and represent the person's attitude), but if the person does not notice this reaction or understand its source, or questions its validity, this negative reaction might be overridden by positive feelings from the environment, and the person would report a favorable evaluation.

Rather than assuming that implicit measures are needed to assess the real attitude, another point of view on implicit–explicit discrepancies is that (putting lying aside) the person has two attitudes and both are meaningful. On the one hand, there is the attitude that the person acknowledges and can report; on the other hand, there is an automatic and more hidden attitude. In essence, this view argues that people can hold separate explicit and implicit attitudes, the first of which is open to conscious awareness, whereas the second is not (e.g., Greenwald & Banaji, 1995; Wilson, Lindsey, & Schooler, 2000). Although there are several versions of this *dual-attitudes* approach, one or more of the following assumptions are commonly made (see Petty & Briñol, 2009; Petty, Briñol, & DeMarree, 2007). First, the dual attitudes are thought to have separate mental representations that could be stored in separate brain regions (e.g., see DeCoster, Banner, Smith, & Semin, 2006). A second common assumption is that the two attitudes stem from distinct mental processes. Implicit attitudes are said to result from relatively automatic associative processes, whereas explicit attitudes stem from more deliberative propositional processes (e.g., Rydell, McConnell, Mackie, & Strain, 2006). Third, implicit and explicit attitudes are postulated to be relatively independent and to operate in different situations, such that explicit attitudes operate primarily when people are being thoughtful, but implicit attitudes operate when people are being spontaneous (see Dovidio, Kawakami, Johnson, Johnson, & Howard, 1997). When considering all of these assumptions together, the dual-attitudes framework suggests that the attitudes people explicitly report holding versus those that come to mind automatically can be quite different.

Explicit versus Implicit Attitudes and Ambivalence

A third point of view on explicit–implicit discrepancies comes from the metacognitive model of attitude structure (MCM; Petty & Briñol, 2006; Petty, Briñol, & DeMarree, 2007). The MCM shares some features with each of the two approaches just described, but it also has some differences. In brief, the MCM holds that attitude objects can be linked in memory to both positive and negative evaluations that spring to mind automatically, but that these evaluations can differ in the extent to which they are explicitly endorsed. When both positive and negative evaluations come to mind automatically and are endorsed (i.e., a person believes these represent his or her true assessments), the person's attitude is best described as being *explicitly ambivalent*. On a bipolar measure, an ambivalent person might appear to endorse a moderate or neutral attitude that represents his or her attempt to integrate both positivity and negativity. Because of this, it is sometimes useful to assess the positivity and negativity of underlying attitudes separately and calculate an objective ambivalence score (e.g., Kaplan, 1972). When people are aware of holding opposing positive and negative reactions to an attitude object, they report feeling conflicted, confused, torn, and mixed about the object (e.g.,Priester & Petty, 1996; Thompson, Zanna, & Griffin, 1995). This conflict is especially apparent when people are about to make an attitude-relevant decision (van Harreveld, van der Pligt, & de Liver, 2009).

In addition to this intrapersonal discrepancy, interpersonal factors also contribute to feelings of ambivalence. In particular, when people believe that their attitudes are discrepant from those of liked others, there are feelings of conflict (Priester & Petty, 2001). One reason for this is that people want to agree with people they like, as specified by balance theory (Heider, 1958), and when they do not, they feel some tension. In addition, disagreement with liked others can indicate that one's attitude is incorrect (Festinger, 1954), which is also troublesome. Research has extended the causes of subjective ambivalence to include concerns about conflicting information that might exist but to which individuals have not yet been exposed (Priester, Petty, & Park, 2007) and to discrepancies between individuals' actual attitudes and the attitudes they would ideally like to possess (DeMarree, Wheeler, Briñol, & Petty, 2011). We discuss the latter in more detail later in this chapter.

When the cause of the conflict is explicit, people report being ambivalent, and the uncomfortable feeling that results from this state produces a number of important outcomes. For example, the more ambivalence people experience regarding an object, the slower they are to report their attitudes (Bargh, Chaiken, Govender, & Pratto, 1992) and the less functional the attitudes become in guiding behavior (Armitage & Conner, 2000; Sparks, Harris, & Lockwood, 2004). Given that subjective ambivalence tends to be a negative state, people are motivated to reduce it. The motivation to reduce ambivalence can lead people to pay careful attention to and think about information that might help them to resolve their conflict (e.g., Clark, Wegener, & Fabrigar, 2008; Maio, Bell, & Esses, 1996).

According to the MCM, in addition to the explicit ambivalence people report and feel when they acknowledge the source of the conflict (e.g., there are both positive and negative aspects to some object; "I disagree with my parents about this"), a more subtle kind of conflict, called *implicit ambivalence* can occur when people are not fully aware of an explicit conflict. For example, implicit ambivalence occurs if both positive and negative reactions to an object automatically come to mind, but one of these is endorsed as one's attitude and the other is rejected (Petty, Tormala, Briñol, & Jarvis, 2006). A rejected evaluation might be a past attitude that still comes to mind when the object is present (e.g., "I used to like smoking, but now I want to quit"), an association that was never endorsed but nonetheless comes to mind due to one's culture (e.g., from continuous depictions of a minority group and criminal activity in the media), or simply a vague feeling of unknown origin. In cases of implicit ambivalence, even though the person does not endorse opposite evaluations of the attitude object, he or she can nevertheless feel uncomfortable when considering the object because unendorsed gut feelings conflict with endorsed evaluations (see Epstein, 2003; Petty & Briñol, 2009; Rydell et al., 2008).

In a series of studies, Briñol, Petty, and Wheeler (2006) have shown that discrepancies between automatic and deliberative measures can tap into this implicit ambivalence and are consequential. As noted earlier, one documented consequence of the doubt that emerges from explicit ambivalence is that it leads to enhanced information processing in a presumed attempt to resolve the ambivalence. In one study testing the notion that explicit–implicit attitude discrepancies can lead to enhanced information processing (Briñol et al., 2006, Experiment 4), undergraduates' self-evaluations (self-esteem) were assessed with both automatic and deliberative measures, then the absolute value of the difference between the two standardized measures was calculated as the index of discrepancy. Next, participants were exposed to either a strong or weak message about eating vegetables that was framed as self-relevant or not. The degree to which participants processed the message information was assessed by examining the extent to which the quality of the arguments affected postmessage attitudes toward vegetables (see Petty & Cacioppo, 1986). The more people process a message carefully, the more argument strength affects their evaluations.

The results of this study revealed that when the message was framed as self-relevant (i.e., relevant to one's personal life and thus relevant to the discrepancy), the extent of explicit–implicit discrepancy interacted with argument quality to affect attitudes. Specifically, the greater this discrepancy, the more participants differentiated strong from weak arguments. However, when the same strong and weak messages were framed as irrelevant to the self (i.e., the message was said to be about the properties of vegetables), explicit–implicit discrepancy did not interact with argument quality to predict attitudes. This suggests that explicit–implicit discrepancies do not lead to motivation to process all information—only information relevant to the object for which the discrepancy occurs.

In addition to examining implicit–explicit discrepancies that already existed, Petty and his colleagues (2006) also investigated discrepancies created in the laboratory. In one study, college students were first classically conditioned to like or dislike a target individual in order to create an initial attitude toward the target. Then, the participants received explicit information about the target individual that led them either to maintain their initially reported attitude or to change it. Next, participants were told that the target person was a candidate for a job at their university. To evaluate the candidate, they were provided with either a strong or a weak resumé to examine.

The key result was that participants' explicit attitudes toward the target person were more influenced by resumé quality in the condition when attitudes were changed than when attitudes toward the candidate had not been changed; that is, even though people whose attitudes were changed now held the same explicit attitude toward the target as people whose attitudes had not changed, they engaged in greater scrutiny of the resumé as if they were attempting to resolve some underlying ambivalence about the candidate. In this case, the implicit ambivalence stemmed from a conflict between the old attitude (which was still automatically activated) and the new one. These individuals did not report being ambivalent about the target person because they only endorsed their new attitude. Nonetheless, the fact that the old attitude did not disappear led them to feel conflicted, and they therefore engaged in greater processing of information about the person (see also Rydell, McConnell, & Mackie, 2008).

Knowing What Our Attitudes Are: Summary

In conclusion, what does the work on implicit versus explicit attitude measures tell us about whether people have knowledge of their attitudes? First, it is clear that when both deliberative and automatic assessments of attitudes agree, it suggests that people are aware of their attitudes and can report them rather easily. The fact that implicit and explicit measures of attitudes often *do* agree across a wide variety of attitude objects suggests that people typically are aware of their attitudes (Greenwald et al., 2009). This makes sense, of course, because if people were not aware of their attitudes, they would not know how to behave, or their behavior would be wildly inconsistent across time, but this is not the case.

However, we have seen that automatic and deliberative measures of attitudes do not always agree, and we have provided three different conceptualizations of this. Our own view, captured by the MCM, is that when there is *genuine divergence* in the valence of what implicit and explicit attitude measures indicate (i.e., the person is not attempting to be deceptive on either measure), then the attitude object is linked to both positivity and negativity in memory and for some reason one of these associations is not accepted; that is, the person's theory about the unendorsed valence, if it is perceived at all, is that it either does not stem from the attitude object or it stems from the attitude object but is invalid to consider for some reason (e.g., it represents an old attitude or is an association from the culture). Because one valence is rejected, the person will not report being ambivalent, but may nonetheless experience discomfort when the attitude object is brought to mind. When deliberating about how to act, people generally behave in accord with what they believe their attitudes to be, as assessed by explicit measures. However, when people are acting more spontaneously without reflection, then automatic evaluative associations, as assessed with implicit measures, are more likely to have an impact (Dovidio et al., 1997; see Olson & Fazio, 2003). Finally, we have seen that both implicit and explicit attitudes can jointly influence information processing when these evaluations are in conflict.

Knowing How Much Knowledge We Have

Even though people are often aware of what their attitudes are, they are not necessarily aware of *why* they hold the attitudes they do (Fox, Ericsson, & Best, 2011; Nisbett & Wilson, 1977; Wilson & Hodges, 1992); that is, people might or might not know what underlies their attitudes. This, however, does not prevent people from having naive theories about the bases of their attitudes, which are consequential even though these naive theories do not necessarily correspond with reality.

First, consider what people know about how much knowledge they have on an attitude issue. People make decisions based on not only what they actually know (objective amount of knowledge; see Wood et al., 1995) but also on what they think they know (subjective amount of knowledge); that is, regardless of its accuracy, subjective knowledge has been documented to have important consequences. For example, Radecki and Jaccard (1995) measured participants' knowledge of nutrition with a self-report questionnaire (subjective knowledge), as well as their performance on a multiple-choice test (objective knowledge). After the researcher controlled for objective knowledge, subjective knowledge predicted information search, such that participants with less subjective knowledge requested more information on the issue than did participants with more subjective knowledge (see also Brucks, 1985). This research suggests that the more people think they know about something, the less likely they are to expend resources on processing or seeking additional information on that topic. Research suggests that the more knowledge on which people think their attitudes are based, the more certain they are about the validity of those attitudes (see Rucker, Petty, & Briñol, 2008), and the more certain they are about their current attitudes, the less people believe it is necessary to consider additional information (e.g., Briñol, Petty, Gallardo, & DeMarree, 2007; Horcajo, Petty, & Briñol, 2010).

Despite the importance of subjective knowledge, relatively little research has examined the relationship between objective and subjective knowledge. Although some research suggests that increases in perceived knowledge accompany increases in actual knowledge (e.g., Smith, Fabrigar, MacDougall, & Wiesenthal, 2008), other research shows that people often have a poorly calibrated perception of how knowledgeable they are (Alba & Hutchinson, 2000; Dunning, Heath, & Suls, 2004). Indeed, it is possible to vary perceptions of knowledge about attitude objects in the absence of any real differences in knowledge. For example, in one study (Tormala & Petty, 2007), students were presented with a large or small amount of positive information about one attitude object (e.g., a person) followed by a moderate amount of positive information about a different attitude object (e.g., a store). When the information about the second object was preceded by a small amount of information about the first object, people felt more knowledgeable about the second object than when it was preceded by a large amount of information about the first object (a contrast effect). Importantly, these perceptions of knowledge in the absence of real knowledge differences led to more favorable attitudes in the condition with greater perceived knowledge, in line with a "more is better" heuristic (Petty & Cacioppo, 1984).

Recent research has even suggested that increasing actual knowledge about an attitude object can sometimes lead to *reductions* in perceived knowledge. In this research (Rucker, Lee, & Briñol, 2011), when people's attention was directed toward the incremental value of new information over the starting point of no knowledge, their perceptions of knowledge increased. However, when attention was directed toward how the new knowledge signaled what else was not known, people showed reduced perceptions of knowledge. Importantly, the extent to which people thought they knew about the attitude object was consequential in terms of processing information relevant to that attitude object. Specifically, the less people thought they knew about the topic, the more processing they did of information relevant to the object.

In closing, we note that perceptions of knowledge can also change as a function of variables unrelated to the presence of new information. For example, in one study (Belding, Briñol, & Petty, 2011), participants were found to feel more knowledgeable and intelligent after they were induced to wear reading glasses versus an item associated with athleticism (i.e., a baseball cap; see also Kellerman & Laird, 1982). Furthermore, participants who were wearing the glasses processed persuasive messages more carefully than participants wearing the cap. Note that this is the opposite effect that perceived knowledge had in the research on processing just described by Rucker and colleagues (2011). We speculate that when people infer that knowledge means that they are intelligent and *capable* of processing (e.g., when wearing glasses), they are more likely to process information, since it fits their momentary self-conception (see Wheeler, DeMarree, & Petty, 2007), but when people infer that knowledge means that they are already certain of their attitude, then they are less likely to process because acquiring new information seems less necessary in the face of an already correct opinion.

Knowing the Affective versus Cognitive Origins of Attitudes

Just as people can reflect upon how much knowledge underlies their attitudes, they can also think about the nature of that information. One important and classic distinction is whether attitudes are based on emotion or cognition (Breckler, 1984; Zanna & Rempel, 1988). A number of studies have shown that it is possible to determine whether a given attitude is actually based on emotion, cognition, or a combination of the two. This can be done, for example, by seeing whether a global measure of people's attitudes (e.g., how people rate an object as good vs. bad) correlates more highly with their ratings of emotion-relevant qualities (e.g., how happy vs. sad the object makes them feel) or cognitive-relevant qualities (e.g., how useful vs. useless the object seems; see Crites, Fabrigar, & Petty, 1994). The underlying cognitive versus affective structural basis of attitudes has been shown to have important consequences. For example, it is generally more effective to change attitudes based on emotion with emotional messages rather than with more cognitive or rational appeals (Edwards, 1990; Fabrigar & Petty, 1999).

Independent of whether attitudes actually are based on affect or cognition, people's perceptions of the basis of their attitudes can be assessed by asking them about the extent to which they believe that their attitudes are cognitively or affectively based (See, Petty, & Fabrigar, 2008). Importantly, individuals' theories about the affective versus cognitive bases of their attitudes predict persuasion independent of the actual (structural) basis of their attitudes; that is, just as it is generally more effective to use emotional appeals for individuals whose attitudes have an affective structural basis, it is also more effective to use an emotional appeal for individuals who perceive their attitudes to be based on affect, whether or not this is true. Additional research has shown that use of persuasion strategies in line with the actual structural bases of attitudes tends to be more effective when people's responses to the message are spontaneous, such as when they are under time pressure, but use of persuasion strategies in line with perceived bases is more effective when people are being deliberative (See et al., 2008).

Why might people not know the bases of their attitudes? With respect to affective–cognitive bases, past research suggests that when people think about their attitudinal bases, what comes to mind may not be representative of the actual structural content of their attitudes. For instance, in one study (Wilson, Dunn, Bybee, Hyman, & Rotondo, 1984), when participants were asked to examine why they liked or disliked an attitude object, they were able to do so, but attitudes assessed shortly after this did not predict behavior very well. Wilson and colleagues (1984) suggested that this was because the reasons people listed as supporting their attitudes were inaccurate or incomplete. In particular, people often underestimated the role of affect in determining attitudes. Moreover, even if people are able to identify a representative sample of the bases of their attitudes (both affective and cognitive), they must also be able to gauge the unique contribution of each basis to their global evaluation in order to have an accurate assessment. This is likely to be a difficult task, particularly in cases in which affect and cognition are evaluatively consistent. Thus, true insight into the actual affective versus cognitive basis of many attitudes could be rare.

Knowing the Consequences of Attitudes

Just as people may not know the actual bases of their attitudes, they are often ignorant of the impact of their attitudes. Attitudes have many consequences, such as guiding perception, information processing, and action (Fazio, 1995), but people do not appear to appreciate this sufficiently. For example, people appear to underestimate how much their attitudes bias their thinking and influence their perception of other objects in an attitude-congruent fashion (Greenwald & Banaji, 1995). Nevertheless, people appear to have at least some recognition of which of their attitudes are more consequential than others.

There are a number of indicators of how consequential or *strong* attitudes are (see Petty & Krosnick, 1995). One that we have discussed already is how much knowledge people have, or perceive themselves to have, about an issue (e.g., Wood, Rhodes, & Biek, 1995). Others include how accessible the attitude is (Fazio, 1995) and how much people have thought about their attitudes (Petty, Haugtvedt, & Smith, 1995). As was the case for attitude knowledge and affective–cognitive bases, for virtually every seemingly objective indicator of an attitude's strength, such as the *actual* speed with which it comes to mind or the *actual* amount of thinking in which people have engaged regarding their attitudes, there is a parallel measure of the *perceived* ease of attitude access or the *perceived* extent of thought (Wegener, Downing, Krosnick, & Petty, 1995). People's perceptions of the qualities of their attitudes can show a reasonable correlation with their objective qualities, though the correlation is far from perfect. For example, in one study, when researchers manipulated the extent of thought by using distraction (Petty, Wells, & Brock, 1976) and personal relevance (Petty & Cacioppo, 1979b), these manipulations affected not only the actual extent of thinking as measured by the number of thoughts listed but also the perceived extent of thinking (see Barden & Petty, 2008). However, this knowledge is incomplete because as we see shortly, the perceived qualities of one's attitudes can be affected in the absence of differences in the real qualities.

Perhaps the most studied subjective indicator of how strong or consequential an attitude is involves the confidence or certainty people have in the validity of their attitudes. Attitude confidence is associated with a number of attitude strength consequences (for reviews, see Petty, Briñol, Tormala, & Wegener, 2007; Tormala & Rucker, 2007; Visser & Holbrook, 2012). For example, attitudes that people hold with high certainty are more resistant to change (e.g., Kiesler, 1971), persistent in the absence of a persuasive attack (Bassili, 1996), and more predictive of behavior (Fazio & Zanna, 1978) than attitudes about which there is doubt. Obviously people can report the certainty with which they hold an attitude, since this is a subjective assessment, but their reasons or theories for why they are certain can be inaccurate. Furthermore, certainty can affect how consequential attitudes are for at least two reasons. First, certainty can make attitudes stronger because the certainty is linked to structural differences in attitudes. For example, attitudes that are thought about more (Barden & Petty, 2008) or that are more accessible (Fazio & Zanna, 1978) are held with greater certainty. If attitudes high in certainty come to mind more readily, they are more able to guide behavior, and thinking about them more helps them resist attack.

Second, attitude certainty can render attitudes more consequential even if the certainty is not tied to any structural differences (Tormala & Petty, 2002). For example, if people are merely led to believe that they have thought a lot about their attitudes (Barden & Petty, 2008) or that they have gained more knowledge supporting their attitudes (Rucker & Petty, 2004; Rucker et al., 2008), they feel more certain. This is important because research shows that attitudes held with greater certainty are more likely to guide behavior, even if these perceptions are not true. Thus, although people can have a sense of which of their many attitudes are consequential (as indexed by certainty), this sense is derived from a combination of verifiable facts (e.g., how much thinking they have actually done) as well as misperceptions (e.g., perceptions of having thought in the absence of real differences). Regardless of the origin, attitude certainty makes attitudes more consequential.

Knowing How to Correct Attitudes for Presumed Biases

In concluding our discussion of people's knowledge about their attitudes, we note that, beginning with Festinger's (1954) classic discussion of social comparison processes, people have been presumed to want to hold subjectively correct attitudes. We have already noted that people typically have good access to their attitudes, but they do not always have good access to the basis of their attitudes. If people do not know what their attitudes are based on, how can they know whether their attitudes are accurate? Festinger proposed that people mostly rely on comparisons with the attitudes of others. To the extent that people agree with others, they can infer that their attitudes are correct. Subsequent research (Goethals & Nelson, 1973) has suggested that people are especially likely to assume validity when the others who agree with their attitudes are similar to them. In matters of fact rather than opinion, however, greater validity comes when dissimilar others agree.

Knowledge about one's attitudes and social consensus do not provide the only cues to validity, however. People also infer validity from numerous other factors, such as how easily their attitudes are retrieved from memory (Haddock, Rothman, Reber, & Schwarz, 1999) or whether their attitudes are perceived to have a moral basis (Wagner, Petty, & Briñol, 2011). Furthermore, if people perceive that there are factors operating that might have biased their attitudes, they take corrective action. These corrections are based on beliefs people have about the magnitude and nature of the bias that has occurred (Petty & Wegener, 1993; Wegener & Petty, 1997; Wilson & Brekke, 1994). If people could accurately diagnose the causes of their attitudes, they could likely correct their attitudes accurately. But since people are often unaware of the real causes of their attitudes, their attempts at correction follow their theories of bias rather than the actual bias that has occurred. Because of this, people sometimes correct for a factor that they believe biased their attitude (since it is consistent with their naive theory of bias) even though it had no effect. In such situations, the factor perceived as biasing can end up producing a reverse bias (e.g., see Petty, Wegener, & White, 1998). For example, if people overestimate the extent to which attending a funny movie with a date has made them like their date for the evening, and they correct their evaluation of the date based on this overestimate, this could lead them to like the date even less than if they had not attended the funny movie at all.

Knowing about Attitude Change

So far, we have focused on what people know about their attitudes, and the bases and consequences of those attitudes. We turn now to the question of attitude change and address issues such as whether, how, and when people know that their attitudes have been changed, and to what extent people know whether, how, and when they can change their own attitudes and those of others.

Do People Know When Their Attitudes Have Changed?

People like to think they are coherent and may believe that people who change their opinions too easily are wishy-washy. As a consequence, research suggests that when people's attitudes have changed as a result of some manipulation, such as writing a counterattitudinal essay (Bem & McConnell, 1970) or participating in a group discussion (Goethals & Reckman, 1973), they often misremember their prechange attitude as being the same as their current attitude. This distortion implies that people are not aware that their attitudes have changed, but are only aware of their current attitude. Then, people assume that they have always felt this way. Even when people acknowledge that their attitudes have changed to some degree, they may underestimate the extent of that change (Wilson, Houston, & Meyers, 1998).

The fact that people misremember their old attitudes as being consistent with their new ones might help to explain why people also can misremember their past behaviors as being consistent with their newly changed attitudes. In one study (Ross, McFarland, & Fletcher, 1981), for example, when students were given a message in favor of toothbrushing, their current attitudes toward the practice became more positive, and they also reported that they brushed their teeth more 2 weeks earlier than those who had received an anti-toothbrushing message. Thus, not only are prior attitudes misremembered to be consistent with current attitudes, but so also are prior behaviors.

The work on misremembering attitudes and attitude-relevant behavior is consistent with a more general phenomenon in which people misremember aspects of their past to make it seem more like the present. For example, in one study (McFarland & Ross, 1987), participants provided ratings of their dating partner over time, then attempted to recall their initial ratings. A key result was that when the relationship improved over time, people misremembered the relationship as initially being better than it was, and when the relationship became worse over time, people misremembered it as initially being worse than it was (see also Ross, 1989).

In many of the studies on recall of past attitudes, the new attitude that was misremembered was invoked externally by another person and may not have been desired. To our knowledge, there is little research examining perceptions of change when the change is desired or self-initiated. Perhaps in such situations people would overestimate the extent of change. In a potentially relevant example, Conway and Ross (1984) asked students in a study skills course to evaluate their progress following completion of the course. Although the course was actually ineffective, it looked useful and participants assumed it was. Thus, in this case, they inferred change in the absence of any real change by exaggerating how bad their study skills were before they took the course. This provided the illusion of change in a desired direction; that is, in this case, people presumably wanted better study skills over time and they misremembered the past to bring about this perception. In a somewhat similar way, people have been shown to recall their past selves as inferior to their current selves so that an image of improvement to a currently desired state, rather than a deterioration from the past, is established (see Wilson & Ross, 2003).

Taken together, the various studies suggest that people can err in either direction—seeing no change in their attitudes or themselves when there actually has been change, and seeing some change when there actually has been none (see Schryer & Ross, 2012, for a review). People's inferences about change appear to be guided by not only a need to be consistent (Cialdini, Trost, & Newsome, 1995), but also a need to hold a positive self-view (Baumeister, 1998) and, ideally, one more positive than that in the past. By believing they did not change their attitudes to a counterposition but did become more effective in their study skills or personal habits, people can maintain a self-enhancing view of themselves as becoming better over time.

Knowing the Attitudes We Want to Have

Just as people's current perceptions of themselves (actual self) can differ from the perceptions they want to have (ideal self; see Higgins, 1987; Markus & Nurius, 1986), the attitudes people currently hold about a wide variety of objects, issues, or other people can be different from the attitudes they would like to possess. For example, a dieter might want to like fast food less and vegetables more, whereas an environmentalist might want to like gas-guzzling SUVs less and bicycling more. Stated simply, people know not only the attitudes they already possess but also that they would like to have different attitudes. In a recent review, Maio and Thomas (2007) suggested that discrepancies between actual and desired opinions often exist, and that people appear to engage in strategies that attempt to bring about change toward the desired opinions.

Recently, DeMarree and colleagues (2011) examined whether discrepancies between actual and desired attitudes could be a source of evaluative conflict, and might therefore account for some of the unexplained variance observed repeatedly in subjective ambivalence research (cf. Priester & Petty, 1996). The unpleasant conflict from not having the attitude one wants could serve as the motivation to change it. In a series of studies, participants indicated their current attitudes toward a diverse number of issues and were asked to report whether they wanted to possess an attitude that differed from the one they just reported, and if so, whether they wanted their attitude to be more positive or negative and how much so. A measure of actual-desired attitude discrepancy was created and then used to predict subjective ambivalence. As hypothesized, actual-desired attitude discrepancies predicted feelings of conflict over and above both intrapersonal and interpersonal ambivalence.

The research on actual-ideal attitude discrepancies raises the possibility that people might want to regulate their attitudes in much the same way they regulate other self-aspects. Furthermore, the prevalence of these discrepancies and the robustness of their association with subjective ambivalence might be surprising. After all, people are presumably free to change their evaluations at any moment. That such discrepancies persist suggests limitations on people's ability to control their own evaluations (see also Wheeler et al., 2007). Perhaps especially when attitudes have an affective basis, it is difficult to create desired attitudes. Imagine a person who for all sorts of rational reasons wants to work things out with a spouse. However, because of the difficulty people have in manufacturing needed emotions, some attitudes are not so easy to change. Indeed, if people could choose whom to fall in love with or choose not to be attracted to someone who isn't their spouse, the divorce rate would be a lot lower. Furthermore, social constraints, reality constraints, personality factors, consistency pressures, goal pursuit, and the like, all can make it difficult to adopt desired attitudes, leading to conflict between one's current evaluations and the ones that are most wanted. It might not be possible ever to eliminate such conflict entirely. Instead, as best they can individuals might hold evaluations that are a tradeoff between these various intrapersonal and interpersonal pressures, resulting in evaluative tension that is invoked whenever the attitude is considered.

Knowing How to Persuade

People have their own naive theories of persuasion—what they think works and what they think does not. Schank and Abelson (1977), in their classic treatise on scripts, plans, and goals, suggested that people have a schema detailing the methods that can be used to influence others (called the *persuade package*). In one of the first empirical investigations of people's persuasion schemas, Rule, Bisanz, and Kohn (1985) found that people reported using persuasion tactics for a wide variety of goals, such as changing other people's opinions and getting others to do things for them. People also reported using a wide variety of influence tactics, such as providing facts and evidence; invoking social norms; and using emotion (e.g., crying), flattery, force, and deception.

Subsequent research has shown that the persuasion theories held by men and women are quite similar and that men and women report using the different persuasion tactics in the same order (i.e., simply ask first and use force last; Bisanz & Rule, 1989). However, the persuasion strategy people think they would use can vary with the specific goals of persuaders, as well as their topic-relevant knowledge (Roskos-Ewoldsen, 1997).

Related to the persuasion schema notion, Friestad and Wright (1994, 1995), in their more recent *persuasion knowledge model*, have suggested that through exposure to persuasion over the lifespan, people develop beliefs about how persuasion works (i.e., the mechanisms of persuasion). For example, people have beliefs about the effectiveness and necessity of factors in advertising, such as attending to, trusting, and remembering the advertisement. Research based on this model has suggested that such beliefs can play an important role in how people respond to persuasion attempts. For example, Campbell and Kirmani (2000) found that consumers viewed a salesperson as less sincere when persuasion knowledge was made accessible than when it was not. Seeing the salesperson as less sincere would presumably make persuasion by that salesperson more difficult.

Not only do people have theories about how to persuade others and the mechanisms of persuasion, but they also have naive theories about how to resist influence. Jacks and Cameron (2003) identified seven resistance strategies that people reported using and found that people were more likely to report using message-related strategies to resist persuasion, such as counterargument, than less socially acceptable strategies, such as source derogation. Furthermore, people reported using different strategies depending on factors such as their issue-relevant knowledge and the importance of the issue.

In addition to their notions of particular strategies of resistance and when they are used, people appear to believe that resistance requires some cognitive effort. This may explain why forewarning people of an impending persuasion attempt leads them to get their guard up (Allyn & Festinger, 1961). In some research, people have engaged in anticipatory counterargument prior to receiving a persuasive message (Petty & Cacioppo, 1979a). In other research (Janssen, Fennis, & Pruyn, 2010), forewarning of persuasion motivated people to conserve their cognitive resources for the upcoming message, and this was reflected in reduced performance on an intermediate self-control task.

Just as metabeliefs about other aspects of attitudes have important cognitive and behavior effects, so too are people's naive theories of resistance consequential. For example, in one study (Rydell, Hugenberg, & McConnell, 2006), people who believed that resistance is good (i.e., implies intelligence) became more certain of the validity of their attitudes following their successful resistance to strong arguments, replicating earlier research (Tormala & Petty, 2002), but people who believed that resistance was bad (i.e., implied closed-mindedness) did not show any increased certainty.

Of course, the possession of theories of persuasion and resistance does not mean that the theories are accurate. There is relatively little work on this topic and what evidence exists presents a mixed picture. For example, some research suggests that people appear to be aware of one tenet of the elaboration likelihood model of persuasion, the notion that people rely on simple cues more than extensive message processing when their motivation or ability to think about a message is reduced (Petty & Cacioppo, 1986). For example, in one study (Vogel, Kutzner, Fiedler, & Freytag, 2010), individuals' naive theories about the simple cue of source attractiveness were investigated. Participants were asked about the extent to which a seller's attractiveness would influence persuasion when the customers were relatively high or low in their motivation or ability to think. Motivation was varied by describing the customers as relatively high or low in their need for cognition (i.e., enjoyment of thinking; Cacioppo & Petty, 1982) and ability was varied by describing the customers as being under time pressure to make a decision or not (e.g., Kruglanski & Webster, 1996). The participants reported that a salesperson's attractiveness would impact persuasion primarily when both motivation and ability to think were low. In other research, people were found to believe generally that individuals who do not like to think are more susceptible to a variety of simple cues used in advertising than are those who like to think (Douglas, Sutton, & Stathi, 2010).

These naive theories about the use of attractiveness and other simple cues appear to be accurate, in that they fit the available data well about how and when people actually respond to simple cues (e.g., Haugtvedt, Petty, & Cacioppo, 1992). Most importantly, perhaps, people use their naive theories of persuasion to guide their own actions. For example, in a series of studies, Vogel and colleagues (2010) found that not only did attractive individuals believe that they were more likely to be effective in influencing people who did not enjoy thinking compared to those who did, but they also were more likely to select customers described as low in motivation to think versus customers described as relatively high in motivation to think.

Although this research suggests that people have some persuasion-relevant knowledge that fits actual findings, other research suggests that people are not always well tuned to the type of appeal that would effectively influence them. For example, in one study (Wilson et al., 1998), students were asked to select one of two messages based on which would influence them the least. The two choices were an explicit speech against their attitudes or a subliminal message. Although the explicit speech was far more effective in producing actual attitude change than the subliminal communication, 69% of the participants chose the speech over the subliminal tape, mistakenly believing that the latter would have the more powerful effect. Additional analyses suggested that people believed that the speech would be easy to counterargue and they selected it for that reason. With respect to the method of resisting persuasion, Jacks and Cameron (2003) found that although people believed that both counterarguing and attitude bolstering would help them resist, and they used both, only the former strategy actually was effective.

In summary, people have naive theories regarding both persuasion and resistance, and those theories, though not completely accurate, can guide how people interact with others. Less research has addressed people's theories about the ways in which they might go about persuading themselves when change is desired. Though not investigating particular strategies of change, some research has examined people's theories about the effort required to produce change in the self versus others (Briñol, McCaslin, & Petty, in press). This research assumes that people hold the reasonable belief that persuading oneself is more difficult when the topic is counterattitudinal rather than proattitudinal, and that people further believe they know their own opinions better than they know the opinions of others (cf. Dunning et al., 2004). Because of this, when the topic of the persuasion task is counterattitudinal, people invest more effort in a message designed to persuade themselves than to persuade another person because they are sure they are opposed but less sure of the opposition of the other. The reverse is the case when the message is proattitudinal. Here, people invest less effort in the message designed to persuade themselves than to persuade another person because they are less sure that the other person agrees already. The extent of actual self-persuasion follows the effort expended in the persuasion task.

Prior research has clearly shown that when people were asked to generate a message with the goal of persuading another person, they themselves often were incidentally changed in the process (e.g., see Janis & King, 1954). The more recent research by Briñol and colleagues (in press) shows that because of people's naive theories about how much effort is necessary to persuade themselves versus another person, depending on the message topic, self-persuasion can be greater if the intended target of the self-generated message is the self rather than another person when the persuasion task is a counterattitudinal one. However, the opposite holds if the task is proattitudinal.

Knowing How Persuadable or Resistant We Are

We have just noted that people have naive theories about what causes persuasion and resistance, and they also have some notion of how much effort might be required to bring about persuasion. This suggests that people have ideas about their own persuadability—how easy or difficult they are to persuade. To provide an explicit exploration of people's theories about their own influenceability, Briñol, Rucker, Tormala, and Petty (2004) developed a Resistance to Persuasion Scale (RPS). The scale contains statements such as "It is hard for me to change my ideas," to which people report the extent of their agreement. Research using the scale has shown that beliefs about resistance to persuasion are consequential for attitude change.

In two studies Briñol and colleagues (2004) predicted and found that individuals exhibited attitude change consistent with their perceptions about their own persuadability when they were not very motivated to think (i.e., were low in need for cognition; Cacioppo & Petty, 1982). Interestingly, when the likelihood of thinking was high (i.e., high need for cognition), they appeared to correct for their persuadability beliefs. Specifically, among low-thinking participants, individuals who believed that they were generally resistant to persuasion showed less attitude change when exposed to various messages than did individuals who believed that they were generally susceptible to persuasion. However, participants high in thinking showed a tendency for a reverse effect, demonstrating more persuasion when they thought they were difficult to persuade. Under high-thinking conditions, people appeared to treat their presumed tendency to be persuaded or resistant as a bias for which they needed to correct by acting in an opposite way. The fact that people correct for bias under high- but not low-thinking conditions is consistent with much other research on correction processes, showing that correction typically requires high thinking and occurs when people become aware of an unwanted influence on their judgments (e.g., see DeSteno, Petty, Rucker, Wegener, & Braverman, 2004; Petty, DeMarree, Briñol, Horcajo, & Strathman, 2008).

Importantly, even two individuals who see themselves as equivalent in resistance to change may believe that they resist influence through very different means. The Bolster–Counterargue Scale (BCS; Briñol et al., 2004) was developed to assess individuals' beliefs about *how* they resist influence. An example item geared toward those who prefer to counterargue is "I take pleasure in arguing with those who have opinions that differ from my own." An item geared toward those who prefer to bolster is "When someone gives me a point of view that conflicts with my attitudes, I like to think about why my views are right for me."

In a study designed to examine the impact of people's perceptions of the strategies they use to resist persuasion, Briñol and colleagues (2004) found that scores on the Bolstering subscale were positively correlated with the number of bolstering thoughts, whereas the Counterarguing subscale was positively correlated with the number of counterarguments generated (but not vice versa). Thus, the spontaneous generation of each type of cognitive response when trying to resist a message can vary from one individual to another, and the BCS seems useful for assessing these individual differences. The predictive utility of the scale, of course, suggests that people have some insight into the strategies they use to resist persuasive messages.

Other lines of research on individual differences suggest that the beliefs people have about their own abilities to defend their attitudes are also consequential in terms of influencing information exposure. For example, according to research on *defensive confidence* by Albarracín and Mitchell (2004), the beliefs people have about their ability to defend their attitudes moderate their approach to attitude-consistent information. Specifically, individuals who feel confident in their ability to defend their beliefs pay more attention to information that threatens their beliefs than individuals who do not feel confident in their ability to defend their abilities.

Summary and Conclusions

In this chapter we have described research regarding what people know about their attitudes, the qualities of their attitudes, what their attitudes do, and whether and how their attitudes can be changed. In the first part of the chapter, we discussed how people generally know what their attitudes are (i.e., whether they like or dislike some attitude object) but sometimes have automatic evaluative reactions that they do not endorse. Furthermore, consistent with literature in other domains, people are generally less aware of *why* they hold the attitudes they do. In particular, the available research has shown that what people actually know about the bases of their attitudes and what they think they know can be two very different things. For example, although people sometimes have good insight into some qualities of their attitudes (e.g., how much thinking they have done), at other times the correlations between objective assessments and subjective assessments hover around zero (e.g., regarding the affective or cognitive bases of attitudes). We also noted that people can acknowledge having evaluative conflict around some issues (explicit ambivalence) but do not acknowledge being conflicted about other issues, though discomfort nevertheless exists (implicit ambivalence). Regardless of whether ambivalence is explicit or implicit, both forms of conflict have important implications for information processing and attitude change.

In the second part of the chapter we described how people sometimes change their attitudes without realizing it, whereas at other times they think they have changed when in fact they have not. Furthermore, sometimes people change without wanting to, whereas other times they try to change intentionally. Of course, just wanting to change does not guarantee that people can change to attain more desired attitudes. We also noted that people have beliefs about how persuasion works, their own persuadability and resistance to change, and they have ideas about how persuasion and resistance are accomplished.

Although people's theories and feelings about their attitudes and susceptibility to change are not always grounded in reality, they can nonetheless be consequential. For example, with respect to the bases of their attitudes, we have seen that (1) feeling conflicted about an attitude or thinking that it is based on little knowledge leads people to be more attentive to attitude-relevant information even if they don't fully understand the basis of the conflict or have an accurate assessment of their amount of knowledge; (2) targeting a message to what people believe their attitude is based on (affect or cognition) can be effective in modifying the attitude, even if the attitude is not really based on that factor; (3) if people come to believe that their attitudes are based on much thought, they are more likely to act on those attitudes, even if that perception has no real basis; and (4) people correct their attitudes for biases they believe have occurred rather than the biases that have actually occurred.

With respect to attitude change, we have seen that people don't always know when their attitudes have changed, and they have theories on how to bring change about in themselves and others. They also have theories about how to resist persuasion. Understanding these theories is important because people act on their theories even if their theories are incorrect. One might imagine that if people became persuasion experts and were aware of the relevant literature on how persuasion works, they could bring about optimal outcomes. However, because social-psychological knowledge on persuasion is aimed at understanding people in general, even the most astute persuasion scholar would not have completely accurate information about him- or herself. Nevertheless, such knowledge is likely to provide a useful guide for suggesting self-relevant hypotheses in everyday life.

REFERENCES

Alba, J. W., & Hutchinson W. (2000). Knowledge calibration: What consumers know and what they think they know. *Journal of Consumer Research, 22,* 62–74.

Albarracín, D., & Mitchell, A. L. (2004). The role of defensive confidence in preference for proattitudinal information: How believing that one is strong can be a weakness. *Personality and Social Psychology Bulletin, 30,* 1565–1584.

Allyn, J., & Festinger, L. (1961). The effectiveness of unanticipated persuasive communication. *Journal of Abnormal and Social Psychology, 62,* 35–40.

Armitage, C. J., & Conner, M. (2000). Attitudinal ambivalence: A test of three key hypotheses. *Personality and Social Psychology Bulletin, 26,* 1421–1432.

Barden, J., & Petty, R. E. (2008). The mere perception of elaboration creates attitude certainty: Exploring the thoughtfulness heuristic. *Journal of Personality and Social Psychology, 95,* 489–509.

Bargh, J. A., Chaiken, S., Govender, R., & Pratto, F. (1992). The generality of the automatic attitude activation effect. *Journal of Personality and Social Psychology, 62,* 893–913.

Bargh, J. A., Chaiken, S., Raymond, P., & Hymes, C. (1996). The automatic evaluation effect: Unconditional automatic attitude activation with a pronunciation task. *Journal of Experimental Social Psychology, 32,* 104–128.

Bassili, J. N. (1996). Meta-judgmental versus operative indices of psychological properties: The case of measures of attitude strength. *Journal of Personality and Social Psychology, 71,* 637–653.

Baumeister, R. F. (1998). The self. In D. Gilbert, S. Fiske, & G. Lindzey (Eds.), *The handbook of social psychology* (4th ed., Vol. 2, pp. 680–740). New York: McGraw-Hill.

Belding, J., Briñol, P., & Petty, R. E. (2011). *Priming through embodiment: External objects influence information processing and attitudes.* Unpublished manuscript, Ohio State University.

Bem, D. J., & McConnell, H. K. (1970). Testing the self-perception explanation of dissonance phenomena: On the salience of premanipulation attitudes. *Journal of Personality and Social Psychology, 14,* 23–31.

Bisanz, G. L., & Rule, B. G. (1989). Gender and the persuasion schema: A search for cognitive invariants. *Personality and Social Psychology Bulletin, 15,* 4–18.

Breckler, S. J. (1984). Empirical validation of affect, behavior, and congtion as distinct components of attitudes. *Journal of Personality and Social Psychology, 47,* 1191–1205.

Briñol, P., McCaslin, M. J., & Petty, R. E. (in press). Self-generated persuasion: Effects of the target and direction of arguments. *Journal of Personality and Social Psychology.*

Briñol, P., Petty, R. E., Gallardo, I., & DeMarree, K. G. (2007). The effects of self-affirmation in non-threatening persuasion domains: Timing affects the process. *Personality and Social Psychology Bulletin, 33*, 1533–1546.

Briñol, P., Petty, R. E., & Wheeler, S. C. (2006). Discrepancies between explicit and implicit self-concepts: Consequences for information processing. *Journal of Personality and Social Psychology, 91*, 154–170.

Briñol, P., Rucker, D. D., Tormala, Z. L., & Petty, R. E. (2004). Individual differences in resistance to persuasion: The role of beliefs and meta-beliefs. In E.S. Knowles & J.A. Linn (Eds.), *Resistance and persuasion* (pp. 83–104). Mahwah, NJ: Erlbaum.

Brucks, M. (1985). The effects of product class knowledge on information search behavior. *Journal of Consumer Research, 12*, 1–16.

Cacioppo, J. T., & Petty, R. E. (1982). The need for cognition. *Journal of Personality and Social Psychology, 42*, 116–131.

Campbell, M. C., & Kirmani, A. (2000). Consumers' use of persuasion knowledge: The effects of accessibility and cognitive capacity on perceptions of an influence agent. *Journal of Consumer Research, 27*, 69–83.

Cialdini, R. B., Trost, M. R., & Newsome, J. T. (1995). Preference for consistency: The development of a valid measure and the discovery of surprising behavioral implications. *Journal of Personality and Social Psychology, 69*, 318–328.

Clark, J. K., Wegener, D. T., & Fabrigar, L. R. (2008). Attitudinal ambivalence and message-based persuasion: Motivated processing of proattitudinal information and avoidance of counterattitudinal information. *Personality and Social Psychology Bulletin, 34*, 565–577.

Conway, M., & Ross, M. (1984). Getting what you want by revising what you had. *Journal of Personality and Social Psychology, 47*, 738–748.

Crites, S., Fabrigar, L., & Petty, R. E. (1994). Measuring the affective and cognitive properties of attitudes: Conceptual and methodological issues. *Personality and Social Psychology Bulletin, 20*, 619–634.

DeCoster, J., Banner, M. J., Smith, E. R., & Semin, G. R. (2006). On the inexplicability of the implicit: Differences in the information provided by implicit and explicit tests. *Social Cognition, 24*, 5–21.

DeMarree, K. G., Wheeler, C., Briñol, P., & Petty, R. E. (2011). *Wanting other attitudes: Actual-desired attitude discrepancies predict feelings of ambivalence*. Unpublished manuscript, Ohio State University.

DeSteno, D., Petty, R. E., Rucker, D. D., Wegener, D. T., & Braverman, J. (2004). Discrete emotions and persuasion: The role of emotion-induced expectancies. *Journal of Personality and Social Psychology, 86*, 43–56.

Dijksterhuis, A., Albers, L. W., & Bongers, K. C. A. (2009). Digging for the real attitude: Lessons from research on implicit and explicit self-esteem. In R. E. Petty, R. H. Fazio, & P. Briñol (Eds.), *Attitudes: Insights from the new implicit measures* (pp. 229–250). New York: Psychology Press.

Douglas, K. M., Sutton, R. M., & Stathi, S. (2010). Why I am persuaded less than you: People's intuitive understanding of the psychology of persuasion. *Social Influence, 5*, 133–148.

Dovidio, J. F., Kawakami, K., Johnson, C., Johnson, B., & Howard, A. (1997). The nature of prejudice: Automatic and controlled processes. *Journal of Experimental Social Psychology, 33*, 510–540.

Dunning, D., Heath, C., & Suls, J. M. (2004). Flawed self-assessment: Implications for health, education, and the workplace. *Psychological Science in the Public Interest, 5*, 69–106.

Edwards, K. (1990). The interplay of affect and cognition in attitude formation and change. *Journal of Personality and Social Psychology, 59*, 202–216.

Epstein, S. (2003). Cognitive-experiential self-theory of personality. In T. Millon & M. Lerner

(Eds.), *Handbook of psychology: Personality and social psychology* (Vol. 5, pp. 159–184). Hoboken, NJ: Wiley.

Fabrigar, L. R., & Petty, R. E. (1999). The role of the affective and cognitive bases of attitudes in susceptibility to affectively and cognitively based persuasion. *Personality and Social Psychology Bulletin, 25*, 363–381.

Fazio, R. H. (1995). Attitudes as object-evaluation associations: Determinants, consequences, and correlates of attitude accessibility. In R. E. Petty & J. A. Krosnick (Eds.), *Attitude strength: Antecedents and consequences* (pp. 247–282). Mahwah, NJ: Erlbaum.

Fazio, R. H., Jackson, J. R., Dunton, B. C., & Williams, C. J. (1995). Variability in automatic activation as an unobtrusive measure of racial attitudes: A bona fide pipeline? *Journal of Personality and Social Psychology, 69*, 1013–1027.

Fazio, R. H., Sanbonmatsu, D. M., Powell, M. C., & Kardes, F. R. (1986). On the automatic activation of attitudes. *Journal of Personality and Social Psychology, 50*, 229–238.

Fazio, R. H., & Zanna, M. P. (1978). Attitudinal qualities relating to the strength of the attitude–behavior relationship. *Journal of Experimental Social Psychology, 14*, 398–408.

Festinger, L. (1954). A theory of social comparison processes. *Human Relations, 7*, 117–140.

Fox, M. C., Ericsson, K. A., & Best, R. (2011). Do procedures for verbal reporting of thinking have to reactive?: A meta-analysis and recommendations for best reporting methods. *Psychological Bulletin, 137*, 316–344.

Friestad, M., & Wright, P. (1994). The Persuasion Knowledge Model: How people cope with persuasion attempts. *Journal of Consumer Research, 21*, 1–31.

Friestad, M., & Wright, P. (1995). Persuasion knowledge: Lay peoples and researchers beliefs about the psychology of advertising. *Journal of Consumer Research, 22*, 62–74.

Gawronski, B., & Bodenhausen, G. V. (2006). Associative and propositional processes in evaluation: An integrative review of implicit and explicit attitude change. *Psychological Bulletin, 132*, 692–731.

Goethals, G. & Nelson, R. E. (1973). Similarity in the influence process: The belief–value distinction. *Journal of Personality and Social Psychology, 25*, 117–122.

Goethals, G. R., & Reckman, R. F. (1973). The perception of consistency in attitudes. *Journal of Experimental Social Psychology, 9*, 491–501.

Greenwald, A. G., & Banaji, M. (1995). Implicit social cognition: Attitudes, self-esteem, and stereotypes. *Psychological Review, 102*, 4–27.

Greenwald, A. G., McGhee, D. E., & Schwartz, J. L. K. (1998). Measuring individual differences in implicit cognition: The Implicit Association Test. *Journal of Personality and Social Psychology, 74*, 1464–1480.

Greenwald, A. G., Poehlman, T. A., Uhlmann, E. L., & Banaji, M. R. (2009). Understanding and using the Implicit Association Test: III. Meta-analysis of predictive validity. *Journal of Personality and Social Psychology, 97*, 17–41.

Haddock, G., Rothman, A. J., Reber, R., & Schwarz, N. (1999). Forming judgments of attitude certainty, intensity, and importance: The role of subjective experiences. *Personality and Social Psychology Bulletin, 25*, 771–782.

Haugtvedt, C. P., Petty, R. E., & Cacioppo, J. T. (1992). Need for cognition and advertising: Understanding the role of personality variables in consumer behavior. *Journal of Consumer Psychology, 1*, 239–260.

Heider, F. (1958). *The psychology of interpersonal relations*. New York: Wiley.

Higgins, E. T. (1987). Self-discrepancy: A theory relating self and affect. *Psychological Review, 94*, 319–340.

Horcajo, J., Petty, R. E., &, Briñol, P. (2010). The effects of majority versus minority source status on persuasion: A self-validation analysis. *Journal of Personality and Social Psychology, 99*, 498–512.

Jacks, J. Z., & Cameron, K. A. (2003). Strategies of resisting persuasion. *Basic and Applied Social Psychology, 25*, 145–161.

Janis, I. L., & King, B. T. (1954). The influence of role-playing on opinion change. *Journal of Abnormal and Social Psychology, 49*, 211–218.

Janssen, L., Fennis, B. M., & Pruyn, A. T. H. (2010). Forewarned is forearmed: Conserving self-control strength to resist social influence. *Journal of Experimental Social Psychology, 46*, 911–921.

Jarvis, W. B. G., & Petty, R. E. (1996). The need to evaluate. *Journal of Personality and Social Psychology, 70*, 172–194.

Jordan, C. H., Whitfield, M., & Zeigler-Hill, V. (2007). Intuition and the correspondence between implicit and explicit self-esteem. *Journal of Personality and Social Psychology, 93*, 1067–1079.

Kaplan, K. J. (1972). On the ambivalence–indifference problem in attitude theory and measurement: A suggested modification of the semantic differential technique. *Psychological Bulletin, 77*, 361–372.

Kellerman, J., & Laird, J. D. (1982). The effect of appearance on self-perceptions. *Journal of Personality, 50*, 296–315.

Kiesler, C. A. (1971). *The psychology of commitment: Experiments linking behavior to beliefs*. New York: Academic Press.

Kruglanski, A. W., & Webster, D. M., (1996). Motivated closing of the mind: Seizing and freezing. *Psychological Review, 103*, 263–283.

Loersch, C., McCaslin, M., & Petty, R. E. (2011). Exploring the impact of social judgeability concerns on the interplay of associative and deliberative attitude processes. *Journal of Experimental Social Psychology, 47*, 1029–1032.

Maio, G. R., Bell, D. E., & Esses, V. M. (1996). Ambivalence and persuasion: The processing of messages about immigrant groups. *Journal of Experimental Social Psychology, 32*, 513–536.

Maio, G. R., & Thomas, G. (2007). The epistemic–teleological model of self persuasion. *Personality and Social Psychology Review, 11*, 1–22.

Markus, H., & Nurius, P. (1986). Possible selves. *American Psychologist, 41*, 954–969.

McFarland, C., & Ross, M. (1987). The relation between current impressions and memories of self and dating partners. *Personality and Social Psychology Bulletin, 13*, 228–238.

Nisbett, R. E., & Wilson, T. D. (1977). Telling more than we can know: Verbal reports on mental processes. *Psychological Review, 84*, 231–259.

Olson, M. A., & Fazio, R. H. (2003). Relations between implicit measures of racial prejudice: What are we measuring? *Psychological Science, 14*, 636–639.

Olson, M. A., & Fazio, R. H. (2009). Implicit and explicit measures of attitudes: The perspective of the MODE model. In R. E. Petty, R. H. Fazio, & P. Briñol (Eds.), *Attitudes: Insights from the new implicit measures* (pp. 19–64). New York: Psychology Press.

Petty, R. E., & Briñol, P. (2006). A meta-cognitive approach to "implicit" and "explicit" evaluations: Comment on Gawronski and Bodenhausen (2006). *Psychological Bulletin, 132*, 740–744.

Petty, R. E., & Briñol, P. (2009). Implicit ambivalence: A meta-cognitive approach. In R. E. Petty, R. H. Fazio, & P. Briñol (Eds.), *Attitudes: Insights from the new implicit measures* (pp. 119–161). New York: Psychology Press.

Petty, R. E., Briñol, P., & DeMarree, K. G. (2007). The meta-cognitive model (MCM) of attitudes: Implications for attitude measurement, change, and strength. *Social Cognition, 25*, 657–686.

Petty, R. E., Briñol, P., Tormala, Z. L., & Wegener, D. T. (2007). The role of metacognition in social judgment. In E. T. Higgins & A. W. Kruglanski, (Eds.), *Social psychology: A handbook of basic principles* (2nd ed., pp. 254–284). New York: Guilford Press.

Petty, R. E., & Cacioppo, J. T. (1979a). Effects of forewarning of persuasive intent on cognitive responses and persuasion. *Personality and Social Psychology Bulletin, 5*, 173–176.

Petty, R. E., & Cacioppo, J. T. (1979b). Issue-involvement can increase or decrease persuasion by enhancing message-relevant cognitive responses. *Journal of Personality and Social Psychology, 37*, 1915–1926.

Petty, R. E., & Cacioppo, J. T. (1984). The effects of involvement on responses to argument quantity and quality: Central and peripheral routes to persuasion. *Journal of Personality and Social Psychology, 46*, 69–81.

Petty, R. E., & Cacioppo, J. T. (1986). *Communication and persuasion: Central and peripheral routes to attitude change*. New York: Springer-Verlag.

Petty, R. E., DeMarree, K. G., Briñol, P., Horcajo, J., & Strathman, A. J. (2008). Need for cognition can magnify or attenuate priming effects in social judgment. *Personality and Social Psychology Bulletin, 34*, 900–912.

Petty, R. E., Fazio, R. H., & Briñol, P. (2009). The new implicit measures: An overview. In R. E. Petty, R. H. Fazio, & P. Briñol (Eds.), *Attitudes: Insights from the new implicit measures* (pp. 3–18). New York: Psychology Press.

Petty, R. E., Haugtvedt, C., & Smith, S. M. (1995). Elaboration as a determinant of attitude strength: Creating attitudes that are persistent, resistant, and predictive of behavior. In R. E. Petty & J. A. Krosnick (Eds.), *Attitude strength: Antecedents and consequences* (pp. 93–130). Mahwah, NJ: Erlbaum.

Petty, R. E., & Krosnick, J. A. (Eds.). (1995). *Attitude strength: Antecedents and consequences*. Mahwah, NJ: Erlbaum.

Petty, R. E., Tormala, Z. L., Briñol, P., & Jarvis, W. B. G. (2006). Implicit ambivalence from attitude change: An exploration of the PAST model. *Journal of Personality and Social Psychology, 90*, 21–41.

Petty, R. E., & Wegener, D. T. (1993). Flexible correction processes in social judgment: Correcting for context-induced contrast. *Journal of Experimental Social Psychology, 29*, 137–165.

Petty, R. E., Wegener, D. T., & White, P. (1998). Flexible correction processes in social judgment: Implications for persuasion. *Social Cognition, 16*, 93–113.

Petty, R. E., Wells, G. L., & Brock, T. C. (1976). Distraction can enhance or reduce yielding to propaganda: Thought disruption versus effort justification. *Journal of Personality and Social Psychology, 34*, 874–884.

Priester, J. M., & Petty, R. E. (1996). The gradual threshold model of ambivalence: Relating the positive and negative bases of attitudes to subjective ambivalence. *Journal of Personality and Social Psychology, 71*, 431–449.

Priester, J. R., Petty. R. E., & Park, K. (2007). Whence univalent ambivalence: From the anticipation of conflicting reactions. *Journal of Consumer Research, 34*, 11–21.

Priester, J. R., & Petty, R. E. (2001). Extending the bases of subjective attitudinal ambivalence: Interpersonal and intrapersonal antecedents of evaluative tension. *Journal of Personality and Social Psychology, 80*, 19–34.

Radecki, C. M., & Jaccard, J. (1995). Perceptions of knowledge, actual knowledge and information search behavior. *Journal of Experimental Social Psychology, 31*, 107–138.

Ranganath, K. A., Smith, C. T., & Nosek, B. A. (2008). Distinguishing automatic and controlled components of attitudes from direct and indirect measurement methods. *Journal of Experimental Social Psychology, 44*, 386–396.

Roskos-Ewoldsen, D. R. (1997). Implicit theories of persuasion. *Human Communication Research, 24*, 31–63.

Ross, M. (1989). The relation of implicit theories to the construction of personal histories. *Psychological Review, 96*, 341–357.

Ross, M., McFarland, C., & Fletcher, G. J. (1981). The effect of attitude on the recall of personal histories. *Journal of Personality and Social Psychology, 40*, 627–634.

Rucker, D. D., Lee, A., & Briñol, P. (2011). *The aftermath of information acquisition: Sometimes knowing more feels like knowing less.* Unpublished manuscript, Northwestern University.

Rucker, D. D., & Petty, R. E. (2004). When resistance is futile: Consequences of failed counterarguing on attitude certainty. *Journal of Personality and Social Psychology, 86*, 219–235.

Rucker, D. D., Petty, R. E., & Briñol, P. (2008). What's in a frame anyway?: A meta-cognitive analysis of the impact of one versus two sided message framing on attitude certainty. *Journal of Consumer Psychology, 18*, 137–149.

Rule, B., Bisanz, G., & Kohn, M. (1985). Anatomy of persuasion schema: Targets, goals, and strategies. *Journal of Personality and Social Psychology, 48*, 1127–1140.

Rydell, R. J., Hugenberg, K., & McConnell, A. R. (2006). Resistance can be good or bad: How theories of resistance and dissonance affect attitude certainty. *Personality and Social Psychology Bulletin, 32*, 740–750.

Rydell, R. J., & McConnell, A. R. (2006). Understanding implicit and explicit attitude change: A systems of reasoning analysis. *Journal of Personality and Social Psychology, 91*, 995–1008.

Rydell, R. J., McConnell, A. R., & Mackie, D. M. (2008). Consequences of discrepant explicit and implicit attitudes: Cognitive dissonance and increased information processing. *Journal of Experimental Social Psychology, 44*, 1526–1532.

Rydell, R. J., McConnell, A. R., Mackie, D. M., & Strain, L. M. (2006). Of two minds: Forming and changing valence-inconsistent implicit and explicit attitudes. *Psychological Science, 17*, 954–958.

Schank, R. C., & Abelson, R. P. (1977). *Scripts, plans, goals, and understanding: An inquiry into human knowledge structures.* Hillsdale, NJ: Erlbaum.

Schryer, E., & Ross, M. (2012). People's thoughts about their personal past and futures. In P. Briñol & K. G. DeMarree (Eds.), *Social metacognition* (pp. 141–158). New York: Psychology Press.

See, Y. H. M., Petty, R. E., & Fabrigar, L. R. (2008). Affective and cognitive meta-bases of attitudes: Unique effects on information interest and persuasion. *Journal of Personality and Social Psychology, 94*, 938–955.

Smith, S. M., Fabrigar, L. R., MacDougall, B. L., & Wiesenthal, N. L. (2008). The role of amount, cognitive elaboration, and structural consistency of attitude-relevant knowledge in the formation of attitude certainty. *European Journal of Social Psychology, 38*, 280–295.

Sparks, P., Harris, P. R., & Lockwood, N. (2004). Predictors and predictive effects of ambivalence. *British Journal of Social Psychology, 43*, 371–383.

Thompson, M. M., Zanna, M. P., & Griffin, D. W. (1995). Let's not be indifferent about (attitudinal) ambivalence. In R. E. Petty & J. A. Krosnick (Eds.), *Attitude strength: Antecedents and consequences* (pp. 361–386). Hillsdale, NJ: Erlbaum.

Tormala, Z. L., & Petty, R. E. (2002). What doesn't kill me makes me stronger: The effects of resisting persuasion on attitude certainty. *Journal of Personality and Social Psychology, 83*, 1298–1313.

Tormala, Z. L., & Petty, R. E. (2007). Contextual contrast and perceived knowledge: Exploring the implications for persuasion. *Journal of Experimental Social Psychology, 43*, 17–30.

Tormala, Z. L., & Rucker, D. D. (2007). Attitude certainty: A review of past findings and emerging perspectives. *Social and Personality Psychology Compass, 1*, 469–492.

van Harreveld, F., van der Pligt, J., & de Liver, Y. N. (2009). The agony of ambivalence and ways to resolve it: Introducing the MAID model. *Personality and Social Psychology Review, 13*, 45–61.

Visser, P. S., & Holbrook, A. L. (2012). Metacognitive determinants of attitude strength. In P. Briñol & K. G. DeMarree (Eds.), *Social metacognition* (pp. 21–42). New York: Psychology Press.

Vogel, T., Kutzner, F., Fiedler, K., & Freytag, P. (2010). Exploiting attractiveness in persuasion: Senders' implicit theories about receivers' processing motivation. *Personality and Social Psychology Bulletin, 36*, 830–842.

Wagner, B. C., Petty, R. E., & Briñol, P. (2011). *Are morally-based attitudes particularly strong?: The impact of moral attitudinal basis on attitude strength indicators and consequences*. Unpublished manuscript, Ohio State University.

Wegener, D. T., Downing, J., Krosnick, J. A., & Petty, R. E. (1995). Measures and manipulations of strength related properties of attitudes: Current practice and future directions. In R. E. Petty & J. A. Krosnick (Eds.), *Attitude strength: Antecedents and consequences* (pp. 455–488). Mahwah, NJ: Erlbaum.

Wegener, D. T., & Petty, R. E. (1997). The flexible correction model: The role of naive theories of bias in bias correction. In M. P. Zanna (Ed.), *Advances in experimental social psychology* (Vol. 29, pp. 141–208). Mahwah, NJ: Erlbaum.

Wheeler, S. C., DeMarree, K. G., & Petty, R. E. (2007). Understanding the role of the self in prime-to-behavior effects: The active self account. *Personality and Social Psychology Review, 11*, 234–261.

Wilson, A. E., & Ross, M. (2003). Autobiographical memory and self-identity. *Memory, 11*, 137–149.

Wilson, T. D., & Brekke, N. (1994). Mental contamination and mental correction: Unwanted influences on judgments and evaluations. *Psychological Bulletin, 116*, 117–142.

Wilson, T. D., Dunn, D. S., Bybee, J. A., Hyman, D. B., & Rotondo, J. A. (1984). Effects of analyzing reasons on attitude–behavior consistency. *Journal of Personality and Social Psychology, 47*, 5–16.

Wilson, T. D., & Hodges, S. D. (1992). Attitudes as temporary constructions. In L.L. Martin & A. Tesser (Eds.), *The construction of social judgments* (pp. 37–65). Hillsdale, NJ: Erlbaum.

Wilson, T. D., Houston, C. E., & Meyers, J. M. (1998). Choose your poison: Effects of lay beliefs about mental processes on attitude change. *Social Cognition, 16*, 114–132.

Wilson, T. D., Lindsey, S., & Schooler, T. Y. (2000). A model of dual attitudes. *Psychological Review, 107*, 101–126.

Wood, W., Rhodes, N., & Biek, M. (1995). Working knowledge and attitude strength: An information processing analysis. In R. E. Petty & J. A. Krosnick (Eds.), *Attitude strength: Antecedents and consequences* (pp. 283–314). Hillsdale, NJ: Erlbaum.

Zanna, M. P., & Rempel, J. K. (1988). Attitudes: A new look at an old concept. In D. Bar-Tal & A. W. Kruglanski (Eds.), *The social psychology of knowledge* (pp. 315–334). Cambridge, UK: Cambridge University Press.

CHAPTER 11

Self-Knowledge, Unconscious Thought, and Decision Making

MAARTEN W. BOS
AP DIJKSTERHUIS

Imagine you had to make a decision: Blond or brunette? You chose blond because, considering all the information you had at that moment, blond seemed to be the most attractive option. Later, however, it turned out that blond did not leave you all that satisfied. But what happened? How, having carefully looked over all the available information, was it possible that your choice to dye your hair blond did not make you happy?

We face many decisions in our lives, ranging from important matters, such as which job we should accept, to mundane choices, such as what shampoo to buy. Making decisions is not always easy, and indeed, making complex decisions with far-reaching consequences can be quite a challenge (Germeijs, & De Boeck, 2002; Rassin & Muris, 2005; Rettinger & Hastie, 2001), although this is more true for some people than for others (Frost & Shows, 1993; Schwartz et al., 2002; Webster & Kruglanski, 1994).

Whereas mundane decisions are usually made relatively quickly and without much effort or thought (Finucane, Alhakami, Slovic, & Johnson, 2000; Gladwell, 2005), complex decisions can take a long time and a great deal of deliberation (Greenleaf & Lehmann, 1995; Johnson & Payne, 1985; Payne, Bettman, & Johnson, 1993). As decisions often fail to lead to satisfactory outcomes (e.g., Tsiros & Mittal, 2000), the question of how we should approach complex decisions arises.

Researchers and theorists have identified various decision-making strategies: Some include thorough conscious deliberation, others focus on intuitive strategies, and still others are mere variations of flipping a coin. Although the latter probably does not rank highly on most people's list of appropriate decision-making strategies, complex decisions sometimes leave us so dissatisfied (Tsiros & Mittal, 2000) that, in retrospect, flipping a coin may not seem like such a bad idea (Ratliff, 1999).

Few people would subscribe to this idea though. In fact, common sense dictates that thorough conscious deliberation leads to the best outcomes when we are faced with a complex decision. Although this is sometimes true, there are important exceptions.

Contrary to common sense, not consciously thinking about a complex decision problem sometimes leads to better results than does conscious thought (Dijksterhuis & Nordgren, 2006; Wilson & Schooler, 1991). Still, people do rely more on conscious thought, especially when a task is complex (Inbar, Cone, & Gilovich, 2010). This reliance on conscious thought is a direct result of the reputation of both consciousness—as reliable and rational—and unconscious and automatic processes—as crude, irrational, and sometimes sloppy.

But what exactly is so rational about the outcomes of conscious thought processes? When making a decision, we like to rely on conscious thought because we think we know what attributes are important for us. That is, we think we have enough self-knowledge to weight attributes of a decision adequately as long as we think consciously. Our strong reliance on conscious thought is reinforced by economic theories. There are various normative decision-making strategies that rely on applying a sophisticated conscious weighting strategy (Baron, 2000). However, the truth is that we often have very little conscious insight into the reasons for our feelings and behavior (e.g., Nisbett & Wilson, 1977), and this hinders us in making decisions with satisfactory outcomes.

We argue that thinking consciously does not necessarily lead to rational decisions for at least two reasons. First, when making decisions consciously, self-knowledge is imperative if we are to weight the attributes of decision alternatives. If we do not know what we think is important, we weight all positive and negative attributes of a choice option equally. Usually, not every attribute is of equal importance, and some weighting of attributes is often necessary (e.g., when buying a car, the amount of cup holders should generally not be weighted equally with safety).

Second, even if people know how best to weight attributes, they may not have the conscious capacity to do so, especially when faced with multiple attributes and multiple decision alternatives. In contrast, weighting of attributes is something at which the unconscious is actually quite good. We argue that, quite often, we have neither the self-knowledge nor the capacity to assign appropriate weight consciously to attributes of a decision option. Let us first look into some decision-making strategies to see the demands they make on conscious processes and self-knowledge.

Normative Decision-Making Strategies

There is a long list of strategies people supposedly use when making a decision. The same problem can lead to different decisions, depending on the strategy the decision maker uses to arrive at a solution.

The equal weight heuristic (EQW) is a "tally" strategy. It ignores the relative importance of attributes and instead just looks at which option has the highest ratio of good to bad features (Payne et al., 1993). EQW does not rely on weighting and, hence, self-knowledge about which attributes are most important to us is hardly necessary. It is relatively easy to perform, since all one has to do is count good and bad attributes of each decision alternative to come to a decision. This, then, can easily be done consciously. However, the benefit of little effort can come at the cost of decision quality, and weighting of attributes is often necessary.

Another relatively simple strategy is the strict lexicographic rule (LEX). When this strategy is applied, the most important attribute is determined and the choice option that scores highest on this attribute is selected. Here, some weighting is necessary (i.e., one has to determine what the most important attribute is), but it is rather simple. This strategy can probably be done consciously.

A more complex decision-making strategy is the weighted adding strategy (WADD; e.g., Bettman, Luce, & Payne, 1998; Edwards, 1961; Janis & Mann, 1977), in which the relative importance (also called *utility*) of various attributes of choice options is weighted. There are several pitfalls to this strategy. To name a few: The value of attributes may differ from one situation to another; we may not always be knowledgeable enough to judge the utility of an attribute; attributes may be interdependent (for an apartment, the attribute "penthouse of a 22-story building" seems of a high value, but may be less so when another attribute is "22-story building lacks elevator"); and so on. As it turns out, even when we try to use this strategy, which we rarely do, we are not very good at it (e.g. Dawes, 1979; Swets, Dawes, & Monahan, 2000).

Multi-attribute utility theory (MAUT) answers some of the issues of WADD strategies, stating, for instance, that every attribute needs to be independent. Making decisions according to MAUT has its problems too, however. One of these problems is that MAUT, like all WADD strategies depends fully on self-reported indications of attribute values. This means that to apply WADD strategies successfully we have to have a sufficient amount of self-knowledge and be able to rely on introspection. Introspection, regretfully, is a notoriously bad indicator of motives (e.g., Nisbett & Wilson, 1977) and relative personal value. A bigger problem is the fact that most people do not know how to use MAUT, and therefore refrain from using it (e.g., Dawes, 1979; Swets et al., 2000).

The decision strategies described earlier all follow certain decision rules. Interestingly enough, they often appear not to come close to the way people actually make decisions. Some strategies describe optimal decision making, but in truth, people do not often make lists or write down the weights of various attributes of decision options, and even if they do, it appears close to impossible to compare values of attributes or even truly to know the subjective value of an attribute. Of course, many of these models are only normative. It is now generally assumed that real-life decision making does not conform to these models. The problem is that due to the limited capacity of conscious processing, we cannot conform to these models, regardless of how much time and effort we put into a decision. So, in fact, many decision theories paint a pretty picture of a nonexistent reality. That we do not achieve this reality appears to be because we not only do not try but we also are simply unable to do so.

The main point, implicit in the theory behind these models, is that thorough conscious thought leads to optimal decision making. MAUT is better than EQW, for instance, and requires a good deal more conscious thought. However, consciously making decisions is, in fact, hard.

Conscious Thought in Decision Making

There is a history of admiration for consciousness. Descartes so eloquently said: "I think therefore I am" (*Cogito ergo sum*; Descartes, 1664), and his views seem to be shared by, among other scholars, a host of economists and decision-making theorists. The more complex normative strategies (e.g., MAUT) assume clever conscious processes and suggest that thinking consciously helps to assign appropriate weights to aspects and attributes of a decision. If only it were that simple. Numerous studies show that, in fact, conscious thought does not help to assign appropriate weights. Let us first look at some of the errors we make and biases we encounter when making decisions.

Decision making falls prey to various errors. There are reasons why we are not very good at weighting various attributes of a choice option. A very prominent reason is that context influences us, such that the value or weight of an attribute varies from one situation to another. This leads to a problem because when we are asked to assign value to an attribute, we often do not realize this. Instead, we judge the attribute solely by our evaluation in the specific context in which we find ourselves. However, the context in which we judge an attribute may be very different from the context in which the results of our decision matter. If we go shopping for dinner just *before* we have lunch, we buy much more food than if we go shopping for dinner just *after* we have lunch (Nisbett & Kanouse, 1969). This occurs because we are in a "hot" state of hunger (Loewenstein, 1996). Also, quitting smokers judge their ability to stop smoking much higher just after they had a (presumably last) cigarette. The same effect occurs for dieting (Nordgren, van der Pligt, & van Harreveld, 2006, 2008) and other impulsive behaviors (Ariely & Loewenstein, 2006; Nordgren et al., 2008; Sayette, Loewenstein, Griffin, & Black, 2008; Van Boven, Loewenstein, & Dunning, 2005). In short, we are generally not very good at judging how we will behave in a situation that differs from the one we are in (Loewenstein, 1996; Loewenstein, Nagin, & Paternoster, 1997; Nordgren et al., 2006, 2007, 2008, 2009; Read & van Leeuwen, 1998; Van Boven & Loewenstein, 2003).

Similarly, values are influenced by context. Research has shown that people are more willing to make an extra trip to save $5 when the total price is low than when the total price is high. When buying a $15 calculator, people are more willing to make an extra trip for a $5 discount than when buying a $125 calculator. The same $5 (and this is the exact same $5) appears to have a different value dependent on the context, or the *framing* (Tversky & Kahneman, 1981). When buying a house, $5 or even $1,000 may seem like a ridiculous amount to negotiate, but these are the same dollars that make you take a detour to a gas station to get a $5 discount over the course of a year, or make you decide not to buy that suit you liked so much. So even comparing money to money seems to become difficult when the context is different. Despite these fluctuations, people are no less certain of their decisions.

When people are asked to estimate how many people die of AIDS, traffic accidents, or homicide, they tend to overestimate the number of deaths from homicide and underestimate the number of AIDS-related deaths. This is caused by the information they have available, and newspapers cover more homicides than AIDS-related deaths. The heuristic they apply, called the *availability heuristic*, is a well-studied phenomenon (e.g. Combs & Slovic, 1979). It describes how we tend to base the estimate of the prevalence of something (e.g., plane crashes) on the ease with which previous occurrences come to mind (Tversky & Kahneman, 1973). As it turns out, thinking more in this case results in more bias from this heuristic. When people were given 12 seconds to answer this question, the bias was smaller than when people were asked to think carefully before answering and given 45 seconds to answer (Dijksterhuis, 2003). More thinking led to more bias because people used the wrong kind of weighting. Availability alone is obviously not sufficient cause to judge a weight.

As demonstrated in the previous examples, various errors pervade decision making. We intuitively blame such errors on people's lack of motivation to engage in serious conscious thought. Can't we avoid such errors if we just deliberate a little more? We think that thorough conscious thought will help us make good decisions. However, assigning values to attributes of choice options is very difficult, and finding an objective standard of the value of an attribute seems almost impossible. Let us now look at some empirical demonstrations of weighting biases when applying conscious thought to a decision, leading to a decrease in decision performance.

Wilson and colleagues (1993) compared postchoice satisfaction of people who chose from five different art posters. Some participants were merely asked to choose, whereas others were asked to deliberate. More specifically, they were asked to scrutinize the reasons for their preference carefully. The expectations of the experimenters were confirmed a few weeks later when postchoice satisfaction was assessed. People who engaged in thorough conscious thought were less happy with their choice. Conscious contemplation seems to disturb what Wilson and colleagues called "natural weighting schemes" (e.g., Wilson & Schooler, 1991; Wilson et al., 1993; see also Levine, Halberstadt, & Goldstone, 1996) because conscious thought leads people to put disproportionate weight on attributes that are accessible, plausible, and easy to verbalize (see also Schooler, Ohlsson, & Brooks, 1993).

Basically, we just don't know ourselves well enough to arrive reliably at good decisions when thinking consciously. Although it is certainly true that conscious thought can help to prevent some pitfalls in decision making, the general rule that conscious thought makes choices and decisions better, intuitive as it may sound, is wrong. More motivation to think about a decision may occasionally help (e.g., for easy decisions), but often it just leads to more enthusiastic application of a suboptimal strategy, leading to suboptimal outcomes (e.g., Arkes, Dawes, & Christensen, 1986). For instance, the more people are motivated to deliberate about a choice, the bigger framing effects become (Igou & Bless, 2007).

Although Descartes' idea was an interesting notion at the very least, it has arguably been the start of centuries of neglect and disregard of smart automatic processes (Damasio, 1994; Koestler, 1964; Wilson, 2002). Many economic theorists and judgment and decision-making experts would have us believe that although conscious thought does not always lead to optimal decision making (e.g. Baron, 2000), other decision styles, among which are more intuitive decision styles, are not likely to be better, and they state so without citing research supporting this claim (e.g., see Baron, 2000, p. 333). So what do we do when we have a decision that is more complex than choosing between one towel or another? We know that using conscious thought leads to biases, so is there a way to arrive at good outcomes when faced with a complex decision?

Self-Knowledge and Decision Making

The research we have discussed so far states that the limitations on what we know of ourselves negatively influences decisions based on conscious thought. A certain amount of self-knowledge is necessary to make good decisions, of course, but regretfully we often have difficulty consciously accessing our motives and attribute preferences.

In the "poster study" by Wilson and colleagues (1993), the role of self-knowledge in decision making was investigated. Some participants were instructed to think about reasons why they preferred one poster over the other; others were not given this instruction. Participants who were instructed to think about their reasons indicated less satisfaction with their choice when asked 3 weeks later. What went wrong here? Does making participants indicate what they think is important actually decrease satisfaction? It seemed that the manipulation used by Wilson and colleagues did not increase self-knowledge. Or maybe it did, but only for a subset of the information. Conscious thought, or in this case reasons analysis, leads people to put disproportionate weight on attributes that are accessible and easy to verbalize (see also Schooler et al., 1993). Not all important attributes of a choice option are easy to verbalize, so this method may not work for complicated decisions. We simply do not have enough self-knowledge to be able to make good decisions consciously when decisions become more complex than buying one toothbrush or another.

A study by Nordgren and Dijksterhuis (2009) showed that when thinking consciously, people also become more inconsistent over time. Participants in this study were asked to make a variety of judgments, such as about the extraversion of people on the basis of their faces and the attractiveness of Chinese ideograms. Participants judged every stimulus twice. Some participants were asked to judge quickly; others were asked to think thoroughly and consciously. People who engaged in conscious thought showed more inconsistency (also see Levine et al., 1996). Quick "gut" judgments were clearly more consistent over time than judgments made after conscious deliberation. Chinese ideograms have no meaning to participants who do not read Chinese, so some inconsistency should not matter. Rating the extraversion of faces is somewhat different, however. Were conscious thinkers perhaps more inconsistent because their judgments simply improved over time? Let's have a look at normative judgments.

In one experiment by Nordgren and Dijksterhuis (2009) participants were asked to judge the quality of various pieces of art. Some of the art was taken from the MOMA (Museum of Modern Art in New York), and other art was taken from the MOBA (Museum of Bad Art in Boston). As in the experiment with the Chinese ideograms, conscious thinkers were less consistent over time. Moreover, their evaluations of the art did not become more accurate, in that over time, conscious thinkers did not become better at distinguishing good art from bad art.

Let's go back to the poster study. What if we do know what is important to us? What if we were able to verbalize all attributes? Would that help us make a good decision? Wilson and colleagues (1993) found that experts were not hindered by presenting reasons why they chose a poster. This is most likely the case because they can access (and verbalize) what information is important when making a decision.

One study examined the role of expertise in unconscious thought (thinking while conscious attention is distracted). After unconscious thought, soccer experts were better at predicting match outcomes than after conscious thought (Dijksterhuis, Bos, Van der Leij, & Van Baaren, 2009). It seemed that after conscious thought, experts tried to (unsuccessfully) include several pieces of information that were not relevant to their predictions. After unconscious thought, precisely the information that was relevant for their prediction was more accessible. So judging from the soccer experiments, expertise does help when making a decision: One could say that after unconscious thought, experts used those pieces of information that at an unconscious level they realized were important.

Basically, when thinking consciously, we are not able to adequately weight relevant information and we even become inconsistent over time. Even when we try to use self-knowledge (by using conscious thought) or increase our self-knowledge (by thought listing) we do not make better decisions. Worse, work by Dijksterhuis and Van Olden (2006) shows that decisions we make after conscious thought leave us less satisfied. Does this mean we are unable to make complex decisions in line with our preferences? Thankfully, such a gloomy conclusion is not necessary. Conscious thought relies on self-knowledge to make a decision. Luckily, we can make decisions based on our preferences without the burden of a limited amount of self-knowledge, using unconscious thought.

Unconscious Thought Theory

Unconscious thought theory is based on six principles (Dijksterhuis & Nordgren, 2006). These principles contrast unconscious thought with conscious thought. The unconscious thought principle states that there are two modes of thought: conscious thought and unconscious thought. The two modes have different characteristics, making them differentially applicable to different situations. The capacity principle states that since unconscious thought makes use of the large capacity of the unconscious, unconscious thought can handle greater amounts of information than conscious thought, which uses the relatively small capacity of consciousness. The bottom-up versus top-down principle states that conscious thought works top-down, applying schemas when we come to a decision. Unconscious thought works bottom-up, allowing it to come to decisions that do not fit a schema, and taking into account information that does not fit prior knowledge (Bos & Dijksterhuis, 2011). The weighting principle states that unconscious thought is better at assigning appropriate weights to information. The rule principle states that conscious thought is rule-based. When making a decision, conscious thought can apply strict rules and is very precise, whereas unconscious thought only gives rough estimates. The convergence versus divergence principle states that conscious thought searches memory in a more focused manner, whereas unconscious thought searches memory in a more divergent manner, allowing it to be more creative for instance (Dijksterhuis & Nordgren, 2006).

Unconscious thought can be defined as a cognitive process in the absence of conscious attention (Dijksterhuis & Nordgren, 2006). It is different from snap judgments in that unconscious thought requires time, whereas snap judgments do not. In a typical unconscious thought experiment, participants are given information about a decision problem. Some participants are asked to think consciously about the information, whereas others are given a distraction task (and presumably engage in unconscious thought). The common finding is that unconscious thought leads to better decisions (Bos, Dijksterhuis, & Van Baaren, 2008; Dijksterhuis, 2004; Dijksterhuis, Bos, Nordgren, & Van Baaren, 2006c; Dijksterhuis et al., 2009; Dijksterhuis & Meurs, 2006; Ham, Van den Bos, & Van Doorn, 2009; Lerouge, 2009). However, not all researchers find clear benefits for unconscious thought. Some research points to a benefit for conscious thought under certain circumstances (e.g., when a decision is not complex), whereas other researchers fail to find a difference between conscious and unconscious thought (Newell, Wong, Cheung, & Rakow, 2009; Payne, Samper, Bettman, & Luce, 2008; see also Bekker, 2006; Shanks, 2006; but see Dijksterhuis, Bos, Nordgren, & Van Baaren, 2006a, 2006b). A recent meta-analysis of more than 80 studies, however, indicates that, overall, there is a benefit for unconscious thought in decision making, although the overall effect size is small (for more information, see Strick et al., 2011).

Unconscious Thought in Decision Making

Let us review some studies showing that unconscious thought can help in decision making. To what extent can we make decisions that are in line with our own, personal preferences, without the burden of limited self-knowledge? Can we automatically apply our own personal weighting scheme without intervention of conscious thought, with its limited capacity?

A study by Dijksterhuis and Van Olden (2006) replicated and extended the Wilson and colleagues' (1993) poster study. Participants in this study chose a poster (out of five) to take home under one of three different conditions. They chose after looking at the posters briefly, or after looking at them and then thinking about them for 9 minutes, or after a 9-minute distraction task following a brief look. That is, people chose immediately, after conscious thought, or after unconscious thought. Participants took their chosen poster home and were called after a few weeks. Participants who had thought unconsciously indicated that they were happier with their poster than participants in the other two conditions. In addition, when asked for what amount of money they would be willing to sell their poster, unconscious thinkers indicated a sum twice as high as that of conscious thinkers (Dijksterhuis & Van Olden, 2006).

Weighting relevant aspects correctly is important when making a decision. In a series of studies we showed that unconscious thought helps with weighting the importance of attributes (Bos, Dijksterhuis, & Van Baaren, 2011). Participants were given a decision task. They were presented with the attributes of four cars that were described by either a lot of positive but unimportant aspects and a few negative but important aspects ("frequency cars") or by a few positive but important aspects and a lot of negative but unimportant aspects ("quality cars"). Compared to participants deciding immediately, participated who were first distracted before making a choice (the unconscious thinkers) showed a stronger preference for the quality cars. It seems that, at an unconscious level, we do know what is important when making a decision. Unconscious thought indeed evokes an automatic weighting process (Bos et al., 2011), which helps when making a decision when there is one normatively best option. But is there also a benefit for unconscious thought when making a subjective decision?

The art poster study (Wilson et al., 1993) we described, in which thinkers were more satisfied with their decisions after unconscious thought, may be seen as an answer to this question. In another study (Dijksterhuis, 2004), participants were asked to decide among three roommates. All roommates were described on 12 dimensions. Participants' preference for each roommate was measured, as well as their rating for each of the 12 dimensions. Correlations were calculated between participants' preference for each of the roommates and what would be predicted from their subjective perspective, based on their ratings of the 12 dimensions (it may strike the reader as strange to rely on participants' personal ratings after we have argued that people are not good at consciously evaluating the relative importance of attributes. In this decision problem, the attributes were constructed to be as independent as possible. And, regretfully, it's the best we have). Conscious thinkers did not show a significant correlation between their preference in the decision task and what they indicated were important dimensions when choosing a roommate. Unconscious thinkers, however, did show such a correlation, indicating that after unconscious thought, choices were in line with their subjective preferences and their personal weighting scheme.

Do we need more self-knowledge to make good decisions? The answer is: not really. Although it is a tempting idea, the problem is not just the amount of self-knowledge we have. The problem is that not all information that is important for a decision can be weighted by our conscious mind. One reason is that we cannot verbalize all information that is important. Another reason is that consciously we do not have the capacity to weight all information, even if we could know everything about what we find important.

How to decide between blond and brunette? A choice like this is complicated. What will our friends think? How quickly will we get bored by one or the other? It seems that, unconsciously, we have better access to what is important to us. Thinking unconsciously can often lead to more optimal choices from a normative perspective (e.g. Bos et al., 2008, 2011; Dijksterhuis, 2004; Dijksterhuis et al., 2006c; but see Acker, 2008; Gonzalez-Vallejo, Lassiter, Belezza, & Lindberg, 2008; Lassiter, Lindberg, Gonzalez-Vallejo, Belleza, & Phillips, 2009; Newell, Wong, Cheung, & Rakow, 2009), but more importantly, thinking unconsciously can lead to more optimal decisions from a subjective perspective, in that it leads to more satisfaction (Dijksterhuis, 2004; Dijksterhuis et al., 2006c; Dijksterhuis & Van Olden, 2006). To come to good decisions, what we need is not more self-knowledge. Well, maybe one very simple piece of self-knowledge: To know that when we have a complex decision to make, we do not have to rely on conscious thought. What we need is to encode all information about a decision problem we face and then trust our unconscious to make a good decision (and always choose brunette).

REFERENCES

Acker, F. (2008). New findings on unconscious versus conscious thought in decision making: Additional empirical data and meta-analysis. *Judgment and Decision Making, 3,* 292–303.

Ariely, D., & Loewenstein, G. (2006). The heat of the moment: The effect of sexual arousal on sexual decision making. *Journal of Behavioral Decision Making, 19,* 87–98.

Arkes, H. R., Dawes, R. M., & Christensen, C. (1986). Factors influencing the use of a decision rule in a probabilistic task. *Organizational Behavior and Human Decision Processing, 37,* 93–110.

Baron, J. (2000). *Thinking and deciding* (3rd ed.). New York: Cambridge University Press.

Bekker, H. L. (2006). Making choices without deliberating. *Science, 312,* 1472.

Bettman, J. R., Luce, M. F., & Payne, J. W. (1998). Constructive consumer choice processes. *Journal of Consumer Research, 25,* 187–217.

Bos, M. W., & Dijksterhuis, A. (2011). Unconscious thought works bottom-up and conscious thought works top-down when forming an impression. *Social Cognition, 29*(6), 727–737.

Bos, M. W., Dijksterhuis, A., & Van Baaren, R. B. (2008). On the goal-dependency of unconscious thought. *Journal of Experimental Social Psychology, 44,* 1114–1120.

Bos, M. W., Dijksterhuis, A., & Van Baaren, R. B. (2011). The benefits of "sleeping on things": Unconscious thought leads to automatic weighting. *Journal of Consumer Psychology, 21,* 4–8.

Combs, B., & Slovic, P. (1979). Newpaper coverage of causes of death. *Journalism Quarterly, 56*(4), 837–843.

Damasio, A. R. (1994). *Descartes error: Emotion, reason and the human brain.* New York: Putnam.

Dawes, R. M. (1979). The robust beauty of improper linear models in decision making. *American Psychologist, 34,* 571–582.

Descartes, R. (1664). Cogito ergo sum. *Philosophica Naturalis, 10,* 150–151.

Dijksterhuis, A. (2003). *Conscious thought and the availability heuristic.* Unpublished dataset, Radboud University, Nijmegen.

Dijksterhuis, A. (2004). Think different: The merits of unconscious thought in preference development and decision making. *Journal of Personality and Social Psychology, 87,* 586–598.

Dijksterhuis, A., Bos, M. W., Nordgren, L. F., & Van Baaren, R. B. (2006a). Complex choices better made unconsciously? *Science, 313,* 760–761.

Dijksterhuis, A., Bos, M. W., Nordgren, L. F., & Van Baaren, R. B. (2006b). Making choices without deliberating. *Science, 312,* 1472.

Dijksterhuis, A., Bos, M. W., Nordgren, L. F., & Van Baaren, R. B. (2006c). On making the right choice: The deliberation-without-attention effect. *Science, 311,* 1005–1007.

Dijksterhuis, A., Bos, M. W., Van der Leij, A., & Van Baaren, R. B. (2009). Predicting soccer matches after unconscious and conscious thought as a function of expertise. *Psychological Science, 20*(11), 1381–1387.

Dijksterhuis, A., & Meurs, T. (2006). Where creativity resides: The generative power of unconscious thought. *Consciousness and Cognition, 15,* 135–146.

Dijksterhuis, A., & Nordgren, L. F. (2006). A theory of unconscious thought. *Perspectives on Psychological Science, 1,* 95–109.

Dijksterhuis, A., Smith, P. K., Van Baaren, R. B., & Wigboldus, D. H. J. (2005). The unconscious consumer: Effects of environment on consumer behavior. *Journal of Consumer Psychology, 15,* 193–202.

Dijksterhuis, A., & Van Olden, Z. (2006). On the benefits of thinking unconsciously:

Unconscious thought can increase post-choice satisfaction. *Journal of Experimental Social Psychology, 42,* 627–631.

Edwards, W. (1961). Behavioral decision theory. *Annual Review of Psychology, 12,* 473–498.

Finucane, M. L., Alhakami, A., Slovic, P., & Johnson, S. M. (2000). The affect heuristic in judgments of risks and benefits. *Journal of Behavioral Decision Making, 13*(1), 1–17.

Frost, R. O., & Shows, D. L. (1993). The nature and measurement of compulsive indecisiveness. *Behaviour Research and Therapy, 31,* 683–692.

Germeijs, V., & De Boeck, P. (2002). A measurement scale for indecisiveness and its relationship to career indecision and other types of indecision. *European Journal of Psychological Assessment, 18*(2), 113–122.

Gladwell, M. (2005). *Blink: The power of thinking without thinking.* New York: Time Warner.

Gonzalez-Vallejo, C., Lassiter, G. D., Belezza, F. S., & Lindberg, M. (2008). "Save angels perhaps": A critical examination of unconscious thought theory and the deliberation-without-attention effect. *Review of General Psychology, 12*(3), 282–296.

Greenleaf, E. A., & Lehmann, D. R. (1995). Reasons for substantial delay in consumer decision making. *Journal of Consumer Research, 22*(2), 186–199.

Ham, J., Van den Bos, K., & Van Doorn, E. (2009). Lady Justice thinks unconsciously: Unconscious thought can lead to more accurate justice judgments. *Social Cognition, 27*(4), 509–521.

Igou, E. R., & Bless, H. (2007). On undesirable consequences of thinking: Framing effects as a function of substantive processing. *Journal of Behavioral Decision Making, 20*(2), 125–142.

Inbar, Y., Cone, J., & Gilovich, T. (2010). People's intuitions about intuitive insight and intuitive choice. *Journal of Personality and Social Psychology, 99*(2), 232–247.

Janis, I. L., & Mann, L. (1977). *Decision making: A psychological analysis of conflict, choice, and commitment.* New York: Free Press.

Johnson, E. J., & Payne, J. W. (1985). Effort and accuracy in choice. *Management Science, 31*(4), 395–414.

Koestler, A. (1964). *The act of creation.* New York: Macmillan.

Lassiter, G. D., Lindberg, M. J., Gonzalez-Vallejo, C., Belleza, F. S., & Phillips, N. D. (2009). The deliberation-without-attention effect: Evidence for an artifactual interpretation. *Psychological Science, 20,* 671–675.

Lerouge, D. (2009). Evaluating the benefits of distraction on product evaluations: The mindset effect. *Journal of Consumer Research, 36*(3), 367–379.

Levine, G. M., Halberstadt, J. B., & Goldstone, R. L. (1996). Reasoning and the weighting of attributes in attitude judgments. *Journal of Personality and Social Psychology, 70,* 230–240.

Loewenstein, G. (1996). Out of control: Visceral influences on behavior. *Organizational Behavior and Human Decision Processes, 65,* 272–292.

Loewenstein, G., Nagin, D., & Paternoster, R. (1997). The effect of sexual arousal on predictions of sexual forcefulness. *Journal of Crime and Delinquency, 32,* 443–473.

Newell, B. R., Wong, K. Y., Cheung, J. C. H., & Rakow, T. (2009). Think, blink or sleep on it?: The impact of modes of thought on complex decision making. *Quarterly Journal of Experimental Psychology, 62,* 707–732.

Nisbett, R. E., & Kanouse, D. (1969). Obesity, food deprivation and supermarket shopping behavior. *Journal of Personality and Social Psychology, 12,* 289–294.

Nisbett, R. E., & Wilson, T. D. (1977). Telling more than we can know: Verbal reports on mental processes. *Psychological Review, 84*(3), 231–259.

Nordgren, L. F., & Dijksterhuis, A. (2009). The devil is in the deliberation: Thinking too much reduces judgmental consistency. *Journal of Consumer Research, 36*, 39–46.

Nordgren, L. F., van der Pligt, J., & van Harreveld, F. (2006). Visceral drives in retrospect: Explanations about the inaccessible past. *Psychological Science, 17*, 636–640.

Nordgren, L. F., van der Pligt, J., & van Harreveld, F. (2007). Evaluating Eve: Visceral states influence the evaluation of impulsive behavior. *Journal of Personality and Social Psychology, 93*, 75–84.

Nordgren, L. F., Van der Pligt, J., & Van Harreveld, F. (2008). The instability of health cognitions: Visceral states influence self-efficacy and related health beliefs. *Health Psychology, 27*(6), 722–727.

Nordgren, L. F., Van der Pligt, J., & Van Harreveld, F. (2009). The restraint bias: How the illusion of self-restraint promotes impulsive behavior. *Psychological Science, 20*(12), 1523–1528.

Payne, J. W., Bettman, J. R., & Johnson, E. J. (1993). *The adaptive decision maker.* New York: Cambridge University Press.

Payne, J. W., Samper, A., Bettman, J. R., & Luce, M. F. (2008). Boundary condition on unconscious thought in complex decision making. *Psychological Science, 19*, 1118–1223.

Rassin, E., & Muris, P. (2005). To be or not to be . . . indecisive: Gender differences, correlations with obsessive–compulsive complaints, and behavioural manifestation. *Personality and Individual Differences, 38*, 1175–1181.

Ratliff, A. (1999). What is a good decision? *Effective Clinical Practice, 2*(4), 185–186.

Read, D., & van Leeuwen, B. (1998). Time and desire: The effects of anticipated and experienced hunger and delay to consumption on the choice between healthy and unhealthy snack food. *Organizational Behavior and Human Decision Processes, 76*, 189–205.

Rettinger, D. A., & Hastie, R. (2001). Content effects on decision making. *Organizational Behavior and Human Decision Processes 85*(2), 336–359.

Sayette, M. A., Loewenstein, G., Griffin, K. M., & Black, J. (2008). Exploring the cold-to-hot empathy gap in smokers. *Psychological Science, 19*, 926–932.

Schooler, J. W., Ohlsson, S., & Brooks, K. (1993). Thoughts beyond words: When language overshadows insight. *Journal of Experimental Psychology: General, 122*, 166–183.

Schwartz, B., Ward, A., Monterosso, J., Lyubomirsky, S., White, K., & Lehman, D. R. (2002). Maximizing versus satisficing: Happiness is a matter of choice. *Journal of Personality and Social Psychology, 83*(5), 1178–1197.

Shanks, D. R. (2006). Making choices without deliberating. *Science, 313*, 760–761.

Strick, M., Dijksterhuis, A., Bos, M. W., Sjoerdsma, A., Van Baaren, R. B., & Nordgren, L. F. (2011). A meta-analysis on unconscious thought effects. *Social Cognition, 29*(6), 738–762.

Swets, J. A., Dawes, R. M., Monahan, J. (2000). Psychological science can improve diagnostic decisions. *Psychological Science in the Public Interest, 1*, 1–26.

Tsiros, M., & Mittal, V. (2000). Regret: A model of its antecedents and consequences in consumer decision making. *Journal of Consumer Research, 26* (4), 401–417.

Tversky, A., & Kahneman, D. (1973). Availability: A heuristic for judging frequency and probability. *Cognitive Psychology, 5*(2), 207–232.

Tversky, A., & Kahneman, D. (1981). The framing of decisions and the psychology of choice. *Science, 211*, 453–458.

Van Boven, L., & Loewenstein, G. (2003). Social projection of transient drive states. *Personality and Social Psychology Bulletin, 29*, 1159–1168.

Van Boven, L., Loewenstein, G., & Dunning, D. (2005). The illusion of courage in social prediction: Underestimating the impact of fear of embarrassment on other people. *Organizational Behavior and Human Decision Processes, 96*, 130–141.

Webster, D., & Kruglanski, A. (1994). Individual differences in need for cognitive closure. *Journal of Personality and Social Psychology. 67*(6), 1049–1062.

Wilson, T. D. (2002). *Strangers to ourselves: Discovering the adaptive unconscious.* Cambridge, MA: Harvard University Press.

Wilson, T. D., Lisle, D., Schooler, J. W., Hodges, S. D., Klaaren, K. J., & LaFleur, S. J. (1993). Introspecting about reasons can reduce post-choice satisfaction. *Personality and Social Psychology Bulletin, 19,* 331–339.

Wilson, T. D., & Schooler, J. W. (1991). Thinking too much: Introspection can reduce the quality of preferences and decisions. *Journal of Personality and Social Psychology, 60,* 181–192.

CHAPTER 12

Knowing Our Emotions
How Do We Know What We Feel?

GERALD L. CLORE
MICHAEL D. ROBINSON

When thinking about the world, we recognize that some of our knowledge reflects belief rather than experience (e.g., that Africa is a continent). Because the self is a subjective entity, we may not recognize how beliefs contribute to what we think our experiences are. Yet self-knowledge is likely to have important blind spots. Just as with the blind spot on the retina, missing information is not perceived as missing because it is automatically "filled in" by plausible inferences.

Does the same apply to knowing our emotions? Since emotions are experienced directly, the idea that our beliefs contribute to what we think our emotions are may seem implausible. But even in the case of self-knowledge about emotion, we contend that beliefs subtly enter the picture. More specifically, people sometimes report about their feelings on the basis of beliefs about them rather than experiences of them. We review multiple phenomena consistent with this point. We then introduce an explanation, present research testing the explanation, and discuss implications for understanding how the self functions and the implications for personality–social psychology and other fields that routinely assess how people feel.

Feelings and Beliefs: Two Sources of Information about Emotion

People have both actual feelings and beliefs about their feelings. These sources of information often diverge, and in this chapter, we review research on situations in which this is the case. Specifically, we highlight conditions under which beliefs trump feelings in self-reports of emotion. An example concerns people's reports of their experiences of pleasure when driving a luxury car.

Does Luxury Deliver Pleasure?

Many people want to own luxury cars. Owning and driving such cars would presumably result in more pleasure when driving. Schwarz and Xu (2011) sought to document this belief by asking undergraduates how much they would enjoy driving a BMW (a high-priced car), a Honda Accord (a midpriced car), or a Ford Escort (a low-priced car). As might be expected, respondents expected to feel more pleasant feelings (e.g., happy, thrilled) when driving a more expensive car and more unpleasant feelings (e.g., depressed, frustrated) when driving a cheaper car. The investigators then asked members of a sample of university faculty and staff and another Web-based sample how they generally felt when driving their own cars. The cars were classified into value categories comparable to the BMW, Honda Accord, and Ford Fiesta. These results, too, suggest that there is more joy and satisfaction in driving a luxury car than an economy car, with pleasure varying linearly with the value of the car.

These results sound reasonable, but the picture changes when the reports are based on actual driving episodes. In addition to asking about their usual feelings when driving, the experimenters also asked the university faculty and staff specifically about their feelings while driving to work earlier the same day. Web respondents were asked to recall the most recent trip of 20 minutes or more in their car. They indicated the purpose of the trip and how they felt while driving. In neither dataset was there any relationship between the pleasantness of the driving experience reported and the value of the car. These results of general and specific reports thus seem to contradict each other.

The key to Schwarz and Xu's (2011) results is that people's reports of their feelings and emotions reflect whatever information is accessible at the time. And since actual subjective experience is ephemeral (Tulving, 1984), it is accessible only as current experiences or recent memories. Such experiential data are not available when reporting how one *expects* to feel or how one *usually* feels. This general conclusion about the relative accessibility of feelings and feeling-relevant beliefs turns out to be a powerful one, applying to not only the role of facts about one's car but also facts about oneself, as we see next.

Research on Emotion and Gender

Are women more emotional than men? Responses to general self-report questions about emotion consistently show that they are. Women are more likely to describe themselves as having frequent emotional reactions (Robinson & Johnson, 1997) and as being emotionally expressive (e.g., Kring, Smith, & Neale, 1994). They are more likely to see themselves as emotional individuals (Spence, Helmreich, & Stapp, 1975), to recall emotional memories more quickly and frequently (Davis, 1999), and to report experiencing emotions more intensely (Seidlitz & Diener, 1998). Women also score higher on measures of emotional awareness (Feldman Barrett, Lane, Sechrest, & Schwartz, 2000), and they report ruminating more about negative personal experiences (Nolen-Hoeksema, Parker, & Larson, 1994; Wood, Saltzberg, Neale, Stone, & Rachmiel, 1990). With respect to particular emotions, women report more shame and guilt (Tangney, 1990) and more empathy (Robinson, Robertson, & Syty, 2002), whereas men report more pride (Stapley & Haviland, 1989). Should we conclude from such highly consistent results that women are more emotional than men? Perhaps, but the evidence comes mainly from studies tapping the beliefs that men and women have about themselves, rather than from studies of current, direct experience.

More specific studies of emotion present a very different picture. Although we expect women to be more empathic than men, measurements of actual behavioral and physiological reactions of empathic distress fail to show such stereotypical differences (Eisenberg & Lennon, 1983). Indeed, men often show greater physiological reactivity to current emotional stimuli than do women (LaFrance & Banaji, 1992; Manstead, 1992).

Research has also examined the stereotype that men feel more anger and pride, and women, more guilt and sympathy (Robinson, Johnson, & Shields, 1998). Investigators have compared reports collected immediately after an emotion-inducing task, a week later, or after only imagining doing the task. The results showed that self-reports reflect the relative accessibility of experiential information. Immediately afterward, men and women look the same; a week later they look different. Gender differences also emerged when respondents merely imagined how they would feel. So men's and women's emotions appeared to differ only when actual experiences were relatively inaccessible (a week later) or completely inaccessible (when imagining feelings). More generally, studies show gender differences in emotion mainly in verbal reports as opposed to other measures (LaFrance & Banaji, 1992), in retrospective as opposed to current reports (Shields, 1991), and in answers to general rather than specific questions (Eisenberg & Lennon, 1983). Global self-reports show large gender differences in emotionality, emotional intensity, openness to emotion, anxiety, and interpersonal warmth (Feldman Barrett, Robin, Pietromonaco, & Eyssell, 1998), but daily reports right after emotional events show no gender differences at all.

Other Individual Differences

Studies have also examined other individual differences by comparing online and retrospective reports. The general conclusion is that retrospective reports appear to be contaminated by beliefs about the self relative to *actual* experiences in everyday life. For example, Larsen (1992) found that the trait of neuroticism predicted retrospective reports of somatic distress to a greater extent than online reports of somatic distress. Feldman Barrett (1997) found that neuroticism predicted retrospective reports of negative emotion to a greater extent than experience-sampled reports of negative emotion. Oishi (2002) found that Asian Americans reported less positive emotion than European Americans in retrospective reports but not in online reports. Other findings of this type may be cited (Robinson & Clore, 2002a), but they converge on similar conclusions.

Recently, clinical psychologists have also become interested in such dissociations. In an empirical review, Strauss and Gold (2011) examined the idea that people with schizophrenia are emotionally *anhedonic*—that is, deficient in their emotional reactions. They found that this appeared to be true when research designs asked people with schizophrenia to report retrospectively on their emotions, to report their emotions in trait terms, or to report their emotions in response to hypothetical scenarios. Yet this apparent deficiency in emotional reactivity was largely if not completely absent in studies in which people with schizophrenia were asked to report their momentary emotional experiences. The authors thus questioned the widespread view that schizophrenia is *actually* associated with anhedonia.

Further Considerations

People seem to possess some beliefs about their happiness that are not supported by empirical research. For example, people say when asked that they would be happier if they lived in states associated with mild climates (e.g., California) relative to colder climates (e.g., the Midwest). Participants reported that they would, but in fact life satisfaction does not vary as a function of such climates (Schkade & Kahneman, 1998). In another study, individuals were asked to report how happy they would be (prospective reports), were (online reports), and had been (retrospective reports) when on vacations (Mitchell, Thompson, Peterson, & Cronk, 1997). It was quite clear that vacations were less pleasant when actually experienced than beforehand, when the vacation was anticipated or when reports were retrospective. Similar dissociations have been reported in the affective forecasting literature (Wilson & Gilbert, 2005).

As is well known, Bartlett (1932) suggested that memory is reconstructive. With the passage of time, a shift from relatively veridical memories to relatively schematic or stereotypical ones can be observed. Recent cognitive literatures have converged on Bartlett's insights. After trying for many years to bypass general knowledge structures in characterizing memory, investigators were forced to admit defeat (McClelland, McNaughton, & O'Reilly, 1995). They came to the conclusion that there are two memory systems, one centered in the hippocampus and another in the prefrontal cortex. The hippocampal memory system is good at storing recent experiences, but poor in characterizing long-term trends in experience. The prefrontal cortex memory system has the opposite set of characteristics (e.g., it is slow to update). The schematic "fill-in" processes posited by Bartlett have been documented in recent neuroimaging studies (e.g., Smith & Muckli, 2010). In relation to such findings, we suggest, it may be naive to assume that self-reports of emotion over long time frames or "in general" are veridical. It is quite likely that they are not.

An Accessibility Model of Emotion Reporting

Robinson and Clore (2002a) reviewed multiple literatures and suggested that they seemed to converge on a simple accessibility model. To the extent that individuals are asked to report on concurrent reactions, their emotion reports are likely based on experiential sources of knowledge (i.e., *feelings*). On the other hand, to the extent that individuals are asked to report on feelings that are not concurrent (e.g., in relation to trait, hypothetical, prospective, or retrospective reports), their emotion reports are likely to be more driven by *beliefs* about their feelings. The model is parsimonious in highlighting these two influences (see Figure 12.1). Beliefs about emotion come from three primary sources:

```
┌─────────┐
│ Belief  │──┐
└─────────┘  │   ┌─────────┐
             ├──▶│ Report  │
┌─────────┐  │   └─────────┘
│Experience│─┘
└─────────┘
```

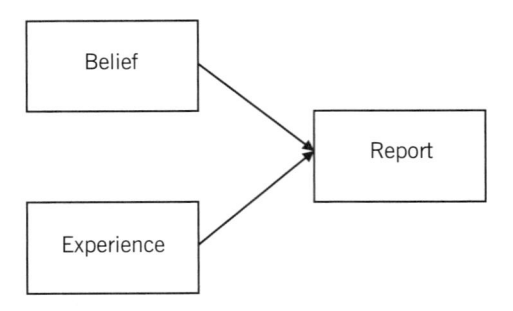

FIGURE 12.1. Two broad influences on emotion reports.

- Beliefs about the influence of particular situations (e.g., insults are angering, birthdays are happy)
- Generalized beliefs about the self (e.g., as captured by trait measures of extraversion or neuroticism)
- Social stereotypes incorporated into the self-concept (e.g., women are emotional)

The model can be further described in terms of three principles, as defined in Table 12.1. The first principle is that emotion reports tend to be made on the basis of the most accessible source of information. The second is that when multiple sources of information are accessible, the most specific source of information will be accorded more weight. Thus, individuals should generally prefer to base their reports on feelings rather than beliefs about feelings, and prefer more specific beliefs (e.g., about the influence of situations) to more generalized beliefs (e.g., about group membership). The third principle is that experience is transitory and fleeting; thus, this source of information—although preferred—is often not available.

This account makes assumptions consistent with "race" models, which have figured prominently in cognitive psychology (e.g., Logan, 2002). The fastest retrieved information tends to win, just as on television game shows (e.g., *Jeopardy*) in which the fastest contestant wins the round. Emotion reports, from this perspective, are not typically based on a careful calculus of all sources of information, but are rather based on a source of information readily retrieved that seems sufficient for making the judgment. We revisit such race model considerations later in this chapter.

TABLE 12.1. The Model's Three Principles

- *Relative accessibility*—The relative accessibility of sources of information will determine their influence on self-reports of emotion.
- *Dominance*—When multiple sources of information are equally accessible, more specific sources of information dominate.
- *Evanescence*—Feelings are transitory and cannot be stored in memory, at least not in a manner available for intentional recall.

Explanatory Value of the Model

We suggest that the findings of Schwarz and Xu (2011) represent a classic case in which situation-specific beliefs (i.e., that driving a luxury car will bring pleasure) are apparently erroneous when actual experiences are assessed. In the latter case, feelings are multiply determined and likely to be based on more pertinent factors (e.g., purpose of the trip) rather than the car one is driving. We interpret the dissociations concerning the pleasure of living in warm climates (Schkade & Kahneman, 1998), the enjoyment of vacations (Mitchell et al., 1997, and affective forecasts (Wilson & Gilbert, 2005) in a similar manner.

The model further suggests that generalized beliefs about the self are likely to be more influential in retrospective reports than in online reports. A number of studies have confirmed this point. For example, individual differences in neuroticism can be defined in terms of beliefs concerning one's negative emotionality (Robinson & Sedikides, 2009). It is thus telling that studies have shown that neuroticism is a better predictor of retrospective distress reports than online reports of distress (Feldman Barrett, 1997; Brown & Moskowitz, 2007; Larsen, 1992). Furthermore, it appears that neuroticism is a weak predictor of disease states and a much stronger predictor of self-reported somatic complaints, likely reflecting belief-driven biases associated with this trait (Watson & Pennebaker, 1989).

The model finally suggests that some group-based stereotypes of emotion may be exaggerated at best and false at worst. The findings reviewed in relation to sex differences in emotion (e.g., Feldman Barrett et al., 1998) and cultural differences in emotion (e.g., Oishi, 2002) are consistent with this point. Again, people live their lives not as stereotypical creatures, but as real human beings whose feelings are much more contextual in nature than can be appreciated on the basis of retrospective or trait reports of emotion.

Tests of the Model

As indicated earlier, a review of the multiple sources of cognitive data (McClelland et al., 1995) pointed to two memory systems in the brain—one that preserves episodic details (the hippocampus) and another that does not (the prefrontal cortex). Furthermore, biological sources of data suggest that the episodic memory system preserves episodic memories for approximately 2 weeks. Accordingly, time frames shorter than 2 weeks should be associated with attempts to recall feelings, but time frames longer than 2 weeks should result in more belief-driven reporting.

To test this idea, we asked people to report on their emotions over seven time frames—right now, last few hours, last few days, last few weeks, last few months, last few years, and in general (Robinson & Clore, 2002b). The first of three studies found that longer time frames were associated with longer latencies of emotion reporting, but only up to the time frame "last few weeks" (see top panel, Figure 12.2). Study 2 found that time frames longer than the last few weeks were associated with significant trial-to-trial priming effects, whereas this was not true for time frames shorter than the last few weeks (see bottom panel, Figure 12.2). Thus, retrieving general semantic knowledge about feelings on one trial facilitates responses on the next trial if it draws on the same semantic knowledge. Such cognitive sources of data are

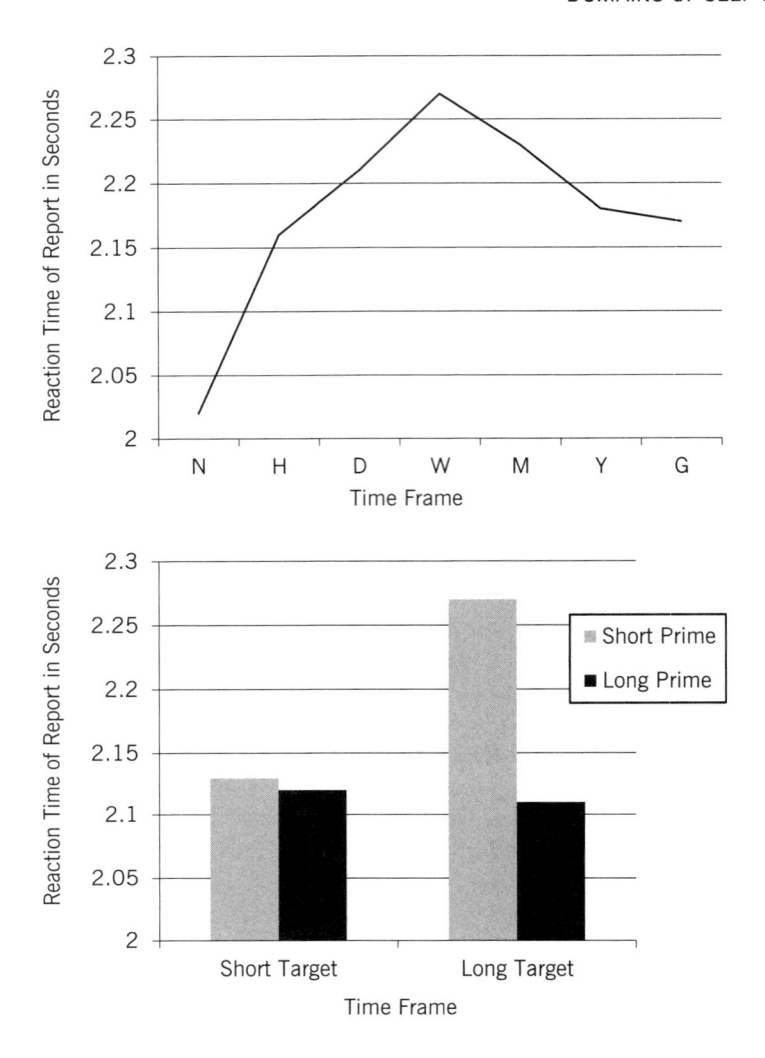

FIGURE 12.2. *Top panel:* Emotion report reaction times by time frame (N = right now; H = last few hours; D = last few days; W = last few weeks; M = last few months; Y = last few years; G = in general). *Bottom panel:* Trial-to-trial priming effects as a function of time frame (short = N, H, and D; long = M, Y, and G; target = trial N; prime = trial N–1).

important in that they suggest that individuals typically abandon attempts to retrieve experiential information when asked to report on their emotions over time frames longer than the last few weeks.

The model suggests that reports of emotion over long time frames, but not short time frames, should be assimilated to accessible beliefs. To test this prediction, Study 3 of Robinson and Clore (2002b) primed gender stereotypes by randomly assigning some individuals to think about how they are different from members of the opposite sex. The other condition was a control condition. As hypothesized, the priming manipulation led women to report that they were more emotional (i.e., to report higher ratings of emotionality) than men, but only for time frames longer than the "last few weeks." Accessible beliefs about emotion, thus, trump actual emotional experience when reporting over longer time frames, but they are apparently discounted when reporting emotions over shorter time frames. The beliefs are discounted in the short time frames because more relevant sources of experiential information (i.e., feelings) are easily accessible. Strictly speaking, our model (Robinson & Clore, 2002a) assumes that experiences are quite momentary and transitory in nature (see Table 12.1). However, the brain does tend to preserve a record of recent encounters for approximately 2 weeks (McClelland et al., 1995). We emphasize that such records are memories, not experiences, and may thus be susceptible to shorter-term episodic memory biases of the sort emphasized by Kahneman (1999). Of more importance to our model, retrieving such records should be somewhat effortful in nature. Accordingly, to the extent that effortful retrieval is disrupted, even shorter-term belief driven biases may be evident.

Three studies examined this prediction (Van Boven & Robinson, 2012). In each experiment, individuals were exposed to emotion inductions (e.g., film clips) lasting about 5 minutes. After distracter tasks, they were asked to recall their emotional reactions to the emotion inductions approximately 20 minutes later. To disrupt episodic retrieval, individuals in all studies were randomly assigned to rehearse and memorize low-load (e.g., BBBBB) versus high-load (e.g., GTPWL) letter strings while recalling their earlier emotional reactions.

The first study found that women reported stronger emotional reactions than men, particularly in the high-load condition. Such findings are consistent with predictions of the accessibility model (Robinson & Clore, 2002a) that disrupting episodic retrieval processes should result in more belief-driven, gender-stereotypical emotional recall. Study 2 replicated Study 1 and found that women were more likely to exaggerate their prior reactivity, consistent with gender stereotypes. Study 3 primed such stereotypes, in addition to manipulating cognitive load, and found that both caused women to report more intense emotional reactions than they otherwise would have. From their results, the authors concluded that even short-term, episodic memories of emotions can be biased in a belief-driven direction when being cognitively busy hampers efforts at episodic retrieval (Van Boven & Robinson, 2012).

Extensions

The phenomenon of self-stereotyping has been a neglected topic relative to other-stereotyping. We hope that the experimental manipulations highlighted earlier may provide a road map for future studies; that is, self-stereotyping should be particularly evident for time frames longer than the last few weeks (Robinson & Clore, 2002a, Study 1). In addition, self-stereotypes can be primed (Robinson & Clore, 2002a, Study 3), and self-stereotyping increases under cognitive load (Van Boven & Robinson, 2012). We expect such experimental manipulations to be useful in understanding self-stereotyping as a function of situation-specific beliefs and individual differences due to personality, mental health diagnoses, and cultural identities.

In our own work, we became interested in the relevance of the two-process model for understanding personality processes. Personality trait measures, we contend, assess generalized beliefs about the self. Furthermore, according to our two-process reporting model, such beliefs about the self are more likely to affect emotion (and symptom) reporting to the extent that episodic (event-specific) information is relatively inaccessible. Moderators of trait–state relations have often been proposed, but not with respect to the roles of the two processes of concern in our two-process model. But, the logic of the model implies that some individuals may be much more "traited" than others.

Basic choice reaction time tasks assess the speed with which particular cognitive events are recognized and accorded meaning (Sanders, 1998). Of importance for our purposes, there are pronounced individual differences in reaction time (Jensen, 1993) that, we suggest, tap a basic skill in ascribing meaning to events as they occur. Slow categorizers are those who display difficulties in assigning meaning to stimuli in our choice reaction tasks. To the extent that they have the same difficulties in assigning meaning to the transitory events in their lives, they may be more likely to fall back on trait self-knowledge when reporting on their experiences. A series of studies has examined this idea.

In one series of four studies, we (Robinson & Clore, 2007) examined relations between trait assessments of neuroticism and somatic symptom reports. It is widely thought that the relation between neuroticism and somatic symptoms is belief-driven (Watson & Pennebaker, 1989). In these studies, participants reported on their levels of neuroticism and completed several different choice reaction time tasks. Thus, a large number of objects were categorized as me (e.g., *self*) versus not me (e.g., *them*), feminine (e.g., *gentle*) versus masculine (e.g., *rational*), vegetable (e.g., *broccoli*) versus fruit (e.g., *peach*), unpleasant (e.g., *dirt*) versus pleasant (e.g., *smile*), and so on. There was a great deal of individual variability in reaction times, but the reliability of the reaction times across items was very high in each study (average $\alpha = .90$). The same individuals also reported on their somatic symptoms (experiences of aches, pains, breathing difficulties, dizziness, etc.).

In three studies (Robinson & Clore, 2007), individual differences in categorization speed moderated relations between neuroticism (the belief measure) and somatic symptom reports. The fourth study focused on daily neurotic behaviors instead. In all cases, the results were the same. Among fast categorizers (−1 *SD* below the RT mean), neuroticism did not predict such outcomes. Among slow categorizers (+1 *SD* above the RT mean), neuroticism was a strong predictor of such outcomes. A representative result is shown in the top panel of Figure 12.3. Such results are important to the personality literature, and they are novel in suggesting that personality traits may be more consequential for some individuals (i.e., those slow to assign meaning to events as they occur) relative to others (i.e., those fast to assign meaning to events as they occur).

Another related project concerned not neuroticism but extraversion. In general, higher extraversion scores are correlated with greater life satisfaction and happiness, though such relations are moderate (Diener, Suh, Lucas, & Smith, 1999). To see whether our model might shed some light on this relationship, three studies were conducted (Robinson & Oishi, 2006). The studies assessed generalized beliefs about the self with respect to extraversion by giving a standard extraversion scale and also assessed individual differences in categorization speed, which were again pronounced. In all three studies, the relationship between extraversion and life satisfaction or happiness was stronger among slow categorizers than fast categorizers.

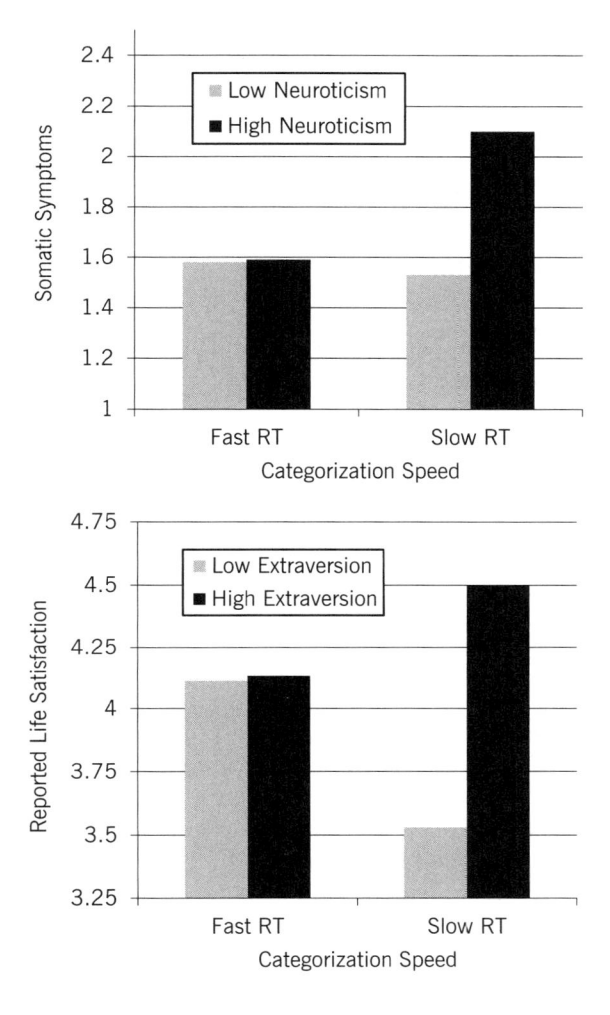

FIGURE 12.3. *Top panel:* Somatic symptom reports as a function of neuroticism and categorization speed. *Bottom panel:* Life satisfaction as a function of extraversion and categorization speed.

Furthermore, among fast categorizers (–1 *SD* below the RT mean), there was no relationship between individual differences in extraversion and life satisfaction. The bottom panel of Figure 12.3 reports a representative result from this series of studies.

The findings of these two sets of studies (Robinson & Clore, 2007; Robinson & Oishi, 2006) are unique, but conceptual parallels can be found in other recent literature. Whether because they are neurotic, worried, or depressed, it is clear that some individuals, relative to others, are much more prone to states of distress in everyday life (Widiger, Verheul, & van den Brink, 1999). Such distress proneness is more consequential to the extent that the individual is "mindless" (i.e., less attuned to present-moment reality) (Fetterman, Robinson, Ode, & Gordon, 2010; Fetterman & Robinson, 2010). Furthermore, the clinical literature has shown that constructs defined in terms of disengagement from present moments of experience—such as experimental avoidance (Hayes, 2004), rumination (Nolen-Hoeksema, 1991), worry

(Borkovec & Sharpless, 2004), and overgeneral autobiographical memory (Healey & Williams, 1999)—exacerbate distress among distress prone individuals. Finally, the clinical literature has shown several times now that mindfulness meditation practices, which train individuals to attend to present-moment experiences, are therapeutic for distress-prone individuals (e.g., Teasdale et al., 2000).

Other Roles for Emotion Beliefs

In this chapter, we have implied that reliance on belief is a shortcoming, a symptom that a person is cognitively and emotionally challenged. We noted that when experiential information is inaccessible, emotional experiences reflect situational and self-beliefs rather than actual experiences. But before concluding, we should note that beliefs about emotion can also play more constructive roles. We discuss two such roles.

Once activated, a stereotypical self-belief might inspire or motivate belief-consistent behavior. This possibility is illustrated in a study of empathic accuracy (Hodges & Klein, 2001). Men and women were initially given a self-report measure of empathic concern and then attempted to infer accurately what a target was thinking or feeling. After this stereotypical gender concern had been activated by the questionnaire, women outperformed men on the empathic accuracy task. But when that concern had not first been cued by the questionnaire, men and women were equally accurate. The belief that women are more empathic, then, may not only contaminate reports of actual empathic feeling but also motivate empathic concern. Thus, in addition to serving a fill-in role when feelings are not accessible, self-stereotyping might also motivate belief-consistent behavior to create a self-fulfilling prophecy.

Another positive role played by emotion beliefs might be to provide coherence to otherwise discrete events. We discussed how people asked about their vacations before or afterward give more glowing accounts than if asked during their vacations (Mitchell et al., 1997). Because online experiences are relatively inaccessible afterward and completely inaccessible beforehand, people necessarily draw on beliefs about vacations, and about their vacation in particular. Such general beliefs are a poor proxy for actual experience because they may have little basis in experience and because they cannot be responsive to the variation inherent in experience.

Similar concerns led Kahneman (1999) to criticize research that asks general questions about subjective well-being because he assumed that people's answers would be biased by the intrusion of their beliefs. He proposed instead a program of research on what he called "objective well-being," which would sample online experiences. He reasoned that a better estimate of one's true well-being would be provided by assessments over time of momentary feelings. His proposal has not been widely accepted, and perhaps for good reason.

The problem is that, in addition to playing a fill-in role (which is what we have emphasized), beliefs also frame and give meaning to online experience. The idea that the value of a vacation, for example, should be reduced to the sum of vacationers' responses to assessments of momentary feelings during their vacation is, we think, likely to throw the baby out with the bath water. A person with a lifelong dream to see the Eiffel Tower, for example, despite moments of distress at the crowds, the expense, and the effort required, is nevertheless likely to be pleased at having traveled to see it. Moreover, it seems unlikely that, if Kahneman confronted vacationers with the various ratings of negative affect they had given along the way, they would decide that their vacation had been a mistake. The point is that when framed as part of the task of reaching a goal, various aspects of the trip may become meaningful parts of the whole in a way that would not be captured by adding up the affective reactions to each part. Thus, neither Kahneman nor the rest of us are likely to stop taking vacations after reading the vacation diary study. Why? Because our general beliefs not only fill-in for feelings but they also organize and give meaning and value to them. Psychologists have long had a bottom-up bias in their accounts of behavior, but phenomena of psychological interest are rarely well captured by the sum of their parts. We suggest, then, that beliefs about our experiences, while they can be problematic when masquerading *as* experiences, also play other important roles, one of which is that beliefs provide the glue that makes experiences something more.

Discussion

The editors posed several excellent questions for authors. Although we discussed preliminary answers to such questions earlier, we deemed it useful to address them more directly in our discussion section:

1. *What do people know about themselves, and what are the limits of self-knowledge in this area of research?* There are two emotional selves: one that exists in the moment, and another that exists as a set of beliefs about one's emotions. These two emotional selves sometimes appear to be dissociated, so that reports of experience based on the kinds of self-views captured on self-report personality scales may not coincide with actual experience (Robinson & Clore, 2002a).

2. *Why do these limits exist?* These limits exist because experiences are transitory in nature. By contrast, beliefs about emotion are quite stable because they are central to how individuals conceptualize the self in general (Robinson & Clore, 2002a). For this reason retrospective and trait-based reports of emotion, while they may be either accurate or inaccurate in themselves, may fail to capture life as it is lived (Conner, Tennen, Fleeson, & Feldman Barrett, 2009).

3. *What are the implications of this presence or lack of self-knowledge?* A primary implication is that when people answer questions about their emotions to themselves or others, it may be unclear when beliefs are filling in for actual experience. Thus, for example, people who believe themselves to be thoughtful may fail to see occasions of their thoughtlessness, or people who think of themselves as socially anxious may fail to note experiences of their own social grace. Such beliefs may be consequential, leading to poor decision making. Thus, some individuals may be more "traited" than others to the extent that they have difficulty assigning meaning to events quickly, as they occur, and rely on more general self-beliefs.

4. *How can self-knowledge in this area be improved?* It can be improved to the extent that individuals attend to events as they occur. Doing so allows lives to be lived in more nuanced and state-dependent terms (Robinson & Clore, 2007; Robinson & Oishi, 2006). In confirmation of this point, several treatment literatures have shown

that mindfulness training mitigates the distress of distress-prone individuals (Hayes, 2004), helping them focus on current experience rather than living in the future, in the past, or in an unchanging personal narrative.

5. What are the methodological issues of measuring self-knowledge in this area of research? The major implication of our model is that trait and retrospective reports of emotion should *not* automatically be viewed as veridical. Rather, our model encourages more state-related assessments of the individual, such as those seen in experience-sampling studies (Connor et al., 2009). We do not suggest that momentary assessments of emotion can replace trait assessments of personality, but we contend that it is important to recognize that trait and state assessments are not interchangeable and likely reflect different sources of self-knowledge.

ACKNOWLEDGMENTS

Support is acknowledged from National Institute of Mental Health Grant No. MH 50074 to Gerald L. Clore and National Science Foundation Grant No. BCS 0843982 to Michael D. Robinson.

REFERENCES

Bartlett, F. C. (1932). *Remembering: A study in experimental and social psychology*. Cambridge, UK: Cambridge University Press.

Borkovec, T. D., & Sharpless, B. (2004). Generalized anxiety disorder: Bringing cognitive behavioral therapy into the valued present. In S. C. Hayes, V. M. Follette, & M. M. Linehan (Eds.), *Mindfulness and acceptance: Expanding cognitive-behavioral tradition* (pp. 209–242). New York: Guilford Press.

Brown, K. W., & Moskowitz, D. S. (1997). Does unhappiness make you sick?: The role of affect and neuroticism in the experience of common physical symptoms. *Journal of Personality and Social Psychology, 72*, 907–917.

Conner, T. S., Tennen, H., Fleeson, W., & Feldman Barrett, L. (2009). Experience sampling methods: A modern idiographic approach to personality research. *Social and Personality Psychology Compass, 3*, 1–22.

Davis, P. J. (1999). Gender differences in autobiographical memory for childhood emotional experiences. *Journal of Personality and Social Psychology, 76*, 498–510.

Diener, E., Suh, E., Lucas, R. E., & Smith, H. L. (1999). Subjective well-being: three decades of progress. *Psychological Bulletin. 125*, 276–302.

Eisenberg, N., & Lennon, R. (1983). Sex differences in empathy and related constructs. *Psychological Bulletin, 94*, 100–131.

Feldman Barrett, L. (1997). The relationships among momentary emotion experience, personality descriptions, and retrospective ratings of emotion. *Personality and Social Psychology Bulletin, 23*, 1100–1110.

Feldman Barrett, L., Robin, L., Pietromonaco, P. R., & Eyssell, K. M. (1998). Are women the "more emotional" sex?: Evidence from emotional experiences in social context. *Cognition and Emotion, 12*, 555–578.

Feldman Barrett, L., Lane, R. D., Sechrest, L., & Schwartz, G. E. (2000). Sex differences in emotional awareness. *Personality and Social Psychology Bulletin, 26*, 1027–1035.

Fetterman, A. K., & Robinson, M. D. (2010). Contingent self-importance among pathological narcissists: Evidence from an implicit task. *Journal of Research in Personality, 44,* 691–697.

Fetterman, A. K., Robinson, M. D., Ode, S., & Gordon, K. H. (2010). Neuroticism as a risk factor for behavioral dysregulation: A mindfulness-mediation perspective. *Journal of Social and Clinical Psychology, 29,* 301–321.

Hayes, S. C. (2004). Acceptance and commitment therapy and new behavior therapies: Mindfulness, acceptance, and relationship. In S. C. Hayes, V. M. Follette, & M. M. Linehan (Eds.), *Mindfulness and acceptance: Expanding the cognitive-behavioral tradition* (pp. 1–29). New York: Guilford Press.

Healy, H., & Williams, J. M. G. (1999). Autobiographical memory. In T. Dagleish & M. J. Power (Eds.), *Handbook of cognition and memory* (pp. 229–242). Chichester, UK: Wiley.

Hodges, S. D., & Klein, K. J. K. (2001). Regulating the costs of empathy: The price of being human. *Journal of Socio-Economics, 30,* 437–452.

Jensen, A. R. (1993). Why is reaction time correlated with psychometric g? *Current Directions in Psychological Science, 2,* 53–56.

Kahneman, D. (1999). Objective happiness. In D. Kahneman, E. Diener, & N. Schwarz (Eds.), *Well-being: The foundations of hedonic psychology* (pp. 85–105). New York: Russell Sage Foundation.

Kring, A. M., Smith, D. A., & Neale, J. M. (1994). Individual differences in dispositional expressiveness: Development and validation of the Expressiveness Scale. *Journal of Personality and Social Psychology, 66,* 934–949.

LaFrance, M., & Banaji, M. (1992). Towards a reconsideration of the gender–emotion relationship. In M. S. Clark (Ed.), *Emotion and social behavior: Vol. 14. Review of personality and social psychology* (pp. 178–201). Newbury Park, CA: Sage.

Larsen, R. J. (1992). Neuroticism and selective encoding and recall of symptoms: Evidence from a combined current–retrospective study. *Journal of Personality and Social Psychology, 62,* 480–488.

Logan, G. D. (2002). An instance theory of attention and memory. *Psychological Review, 109,* 376–400.

Manstead, A. S. R. (1992). Gender differences in emotion. In M. A. Gale & M. W. Eysenck (Eds.), *Handbook of individual differences: Biological perspectives* (pp. 355–387). Chichester, UK: Wiley.

McClelland, J. L., McNaughton, B. L., & O'Reilly, R. C. (1995). Why there are complementary learning systems in hippocampus and neocortex: Insights from the successes and failures of connectionist models of learning and memory. *Psychological Review, 102,* 419–457.

Mitchell, T. R., Thompson, L., Peterson, E., & Cronk, R. (1997). Temporal adjustments in the evaluation of events: The "rosy view." *Journal of Experimental Social Psychology, 33,* 421–448.

Nolen-Hoeksema, S. (1991). Responses to depression and their effects on the duration of depressive episodes. *Journal of Abnormal Psychology, 100,* 569–582.

Nolen-Hoeksema, S., Parker, L., & Larson, J. (1994). Ruminative coping with depressed mood following loss. *Journal of Personality and Social Psychology, 67,* 92–104.

Oishi, S. (2002). The experiencing and remembering of well-being: A cross-cultural analysis. *Personality and Social Psychology Bulletin, 28,* 1398–1406.

Robinson, M. D., & Clore, G. L. (2002a). Beliefs, situations, and their interactions: Towards a model of emotion reporting. *Psychological Bulletin, 128,* 934–960.

Robinson, M. D., & Clore, G. L. (2002b). Episodic and semantic knowledge in emotional self-report: Evidence for two judgment processes. *Journal of Personality and Social Psychology, 83,* 198–215.

Robinson, M. D., & Clore, G. L. (2007). Traits, states, and encoding speed: Support for a top-down view of neuroticism/state relations. *Journal of Personality, 75*, 95–120.

Robinson, M. D., & Johnson, J. T. (1997). Is it emotion or is it stress?: Gender stereotypes and the perception of subjective experience. *Sex Roles, 36*, 235–258.

Robinson, M. D., Johnson, J. T., & Shields, S. A. (1998). The gender heuristic and the database: Factors affecting the perception of gender related differences in the experience and display of emotions. *Basic and Applied Social Psychology, 20*, 206–219.

Robinson, M. D., & Oishi, S. (2006). Trait self-report as a "fill in" belief system: Categorization speed moderates the extraversion/life satisfaction relation. *Self and Identity, 5*, 15–34.

Robinson, M. D., Robertson, D. A., & Syty, N. A. (2002). *Personality as belief: Evidence for situation-contingent activation.* Unpublished manuscript, North Dakota State University.

Robinson, M. D., & Sedikides, C. (2009). Traits and the self: Toward an integration. In P. J. Corr & G. Matthews (Eds.), *The Cambridge handbook of personality psychology* (pp. 457–472). Cambridge, UK: Cambridge University Press.

Sanders, A. F. (1998). *Elements of human performance.* Mahwah, NJ: Erlbaum.

Schkade, D. A., & Kahneman, D. (1998). Does living in California make people happy?: A focusing illusion in judgments of life satisfaction. *Psychological Science, 9*, 340–346.

Schwarz, N., & Xu, J. (2011). Why don't we learn from poor choices?: The consistency of expectation, choice, and memory clouds the lessons of experience. *Journal of Consumer Psychology 21*, 142–145.

Seidlitz, L., & Diener, E. (1998). Sex differences in the recall of affective experiences. *Journal of Personality and Social Psychology, 74*, 262–271.

Shields, S. A. (1991). Gender in the psychology of emotion: A selective research review. In K. T. Strongman (Ed.), *International review of studies on emotion* (Vol. 1, pp. 227–245). New York: Wiley.

Smith, F. W., & Muckli, L. (2010). Nonstimulated early visual areas carry information about surrounding context. *Proceedings of the National Academy of Sciences USA, 107*(46), 20099–20103.

Spence, J. T., Helmreich, R., & Stapp, J. (1975). Ratings of self and peers on sex role attributes and their relation to self-esteem and conceptions of masculinity and femininity. *Journal of Personality and Social Psychology, 32*, 29–39.

Stapley, J. C., & Haviland, J. M. (1989). Beyond depression: Gender differences in normal adolescents' emotional experiences. *Sex Roles, 20*, 295–308.

Strauss, G. P., & Gold, J. M. (2011). *A new perspective on anhedonia in schizophrenia: The accessibility model of emotional self-report explains the discrepancy among different methods of measurement.* Unpublished manuscript, University of Maryland School of Medicine.

Tangney, J. P. (1990). Assessing individual differences in proneness to shame and guilt: Development of the Self-Conscious Affect and Attribution Inventory. *Journal of Personality and Social Psychology, 59*, 102–111.

Teasdale, J. D., Segal, Z. V., Williams, J. M. G., Ridgeway, V., Soulsby, J., & Lau, M. (2000). Prevention of relapse/recurrence in major depression by mindfulness-based cognitive therapy. *Journal of Consulting and Clinical Psychology, 68*, 615–623.

Tulving, E. (1984). Précis of elements of episodic memory. *Behavioral and Brain Sciences, 7*, 223–268.

Van Boven, L., & Robinson, M. D. (2012). Boys don't cry: Cognitive busyness increases gender stereotypic emotion memory. *Journal of Experimental Social Psychology, 48*, 303–309.

Watson, D., & Pennebaker, J. W. (1989). Health complaints, stress, and disease: Exploring the central role of negative affectivity. *Psychological Review, 96,* 234–254.

Widiger, T. A., Verheul, R., & van den Brink, W. (1999). Personality and psychopathology. In L. A. Pervin & O. P. John (Eds.), *Handbook of personality psychology: Theory and research* (2nd ed., pp. 347–366). New York: Guilford Press.

Wilson, T. D., & Gilbert, D. T. (2005). Affective forecasting: Knowing what to want. *Current Directions in Psychological Science, 14,* 131–134.

Wood, W., Saltzberg, J. A., Neale, J. M., Stone, A. A., & Rachmiel, T. B. (1990). Self-focused attention, coping responses, and distressed mood in everyday life. *Journal of Personality and Social Psychology, 58,* 1027–1036.

CHAPTER 13

On (Not) Knowing and Feeling What We Want and Like

GALIT HOFREE
PIOTR WINKIELMAN

Knowing what we like and want seems an integral part of our everyday experience. We feel intimately familiar with our preferences and motivations, and view them as stable aspects of our selves. Rational theories of preferences assume that our choice behavior is coherent—reflective of the utility we will gain from the outcome of our choice (Gilboa, 2009). The same is true of classic expectancy-value theories in psychology and attributional theories of motivation (Weiner, 2012). People, more or less, desire, choose, and pursue what they (expect to) like and reasonably expect to get.

However, these assumptions fall short of explaining many curious behaviors we observe in everyday life. For example, why do we put great effort into obtaining "rewards" that we do not really enjoy all that much at the end? (Writing a chapter comes to mind.) Why is a dieter compelled to eat that chocolate cake, even after sampling it and discovering that it is not very tasty? Why do we need others (e.g., therapists) to tell us what we like and desire? Why do we buy too much on an empty stomach? Why do we fail to predict how we will feel about the hot date the next morning?

In this chapter we review research showing that we can be unaware of some of the core processes that underlie our feelings, desires, and choices. These low-level biological processes enable useful, flexible, and quick behaviors. Yet because such processes are often subconscious, they can generate preferences, desires, and behaviors that are inconsistent, or even in direct conflict with our conscious beliefs. This conflict sometimes leads to seemingly irrational behaviors, as described earlier.

In this context, we discuss evidence for situations in which core liking and wanting can be manipulated at a subconscious level, causing situations such as wanting something one doesn't really like. We also present neuroscience research supporting the distinction between wanting and liking. In addition, we review different levels on which our conscious knowledge of what we want and like can diverge from unconscious processing. We go on to examine processes underlying separation of affective and motivational systems in humans. Finally, we discuss how our subconscious wanting and liking processes influence our predictions for future behavior.

Liking and Wanting

Our world is filled with attractive objects, whether they are tasty foods, desirable mates, beautiful paintings, exotic vacations, or prestigious chapter publications. People like these things, want these things, choose them, and work for them. Yet, surprisingly, research in neuroscience shows that our motivation for obtaining such rewards, and our actual enjoyment of them, are not necessarily coupled, and can be influenced separately.

Definitions of Wanting and Liking

Let us take a closer look at the concepts of wanting and liking. The terms *wanting* and *liking* have familiar meanings in everyday language—equivalent, more or less, to the terms *conscious desire* and *conscious pleasure*. Our use of these terms corresponds to the usage common in the biopsychology literature, where they have slightly different meanings that are grounded in modern approaches to motivation.

Historically, theories of motivation postulated that behavior toward valued stimuli was driven by desires—subjectively represented need states (Hull, 1951). For example, people drink to reduce the unpleasant desire for liquid ("feeling thirsty"), and they seek mating opportunities when they experience the state of sexual desire ("feeling horny"). In contrast, modern theories of motivation posit that hedonic behavior is also determined by the stimulus's incentive value: The stimulus directly promotes approach–avoidance motivation through changes in its perceived value (Toates, 1986). Motivational states, such as thirst or sexual needs, are still important, but they work by directly influencing affective and motivational responses to the relevant features of the stimulus. This influence can be observed in a phenomenon known as *alliesthesia*—change in incentive value as a function of a relevant motivational state (Cabanac, 1971). For example, a functional value of, say, a hot drink depends on whether one just returned from the freezing cold or from a sauna. More interestingly, the very perception of how attractive and desirable something is depends on a motivational state. For example, people perceive the taste of water more favorably when they are thirsty (Rolls, Rolls, & Rowe, 1983). Interestingly, this need-based modulation of value does not require that the need (e.g., thirst) becomes conscious, suggesting that core motivational processes directly regulate perceptual salience and value. Similarly, sexual motivation can directly increase how attractive (appealing or interesting) a mate appears, without necessarily manifesting in a subjective experience of "horniness." For example, ovulatory cycle shifts women's receptivity to sexual advances, and evaluation of different kinds of mates, without manifesting as a state of desire (e.g., Gangestad, Garver-Apgar, Simpson, & Cousins, 2007).

One particularly influential modern conceptualization of liking and wanting comes from the writing of two neuroscientists—Kent Berridge and Terry Robinson

(Berridge, 1996; Berridge & Robinson, 1995). They define *wanting* as the motivation to acquire the reward driven by the incentive value that the stimulus possesses. This incentive value, its magnet-like properties, determines how hard organisms will work to obtain this reward. *Liking*, on the other hand, is the hedonic pleasure experienced when actually receiving the reward (Berridge, 1996; Winkielman & Berridge, 2003).

The distinction between liking and wanting was originally made in studies on rats. One such study examined how damage to so-called "reward" pathways influences these two processes. Interestingly, when dopamine-releasing brain areas were lesioned, rats made no efforts to acquire food readily available to them, yet they still produced negative and positive taste reactions (Berridge, Venier, & Robinson, 1989). This study suggests that while these dopaminergic brain regions are necessary for motivated appetitive behavior (wanting), they have little or no influence on liking.

Researchers have begun to explore these processes in humans. One interesting approach explores responses to beautiful faces (Aharon et al., 2001). Heterosexual males viewed both male and female faces of either high or average attractiveness. Subjects rated both beautiful male and beautiful female faces as equally attractive, or pleasant to look at, presumably reflecting equal liking. However, subjects were willing to put significantly more effort via keypress in order to view attractive female faces for a longer duration than equally attractive male faces, presumably reflecting greater wanting for attractive females. In other words, heterosexual males might "like" attractive faces in general, hence rating them similarly, yet beautiful female faces represent a higher incentive for heterosexual males, and are therefore "wanted" more than male faces, which do not present any such incentives.

Dissociation of Wanting from Liking: The Incentive Salience Hypothesis

The example of beautiful faces illustrates that sometimes an object (e.g., a male face for heterosexual males) may be liked without being really wanted. This situation represents a mild form of liking–wanting dissociation. But can we find stronger examples? Furthermore, can such dissociations go in the opposite direction—wanting without liking? Recall the example of a dieter confronted with a piece of chocolate cake that she consumes but does not enjoy. There are many such cases where wanting appears to exceed liking, to the point that sometimes people crave and put serious effort to pursue things they don't savor to the same extent. An extreme case of this is addiction.

Drug addiction causes people to behave in ways that are detrimental to their health, work, and social relations. Furthermore, addicts spent all sort of resources supporting their habit. Nevertheless, one might consider addicts' behavior to be rational by assuming that for them drugs produce such an intense hedonic experience that it is "worth their effort" (e.g., Becker & Murphy, 1988). However, through processes of drug tolerance, the drug's effect on hedonic experiences lessens over time, and addicts experience less and less pleasure when taking them. So why would they continue to sacrifice other pleasures (family, career, relationships, health) and exert great effort to obtain a drug that is not actually causing them much pleasure? One explanation of this behavior is offered by incentive sensitization theory, which posits that a combination of associative learning and neuronal sensitization processes enhance the incentive value of the drug and related cues (Berridge & Robinson, 1995; Robinson & Berridge, 1993). According to this theory, neural systems, especially within the dopaminergic pathway, that are specifically associated with wanting processes (e.g., assigning incentive value to stimuli) undergo sensitization through the repeated pairing of the drug with the positive hedonic responses. Over time, this sensitization produces an amplified response to the drug and drug-related cues, increasing their "motivational pull," wanting—hence, the behavioral effects observed in addicts. Curiously, the increase in desire for the drug does not influence liking of the drug, which actually may lessen over time (through parallel process of habituation).

Addicts are not necessarily aware of the discrepancies between the systems. An experiment by Lamb and colleagues (1991) beautifully illustrates this. In this experiment, recovering heroin addicts were given the opportunity to press a lever in order to receive an injection that contained varying doses of morphine or saline solution (a placebo). Subjects were later requested to rate the drug they received according to how much they liked it. Not surprisingly, subjects rated saline injections as worthless and quickly stopped working to receive these injections. In addition, high doses of morphine were rated as very pleasant, and addicts exerted a lot of effort in order to obtain them. Their responses to the low doses of morphine were much more intriguing. In these situations, addicts rated the injections just as worthless as those of saline solution, yet many of these addicts continued to exert the same effort (by pressing the lever) to receive the injections as they did for injections of high doses of morphine.

In addition to the dissociation between the wanting and liking system, the example of drug addiction also illustrates a somewhat counterintuitive point about motivation and the concept of "reward." Specifically, states, such as drug craving, hunger, and thirst are in some sense negative, as they are associated with deprivation and a disturbance of homeostasis. But they induce motivation through the attribution of positive value to the stimulus. The action based on this high incentive value alleviates this negative state and returns the body to homeostasis. Thus, the concept of reward encompasses both stimuli that alleviate a negative state and those that induce a positive one.

Separate Neural Systems for Wanting and Liking

As briefly indicated earlier, researchers were able to tease apart the underlying neural systems that correspond to the psychological constructs of liking and wanting. This was mostly achieved through studies conducted on rats and food rewards. The mesotelencephalic dopaminergic system has been identified as a candidate for a neural wanting system. This system includes various nuclei from the brainstem, all the way up to the frontal cortex, among which are the nucleus accumbens, amygdala, and the ventral pallidum (Berridge, 2007, 2009; Berridge & Robinson, 1998; Smith, Tindell, Aldridge, & Berridge, 2009). Lesions to these areas causes a decrease in wanting. An elevated level of activation in the wanting system can also be elicited through neurochemical manipulations (Wan & Peoples, 2008; Wyvell & Berridge, 2000).

Liking has been associated with opioid, endocanabinoid, and benzodiazepine/gamma-aminobutyric acid (GABA) neurotransmitter "hotspots" in the forebrain (Berridge, 2009; Mahler, Smith, & Berridge, 2007; Peciña, 2008). It is important to note that though these systems are separable, they usually work together closely, ensuring that liking and wanting processes coherently support goals and needs in "normal" organisms.

Psychological Factors Involved in Dissociations of Liking and Wanting

As mentioned, the function of the wanting system is to attach incentive value to stimuli. This process usually occurs through conditioning with hedonically rewarding stimuli. However, conditional learning acts not only upon the actual reward but also on a variety of stimuli associated with receiving such a reward. This raises the possibility that conditioned cues can activate wanting, even when such conditioned stimuli are no longer predictive of the reward. For example, as a treat, American parents sometimes give their children and their friends a trip to McDonald's. Later in life, when the now-adult children see a McDonald's, they may feel strong urge to eat there, although they have no expectation of being socially rewarded for it, and if they actually do it, they may not enjoy it. Indeed, research have shown that a conditioned stimulus can activate the wanting system, even when it no longer predicts the reward (Berridge, 1996).

Goal obstruction can also intensify wanting, but not liking. Interestingly, this dissociation is related to individual differences in the intensity of affective responses (Beaver et al., 2006; Cohen et al., 2005; Litt, Khan, & Shiv, 2010). One study (Litt et al., 2010) examined how being "jilted" (i.e., being thwarted from obtaining a desired outcome) can increase desire to obtain the outcome (wanting), yet also decrease the pleasure received from that outcome (liking). In the experiment, subjects were offered a specific prize for winning a game. Those in the jilted condition "lost" the game, and therefore did not receive the prize. Subjects in this condition, who scored low on the Affect Intensity Measure (AIM) scale (Larsen & Diener, 1987), were willing to pay more in order to receive this prize, yet when they actually received this prize, they were more willing to exchange it for another, similar product than those who were not jilted. One explanation for this, according to the authors, could be that wanting and liking disassociations are more prone to happen at low affect intensity, as opposed to high affect intensity. An intense reaction to a stimulus may cause wanting to go along with liking (e.g., a disgust reaction to food will severely decrease hunger reactions). On the other hand, less extreme changes in liking, such as those hypothesized to be experienced by subjects rating low on the AIM scale in the experiment, might not exert a strong enough influence on wanting processes, therefore enabling a disassociation to take place. However, further research on how these systems vary across individuals should be conducted in order to broaden our understanding of how they interact.

What Do We Know about What We Like or Want?

Conscious Components of the Process in Humans

The majority of research on the biopsychological processing that underlies wanting and liking has been carried out on animals. A question thus arises as to what role consciousness plays in these processes. Are human beings aware of their "likes and wants," their causes, their separate nature, and that these processes might not necessarily work together? Here we discuss evidence for unconscious liking and wanting by presenting research on (1) unconscious causes of hedonic states, (2) how hedonic states can themselves be unconscious, and (3) how people can be wrong about linking affective states and their causes.

Processing of Unconscious or Unattended Stimuli

We attend to a wide variety of stimuli throughout our everyday experiences, yet we are not always aware of the specific stimuli that elicit an affective response in us. Research on the influence of subliminal priming on mood and choice illustrates this point. In Zajonc's classic priming studies, subjects were requested to evaluate affectively ambiguous stimuli (such as Chinese ideographs). Unbeknownst to them, each stimulus was preceded by a subliminal presentation of either a happy or an angry face. Although they were not aware that they had seen these faces, subjects made affective judgments based on them—they preferred those stimuli preceded by happy faces more than those preceded by angry faces (Murphy & Zajonc, 1993).

Additional evidence for affective processing of stimuli that do not reach awareness is found in the remarkable case of affective blindsight. *Blindsight* is a phenomenon that occurs in people who are blind due to damage to their visual cortex. These people cannot see or describe anything presented visually to them, yet they are able to guess certain features of stimuli, such as angle or shape, above chance. Affective blindsight describes a similar phenomenon, in which cortically blind subjects were able to guess above chance whether a face presented to them was either happy or angry, although they claimed they were unable to see the face at all (de Gelder, Pourtois, van Raamsdonk, Vroomen, & Weiskrantz, 2001; Hamm et al., 2003).

These examples suggest that affective processing of stimuli may occur automatically and during early stages of perception, before people are consciously aware of the stimuli. It is therefore the case that we may at times be totally unaware of the cause of our affective responses. But what about the affective response itself?

Awareness of Affective Response

It is hard to imagine going through an emotional episode without being aware of it. Indeed, we are usually conscious of our emotions and our affective reactions to stimuli. However, hedonic processes may also be expressed in perception and behavior before they reach consciousness, or even without people ever becoming aware of them. This idea may initially sound paradoxical. After all, it suggests that there are emotions that are not being felt. However, note that the conscious analysis of emotional stimuli and the generation of conscious feelings are relatively slow and sometimes effortful processes. In contrast, much of the business of daily emotional responding to threats and dangers, as well as enticements and rewards, is done by quick, automatic affective responses. These unconscious processes might be predecessors of our more complex emotions that enable goal-directed behavior (Berridge, 1996; LeDoux, 1996).

Similar processes can be found in many animals in which conscious awareness is debatable. For example, decorticated rats can show both hedonic response to sweets and aversive response to bitter tastes (Berridge, 1996). Such reactions are also found in anencephalic babies. These babies are born with a congenital disorder in which the neural tube fails to close, so that they are missing a large portion of the brain. Importantly, these babies are missing most of their cortex and are assumed to lack consciousness. Nevertheless, they show positive facial reactions to hedonic stimuli and negative facial reactions to aversive stimuli (Steiner, 1973).

As mentioned previously, circuitry involved in reward processing involves a complex system of projections that start at the brainstem and continue to the mesolimbic areas, as well as many parts of the cortex. Wanting and liking processes interact with perception at many levels of stimuli processing. Basic affective processing precedes attention, as well as other higher-level cognitive processes, as mentioned before, and can therefore occur at a subconscious level.

Intriguing evidence for this are studies in which people are guided in their behavior by subliminal stimuli, yet do not seem to be aware of any change in their affective experience. Winkielman, Berridge, and Wilbarger (2005) conducted several studies in which subjects were presented happy, angry or sad faces subliminally, and were then requested to evaluate a novel beverage (Kool-Aid). They were requested not only to evaluate the drink but also to pour themselves as much as they wanted and drink it. The amount poured and consumed was monitored, as well as participants' initial state of thirst. Thirsty participants not only rated drinks preceded by happy faces as more appealing than those preceded by sad or angry faces but they also poured and consumed more of the beverage in these conditions. However, when requested to rate their conscious feelings toward the drinks, participants showed no difference in ratings following the differently valenced faces.

Importantly, this failure to access the underlying affective change is not due to inattention to the internal state. In fact, even when subjects are explicitly forewarned that their affect may vary as a function of a facial prime, they still fail to report changes in subjective feelings (Winkielman, Zajonc, & Schwarz, 1997). Participants also cannot access such changes in subjective feelings even when they are motivated to do so and are explicitly told that "listening to feelings" might help them succeed in a task, such as detecting the valence of subliminally presented faces (Bornemann, Winkielman, & van der Meer, in press). Critically, these failures of introspection are not due to the weakness of affective responses. In several studies, we found robust congruent facial electromyographical (EMG) responses, such as frowning in response to subliminally presented angry faces (e.g., Bornemann et al., in press). We also found emotion-congruent modulation of the postauricular startle response to the same emotional faces (Starr, Linn, & Winkielman, 2007). These findings clearly indicate the presence of an affective response on a physiological level, even if the response is not present on the phenomenological level.

Overall, these and other studies suggest that unconscious affective processes may influence our behavior. In the case of the Kool-Aid study, these effects were mostly short-lived, yet they generated a sizable difference in behavior between conditions. Interestingly, both wanting and liking were influenced by affective stimuli (i.e., ratings of taste and amount of consumption were increased for positive stimuli and decreased for negative stimuli). This suggests that both liking and wanting processes can take place without awareness.

Finally, it is worth emphasizing the limits of the notion of unconscious liking and wanting. Conceptually, it makes sense for the affective and motivational systems not only to be able to run unconsciously but also to produce conscious output, in the sense of feeling and desires. After all, consciousness allows us to go beyond simple, habitual reactions and design novel, complex, context-sensitive forms of responding (Winkielman & Schooler, 2011). Consciousness also allows control. The organism can stop undesirable responses and promote the desirable ones, deciding how and when to respond. Conscious access to feelings and desires also plays a communicative and motivational function. Thus, conscious feelings give internal feedback about how well the organism is doing with the current pursuits, telling it to maintain or change its path. More importantly, being aware of one's emotion and being able to communicate this to others seems crucial for basic social coordination. Thus, pangs of guilt propel us to make amends, whereas green eyes of jealousy alert us to trespasses of our mates (Frank, 1998). Consistent with these ideas, there are many reports in the emotion literature where "it all hangs together"—emotion is conscious and coheres with its physiological representation (e.g., Mauss, Levenson, McCarter, Wilhelm, & Gross, 2005).

Awareness of the Causal Relationship between Stimuli and Feelings

One of the central elements of any affective experience is an awareness of the object that brought it about (Clore & Huntsinger, 2009). We rarely feel "just happy"; we typically feel happy about something, and because of something. Yet the process by which we infer objects and causes of emotions is not flawless. As mentioned earlier, we might be unaware of emotionally relevant stimuli—"blaming" Kool-Aid for a negative reaction to an unconscious angry face. But even in situations in which we are fully aware of the surrounding stimuli, we might not manage to select correctly the stimulus that brought about our emotional reaction (Nisbett & Wilson, 1977). The classic demonstration comes from Dutton and Aron's study (1974). Males approached by a female interviewer while on a fear-inducing suspension bridge were more likely to call the interviewer to ask her out than those who crossed a more stable "control bridge." This "excitation transfer" presumably reflects a mistaken "use" of one's own arousal as information about the value or importance of the stimulus (Storbeck & Clore, 2008). Note, though, that it is often unclear at which level such transfer processes occur. For example, in the classic suspension bridge situation the "arousal transfer" could reflect a strategic inferential attributional process ("I am aroused. It must be her who caused it. I am in love"), in accordance with two-factor theory of emotions (Schachter & Singer, 1962). But this could also reflect a simple "incentive assignment" process by which the female research assistant actually looked "hotter" when subjects were aroused.

The best-known model that assumes strategic use of informational value of conscious affective states is the feelings-as-information hypothesis (Schwarz & Clore, 1983, 2007). The model suggests that when we are evaluating an ambiguous or complex object, we sometimes simplify the task into the question "How do I feel about it?" (Schwarz & Clore, 1988). This simplification can be considered a heuristic, enabling us to reach a conclusion in a quicker and more efficient manner than if we were to conduct a slow and effortful examination of all the relevant information. However, the heuristic can lead to errors and being mistaken about what one "likes and wants," such as when feelings are not actually caused by what we are evaluating but by some irrelevant factor (e.g., weather). As a result, the person may end up with a series of mistaken beliefs of what he or she likes and wants.

Finally, it is important to note that the act of attribution itself may distort hedonic experience. In a study investigating the influence of such processes, subjects listened to musical excerpts from Stravinsky's *The Rite of Spring,* and evaluated their state of happiness either throughout the episode or only at the end. Those who were continuously monitoring their affective state rated their happiness below those who only evaluated it at the end of the musical piece (Schooler, Ariely, & Loewenstein, 2003). In short, by trying to understand why we like something, we may destroy the liking itself. We may also get ourselves confused and focus on the wrong reasons why we engaged in the experience in the first place (e.g., Wilson & Kraft, 1993).

Overall, these findings suggest that processes of affective attribution can be complex and prone to irrelevant influences, especially in cases where irrelevant ambiguous stimuli are made salient and the true causes of our affective states are unclear. In these situations, we might end up wanting and pursuing objects we actually have little interest in and do not necessarily like. Of course, it is a question of debate how often this is normally the case. After all, our affective states are typically informative and aid us in responding effectively to surrounding stimuli (Clore & Huntsinger, 2009). And, as with all heuristics, they tend be reasonably matched to the environment (Gigerenzer, 2007). Finally, there is always a tricky possibility that misattribution processes can create real affects. For example, it is possible that participants in the Dutton and Aron (1974) study, after misattributing their arousal to attraction to the woman, genuinely liked her. Future research should explore when or whether misattributed feelings are any less "genuine" than correctly attributed ones.

Related Phenomena in Social Psychology: The Ability to Predict Future Wanting and Liking

Successful and happy life (or at least a reasonable marriage) requires the ability to know what we like and want now, and to foresee what we will want, like, and choose in the future. This problem can be expressed in decision-making parlance. Kahneman and Snell (1992) distinguish between decision utility, experienced utility, and predicted utility of outcomes. *Decision utility* refers to the value (or weight) that a specific outcome has in determining our actual decision. *Experienced utility* refers to the actual hedonic experience we receive from that outcome. Finally, *predicted utility* refers to our prediction for future experienced utility of that outcome. These easily map onto our concepts of wanting and liking: Decision utility corresponds to the incentive value of the outcome. Experienced utility refers to our hedonic experience. While we may assume that predicted utility matches experienced utility, there is abundant evidence that this is not the case—people are often inaccurate at predicting how they will feel, what they will want, and what they will chose (Gilbert & Wilson, 2007). Interestingly, some prediction errors reflect the dissociations between future liking and wanting. People make different predictions about how they will *feel* in a future situation, or future attitudes, and predictions about their future *behavior*, such as choice and preferences (Van Boven & Kane, 2006). This discrepancy is due to our different assumptions regarding the dynamics of hedonic experience and preference behavior. Specifically, people are well aware that their feelings change (e.g., their mood today does not predict their mood a week from now). However, they usually assume that their actual preference behavior is fairly stable.

One specific example of our misperceptions regarding future feelings is the impact bias. We are aware that emotions and feelings tend to fluctuate, to the point that we sometimes overestimate this fluctuation (Wilson & Gilbert, 2003). Yet we are unaware that underlying psychological processes, such as dissonance reduction processes, sense-making processes, and others, are at work in order to enable us to recover to a relatively stable affective state after an emotional episode. These processes also underlie our inability to predict emotional effects of inaction, or "opting out." Andrade and Van Boven (2010) examined how participants predicted their reactions and their actual affective experience to the outcome of a gamble in which they chose not to participate. In this study, participants were presented with a gamble with a negative expected outcome, such that it was unappealing to almost all participants, and therefore most chose to reject the gamble. Participants underestimated their future reactions to both a forgone loss and a forgone gain, when compared to their ratings after the event. We underestimate in such situations the ease of making counterfactual comparisons, such that a forgone gain might cause us significant regret. It is easier for us to think about reactions to actions we take than to actions we don't take; therefore, we don't take these into account.

When predicting future choices and preferences, we are under the assumption that these are stable constructs that reflect our personality, and we therefore do not expect them to change by much over time and under various situations (Dunning, 2005; Quoidbach & Dunn, 2010). However, as detailed below, processes underlying preferences and motivation are susceptible to habituation and sensitization processes, as well as fluctuations in arousal states. This susceptibility may render our perceptions of future choices at odds with actual behavior in these situations.

Processes Underlying Mispredictions of Wanting and Liking

Several recent lines of research have looked specifically at one set of factors that can lead to a mismatch between how liking and wanting processes really work "under the hood"—the automatic operation of sensitization and habituation. Such processes take place at both a biophysiological and cognitive levels. Biopsychologically, as described in the section on the incentive sensitization theory, repeated exposure to a strong reward (e.g., drug) may paradoxically causes sensitization processes in the wanting system to the point that it is decoupled from liking (Berridge & Robinson, 1995). On the habituation side, recent research suggest that automatic processes of satiation work quickly and similarly across cognitive and affective stimuli: People quickly lose access to the affective meaning of a repeated stimulus, just as they lose accesses to a semantic meaning of an overexposed word (Irwin, Huber, & Winkielman, 2010). Importantly, there is evidence that these habituation processes can specifically influence our preferences, altering the incentive value of a stimulus without affecting the pleasure derived from it (Morewedge, Huh, & Vosgerau, 2010). One result of people's poor access and understanding of their own dynamics of sensitization and habituation is that they make suboptimal choices about interruption of experience in many domains, some as common as television viewing (Nelson & Meyvis, 2008; Nelson, Meyvis, & Galak, 2009).

One of the most curious reasons for failures of self-prediction is a difficulty in imagining ourselves in future "hot" affective state while we are currently in a "cold state." Thus, when we are sated, calm, and unaroused, it is hard for us to imagine how we will feel and act when we are very hungry, upset, or sexually excited. Accordingly, we do not take into sufficient consideration how a change in these states will influence our future experience and behavior. Loewenstein (1996) states that our memory for visceral experience is qualitatively different from other forms of memory, in that it is for the most part less accessible for decision making and future predictions. The consideration of the liking and wanting system dynamics adds another dimension. As we discussed earlier, some situations and cues can cause the wanting system to become hyperactive, eliciting desires that do not necessarily correspond to liking. Thus, we may actually correctly predict how we will "feel" in a hot state but fail to predict what we will want.

Evidence for these gaps in experience can be seen in various studies that examine decision-making behavior under various states of visceral arousal, specifically sexual arousal. Knutson, Wimmer, Kuhnen, and Winkielman (2008) showed that male subjects switched from low-risk to high-risk gambles after viewing erotic pictures. This change was mediated by the activation of the nucleus accumbens, which, as mentioned, is a part of the wanting system. Importantly, subjects who under sexual arousal chose more risky choices knew that the frisky pictures were irrelevant to the task, and claimed afterwards that the pictures didn't influence their financial choices. Thus, they failed to appreciate how their visceral states changed their perception of the gamble.

Ditto, Pizarro, Epstein, Jacobson, and MacDonald (2006) compared risk-taking behavior in subjects who were either under visceral influences, such as the smell of freshly baked cookies, or in a neutral state. In the first study, subjects were willing to engage in more risk to receive the cookies they smelled, and in the second study, after exposure to an erotic movie, subjects expressed greater likelihood in engaging in unprotected sex. Ariely and Loewenstein (2006) compared college-age males' sexual preferences and decisions in a state of heightened sexual arousal with a neutral state, and found that sexually aroused subjects were more willing to engage in morally questionable sexual behavior. Both these experiments further demonstrate that actual preferences during a "hot" state may differ greatly from our predictions in a neutral state, even to the point where we might find ourselves crossing our own moral boundaries.

Even young children (ages 3–5) show similar biases in prediction of future preferences, regardless of whether they fully grasp the meaning of "tomorrow" (Atance & Meltzoff, 2006). Although a majority of children prefer pretzels to water, thirsty preschoolers preferred water to pretzels not only as their present choice but also for future encounters. This suggests that such "hot"–"cold" gaps are not necessarily accessible to regulation by higher-level cognitive processes that characteristically develop between the ages of 3 and 5.

In summary, these phenomena illustrate how underlying wanting and liking processes interact with our thoughts and expectations of our future behavior. Specifically, they demonstrate the instability of our preferences across various visceral states, in that what we value in a "hot" state can vary greatly from what we value at a "cold" state. Critical to our biases in prediction is the fact that many of these processes are at least partly subconscious and inaccessible for decision making. Our limited understanding of how our affective system responds in various situations creates consistent biases in our predictions, rendering our actual behavior and experience at odds with our expectations.

Summary

It has been traditionally assumed that our preferences (liking) are stable, and that wanting naturally and coherently follows from liking. In addition, it has been assumed that liking and wanting are consciously experienced—internally sensed as pleasure and desire. Yet evidence from current research on affect and motivation challenges all these assumptions. Hedonic pleasure from reward (liking) and motivation for obtaining it (wanting) appear to be two different processes that can be dissociable in certain situations. Critically, both processes can sometimes operate on a subconscious level and are subject to a host of biological and cognitive manipulations that can "tweak" them without our knowledge.

The inaccessibility of our internal affective processes is linked to biases in affective forecasting, or how we make predictions of our own future emotional experience and behaviors. While these subconscious reward processes may lead us to make disadvantageous decisions in certain situations, they usually produce adaptive behavior. In addition, these affective processes do interact with conscious processes, so that we are not always completely in the dark as to our affective state. Nevertheless, awareness of our affective and motivational "blind spots" might enable us to understand our limits and live with that extra cookie we ate.

ACKNOWLEDGMENT

We thank the editors for their remarkably generous and thoughtful comments.

REFERENCES

Aharon, I., Etcoff, N., Ariely, D., Chabris, C. F., O'Connor, E., & Breiter, H. C. (2001). Beautiful faces have variable reward value: fMRI and behavioral evidence. *Neuron, 32*(3), 537–551.

Andrade, E. B., & Van Boven, L. (2010). Feelings not forgone. *Psychological Science, 21*(5), 706–711.

Ariely, D., & Loewenstein, G. (2006). The heat of the moment: The effect of sexual arousal on sexual decision making. *Journal of Behavioral Decision Making, 19*(2), 87–98.

Atance, C. M., & Meltzoff, A. N. (2006). Preschoolers' current desires warp their choices for the future. *Psychological Science, 17*(7), 583–587,

Beaver, J. D., Lawrence, A. D., van Ditzhuijzen, J., Davis, M. H., Woods, A., & Calder, A. J. (2006). Individual differences in reward drive predict neural responses to images of food. *Journal of Neuroscience, 26*(19), 5160–5166.

Becker, G. S., & Murphy, K. M. (1988). A theory of rational children. *Journal of Political Economy, 96*(1), 675–700.

Berridge, K. C. (1996). Food reward: Brain substrates of wanting and liking. *Neuroscience and Biobehavioral Reviews, 20*(1), 1–25.

Berridge, K. C. (2007). The debate over dopamine's role in reward: The case for incentive salience. *Psychopharmacology, 191*(3), 391–431.

Berridge, K. C. (2009). "Liking" and "wanting" food rewards: Brain substrates and roles in eating disorders. *Physiology and Behavior, 97*(5), 537–550.

Berridge, K. C., & Robinson, T. E. (1995). The mind of an addicted brain: Neural sensitization of wanting versus liking. *Current Directions in Psychological Science, 4*(3), 71–76.

Berridge, K. C., & Robinson, T. E. (1998). What is the role of dopamine in reward: Hedonic impact, reward learning, or incentive salience? *Brain Research Reviews, 28*(3), 309–369.

Berridge, K. C., & Robinson, T. E. (2003). Parsing reward. *Trends in Neurosciences, 26*(9), 507–513.

Berridge, K. C., Venier, I. L., & Robinson, T. E. (1989). Taste reactivity analysis of 6-hydroxydopamine-induced aphagia: Implications for arousal and anhedonia hypotheses of dopamine function. *Behavioral Neuroscience, 103*(1), 36–45.

Bornemann, B., Winkielman, P., & van der Meer, E. (in press). Can you feel what you don't see?: Using internal feedback to detect briefly presented emotional stimuli. *International Journal of Psychophysiology.*

Cabanac, M. (1971). Physiological role of pleasure. *Science, 173*(2), 1103–1107.

Clore, G. L., & Huntsinger, J. R. (2009). How the object of affect guides its impact. *Emotional Review, 1*, 39–54.

Cohen, M. X., Young, J., Baek, J.-M., Kessler, C., & Ranganath, C. (2005). Individual differences in extraversion and dopamine genetics predict neural reward responses. *Cognitive Brain Research, 25*(3), 851–861.

de Gelder, B., Pourtois, G., van Raamsdonk, M., Vroomen, J., & Weiskrantz, L. (2001). Unseen stimuli modulate conscious visual experience: Evidence from inter-hemispheric summation. *NeuroReport, 12*(2), 385–391.

Ditto, P. H., Pizarro, D. A., Epstein, E. B., Jacobson, J. A., & MacDonald, T. K. (2006). Visceral influences on risk-taking behavior. *Journal of Behavioral Decision Making, 19*(2), 99–113.

Dunning, D. A. (2005). *Self-insight: Roadblocks and detours on the path to knowing thyself.* New York: Psychology Press.

Dutton, D. G., & Aron, A. P. (1974). Some evidence for heightened sexual attraction under conditions of high anxiety. *Journal of Personality and Social Psychology, 30*(4), 510–517.

Frank, S. A. (1998). *Foundations of social evolution.* Princeton, NJ: Princeton University Press.

Gangestad, S. W., Garver-Apgar, C. E., Simpson, J. A., & Cousins, A. J. (2007). Changes in women's mate preferences across the ovulatory cycle. *Journal of Personality and Social Psychology, 92*(1), 151–163.

Gigerenzer, G. (2007). *Gut feelings: The intelligences of the unconscious.* New York: Viking.

Gilbert, D. T., & Wilson, T. D. (2007). Prospection: Experiencing the future. *Science, 317,* 1351–1354.

Gilboa, I. (2009). *Theory of decision under uncertainty.* Cambridge, UK: Cambridge University Press.

Hamm, A. O., Weike, A. I., Schupp, H. T., Treig, T., Dressel, A., & Kessler, C. (2003). Affective blindsight: Intact fear conditioning to a visual cue in a cortically blind patient. *Brain, 126*(2), 267–275.

Hull, C. L. (1951). *Essentials of behavior*. New Haven, CT: Yale University Press.

Irwin, K. R., Huber, D. E., & Winkielman, P. (2010). Automatic affective dynamics: An activation–habituation model of affective assimilation and contrast. *Modeling Machine Emotions for Realizing Intelligence, 1*, 17–34.

Kahneman, D., & Snell, J. (1992). Predicting a changing taste: Do people know what they will like? *Journal of Behavioral Decision Making, 5*(3), 187–200.

Knutson, B., Wimmer, G. E., Kuhnen, C. M., & Winkielman, P. (2008). Nucleus accumbens activation mediates the influence of reward cues on financial risk taking. *NeuroReport, 19*(5), 509–513.

Lamb, R. J., Preston, K. L., Schindler, C. W., Meisch, R. A., Davis, F., Katz, J. L., et al. (1991). The reinforcing and subjective effects of morphine in post-addicts: A dose–response study. *Journal of Pharmacology and Experimental Therapeutics, 259*(3), 1165–1173.

Larsen, R. J., & Diener, E. (1987). Affect intensity as an individual difference characteristic: A review. *Journal of Research in Personality, 21*(1), 1–39.

LeDoux, J. (1996). *The emotional brain: The mysterious underpinnings of emotional life*. New York: Simon & Schuster.

Litt, A., Khan, U., & Shiv, B. (2010). Lusting while loathing. *Psychological Science, 21*(1), 118–125.

Loewenstein, G. (1996). Out of control: Visceral influences on behavior. *Organizational Behavior and Human Decision Processes, 65*(3), 272–292.

Mahler, S. V., Smith, K. S., & Berridge, K. C. (2007). Endocannabinoid hedonic hotspot for sensory pleasure: Anandamide in nucleus accumbens shell enhances "liking" of a sweet reward. *Neuropsychopharmacology, 32*(11), 2267–2278.

Mauss, I. B., Levenson, R. W., McCarter, L., Wilhelm, F. H., & Gross, J. J. (2005). The tie that binds?: Coherence among emotion experience, behavior, and physiology. *Emotion, 5*(2), 175–190.

Morewedge, C. K., Huh, Y. E., & Vosgerau, J. (2010). Thought for food: Imagined consumption reduces actual consumption. *Science, 330*, 1530–1533.

Murphy, S. T., & Zajonc, R. B. (1993). Affect, cognition, and awareness: Affective priming with optimal and suboptimal stimulus exposures. *Journal of Personality and Social Psychology, 64*, 723–729.

Nelson, L. F., & Meyvis, T. (2008). Interrupted consumption: Disrupting adaptation to hedonic experience. *Journal of Marketing Research, 45*, 654–664.

Nelson, L. F., Meyvis, T., & Galak, J. (2009). Enhancing the television viewing experience through commercial interruption. *Journal of Consumer Research, 36*(2), 160–172.

Nisbett, R. E., & Wilson, T. D. (1977). Telling more than we can know: Verbal reports on mental processes. *Psychological Review, 84*(3), 231–259.

Peciña, S. (2008). Opioid reward "liking" and "wanting" in the nucleus accumbens. *Physiology and Behavior, 94*(5), 675–680.

Quoidbach, J., & Dunn, E. W. (2010). Personality neglect. *Psychological Science, 21*(12), 1783–1786.

Robinson, T. E., & Berridge, K. C. (1993). The neural basis of drug craving: an incentive-sensitization theory of addiction. *Brain Research Reviews, 18*(3), 247–291.

Rolls, E. T., Rolls, B. J., & Rowe, E. A. (1983). Sensory-specific and motivation-specific satiety for the sight and taste of food and water in man. *Physiology and Behavior, 30*(2), 185–192.

Schachter, S., & Singer, J. (1962). Cognitive, social, and physiological determinants of emotional state. *Psychological Review, 69*(5), 379–399.

Schooler, J. W., Ariely, D., & Loewenstein, G. (2003). The pursuit and assessment of happiness can be self-defeating. In I. Brocas & J. Carrillo (Eds.), *The psychology of economic decisions: Vol. 1. Rationality and well-being* (pp. 41–70). New York: Oxford University Press.

Schwarz, N., & Clore, G. L. (1983). Mood, misattribution, and judgments of well-being: Informative and directive functions of affective states. *Journal of Personality and Social Psychology, 45*(3), 513–523.

Schwarz, N., & Clore, G. L. (1988). How do I feel about it?: The informative function of affective states. In K. Fiedler & J. Forgas (Eds.), *Affect, cognition, and social behavior* (pp. 44–62). Toronto: Hogrefe.

Schwarz, N., & Clore, G. L. (2007). Feelings and phenomenal experiences. In A. W. Kruglanski & E. T. Higgins (Eds.), *Social psychology: Handbook of basic principles* (2nd ed., pp. 385–407). New York: Guilford Press.

Smith, K. S., Tindell, A. J., Aldridge, J. W., & Berridge, K. C. (2009). Ventral pallidum roles in reward and motivation. *Behavioural Brain Research, 196*(2), 155–167.

Starr, M. J., Lin, J., & Winkielman, P. (2007). *The impact of unconscious facial expressions on consumption behavior involves changes in positive affect: Evidence from EMG and appetitive reflex-modulation.* Poster presented at the 47th annual meeting of the Society for Psychophysiological Research, Savannah, GA.

Steiner, J. E. (1973). The gustofacial response: Observation on normal and anencephalic newborn infants. *Symposium on Oral Sensation and Perception, 4,* 254–278.

Storebeck, J., & Clore, G. L. (2008). Affective arousal as information: How affective arousal influences judgments, learning, and memory. *Social and Personality Psychology Compass, 2,* 1824–1843.

Toates, F. M. (1986). *Motivational systems.* Cambridge, UK: Cambridge University Press.

Van Boven, L., & Kane, J. (2006). Predicting feelings versus choices. In L. J. Sanna & E. C. Chang (Eds.), *Judgments over time: The interplay of thoughts, feelings and behaviors* (pp. 67–81). Oxford, UK: Oxford University Press.

Wan, X., & Peoples, L. L. (2008). Amphetamine exposure enhances accumbal responses to reward-predictive stimuli in a Pavlovian conditioned approach task. *Journal of Neuroscience, 28*(30), 7501–7512.

Weiner, B. (2012). An attribution theory of motivation. In P. A. M. van Lange, A. W. Kruglansky, & E. T. Higgins (Eds.), *Handbook of theories of social psychology* (Vol. 1, pp. 135–155). Thousand Oaks, CA: Sage.

Wilson, T., & Gilbert, D. T. (2003). Affective forecasting. *Advances in Experimental Social Psychology, 35,* 345–411.

Wilson, T. D., & Kraft, D. (1993). Why do I love thee?: Effects of introspections about a dating relationship on attributes towards the relationship. *Personality and Social Psychology Bulletin, 19*(4), 409–418.

Winkielman, P., & Berridge, K. C. (2003). Irrational wanting and subrational liking: How rudimentary motivational and affective processes shape preferences and choices. *Political Psychology, 24*(4), 657–680.

Winkielman, P., Berridge, K. C., & Wilbarger, J. L. (2005). Unconscious affective reactions to masked happy versus angry faces influence consumption behavior and judgments of value. *Personality and Social Psychology Bulletin, 31*(1), 121–135.

Winkielman, P., & Schooler, J. W. (2011). Splitting consciousness: Unconscious, conscious, and metaconscious processes in social cognition. *European Review of Social Psychology, 22,* 1–35.

Winkielman, P., Zajonc, R. B., & Schwarz, N. (1997). Subliminal affective priming resists attributional interventions. *Cognition and Emotion, 11*(4), 433–465.

Wyvell, C. L., & Berridge, K. C. (2000). Intra-accumbens amphetamine increases the conditioned incentive salience of sucrose reward: Enhancement of reward "wanting" without enhanced "liking" or response reinforcement. *Journal of Neuroscience, 20*(21), 8122–8130.

CHAPTER 14
Partner Knowledge and Relationship Outcomes

JEFFRY A. SIMPSON
JENNIFER FILLO
JOHN MYERS

Individuals base some of life's most important decisions on the knowledge they have—or *assume* they have—about themselves, close others, and the world around them. Most of the chapters in this book address how knowledge about the self impacts a diverse array of important life outcomes. In this chapter, our primary focus is somewhat different. Instead of focusing on people's beliefs about their *own* traits, attitudes, and emotions, we focus on people's beliefs about the traits, attitudes, and emotions of their romantic partners, which eventually become part of the self, as well as their relationship beliefs, which help to define the self. We review how knowledge about one's current romantic relationship and especially one's romantic partner (e.g., what individuals believe their partner is thinking or feeling during important social interactions) is associated with significant relationship outcomes, such as how satisfied individuals are and whether their relationship is likely to endure. As we shall see, knowledge about partners and relationships exists at different levels, ranging from specific inferences about what one's romantic partner is thinking or feeling at specific moments during a critical discussion to more global assessments of a partner's defining traits and personal attributes. One of our primary goals is to explain how and why accurate versus inaccurate knowledge of the *partner* at different levels of measurement is related to important relationship outcomes.

The chapter has four sections. In the first section, we discuss how people typically acquire knowledge about their partners and relationships, focusing on the concepts of relationship awareness (Acitelli, 2002) and minding in relationships (Harvey & Omarzu, 1997, 1999). In the second section, we review what has been learned about the "knowing process," highlighting recent research on self-expansion processes in close relationships (Aron, Aron, & Norman, 2001). The third section examines the conditions under which accuracy and bias affect partner and relationship knowledge. We focus on the importance of the "global bias, specific accuracy" pattern for good relationship functioning (Neff & Karney, 2002, 2005), as well as how mean-level bias and "tracking accuracy" (Fletcher & Kerr, 2010) can influence relationship outcomes. The fourth section, which is the centerpiece of the chapter, addresses how *empathic accuracy*—the degree to which an individual accurately infers what his or her partner is thinking or feeling during an important social interaction—is linked to relationship outcomes. We review Ickes and Simpson's (1997, 2001) empathic accuracy model, and then discuss several laboratory studies that have tested predictions derived from this model.

Acquiring Relationship Knowledge

Various authors have theorized about the different ways in which individuals acquire knowledge about their partners and relationships. These theoretical approaches incorporate similar components and address similar outcomes, but they vary in their scope and emphasis. In this section, we review two major theories of the relationship knowledge acquisition processes: Acitelli's (2002) model of relationship awareness, and Harvey and Omarzu's (1997) theory of minding.

Relationship Awareness

At its most basic level, relationship awareness involves paying attention to one's relationships by thinking or talking about them with others. In the 1980s, several studies documented positive relations between romantic partners' relationship satisfaction and their self- and partner-related awareness (e.g., Franzoi, Davis, & Young, 1985). Inspired by these preliminary findings, Acitelli (2002) developed a process model to organize existing research linking relationship awareness with satisfaction. Acitelli's model of *relationship awareness* incorporates individual, situational, and sociocultural factors that influence relationship awareness and its connection to relationship satisfaction (see Figure 14.1).

It is easiest to work through the model starting with factors that exist prior to two individuals meeting or interacting, specifically their individual characteristics and predispositions (2A, 2B in Figure 14.1). These individual factors can influence each person's thoughts about the self, the partner, and the relationship (3A, 3B), which in turn can influence the partners' discussions about their relationship (3X). These discussions can also feed back to influence each individual's thoughts (3A, 3B). This tendency to think about the relationship constitutes "relationship awareness." Over time, relationship awareness can impact each individual's satisfaction with the relationship (4A, 4B), which typically influences relationship stability (4X).

This entire relationship awareness process takes place within a broader sociocultural context; that is, sociocultural factors can affect how relationship-oriented discussions feed back on relationship awareness, how relationship awareness is related to satisfaction, or any other processes outlined in the model. Acitelli (2002) describes five sociocultural factors that are most likely to influence relationship awareness: ethnicity, acculturation, sex role ideology, religiosity, and socioeconomic status (1A, 1B

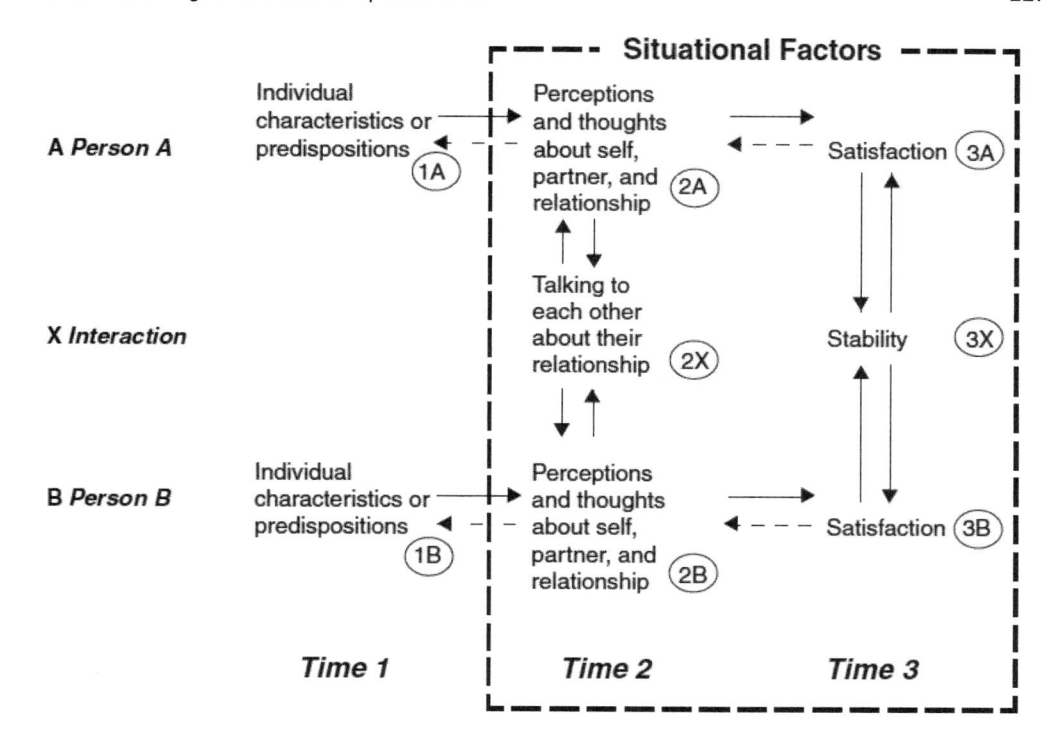

FIGURE 14.1. Acitelli's (2002) model of relationship awareness.

in Figure 14.1). The relative importance of these factors and the degree to which they affect relationship outcomes varies across individuals and relationships.

Working through the entire model (from left to right in Figure 14.1), individuals are raised in certain cultures and are socialized to hold certain values and beliefs (1A, 1B). These sociocultural factors impact individuals' characteristics (2A, 2B) to varying degrees. When two individuals meet, they become aware of their relationship (3A, 3B) and eventually begin to talk about it (3X). These discussions frequently have an impact on the subsequent thoughts that individuals have about themselves, their partner, and/or the relationship (3A, 3B), which contributes to greater relationship awareness. Over time, relationship awareness can affect each individual's satisfaction with the relationship (4A, 4B), which in turn affects the long-term stability of the relationship (4X). This entire process always takes place within a specific sociocultural milieu that can influence one or several steps of the relationship awareness process.

Acitelli and her colleagues have tested various components of the relationship awareness model. Most of this research, however, has focused on one individual factor: gender. For example, Acitelli (1988) has found that women view relationship-oriented discussions as serving different functions and purposes than men do; women value talking about their relationships in pleasant and unpleasant situations, whereas men value relationship talk only as an instrumental means to solve problems. This gender difference may explain why women are generally more aware of their relationships than most men are (Acitelli & Holmberg, 1993). Research has also revealed that relational variables, especially relationship-oriented talk, are more important to women's than to men's well-being and relationship satisfaction (Acitelli & Antonucci, 1994). However, the link between relationship awareness and relationship satisfaction tends to be driven more by relational identity than by biological sex (Acitelli, Rogers, & Knee, 1999). Therefore, this link is perhaps stronger for women because they have a more relationship-oriented sense of self (Acitelli & Holmberg, 1993).

The proposition that women are more aware of their relationships is somewhat at odds with other theorizing and research on relationship and partner knowledge. Harvey and Omarzu (1999), for example, do not think that there are overall differences between men and women in minding activities. Additionally, Ickes (2003) has not found consistent gender differences in his extensive research on empathic accuracy. Indeed, some of the gender differences found by Acitelli and colleagues may be a by-product of the specific types of behaviors they have measured rather than global differences in relationship awareness. Acitelli and colleagues have typically defined *attending* to one's relationship as talking or thinking about the relationship. Men, however, may attend to their relationships through shared activities with their partners (Wood & Inman, 1993). By broadening their exploration of relationship awareness to include shared activities, Acitelli and Carlson (1997) found that attending to the relationship was associated with positive relationship outcomes for both sexes. Therefore, it appears that both men and women are aware of their relationships; they may just go about achieving this awareness in different ways.

Minding in Relationships

Whereas Acitelli's (2002) relationship awareness model incorporates both the predictors and consequences of *relationship-oriented* thoughts and discussions, Harvey and Omarzu's (1997, 1999) theory of minding focuses specifically on *partner-oriented* thoughts, attributions, and behaviors. Harvey and Omarzu (1997, p. 224) define *minding* as a "reciprocal knowing process" in relationships, one that incorporates thoughts, feelings, and behaviors that facilitate closeness and relationship stability. Minding has five components: (1) behaviors facilitating disclosure, (2) relationship-enhancing attributions, (3) acceptance and respect, (4) reciprocity, and (5) continuity.

The first component of minding involves *behaviors that facilitate the knowing process*, particularly those that encourage disclosure on the part of one's partner. By attentively listening and responding to partners when they disclose information, individuals can create an environment that promotes further disclosure, in terms of both the breadth and depth of topics discussed. Self-disclosure, coupled with behaviors that facilitate partner disclosure, ultimately fosters greater intimacy between relationship partners. However, simply gaining knowledge about one's partner does not, by itself, constitute minding.

Individuals must also make *relationship-enhancing attributions* for their partners' statements and behaviors; that is, in well-minded relationships, individuals perceive their partners' relationship-relevant behaviors as being caring and well intentioned. One way to accomplish this is to attribute negative behaviors enacted by one's partner to fleeting, external causes (e.g., "She yelled at me because she had a bad day at work") and to attribute positive behaviors to stable, internal causes (e.g., "He made dinner because he cares about me"; Harvey, Pauwels, & Zickmund, 2002). In well-minded relationships, individuals use their knowledge about their partners in the careful formulation of attributions regarding their partners' behaviors.

Other important aspects of the minding process involve *acceptance* of newly acquired information about one's partner as well as *respect* for the sensitivity and privacy of the information. Sustained self-disclosure relies heavily on trusting one's partner to not take advantage of the disclosed information; therefore, acceptance and respect are especially important early in relationship development. Additionally, the minding process must be *reciprocal*. Continued imbalances between partners in the degree of minding may cause one partner to feel a sense of dependence or obligation and may cause the other partner to feel taken advantage of. An imbalance in minding may also make relationship-enhancing attributions more difficult to do, as one partner may conclude that the other is not motivated or able to engage in minding behaviors. Most importantly, reciprocity facilitates the last component of minding: *continuity*. It usually takes considerable time to establish the minding process and, once established, the process remains ongoing. Because individuals change over time, relationship partners must continually update their knowledge of each other. As Harvey and colleagues (2002) conclude, "minding is a process . . . not an ultimate destination" (p. 429).

Most of the evidence supporting the minding model has been indirect, typically through research exploring concepts related to the five components of minding. For example, Gottman (1994) has found that couples who engage in positive social behaviors tend to be more satisfied in their relationships. This includes respect for and acceptance of partners' thoughts and feelings during social interactions, which can also help prevent the types of negative behaviors that are often destructive to relationships. Indeed, acceptance and respect are the basis for a form of marital therapy known as *acceptance therapy*, which is effective with couples who have been unsuccessful with other forms of therapy (Jacobson & Christensen, 1996). Instead of trying to change behavioral patterns, acceptance therapy focuses on accepting a partner's traits and behaviors that one has found annoying in the past. This technique is consistent with Harvey and Omarzu's (1997) emphasis on accepting partners' flaws and having accurate partner representations. Additionally, the importance of reciprocity in minding is supported by research showing that individuals in inequitable relationships are less satisfied than those who view their relationships as more equitable (Van Yperen & Buunk, 1991). Although Harvey and Omarzu (1999) review other preliminary evidence that supports their model of minding, most hypotheses regarding connections between various components or potential outcomes of minding have not been directly tested.

Outcomes of the Knowing Process

Both Acitelli (2002) and Harvey and Omarzu (1997, 1999) discuss how increased partner- and relationship-oriented knowledge can increase closeness between romantic partners. Once a certain degree of closeness has been achieved, relationships may also begin to affect how individuals perceive themselves. One prominent theoretical model that addresses how and why relationships can affect self-perception processes and vice versa is the self-expansion model (Aron & Aron, 1986; Aron et al., 2001).

The Self-Expansion Model

According to the self-expansion model (Aron & Aron, 1986; Aron et al., 2001), when an individual enters a close relationship, the social, informational, and material qualities of the relationship partner become, in some respects, one's own qualities. According to this model, individuals are motivated in part to forge close relationships because these newly acquired qualities can bolster one's self-efficacy and competence. An unconscious by-product of this blending of resources and qualities is a restructuring of the cognitive system, such that the perspectives and identities of the relationship partner become incorporated into one's *own* self-representation. This phenomenon is called *inclusion of other in the self*. These overlapping cognitive representations between the self and other are a hallmark of close relationships. Indeed, according to the model, this overlap is what it means to be close to another person (Aron & Aron, 1986; Aron, Aron, Tudor, & Nelson, 1991).

Evidence for Self-Expansion

The self-expansion model claims that individuals experience a broadening of the self-concept when a new relationship is formed. This "broadening of the self" often should result in greater self-efficacy and higher self-esteem. To test this premise, Aron, Paris, and Aron (1995) followed individuals who were likely to meet a new partner and fall in love (first-year and second-year undergraduates) for 10 weeks. Aron and his colleagues found that individuals who had fallen in love developed more diverse self-concepts and showed more self-concept change than did those who had not fallen in love. In addition, individuals who had fallen in love experienced increases in self-efficacy and self-esteem.

If people typically experience self-expansion after entering a new romantic relationship, it stands to reason that the self should also "contract" when a close relationship dissolves. Indeed, Lewandowski, Aron, Bassis, and Kunak (2006) found that individuals who had recently lost a self-expanding relationship experienced a considerable contraction of the self-concept. Viewed together, these two lines of research indicate that close relationships can and do play important roles in both the expansion *and* contraction of individuals' self-concepts.

Including the Other in the Self

According to the self-expansion model, closeness blurs distinctions between one's own resources and one's partner's resources. Indeed, research by Aron and colleagues (1991) suggests that individuals tend to forgo personal financial gains in order to allocate money equitably to close others, suggesting that individuals may view the resources of close others as if they are their own resources. They also found that participants allocated equal amounts of money to themselves and their best friends, even when they knew that their friends did not know how the money was divided up and could not reciprocate the gesture.

Additional research suggests that this "blurring of distinction" between self and other is pervasive. In fact, we often perceive the world from the perspective of close others. Aron and his colleagues (1991) tested this hypothesis using a clever noun-recollection paradigm. They reasoned that when individuals perceive the world from the first person (an individual-centered perspective), objects are the figure and they are the ground (e.g., when one imagines oneself holding a cup, one attends to the cup, which is the figure). However, when individuals watch others interacting with objects, the actor and the object are both the figure. Thus, when individuals imagine themselves interacting with objects, their memories for these objects are poorer than their memories for imagined objects interacted with by others. Aron and colleagues reasoned that if individuals view the world from the perspective of their partners, then their recollection of imagined objects interacted with by their partners should be as poor as their recollection for imagined objects interacted with by themselves because, in both cases, the actor should be more ground-like. This is precisely what they found. Thus, individuals tend to view the world through the eyes of close others.

In addition to perceiving the world from the vantage point of close others, individuals may also begin to incorporate their cognitive representations of their partners into their own cognitive representations. One implication of this is that individuals may, at times, confuse themselves with their partners. Consistent with this logic, individuals find it more difficult to identify traits that are distinctive to their partners (i.e., traits their partners have that they themselves do not have) than traits that are distinctive to non-close others (Aron et al., 1991). Mashek, Aron, and Boncimino (2003) asked participants to rate traits according to how well each trait described the self, a close other, and a non-close other. Later, participants were asked to recall which person each trait best described. Individuals displayed more source confusions between the traits of close others and the self (i.e., erroneously claiming that a trait rated as highly descriptive of a close other earlier was descriptive of the self) than between the traits of non-close others and the self. Importantly, closeness, rather than familiarity or similarity, was responsible for these effects.

Accuracy and Bias in Relationship Beliefs

Not all of the information that people acquire about their partners or relationships is accurate. The consequences of holding accurate versus inaccurate representations of one's partner have been hotly debated in the relationships literature. Some researchers have claimed that positive relationship outcomes are associated with accurate perceptions of relationship partners (e.g., Harvey & Omarzu, 1997; Kobak & Hazan, 1991; Swann, De La Ronde, & Hixon, 1994). Others have concluded that harboring "positive illusions" of one's partner is critical to relationship satisfaction (e.g., Murray, Holmes, & Griffin, 1996). Recent work, however, suggests that these two views are not mutually exclusive; both accurate and positively biased partner perceptions may be systematically related to positive relationship outcomes.

Luo and Snider (2009), for example, examined accuracy, similarity bias, and positivity bias in four domains (the Big Five, the Positive and Negative Affect Schedule, emotional expressivity, and attachment styles) as possible determinants of relationship satisfaction. They found that all three perceptual processes contributed to relationship satisfaction. Specifically, positivity bias was associated with greater satisfaction with the self, whereas accuracy and similarity bias predicted both self-satisfaction and the partner's satisfaction. Thus, both accuracy and bias can have beneficial effects on relationship outcomes.

Global Bias, Specific Accuracy

Other researchers have investigated the operation of accuracy and bias at different levels of abstraction. Neff and Karney (2002, 2005), for example, distinguish between accuracy and bias for specific versus global evaluations of one's partner. Adopting this perspective, they have found that individuals in satisfying marriages tend to describe their spouses' positive traits in broader, more global terms. Conversely, happy individuals tend to be more specific when describing their partners' negative qualities. Individuals in satisfying marriages also tend to be more accurate about their partners' specific traits than their global traits (Neff & Karney, 2002).

To investigate the impact that deviation from the "specific accuracy/global bias" pattern has on relationship outcomes, Neff and Karney (2005) followed newlyweds over time. They found that nearly all newlyweds held similarly positive perceptions of their partners' global traits. However, there was more variation in newlyweds' perceptions of their partners' specific traits. For example, wives' (but not husbands') accurate perceptions of their spouses' specific qualities predicted more positive relationship outcomes, such as more supportive behavior and a lower likelihood of eventual divorce. This pattern of results suggests that the most successful relationships are based on global adoration of the relationship partner coupled with a realistic recognition of his or her unique strengths and weaknesses.

Mean-Level Bias and Tracking Accuracy

In a recent meta-analysis, Fletcher and Kerr (2010) distinguish between two independent forms of accuracy: mean-level bias and tracking accuracy. *Mean-level bias* reflects mean differences between the perceived qualities of one's partner and his or her actual qualities. *Tracking accuracy*, in contrast, is the extent to which correlations among a set of qualities are correctly perceived (similar to profile correlations). Consider the following example (adapted from Fletcher, 2002) of a hypothetical couple, Mary and Stephen. On Likert-type scales (where 1 = *not at all like my partner* and 7 = *very much like my partner*), Mary rates Stephen as highly sensitive (7), very warm (6), very sexy (6), and moderately ambitious (5). Now assume that we have another set of valid benchmark ratings of Stephen that represent *perfectly* valid and accurate ratings of him. These benchmark ratings are sensitive (6), warm (5), sexy (5), and ambitious (4). Comparing the two sets of ratings, Mary has a positively biased but fairly accurate view of Stephen; that is, the mean level of Mary's judgments (6) is one unit higher than the mean of the valid benchmark ratings (5), yet her ratings accurately track (perfectly parallel) the benchmark traits ($r = 1.0$). If, however, Mary gave Stephen ratings of 6, 7, 5, and 6, respectively, this would reflect the same level of positivity bias (because the mean level of her judgments are still one unit higher), but no accuracy (because these judgments do not track the relative levels across the different traits).

Using this definition of accuracy and bias, Fletcher and Kerr's (2010) meta-analysis revealed a substantial and reliable effect size of tracking accuracy across

98 studies of relationship partners ($r = .47$). The effect size of positive mean-level bias across 48 studies was also reliable, but somewhat lower ($r = .09$). Fletcher and Kerr also found positive mean-level bias for personality traits as well as relationship-relevant memories and predictions. With respect to individuals' perceptions of their partners' relationship-relevant beliefs, attitudes, and behaviors, they found *negative* mean-level bias. These findings make sense from the perspective of error management theory (Haselton & Buss, 2000), in that people might have more to lose by being positively biased about the degree to which a relationship partner loves them and forgives them for their transgressions. In the case of personality traits, memories, and predictions, there is little to lose (and, in fact, possibly much to gain) by holding such positive biases.

The Fletcher and Kerr (2010) meta-analysis also found that greater positive mean-level bias was associated with more positive perceptions of relationship quality, whereas tracking accuracy was unrelated to perceived relationship quality. This effect, however, was moderated by the stage of the relationship. Specifically, the connection between relationship satisfaction and positive mean-level biases decreased with relationship length. This suggests that when a relationship is blossoming and passion runs high, individuals are more motivated to be positively biased about their partners/relationships. This positive bias early in relationships may serve an adaptive function, insofar as it fosters closer bonds between new partners. However, as the relationship develops and passionate love is displaced by companionate love, positive biases toward the partner/relationship become less critical in maintaining relationship quality.

In summary, the Fletcher and Kerr (2010) meta-analysis reveals that individuals tend to be quite accurate in their perceptions of their relationship partners, at least with regard to the specific relations *among* their partners' traits. A certain degree of bias is also beneficial to relationship outcomes, at least when relationships are new. As relationships develop, however, bias tends to become more weakly related to overall perceptions of relationship quality.

Partner Knowledge in Relationships: Empathic Accuracy

When individuals interact with their romantic partners, the information they usually "act on" is not necessarily what their partners thought, felt, or did; they act on what they *perceive* their partners thought, felt, or did. For this reason, it is important to understand where "partner knowledge" comes from, as well as the circumstances in which it is "acted upon" in relationship contexts.

Empathic accuracy (Ickes, 2001) reflects the extent to which an individual accurately infers what his or her partner is thinking and feeling during a given social interaction. Although greater empathic accuracy tends to be associated with greater relationship satisfaction and stability in situations that pose little or no threat to relationships (e.g., Kahn, 1970; Noller, 1980), empathic accuracy is associated with *less* satisfaction and *less* stability in many relationship-threatening situations (e.g., Sillars, Pike, Jones, & Murphy, 1984; Simpson, Ickes, & Blackstone, 1995). At first blush, these findings seem somewhat counterintuitive given that relationship threats could be more easily defused or better resolved if each partner simply understood what the other was thinking and feeling more accurately.

To resolve this paradox, Ickes and Simpson (1997, 2001) developed a model of how relationship partners "manage" their levels of empathic accuracy in relationship-threatening versus nonthreatening contexts. As we shall see, the model identifies conditions under which (1) empathic accuracy should help relationships (the general rule); (2) empathic accuracy should hurt relationships (the major exception to the rule); and (3) empathic *in*accuracy may buffer individuals and relationships from potential harm (a complement of the exception to the rule).

The Empathic Accuracy Model

According to the empathic accuracy model (Ickes & Simpson, 1997, 2001), the upper and lower limits of empathic accuracy during a specific interaction are constrained by (1) each partner's "readability" (i.e., the degree to which he or she displays cues that reflect his or her true internal states), and (2) each partner's empathic ability (i.e., the degree to which he or she can accurately read his or her partner's valid behavioral cues). Within these boundaries, however, empathic accuracy can be managed differently depending on the context of an interaction. The interaction contexts that are most relevant to the empathic accuracy model are shown in Figure 14.2.

When relationship partners enter a situation, each individual first determines whether it might be a *danger zone* to the relationship. Danger zones are sensitive topic areas to one or both partners. In these areas, insights or revelations that emerge might easily threaten the relationship if a perceiver accurately inferred his or her partner's actual thoughts and feelings.

At the first branching point of the model, perceivers must decide whether a danger zone issue is present or might emerge in the situation. If perceivers believe they will discuss issues that are *not* relationship-threatening (see the right-hand side of Figure 14.2), they should be motivated to be empathically accurate, personal and relational distress should remain low, and the relationship should remain stable. That is, to the extent that (1) mutual understanding facilitates the coordination of joint actions so personal and relational goals can be achieved, and (2) the behaviors needed to achieve accurate understanding have been reinforced over time, most perceivers should be motivated to achieve moderately high levels of empathic accuracy in most non-relationship-threatening situations (see the far right-hand path of Figure 14.2). More specifically, in situations where danger zones are not likely to occur (e.g., during everyday conversations about nonthreatening issues), perceivers should adopt an "accuracy" orientation that allows them to clarify minor misunderstandings, keep disagreements from boiling over, and gain a clearer understanding of their partners' views on these issues. These tendencies, in turn, should maintain or sometimes even enhance relationship satisfaction and stability (see the middle-right portion of Figure 14.2).

However, perceivers are not always motivated to attend to their partner's thoughts and feelings, especially during interactions that are routine and become habitual (Thomas, Fletcher, & Lange, 1997). In these habitual and non-threatening interactions, the perceivers' levels of empathic accuracy should be moderate rather than high (see the lower right-hand side of Figure 14.2). Nonetheless, empathic accuracy should still be associated with greater relationship satisfaction and stability in these

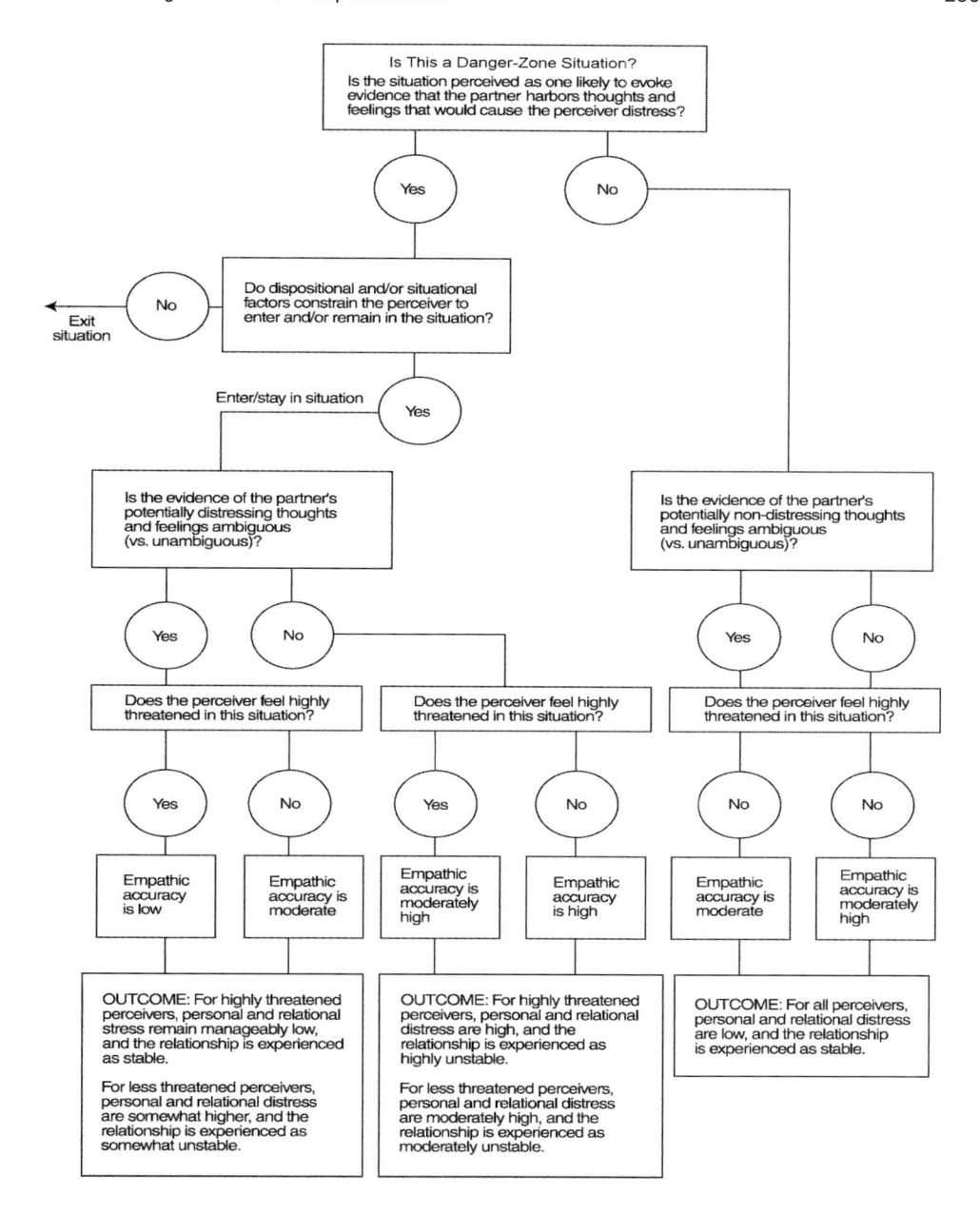

FIGURE 14.2. Ickes and Simpson's (2001) empathic accuracy model.

situations, consistent with the general rule that *greater empathic accuracy should help relationships* in benign, nonthreatening situations.

However, there are times when individuals encounter situations in which danger zone topics or issues could emerge and might destabilize their relationships (see the left-hand side of Figure 14.2). When these situations are encountered, most perceivers should try to avoid or escape from them if they can; that is, averting or escaping from danger zone situations should be the first tactic that most perceivers attempt to use to manage their empathic accuracy because doing so allows perceivers to avoid having to deal with evidence that their partner might be harboring relationship-damaging thoughts or feelings.

Avoiding or escaping danger zone issues, of course, is not always possible (see the left and middle portions of Figure 14.2). When perceivers must remain in a relationship-threatening situation, their second tactic should be *motivated inaccuracy*—a conscious or unconscious failure to infer accurately the potentially harmful thoughts and feelings that their partners might be having. Motivated inaccuracy is most likely to be an effective tactic when relationship threats are temporary or fleeting, they cannot be easily fixed or resolved, and they are unlikely to occur again in the future. The success of this strategy should hinge on the degree to which the cues of the partner's potentially damaging thoughts and feelings are ambiguous versus unambiguous. If the cues are ambiguous (see the middle left-hand side of Figure 14.2), perceivers can use motivated *in*accuracy as a defensive tactic. By disregarding, distorting, or reframing potentially threatening information, or by using other psychological defenses, such as denial, repression, or rationalization, individuals can shelter themselves from the threatening implications of their partners' private thoughts and feelings, resulting in low (and sometimes *very* low) levels of empathic accuracy. The selective use of these defenses may benefit perceivers and their relationships by minimizing personal and relational distress, thereby keeping the relationship more stable over time. The left-hand portion of the model illustrates this logical complement of the major exception to the general rule—that *motivated inaccuracy can sometimes sustain relationships faced with threat.*

Tests of the Empathic Accuracy Model

There have been several formal tests of the empathic accuracy model, the most relevant of which are discussed below. Simpson and colleagues (1995) first documented the use of motivated inaccuracy in relationship-threatening situations. They recruited heterosexual dating couples and asked each individual (partner) to view, rate, and then discuss slides of opposite-sex people on measures of physical attractiveness and sexual appeal *with his or her partner*. Dating partners completed this task while seated next to one another. Half of the couples were randomly assigned to view slides of highly attractive people (the high-threat condition), and half viewed less attractive people (the low-threat condition). After stating the attractiveness and sexual appeal rating of each stimulus person aloud (on a 1- to 10-point scale), the dating partner who made the rating then discussed what he or she liked or disliked about each stimulus person with his or her partner. After the rating and discussion task, each partner watched his or her videotaped session and reported when during the interaction he or she had a specific thought or feeling. The partner then watched the videotape and tried to infer each thought or feeling reported by his or her partner, which was the measure of each partner's level of empathic accuracy during the interaction.

In line with the empathic accuracy model, partners in the high-threat condition were more empathically *in*accurate than those in the low-threat condition. In other words, when confronted with a somewhat ambiguous situation that might pose a threat to their relationships (i.e., rating highly attractive opposite-sex people in the presence of their partner), individuals choose to not "get in the heads" of their partners. Given the temporary and inescapable nature of this threatening situation, individuals reacted as if it were more important to keep the interaction pleasant and amicable rather than recognize the lustful thoughts and feelings that their partners might be having about the highly attractive stimulus persons they were evaluating. Four months later, *all* of the couples in this specific condition were still dating, whereas nearly 30% of the other couples in the study had broken up. Thus, by *in*accurately inferring the relationship-threatening thoughts of their partners, individuals in the high-threat condition were able both to avoid unnecessary unpleasantness in the short run and to keep their relationships stable in the long run.

What happens when individuals are in relationship-threatening situations but cannot use motivated inaccuracy as a tactic to reduce threat? According to the empathic accuracy model (see the middle section of Figure 14.2), when cues signaling the relationship-threatening content of the partner's thoughts and feelings are unambiguous (e.g., the partner states he or she is having an extramarital affair), the sheer clarity of this information should force perceivers to have at least moderately high empathic accuracy, which should be followed by sharp declines in relationship satisfaction and stability. In this situation, greater empathic accuracy should actually harm relationships. However, because perceivers are forced to be accurate by virtue of the clarity of the available information, it is not a case in which *motivated* accuracy hurts relationships.

Motivated accuracy occurs when perceivers have a strong personal need to "know the truth" about what a partner is really thinking and feeling. As we discuss below, individuals who harbor insecurities about their value or worth as romantic partners (e.g., anxiously attached or low self-esteem individuals) should be particularly likely to display motivated accuracy. This special case is not shown in Figure 14.2. Need-based or disposition-based accuracy motives might occasionally override the initial tendency to avoid danger zone issues or to use motivated inaccuracy to dampen short-term relationship threats. These situations are a special case of the major exception to the general rule—that *motivated accuracy can hurt relationships when partners' thoughts and feelings are relationship-threatening*, just as unmotivated (situationally constrained) accuracy can.

The first study to demonstrate motivated accuracy was conducted by Simpson, Ickes, and Grich (1999). After recoding and reanalyzing the Simpson and colleagues (1995) dataset, Simpson and his colleagues (1999) found that more anxiously attached women were the most empathically accurate when their relationships were *most* threatened. Being more empathically accurate at "the worst times" led these women to report and experience the greatest emotional distress. Thus, by failing to rely on a motivated *in*accuracy strategy in this relationship-threatening context, highly anxious women suffered considerable emotional costs.

Other research has confirmed that higher levels of empathic accuracy forecast larger pre- to postdiscussion declines in the feelings of closeness during stressful discussions. Simpson, Oriña, and Ickes (2003) videotaped married couples as they attempted to resolve a nagging problem in their marriage. Consistent with the empathic accuracy model, when the partner's thoughts and feelings were relationship-threatening (rated by both partners and trained observers), heightened empathic accuracy on the part of the perceiver predicted larger pre- to postdiscussion declines in the perceiver's feelings of subjective closeness to his or her partner/relationship. The reverse was true when the partner's thoughts and feelings were nonthreatening.

The tendency to use motivated accuracy or motivated inaccuracy tactics should be associated with certain individual differences, especially anxious and avoidant attachment orientations. Highly avoidant individuals are motivated to maintain independence and autonomy in their close relationships, and one way they do so is by limiting the amount of personal information they know about their romantic partners (Rholes, Simpson, Tran, Martin, & Friedman, 2007). Highly anxious individuals, in contrast, are motivated to become closer and feel more secure in their relationships, which they accomplish by more closely monitoring their romantic partners when they (anxious individuals) feel threatened (Mikulincer & Shaver, 2003).

Simpson and colleagues (2011) conducted two social interaction studies to test how highly anxious and highly avoidant people managed empathic accuracy in discussions that differed in level of threat. In one study, married couples discussed threatening or nonthreatening relationship problems that centered on intimacy or jealousy issues; in the second study, dating couples tried to resolve a major or minor conflict in their relationship. In both studies, highly avoidant people displayed lower levels of empathic accuracy than less avoidant (more secure) people on average. The empathic accuracy levels of some highly avoidant participants, in fact, were barely above zero, reflecting complete inaccuracy. Many avoidant people, in other words, simply refused to "get into the heads" of their partners in order to maintain comfortable psychological distance. Across both studies, highly anxious individuals displayed greater empathic accuracy than less anxious (more secure) individuals, but only when they discussed relationship-threatening issues, illustrating motivated accuracy. Perhaps in an attempt to protect themselves or their relationships from exposure to harmful information, less anxious (more secure) people experienced slight *decreases* in empathic accuracy when relationship-threatening problems were being discussed, illustrating motivated inaccuracy.

Conclusion

In conclusion, what people know—or what they *believe* they know—about their partners and their relationships can have a strong bearing on the quality and stability of their romantic relationships. According to the empathic accuracy model, relationships should be happier and more stable when partners display motivated inaccuracy in *select* situations (Ickes & Simpson, 2001), especially those that pose temporary problems that cannot be "fixed" and are not likely to reoccur (Simpson et al., 1995). Not everyone, however, is able or willing to use this "turn a blind eye" tactic. Motivated accuracy is more likely to be the tactic of choice by some, such as highly anxious individuals, who feel compelled to know exactly what their partners are thinking and feeling, especially in relationship-threatening contexts (Simpson et al., 2011). Across time, we suspect that relationships may benefit the most from a situationally sensitive mix of controlled confrontation and discreet circumvention with respect to what one's partner is thinking and feeling in different situations. Highly secure individuals, who are motivated to build deeper and well-balanced intimacy with their romantic partners, may be most adept at managing this situational mix, knowing when to "turn on" and "turn off" partner monitoring.

REFERENCES

Acitelli, L. K. (1988). When spouses talk to each other about their relationship. *Journal of Social and Personal Relationships, 5,* 185–199.

Acitelli, L. K. (2002). Relationship awareness: Cross the bridge between cognition and communication. *Communication Theory, 12,* 92–112.

Acitelli, L. K., & Antonucci, T. C. (1994). Gender differences in the link between marital support and satisfaction in older couples. *Journal of Personality and Social Psychology, 67,* 688–698.

Acitelli, L. K., & Carlson, C. (1997, July). *Maintaining the relationship by attending to it.* Paper presented at the International Network on Personal Relationships Conference, Oxford, OH.

Acitelli, L. K., & Holmberg, D. (1993). Reflecting on relationships: The role of thoughts and memories. In D. Perlman & W. H. Jones (Eds.), *Advances in personal relationships* (Vol. 4, pp. 71–100). London: Kingsley.

Acitelli, L. K., Rogers, S., & Knee, C. R. (1999). The role of relational identity in the link between relationship thinking and relationship satisfaction. *Journal of Social and Personal Relationships, 16,* 591–618.

Aron, A., & Aron, E. N. (1986). *Love as the expansion of the self: Understanding attraction and satisfaction.* New York: Hemisphere.

Aron, A., Aron, E. N., & Norman, C. (2001). The self expansion model of motivation and cognition in close relationships and beyond. In M. Clark & G. Fletcher (Eds.), *Blackwell handbook of social psychology: Vol. 2. Interpersonal processes* (pp. 478–501). Oxford, UK: Blackwell.

Aron, A., Aron, E. N., Tudor, M., & Nelson, G. (1991). Close relationships as including other in the self. *Journal of Personality and Social Psychology, 60,* 241–253.

Aron, A., Paris, M., & Aron, E. N. (1995). Falling in love: Prospective studies of self-concept change. *Journal of Personality and Social Psychology, 69,* 1101–1112.

Fletcher, G. J. O. (2002). *The new science of intimate relationships.* Mahwah, NJ: Erlbaum.

Fletcher, G. J. O., & Kerr, P. S. G. (2010). Through the eyes of love: Reality and illusion in intimate relationships. *Psychological Bulletin, 136,* 627–658.

Franzoi, S., Davis, M. H., & Young, R. D. (1985). The effects of private self-consciousness and perspective taking on satisfaction in close relationships. *Journal of Personality and Social Psychology, 48,* 1584–1594.

Gottman, J. M. (1994). *What predicts divorce: The relationship between marital processes and marital outcomes.* Hillsdale, NJ: Erlbaum.

Harvey, J. H., & Omarzu, J. (1997). Minding the close relationship. *Personality and Social Psychology Review, 1,* 224–240.

Harvey, J. H., & Omarzu, J. (1999). *Minding the close relationship: A theory of relationship enhancement.* Cambridge, UK: Cambridge University Press.

Harvey, J. H., Pauwels, B. G., & Zickmund, S. (2002). Relationship connection: The role of minding in the enhancement of closeness. In C. R. Snyder & S. J. Lopez (Eds.), *Handbook of positive psychology* (pp. 423–433). New York: Oxford University Press.

Haselton, M. G., & Buss, D. M. (2000). Error management theory: A new perspective on biases in cross-sex mind-reading. *Journal of Personality and Social Psychology, 78*, 81–91.

Ickes, W. (2001). Measuring empathic accuracy. In J. A. Hall & F. J. Bernieri (Eds.), *Interpersonal sensitivity* (pp. 219–241). Mahwah, NJ: Erlbaum.

Ickes, W. (2003). *Everyday mind reading: Understanding what other people think and feel.* Amherst, NY: Prometheus Books.

Ickes, W., & Simpson, J. A. (1997). Managing empathic accuracy in close relationships. In W. Ickes (Ed.), *Empathic accuracy* (pp. 218–250). New York: Guilford Press.

Ickes, W., & Simpson, J. A. (2001). Motivational aspects of empathic accuracy. In G. J. O. Fletcher & M. S. Clark (Eds.), *Interpersonal processes: Blackwell handbook of social psychology: Interpersonal processes* (pp. 229–249). Oxford, UK: Blackwell.

Jacobson, N. S., & Christensen, A. (1996). *Integrative couple therapy: Promoting acceptance and change.* New York: Guilford Press.

Kahn, M. (1970). Nonverbal communication and marital satisfaction. *Family Process, 9*, 449–456.

Kobak, R., & Hazan, C. (1991). Attachment in marriage: Effects of security and accuracy of working models. *Journal of Personality and Social Psychology, 60*, 861–869.

Lewandowski, G. W., Jr., Aron, A., Bassis, S., & Kunak, J. (2006). Losing a self-expanding relationship: Implications for the self-concept. *Personal Relationships, 13*, 317–331.

Luo, S., & Snider, A. G., (2009). Accuracy and biases in newlyweds' perceptions of each other: Not mutually exclusive but mutually beneficial. *Psychological Science, 20*, 1332–1339.

Mashek, D. J., Aron, A., & Boncimino, M. (2003). Confusions of self with close others. *Personality and Social Psychology Bulletin, 29*, 382–392.

Mikulincer, M., & Shaver, P. R. (2003). The attachment behavioral system in adulthood: Activation, psychodynamics, and interpersonal processes. In M. P. Zanna (Ed.), *Advances in experimental social psychology* (Vol. 35, pp. 53–152). New York: Academic Press.

Murray, S. L., Holmes, J. G., & Griffin, D. W. (1996). The benefits of positive illusions: Idealization and the construction of satisfaction in close relationships. *Journal of Personality and Social Psychology, 70*, 79–98.

Neff, L. A., & Karney, B. R. (2002). Judgments of a relationship partner: Specific accuracy but global enhancement. *Journal of Personality, 70*, 1079–1112.

Neff, L. A., & Karney, B. R. (2005). To know you is to love you: Implications of global adoration and specific accuracy for marital relationships. *Journal of Personality and Social Psychology, 88*, 480–497.

Noller, P. (1980). Misunderstandings in marital communication: A study of couples' nonverbal communication. *Journal of Personality and Social Psychology, 39*, 1135–1148.

Rholes, W. S., Simpson, J. A., Tran, S., Martin, A. M., & Friedman, M. (2007). Attachment and information seeking in romantic relationships. *Personality and Social Psychology Bulletin, 33*, 422–438.

Sillars, A. L., Pike, G. R., Jones, T. S., & Murphy, M. A. (1984). Communication and understanding in marriage. *Human Communication Research, 10*, 317–350.

Simpson, J. A., Ickes, W., & Blackstone, T. (1995). When the head protects the heart: Empathic accuracy in dating relationships. *Journal of Personality and Social Psychology, 69*, 629–641.

Simpson, J. A., Ickes, W., & Grich, J. (1999). When accuracy hurts: Reactions of anxious–ambivalent dating partners to a relationship-threatening situation. *Journal of Personality and Social Psychology, 76*, 754–769.

Simpson, J. A., Kim, J., Fillo, J., Ickes, W., Rholes, W. S., Oriña, M. M., et al. (2011). Attachment and the management of empathic accuracy in relationship-threatening situations. *Personality and Social Psychology Bulletin, 37,* 242–254.

Simpson, J. A., Oriña, M. M., & Ickes, W. (2003). When accuracy hurts, and when it helps: A test of the empathic accuracy model in marital interactions. *Journal of Personality and Social Psychology, 85,* 881–893.

Swann, W. B., De La Ronde, C., & Hixon, J. G. (1994). Authenticity and positive strivings in marriage and courtship. *Journal of Personality and Social Psychology, 66,* 857–869.

Thomas, G., Fletcher, G. J. O., & Lange, C. (1997). On-line empathic accuracy in marital interaction. *Journal of Personality and Social Psychology, 72,* 839–850.

Van Yperen, N. W., & Buunk, B. P. (1991). Equity theory and exchange and communal orientation from a cross-national perspective. *Journal of Social Psychology, 131,* 5–20.

Wood, J. T., & Inman, C. (1993). In a different mode: Masculine styles of communicating closeness. *Journal of Applied Communication Research, 21,* 279–295.

CHAPTER 15

Meta-Accuracy
Do We Know How Others See Us?

ERIKA N. CARLSON
DAVID A. KENNY

Trust not yourself, but your defects to know,
Make use of every friend and every foe.
—ALEXANDER POPE (1822)

Very early in life, we realize that others have minds, and we attempt to understand what is going in those minds. Perhaps more than anything else, what we often want to know is how others perceive us. Intuitively, forming beliefs about how others perceive us, called *metaperception* (Laing, Phillipson, & Lee, 1966), seems to require a great deal of mind reading and attention to social cues. Perhaps for this reason, the degree to which metaperceptions are correct, called *meta-accuracy* (Kenny & DePaulo, 1993), has generally been viewed as a form of *social* knowledge. However, in many ways, meta-accuracy is also a form of *self*-knowledge (Vazire & Carlson, 2010). As we show, meta-accuracy often reflects self-knowledge of one's own personality and behavior (Albright, Forest, & Reiseter, 2001; Albright & Malloy, 1999; Kenny & West, 2008), and of how one's behavior differs across social contexts (Carlson & Furr, 2009; Malloy, Albright, Kenny, Agatstein, & Winquist, 1997).

In this chapter, we provide a summary of the findings for meta-accuracy and focus on factors that affect meta-accuracy. First, we define three different types of meta-accuracy and review the results from 26 studies that highlight the bright spots (i.e., when people are meta-accurate) and blind spots (i.e., when they are not) of meta-accuracy research. Next, we explore how people form metaperceptions, and in doing so, identify potential moderators that affect meta-accuracy. Finally, we consider the benefits and costs of meta-accuracy, speculate about how people might become better metaperceivers, and provide suggestions for future research.

Do People Know How They Are Seen by Others?

When examining meta-accuracy, a basic question is do *metaperceivers* hold accurate beliefs about how others, or *judges*, perceive them? Because meta-accuracy can be conceptualized as several conceptually independent questions (Fletcher & Kerr, 2010; Kenny & DePaulo, 1993), the answer is necessarily multifaceted. The first type of meta-accuracy, called *generalized meta-accuracy* (GMA; Kenny, 1994), assesses whether people know how they are perceived by others in general (i.e., do people know their reputation?). The second type, called *dyadic* or *differential meta-accuracy* (DMA; Carlson & Furr, 2009; Kenny, 1994), assesses whether people know the impression they make on a specific person (e.g., do people know how a romantic partner sees them differently than a best friend?). The third type, called *metaperception enhancement* (MPE), assesses whether people consistently over- or underestimate how positively others see them (i.e., do people assume that others see them more positively than they really do?).

Our summary focuses exclusively on meta-accuracy for traits and affect in adults' face-to-face interactions. Specifically, our summary includes studies that have assessed meta-accuracy in first-impression contexts (i.e., laboratory studies in which people meet for the first time) and acquainted contexts (i.e., naturalistic contexts, such as coworkers) but excludes studies that examined metastereotypes (i.e., beliefs of how others stereotype groups of persons; e.g., Frey & Tropp, 2006), hypothetical or computer-mediated interactions (e.g., Hebert & Vorauer, 2003), and studies of children (e.g., Malloy, Albright, & Scarpati, 2007). Based on these criteria, our summary included 26 studies that contain 174 estimates of meta-accuracy effects.[1] Table 15.1 summarizes the meta-analytic averages of generalized and dyadic meta-accuracy for the following traits: the Big Five, leadership, attractiveness, evaluative traits (positive and negative), well-being, needs, and likeability. Table 15.2 summarizes findings for MPE for both traits and affect based on the eight studies from Kenny and DePaulo (1993), and reflect the differences between metaperceptions and the judges' perceptions.

Generalized Meta-Accuracy: Do People Know Their Reputation?

Generalized meta-accuracy (GMA) reflects the degree to which people understand how others generally see them, or whether people know their reputation (Kenny, 1994). GMA is typically assessed in studies that employ a *round-robin* design, where each person in a small group provides ratings for every other group member (i.e., everyone serves both as a metaperceiver and a judge; e.g., Malloy & Janowski, 1992), or a *one-with-many* design, where a metaperceiver guesses how judges perceive him or her and then those judges rate his or her personality (e.g., Carlson & Furr, 2009). In both cases, GMA is measured as the degree to which metaperceivers' average metaperceptions corresponds to the average impression of their judges.

The left three columns of Table 15.1 summarize the GMA findings. GMA is strongest for the Big Five ($r = .38$), especially for Extraversion ($r = .58$), and weaker for evaluative traits (positive: $r = .18$; negative: $r = .20$) and needs ($r = .17$). For first-impression contexts, GMA is especially strong for observable traits, such as Extraversion ($r = .51$). For acquaintances (e.g., friends, family, and coworkers), GMA is strong for most traits

TABLE 15.1. Summary of GMA and DMA

Trait	GMA Overall	GMA First impression	GMA Acquaintance	DMA Overall	DMA First impression	DMA Acquaintance
Big Five						
Extraversion	.58(18)	.51(5)	.63(13)	.28(8)	.21(24)	.35(4)
Agreeableness	.40(15)	.17(2)	.46(13)	.22(9)	.09(5)	.40(4)
Conscientiousness	.29(20)	.06(5)	.42(15)	.19(9)	.09(5)	.32(4)
Emotion stability	.38(18)	.34(5)	.42(13)	.12(7)	.01(3)	.25(4)
Openness	.24(11)	−.02(2)	.31(9)	.37(4)	.42(1)	.34(3)
Mean	.38	.22	.45	.24	.17	.33
Dominance/Leadership						
Leadership	.30(5)	.33(4)	.20(1)	.07(2)	.07(2)	
Assertive	.21(2)	.16(1)	.27(1)			
Competent	.22(1)	.22(1)				
Good at public speaking	.12(1)	.05(1)	.20(1)			
Confident				.19(1)	.19(1)	
Likes to be the center of attention	.41(2)	.31(1)	.51(1)			
Mean	.25	.22	.30	.13	.13	
Attractiveness						
Physically attractive	.32(11)	.28(6)	.37(5)	.20(5)	.11(3)	.42(2)
Sexy	.16(2)	.16(2)		.12(2)	.12(2)	
Mean	.24	.22	.37	.16	.12	.42
Evaluative—positive						
Intelligent	.18(18)	.11(6)	.23(12)	.18(5)	.14(4)	.31(1)
Funny	.17(2)	.02(1)	.31(1)	.25(2)	.20(1)	.30(1)
Honest	.18(2)	.04(1)	.33(1)	.11(2)	−.03(1)	.23(1)
Mean	.18	.06	.29	.18	.10	.28
Evaluative—negative						
Exaggerates his or her skills	.14(2)	.18(1)	.09(1)	.19(2)	.24(1)	.15(1)
Arrogant	.22(2)	.13(1)	.31(1)	.27(2)	.21(1)	.33(1)
Impulsive	.16(2)	.18(1)	.14(1)	.25(2)	.15(1)	.34(1)
Personality pathology	.26(10)		.26(10)			
Mean	.20	.16	.20	.24	.20	.28
Well-being						
Happy	.30(3)	.11(1)	.42(2)			
Depressed	.10(2)	−.07(1)	.27(1)			
Lonely	.34(3)		.34(3)			
High self-esteem	.28(4)	.09(1)	.35(3)			
Mean	.26	.04	.35			
Needs						
Strong drive to achieve	.19(2)	.02(1)	.36(1)			
Strong need to be around others	.06(2)	−.04(1)	.16(1)			
Values power in self and others	.25(2)	.12(1)	.38(1)	.17(2)	.13(1)	.20(1)
Mean	.17	.03	.30	.17	.13	.20
Likeability						
Interesting	.45(1)		.45(1)	.45(1)		.45(1)
Tends to be liked by others	.20(2)	.12(1)	.28(1)			
Likeable	.26(5)	.29(2)	.24(3)	.25(2)	.13(1)	.35(1)
Tends to like others	.22(2)	.04(1)	.40(1)			
Mean	.29	.15	.35	.35	.13	.40

Note. Meta-accuracy for individual traits reflects the meta-analytic average correlation (i.e., the Hunter-Schmidt method; Field & Gillet, 2010). Estimates were based on the number of correlations contained in the subscript. Mean correlations for trait categories were computed by first averaging the Fisher *r*-to-*z*-transformed meta-analytic average correlations and then transforming the averages back into correlations. In addition to computing an overall index of GMA and DMA for each trait (i.e., Overall), we also computed indices of GMA and DMA for first impression and acquaintance (e.g., friends, family, and coworkers) contexts.

TABLE 15.2. MPE and Self-Enhancement for Affect and Traits

Study	MPE Affect	MPE Trait	Self-enhancement Affect	Self-enhancement Trait
Anderson (1984)		0.34		0.80
Curry & Kenny (1974)	0.08			
DePaulo et al. (1987)	−0.38	−0.08		
Kenny & DePaulo (1990)	−0.18	−0.08	0.23	0.10
Malloy & Albright (1990)		0.03	0.26	
Malloy & Janowski (1992)		0.27		0.41
Oliver (1988)	−0.11	0.10	0.04	0.21
Reno & Kenny (1992)	−0.22	0.15	−0.02	0.41
Mean	−0.16	0.11	0.13	0.39

Note. MPE reflects the mean difference between metaperceptions and the judges' actual perceptions. A positive difference indicates overestimation or enhancement whereas a negative difference indicates underestimation or deprecation. Measures are transformed to be on a 7-point scale.

but notably weaker for undesirable traits ($r = .20$). Finally, GMA tends to be weaker in first-impression contexts than among acquaintances, and the differences between contexts are especially strong for internal traits such as well-being (first impression: $r = .04$; acquainted: $r = .35$) and needs (first impression: $r = .03$; acquainted: $r = .30$).

Dyadic Meta-Accuracy: Do People Know the Unique Impressions That They Make?

Dyadic or differential meta-accuracy (DMA) reflects the degree to which people can detect how others uniquely see them. There are two ways to conceptualize DMA: a trait-centered approach and a person-centered approach.[2] The trait-centered approach conceptualizes DMA as the degree to which people can detect who sees them as particularly high or low on a given trait. Like GMA, trait-centered DMA is often assessed using a round-robin or a one-with-many design. The right three columns of Table 15.1 summarize results for trait-centered DMA. As shown, DMA is stronger for likeability ($r = .35$) than for other traits, such as the Big Five ($r = .24$). Interestingly, DMA appears to be stronger for agentic, or "get ahead" traits (Extraversion: $r = .21$; Openness: $r = .42$), than for communal, or "get along" traits (Agreeableness: $r = .09$; tends to like others: $r = .04$), for new acquaintances in a first-impression context. However, the opposite is true for acquaintances (e.g., friends, family, and coworkers)—DMA is somewhat stronger for communal traits (Agreeableness: $r = .40$; tends to like others: $r = .40$) than for agentic traits (Extraversion: $r = .35$; Openness: $r = .34$).

Person-centered DMA reflects the degree to which people can detect which traits a judge perceives as more characteristic of their personality and is generally measured as the profile correlation between metaperceptions and actual impressions across a set of traits (Campbell & Fehr, 1990; Carlson, Furr, & Vazire, 2010; Ohtsubo, Takezawa, & Fukuno, 2009; Snodgrass, 2001). For instance, person-centered DMA reflects people's ability to guess whether a particular friend sees them as more extraverted than agreeable and anxious. After a short conversation with a new acquaintance, people achieve DMA for the Big Five and other traits, such as "honest" (Carlson et al., 2010; Carlson, Vazire, & Furr, 2009; Ohtsubo et al., 2009). Even more impressive, people's confidence in their metaperceptions correlates positively with their meta-accuracy for a new acquaintance, as well as for close others (Carlson et al., 2009, 2010). In other words, people seem to have some self-knowledge about their meta-accuracy or lack thereof.

Metaperception Enhancement: Do People Over- or Underestimate How Others See Them?

MPE reflects the degree to which people over- or underestimate how others see them. For example, do people think they are perceived more positively than they actually are? MPE reflects the mean difference between metaperceptions and the judges' actual perceptions. A positive difference indicates *overestimation*, or *enhancement*, whereas a negative difference indicates *underestimation*, or *deprecation*. Thus, MPE is similar to measures of self-enhancement (SE; Taylor & Brown, 1988) that compare the mean difference between self-perceptions and some measure of personality.

The positive illusions literature generally shows that most people view themselves in overly positive ways (i.e., self-enhancement). Thus, we might expect that metaperceptions are also positively biased. Table 15.2 summarizes the results for MPE. For affect, metaperceptions are less positive than the judges' perceptions (mean MPE = −0.16), suggesting that people underestimate how much others like them. For traits, metaperceptions were more positive than the judge's perceptions (mean MPE = 0.11), suggesting that people overestimate how positively they are seen by others. However, trait MPE was much less than self-enhancement (mean SE = 0.39). Thus, it appears that people's metaperceptions are closer to judges' perceptions than are their self-perceptions.

Summary

Our review revealed several bright spots and blind spots in meta-accuracy. On the bright side, people have insight into how they are generally seen by others on core personality traits: They know who especially likes them, they can detect which traits others perceive as especially characteristic of their personality, and they seem to have some self-knowledge about when their metaperceptions are accurate. On the darker side, people struggle to detect their reputation on evaluative traits and, to some extent, hold overly positive metaperceptions relative to others' impressions. Next, we examine the sources of information that people use to form metaperceptions and how each source might be responsible for the bright spots and blind spots in meta-accuracy that we have just reviewed.

Causes of Metaperception: Searching for Moderators of Meta-Accuracy

Kenny and his colleagues (Kenny, 1994; Kenny & DePaulo, 1993) have discussed three potential sources of information people use to form metaperceptions: feedback from others, self-perceptions of personality, and self-observation of behavior. We propose a fourth source: the use of heuristics. In this section, we review the extent to which each of the four sources is used to form metaperceptions and how each source might aid or hinder meta-accuracy.

Feedback from Others

Intuitively, perceptions of verbal or nonverbal feedback from the other should provide the most diagnostic information about others' actual impressions (Cooley, 1902; Jussim, Soffin, Brown, Ley, & Kohlhepp, 1992; Kenny & DePaulo, 1993; Mead, 1934). For feedback to lead to meta-accuracy, at least two things must occur: (1) The judge must provide valid feedback and (2) the metaperceiver must detect and correctly utilize that information. However, both processes are far from perfect. People often fail to provide feedback (Blumberg, 1972), or they provide feedback that is ambiguous or deceptive (e.g., Swann, Stein-Seroussi, & McNulty, 1992). People also have a difficult time detecting or utilizing feedback even when it is available and unambiguous (Shechtman & Kenny, 1994). For example, generating conversation topics and responding to others prevents people from observing feedback (Kenny & DePaulo, 1993; Liberman & Rosenthal, 2001), and even when people do observe feedback, the motivation to make a desirable impression, to be seen in a positive way, or to be seen as they see themselves, may prevent people from correctly interpreting diagnostic feedback (Kwang & Swann, 2010). These informational and motivational barriers might explain why people who base their metaperceptions primarily on their perceptions of feedback are often less meta-accurate than are people who base their metaperceptions on their self-perceptions (Kaplan, Santuzzi, & Ruscher, 2009). Thus, despite the intuitive appeal of feedback, basing metaperceptions on the feedback from judges seems to hurt more than help meta-accuracy.

Self-Perceptions of Traits

Metaperception seems to require that people somehow peer into the minds of others. In fact, symbolic interactionists call metaperceptions *reflected appraisals* (Felson, 1980), which refers to the process of looking through the eyes of significant others to form self-perceptions (Cooley, 1902; Mead, 1934). Yet several researchers have concluded that people assume others see them as they see themselves, instead of the other way around.

Metaperceptions are strongly correlated with self-perceptions ($r = .87$; Kenny, 1994), which suggests that meta-accuracy might largely depend on the extent to which others actually share one's self-views (i.e., self–other agreement). There is, we believe, strong evidence for the role of self-perception in the formation of metaperceptions. First, self–other agreement is strong for close others and weaker for new acquaintances (Connelly & Ones, 2010; Vazire & Carlson, 2010). GMA and DMA show the same pattern, perhaps because people (correctly) assume that the ones they are closest to see them as they see themselves. Second, self–other agreement is stronger for observable traits but weaker for evaluative traits (John & Robins, 1993). GMA is also stronger for observable traits and weaker for evaluative traits, which provides further evidence that meta-accuracy is strong when self–other agreement is also strong. Together, these results suggest that people rely heavily on their self-perceptions of their personality when forming metaperceptions and that this reliance leads to meta-accuracy.

In general, self-perception appears to be a valid source of information, especially for close others and for observable, nonevaluative traits. However, basing metaperceptions on self-perceptions of personality also explains some inaccuracies of metaperception in several domains. First, even if our global self-perception reflects how we are generally seen, some people are particularly harsh or lenient judges of personality (Srivastava, Guglielmo, & Beer, 2010; Wood, Harms, & Vazire, 2010). Thus, basing metaperceptions on self-perceptions prevents people from detecting the unique impressions they make (Kenny & DePaulo, 1993). This might also explain why DMA is generally weaker than GMA. Second, self–other agreement is often weaker for internal traits because others do not have access to thoughts and emotions, suggesting that meta-accuracy should also be weaker for internal traits than for observable traits when metaperceptions are based on self-perceptions. This might explain why meta-accuracy is relatively weak for traits such as depression and emotional stability. Third, people are generally motivated to see themselves in a positive light, especially on evaluative traits (John & Robins, 1993; Vazire, 2010). This might explain why GMA is weaker for personality pathology than for the Big Five traits.

Self-Observation of Behavior

Although self-perceptions are strongly correlated with metaperceptions, metaperceptions and meta-accuracy are not entirely due to self-perceptions. Specifically, people make valid distinctions between how they see themselves and how others see them, a form of self-knowledge called *meta-insight* (Carlson, Vazire, & Furr, 2011). Moreover, if people relied exclusively on self-perception, they would never detect the unique impressions they made (i.e., there would be no DMA). Instead, it appears that people also use self-perceptions of their behavior to guess how they are seen by others (Felson, 1980). Given that judges generally base their personality judgments on their observations of metaperceivers' behavior, and that judges tend to agree about which behaviors reflect which traits (Funder & Sneed, 1993; Mehl, Gosling, & Pennebaker, 2006), metaperceptions are likely to be correct if they are also based on observing one's own (i.e., the metaperceiver's) behavior. Indeed, there is strong evidence that when we attend to our behavior (Albright et al., 2001) or when we have special access to our behavior (e.g., videotape feedback; Albright & Malloy, 1999), meta-accuracy is strong.

Self-observation of behavior might explain why GMA and DMA are strong for observable traits like extraversion. Self-observation might also explain an interesting pattern of findings for DMA not reported in Table 15.1. Specifically, DMA tends to be weak when assessed for judges who know metaperceivers from a single social context (e.g., roommates; Malloy & Albright, 1990) but stronger when assessed for judges who know metaperceivers from different social contexts (e.g., college friends vs. hometown friends vs. parents; Carlson & Furr, 2009). People tend to behave differently in different situations (Furr & Funder, 2004) and make different impressions on those who know them from different social contexts (Funder, Kolar, & Blackman, 1995). Carlson and Furr (2009) found that people can detect the unique impressions they make across social contexts, suggesting that perhaps people understand how their behavior varies across social contexts. However, the research examining meta-insight discussed earlier found that people do not base their metaperceptions exclusively on their behavior or on context-specific self-perceptions (Carlson et al., 2011). In other words, metaperceptions incorporate valid information other than self-perception of personality and self-observation of behavior.

Despite the apparent boost in meta-accuracy, self-observation of behavior might not always be a path to meta-accuracy because people do not always know very well how they behave (Gosling, John, Craik, & Robins, 1998; Leising, Rehbein, & Sporberg, 2006; Vazire & Mehl, 2008). Metaperceivers and judges have unique perspectives, such that metaperceivers tend to notice and remember more information about their internal experiences (e.g., feelings of nervousness), past behavior, or the judge's behavior, than about their own current behavior (Albright et al., 2001; Chambers, Epley, Savitsky, & Windschitl, 2008; DePaulo, 1992; Malle & Pearce, 2001). For example, a shy person might assume that others perceive his or her lack of talkativeness as shyness when others actually perceive him or her as cold. Thus, we often mistakenly assume that the thoughts and intentions underlying our behavior are apparent to others (Cameron & Vorauer, 2008; Gilovich, Savitsky, & Medvec, 1998; see also Hansen & Pronin, Chapter 21, this volume). We also often fail to notice the extremity of our behavior because we have become accustomed to our own behavioral style (Leising et al., 2006). Additionally, our ability to accurately observe our behavior may also be hindered by self-enhancement motives (Gosling et al., 1998; Hall, Murphy, & Mast, 2007).

Heuristics

A fourth source of information that might drive metaperceptions is the use of heuristics or assumptions that the perceiver makes to guess the judge's metaperception. We discuss three heuristics that drive metaperception: assumed reciprocity, assumed similarity, and normativeness. *Assumed reciprocity* reflects the tendency to assume that others see us as we see them, and it probably has mixed effects on meta-accuracy. Assumed reciprocity should have positive effects for DMA, specifically for traits that tend to show actual reciprocity, such as likeability (e.g., if I think that you are likeable, you are more likely to see me as likeable as well). Yet, for the same traits, assumed reciprocity may have negative effects for GMA because actual reciprocity of liking at the group level tends to be low or even negative (Eastwick, Finkel, Mochon & Ariely, 2007; Kenny, 1994).

Assumed similarity reflects the tendency to assume that others share our personality traits. This can affect meta-accuracy in two ways. First, it can affect the positivity of metaperceptions: If we think that others are similar to us, we assume that others will like us (Newcomb, 1953), and that others will rate us positively. This might explain why mutual liking tends to result in meta-accuracy (Ohtsubo et al., 2009)—the positivity of metaperceptions and judges' actual ratings probably covary with liking. Second, assumed similarity might increase the chance that people base their metaperceptions on self-perceptions: If we think others are like us, we assume that others see us as we see ourselves. Because close others are actually likely to see us similarly to how we see ourselves, assumed similarity likely has positive effects for meta-accuracy among close others but may hinder meta-accuracy in first-impression contexts.

Normativeness reflects information about the typical person. For example, before meeting someone for the first time, we might assume that he or she is more kind than cruel, which is true of most people. Normativeness likely has its greatest effect on meta-accuracy in first-impression contexts because people have little information about judges and believe that judges have little information about them (Ames, 2004; Biesanz, West, & Millevoi, 2007; Kenny, 1994). One way to assess the role of normativeness is to remove the average rating from all observations (i.e., meta-perceptions and actual impressions) before computing meta-accuracy, which removes any potential agreement about what the typical person is like (Cronbach, 1955; Furr, 2008; Kenny & Acitelli, 1994). In first-impression contexts, person-centered DMA decreases substantially when normativeness is removed, suggesting that information about the typical person is a major source of information driving metaperceptions in these situations (e.g., Carlson et al., 2010; Kenny, Snook, Boucher, & Hancock, 2010). We hope that future work will investigate the role of normative information in metaperceptions for close others.

Summary

Overall, it appears that we rely heavily on self-perceptions when forming metaperceptions, and that this strategy seems to help more than hurt meta-accuracy. Yet self-perception is not the whole story, suggesting that self-observations of behavior, feedback, and heuristics are also paths to meta-accuracy. Regardless of the source of information, the two major obstacles we face when it comes to learning how others see us are informational and motivational barriers. For instance, we do not always have access to a judge's reaction to us or to our own behavior (informational barriers), and our desire to be seen in certain ways often lead us to look for certain types of feedback, to see our personality and behavior in certain ways, and to assume that others feel the same way about us as we feel about them (motivational barriers). In summary, the path to meta-accuracy is much more complicated than we might naively think.

Improving Meta-Accuracy: Implications and Future Directions

How might we become better metaperceivers? Given that meta-accuracy is mostly hindered by informational and motivational barriers, improving meta-accuracy might simply require that we process (more) information in an unbiased and nonjudgmental manner. A recent study provides initial support for this possibility. Specifically, people high in trait mindfulness had better meta-accuracy for evaluative traits such as attractiveness and agreeableness (Carlson, Vazire, & Livingston, 2011). *Mindfulness* refers to awareness and attention to the present moment, and nonjudgmental observation of one's experience (Brown & Ryan, 2003). Why might individuals higher in mindfulness be more meta-accurate? One possibility is that these individuals pay more attention in social interactions and, consequently, notice more of their own or others' behavior. Another possibility is that these individuals respond to observations of themselves or others in less defensive or ego-protective ways (see Leary & Toner, Chapter 25, this volume). Future research might identify other moderators of meta-accuracy by taking an approach similar to Funder's (1995) realistic accuracy model (RAM) of personality; that is, like mindfulness, there may be other types of "good metaperceivers," as well as "good judges" (e.g., individuals who are easy to read), "good information" (e.g., less ambiguous feedback), or "good traits." There may also be important interactions between these moderators (e.g., interactions between metaperceivers and traits). For example, narcissists are aware that others see them as narcissistic (Carlson, Vazire, & Oltmanns, 2011) suggesting that perhaps certain types of metaperceivers are skilled at detecting the impressions they make about certain traits.

Interestingly, one relatively unexplored empirical question is whether meta-accuracy is beneficial or costly. There are a few reasons to believe that meta-accuracy is beneficial. First, meta-accuracy probably improves our ability to make important decisions. For example, DMA allows us to select the best person for a professional recommendation and to pursue relationships with people who see us positively, or see us as we see ourselves (Kwang & Swann, 2010). Second, meta-accuracy provides an opportunity to improve self-knowledge. Others know more than we know about certain aspects of our personality (e.g., evaluative traits; Vazire, 2010). Thus, one way to learn more about what we are like is to learn more about how others see us (Vazire & Carlson, 2011; Wilson & Dunn, 2004). This type of self-knowledge allows us to make positive changes in our behavior (e.g., learning that others see us as cold and aloof might prompt us to show more warmth). Of course, meta-accuracy about negative information might initially be costly. For example, the sociometer theory of self-esteem argues that we experience low self-esteem when we believe that we have made negative impressions (Leary, 2005). However, the temporary blow to one's ego is likely outweighed by the fact that meta-accuracy protects us from larger, more negative consequences (e.g., asking the wrong person for a letter of recommendation).

Despite these potential benefits, there are some situations in which people might benefit more from being inaccurate about the impressions they make. We can think of two such examples. First, in many cases, it may be best for people to use role prescriptions to guess how they are seen by others to be accurate (e.g., a supervisor may be better off using a role prescription when guessing how subordinates see him or her; Steiner, 1955). Indeed, individuals in a supervisor role are less meta-accurate than individuals in a subordinate role (Snodgrass, 1992). Second, several findings in the close relationships literature suggest that knowing too well what is going on in one's partner's mind can be harmful to the relationship. For instance, accurately perceiving relationship-threatening thoughts during discussions about relationship problems or accurately inferring romantic partners' thoughts about alternative dating partners results in reduced feelings of closeness (Simpson, Ickes, & Grich, 1999; Simpson, Oriña, & Ickes, 2003; see also Simpson, Fillo, & Myers, Chapter 14, this volume). In fact, being deluded about how much a partner cares about the self (i.e., inferring that he or she cares more than he or she does) is associated with greater relationship satisfaction, as well as more positive thoughts and emotions, and these consequences may actually bolster the partner's caring over time (Lemay & Clark, 2008; Lemay, Clark, & Feeney, 2007). We hope that future research will explore the short- and long-term consequences of meta-accuracy.

In conclusion, although meta-accuracy is often considered to be a form of social knowledge, we suggest that understanding how others perceive us reflects a form of self-knowledge. Our review has revealed that although we have a great deal of self-knowledge about how our personality manifests itself in different contexts, meta-accuracy is far from perfect. Given the role meta-accuracy might play in shedding light on the blind spots in self-knowledge, we hope that future research will explore how meta-accuracy might be improved.

ACKNOWLEDGMENT

We wish to thank Edward Lemay for helpful comments.

NOTES

1. Studies included in the review are noted in the reference section (*).
2. As discussed in Kenny and Winquist (2001), what we call *person-centered* DMA is essentially the same as trait-centered DMA. We also note that GMA correlations tend to be larger than DMA correlation because GMA correlations benefit from the aggregation across judges.

REFERENCES

Asterisks (*) indicate papers included in Tables 15.1 and 15.2.

Albright, L., Forest, C., & Reiseter, K. (2001). Acting, behaving, and the selfless basis of metaperception. *Journal of Personality and Social Psychology, 81*, 910–921.
Albright, L., & Malloy, T. E. (1999). Self-observation of social behavior in metaperception. *Journal of Personality and Social Psychology, 77*, 726–734.
Ames, D. R. (2004). Inside the mind reader's tool kit: Projection and stereotyping in mental state inferences. *Journal of Personality and Social Psychology, 87*, 340–353.
Anderson, R. D. (1984). *Measuring social self-perception: How accurately can individuals predict how others view them?* Unpublished doctoral dissertation, University of Connecticut, Storrs. (*)
Back, M. D., Krause, S., Hirschmüller, S., Stopfer, J. M., Egloff, B., & Schmukle, S. C. (2009). Unraveling the three faces of self-esteem. A new information-processing sociometer. *Journal of Research in Personality, 43*, 933–937. (*)
Biesanz, J. C., West, S. G., & Millevoi, A. (2007). What do you learn about someone over time?: The relationship between length of acquaintance and consensus and self–other agreement in judgments of personality. *Journal of Personality and Social Psychology, 92*, 119–135.
Blumberg, H. H. (1972). Communication of interpersonal evaluations. *Journal of Personality and Social Psychology, 23*, 157–162.
Brown, K. W., & Ryan, R. M. (2003). The benefits of being present: Mindfulness and its role in psychological well-being. *Journal of Personality and Social Psychology, 84*, 822–848.
Cameron, J. J., & Vorauer, J. D. (2008). Feeling transparent: On metaperceptions and miscommunications. *Social and Personality Psychology Compass, 2*, 1093–1108.

Campbell, J. D., & Fehr, B. (1990). Self-esteem and perceptions of conveyed impressions: Is negative affectivity associated with greater realism? *Journal of Personality and Social Psychology, 58*, 122–133.

Carlson, E. N., & Furr, R. M. (2009). Evidence of differential meta-accuracy: People understand the different impressions they make. *Psychological Science, 20*, 1033–1039. (*)

Carlson, E. N., Furr, R. M., & Vazire, S. (2010). Do we know the first impressions we make?: Evidence for idiographic meta-accuracy and calibration of first impressions. *Social Psychological and Personality Science, 1*, 94–98.

Carlson, E. N., Vazire, S., & Furr, R. M. (2009, July). *Moderators of differential meta-accuracy.* Poster presented at the 1st annual conference for the Association for Research in Personality, Chicago.

Carlson, E. N., Vazire, S., & Furr, R. M. (2011). Meta-insight: Do people really know how others see them? *Journal of Personality and Social Psychology, 101*, 831–846.

Carlson, E. N., Vazire, S. & Livingston, J. (2011). Mindfulness as a path to self-knowledge. In C. Carlson & S., Vazire (Chairs), *Minding the self: How mindfulness improves self-reflection and self-knowledge.* Symposium conducted at 12th annual meeting of the Society of Personality and Social Psychology, San Antonio, TX.

Carlson, E. N., Vazire, S., & Oltmanns, T. F. (2011). You probably think this paper's about you: Narcissists' perceptions of their personality and reputation. *Journal of Personality and Social Psychology, 101*, 185–201. (*)

Chambers, J. R., Epley, N., Savitsky, K., & Windschitl, P. D. (2008). Knowing too much: Using private knowledge to predict how one is viewed by others. *Psychological Science, 19*, 542–548.

Christensen, P. N., Stein, M. B., & Means-Christensen, A. (2003). Social anxiety and interpersonal perception: A social relations model analysis. *Behaviour Research and Therapy, 41*, 1355–1371. (*)

Connelly, B. S., & Ones, D. S. (2010). An other perspective on personality: Meta-analytic integration of observers' accuracy and predictive validity. *Psychological Bulletin, 136*, 1092–1122.

Cooley, C. H. (1902). *Human nature and the social order.* New York: Scribner.

Cronbach, L. J. (1955). Processes affecting scores on "understanding of others" and "assumed similarity." *Psychological Bulletin, 52*, 177–193.

Curry, T., & Kenny, D. A. (1974). The effect of perceived and actual similarity in value and personality in the process of interpersonal attraction. *Quantity and Quality, 8*, 27–44.

DePaulo, B. M. (1992). Nonverbal behavior and self-presentation. *Psychological Bulletin, 111*, 203–243.

DePaulo, B. M., Kenny, D. A., Hoover, C. W., Webb, W., & Oliver, P. (1987). Accuracy of person perception: Do people know what kinds of impressions they convey? *Journal of Personality and Social Psychology, 52*, 303–315. (*)

Eastwick, P. W., Finkel, E. J., & Machon, D., & Ariely, D. (2007). Selective versus unselective romantic desire: Not all reciprocity is created equal. *Psychological Science, 18*, 317–319.

Felson, R. B. (1980). Communication barriers and the reflected appraisal process. *Social Psychology Quarterly, 43*, 116–126.

Field, A. P., & Gillet, R. (2010). How to do a meta-analysis. *British Journal of Mathematical and Statistical Psychology, 63*, 665–694.

Fletcher, G. J. O., & Kerr, P. S. G. (2010). Through the eyes of love: Reality and illusion in intimate relationships. *Psychological Bulletin, 136*, 627–658.

Frey, F. E., & Tropp, L. R. (2006). Being seen as individuals versus as group members: Extending research on metaperception to intergroup contexts. *Personality and Social Psychology Review, 10*, 265–280.

Funder, D. C. (1995). On the accuracy of personality judgment: A realistic approach. *Psychological Review, 102*, 652–670.

Funder, D. C., Kolar, D. C., & Blackman, M. C. (1995). Agreement among judges of personality: Interpersonal relations, similarity, and acquaintanceship. *Journal of Personality and Social Psychology, 69*, 656–672.

Funder, D. C., & Sneed, C. D. (1993). Behavioral manifestations of personality: An ecological approach to judgmental accuracy. *Journal of Personality and Social Psychology, 64*, 479–490.

Furr, R. M. (2008). A framework for profile similarity: Integrating similarity, normativeness, and distinctiveness. *Journal of Personality, 76*, 1267–1316.

Furr, R. M., & Funder, D. C. (2004). Situational similarity and behavioral consistency: Subjective, objective, variable-centered, and person-centered approaches. *Journal of Research in Personality, 38*, 421–447.

Gilovich, T., Savitsky, K., & Medvec, V. H. (1998). The illusion of transparency: Biased assessments of others' ability to read one's emotional states. *Journal of Personality and Social Psychology, 75*, 332–346.

Gosling, S. D., John, O. P., Craik, K. H., & Robins, R. W. (1998). Do people know how they behave?: Self-reported act frequencies compared with on-line codings by observers. *Journal of Personality and Social Psychology, 74*, 1337–1349.

Hall, J. A., Murphy, N. A., & Mast, M. S. (2007). Nonverbal self-accuracy in interpersonal interaction. *Personality and Social Psychology Bulletin, 33*, 1675–1685.

Hebert, B. G., & Vorauer, J. D. (2003). Seeing through the screen: Is evaluative feedback communicated more effectively in fact-to-face or computer-mediated exchanges? *Computers in Human Behavior, 19*, 25–38.

John, O. P., & Robins, R. W. (1993). Determinants of interjudge agreement on personality traits: The Big Five domains, observability, evaluativeness, and the unique perspective of the self. *Journal of Personality, 61*, 521–551.

Jussim, L., Soffin, S., Brown, R., Ley, J., & Kohlhepp, K. (1992). Understanding reactions to feedback by integrating ideas from symbolic interactionism and cognitive evaluation theory. *Journal of Personality and Social Psychology, 62*, 402–421.

Kaplan, S. A., Santuzzi, A. M., & Ruscher, J. B. (2009). Elaborative metaperceptions in outcome-dependent situations: The diluted relationship between default self-perceptions and metaperceptions. *Social Cognition, 27*, 601–614.

Kenny, D. A. (1994). *Interpersonal perception: A social relations analysis*. New York: Guilford Press.

Kenny, D. A., & Acitelli, L. K. (1994). Measuring similarity in couples. *Journal of Family Psychology, 8*, 417–431.

Kenny, D. A., Snook, A., Boucher, E. M., & Hancock, J. T. (2010). Interpersonal sensitivity, status, and stereotype accuracy. *Psychological Science, 21*, 1735–1739.

Kenny, D. A., & DePaulo, B. M. (1990). [Applicant–interviewer study]. Unpublished raw data. (*)

Kenny, D. A., & DePaulo, B. M. (1993). Do people know how others view them?: An empirical and theoretical account. *Psychological Bulletin, 114*, 145–161.

Kenny, D. A., & West, T. V. (2008). Self-perception as interpersonal perception. In J. V. Wood, A. Tesser, & J. G. Holmes (Eds.), *The self and social relationships* (pp. 119–137). New York: Psychology Press.

Kenny, D. A., & Winquist, L. (2001). The measurement of interpersonal sensitivity: Consideration of design, components, and unit of analysis. In A. Hall & F. J. Bernieri (Eds.), *Interpersonal sensitivity: Theory and measurement* (pp. 265–302). Mahwah, NJ: Erlbaum.

Kwang, T., & Swann, W. B., Jr. (2010). Do people embrace praise even when they feel unworthy?: A review of critical tests of self-enhancement versus self-verification. *Personality and Social Psychology Review, 14,* 263–280.

Laing, R. D., Phillipson, H., & Lee, A. R. (1966). *Interpersonal perception: A theory and a method of research.* New York: Springer-Verlag.

Leary, M. R. (2005). Sociometer theory and the pursuit of relational value: Getting to the root of self-esteem. *European Review of Social Psychology, 16,* 75–111.

Leising, D., Rehbein, D., & Sporberg, D. (2006). Does a fish see the water in which it swims?: A study of the ability to correctly judge one's own interpersonal behavior. *Journal of Social and Clinical Psychology, 25,* 963–974.

Lemay, E. P., Jr., & Clark, M. S. (2008). "Walking on eggshells": How expressing relationship insecurities perpetuates them. *Journal of Personality and Social Psychology, 95,* 420–441.

Lemay, E. P., Jr., Clark, M. S., & Feeney, B. C. (2007). Projection of responsiveness to needs and the construction of satisfying communal relationships. *Journal of Personality and Social Psychology, 92,* 834–853.

Levesque, M. J. (2007, October). On being a good judge: Gender as a moderator of interpersonal accuracy and meta-accuracy in mixed gender dyads. In J. Spain (Chair), *Interpersonal perception and the eye of the beholder: Understanding the role of personality, gender, and relationship variables in perceiver judgments.* Symposium conducted at the meeting of the Society of Southeastern Social Psychologists, Durham, NC. (*)

Levesque, M. J. (1997). Meta-accuracy among acquainted individuals: A social relations analysis of interpersonal perception and metaperception. *Journal of Personality and Social Psychology, 72,* 66–74. (*)

Liberman, M. D., & Rosenthal, R. (2001). Why introverts can't always tell who likes them: Multitasking and nonverbal decoding. *Journal of Personality and Social Psychology, 80,* 294–310.

Malle, B. F., & Pearce, B. E. (2001). Attention to behavioral events during interaction: Two actor–observer gaps and three attempts to close them. *Journal of Personality and Social Psychology, 81,* 278–294.

Malloy, T. E., & Albright, L. (1990). Interpersonal perception in a social context. *Journal of Personality and Social Psychology, 58,* 419–428. (*)

Malloy, T. E., Albright, L., Diaz-Loving, R., Dong, Q., & Lee, Y. T. (2004). Agreement in personality judgments within and between nonoverlapping social groups in collectivist cultures. *Personality and Social Psychology Bulletin, 30,* 106–117. (*)

Malloy, T. E., Albright, L., Kenny, D. A., Agatstein, F., & Winquist, L. (1997). Interpersonal perception and metaperception in nonoverlapping social groups. *Journal of Personality and Social Psychology, 72,* 390–398. (*)

Malloy, T. E., Albright, L., & Scarpati, S. (2007). Awareness of peers' judgments of oneself: Accuracy and process of metaperception. *International Journal of Behavioral Development, 31,* 603–610.

Malloy, T. E., & Janowski, C. L. (1992). Perceptions and metaperceptions of leadership: Components, accuracy, and dispositional correlates. *Personality and Social Psychology Bulletin, 18,* 700–708. (*)

Mead, G. H. (1934). *Mind, self, and society.* Chicago: University of Chicago Press.

Mehl, M. R., Gosling, S. D., & Pennebaker, J. W. (2006). Personality in its natural habitat: Manifestation and implicit folk theories of personality in daily life. *Journal of Personality and Social Psychology, 90,* 862–877.

Miller, S., & Malloy, T. E. (2003). Interpersonal behavior, perception, and affect in status-discrepant dyads: Social interaction of gay and heterosexual men. *Psychology of Men and Masculinity, 4,* 121–135. (*)

Newcomb, T. M. (1953). An approach to the study of communicative acts. *Psychological Review, 60,* 393–404.

Oliver, P. V. (1989). Effects of need for social approval on first interactions among members of the opposite sex (Doctoral dissertation, University of Connecticut). *Dissertation Abstracts International, 50*(3-B), 1155. (*)

Ohtsubo, Y., Takezawa, M., & Fukuno, M. (2009). Mutual liking and metaperception accuracy. *European Journal of Social Psychology, 39,* 707–718. (*)

Oliver, P. V. (1988). *Effects of need for social approval on first interaction among members of the opposite sex.* Unpublished doctoral dissertation, University of Connecticut, Storrs. (*)

Oltmanns, T. F., Gleason, M. E., Klonsky, E. D., & Turkheimer, E. (2005). Metaperception for pathological personality traits: Do we know when others think that we are difficult? *Consciousness and Cognition, 14,* 739–751. (*)

Peters, S., Kinsey, P., & Malloy, T. E. (2004). Gender and leadership perceptions among African Americans. *Basic and Applied Social Psychology, 26,* 93–101. (*)

Reno, R., & Kenny, D. A. (1992). Effects of self-consciousness on self-disclosure among unacquainted individuals: An application of the social relations model. *Journal of Personality, 60,* 79–94. (*)

Shechtman, Z., & Kenny, D. A. (1994). Metaperception accuracy: An Israeli study. *Basic and Applied Social Psychology, 15,* 451–465. (*)

Simpson, J. A., Ickes, W., & Grich, J. (1999). When accuracy hurts: Reactions of anxiously-attached dating partners to a relationship-threatening situation. *Journal of Personality and Social Psychology, 76,* 754–769.

Simpson, J. A., Oriña, M. M., & Ickes, W. (2003). When accuracy hurts, and when it helps: A test of the empathic accuracy model in marital interactions. *Journal of Personality and Social Psychology, 85,* 881–893.

Snodgrass, S. E. (2001). Correlational method for assessing interpersonal sensitivity within dyadic interaction. In J. A. Hall & F. J. Bernieri (Eds.), *Interpersonal sensitivity: Theory and measurement* (pp. 201–218). Mahwah, NJ: Erlbaum.

Snodgrass, S. E. (1992). Further effects of role versus gender on interpersonal sensitivity. *Journal of Personality and Social Psychology, 62,* 154–158.

Srivastava, S., Guglielmo, S., & Beer, J. (2010). Perceiving others' personalities: Examining the dimensionality, assumed similarity to the self, and stability of perceiver effects. *Journal of Personality and Social Psychology, 98,* 520–534.

Steiner, I. D. (1955). Interpersonal behavior as influenced by accuracy of social perception. *Psychological Review, 62,* 268–274.

Swann, W. B., Stein-Seroussi, A., & McNulty, S. E. (1992). Outcasts in a white-lie society: The enigmatic worlds of people with negative self-concepts. *Journal of Personality and Social Psychology, 62,* 618–624.

Taylor, S. E., & Brown, J. D. (1988). Illusion and well-being: A social psychological perspective on mental health. *Psychological Bulletin, 103,* 193–210.

Vazire, S. (2006). *The person from the inside and outside.* Unpublished doctoral dissertation, University of Texas at Austin. (*)

Vazire, S. (2010). Who knows what about a person?: The Self–Other Knowledge Asymmetry (SOKA) model. *Journal of Personality and Social Psychology, 98,* 281–300.

Vazire, S., & Carlson, E. N. (2011). Others sometimes know us better than we know ourselves. *Current Directions in Psychological Science, 20,* 104–108.

Vazire, S., & Carlson, E. N. (2010). Self-knowledge of personality: Do people know themselves? *Social and Personality Psychology Compass, 4,* 605–620.

Vazire, S., & Mehl, M. R. (2008). Knowing me, knowing you: The accuracy and unique predictive validity of self and other ratings of daily behavior. *Journal of Personality and Social Psychology, 95*, 1202–1216. (*)

Vazire, S., Naumann, L. P., Rentfrow, P. J., & Gosling, S. D. (2008). Portrait of a narcissist: Manifestations of narcissism in physical appearance. *Journal of Research in Personality, 42*, 1439–1447. (*)

Wilson, T. D., & Dunn, E. W. (2004). Self-knowledge: Its limits, value, and potential for improvement. *Annual Review of Psychology, 55*, 493–518.

Wood, D., Harms, P., & Vazire, S. (2010). Perceiver effects as projective tests: What your perceptions of others say about you. *Journal of Personality and Social Psychology, 99*, 174–190.

CHAPTER 16
Knowing Our Pathology

THOMAS F. OLTMANNS
ABIGAIL D. POWERS

Recognition of personal problems and symptoms of illness is one important aspect of self-knowledge. We begin our chapter with a brief review of the literature concerned with deficiencies in self-knowledge as they are observed in several different forms of mental disorder. There is an important need for an integrated conceptual approach to this understudied aspect of psychopathology. The second section of the chapter outlines several important methodological challenges that must be addressed by investigators who hope to expand the base of scientific data in this area. Finally, we summarize evidence that has been generated in two of our own studies regarding self-knowledge and personality disorders.

Overview: Insight and Mental Disorders

Failure to acknowledge the presence, severity, and impact of significant symptoms has traditionally been considered a central feature of several mental disorders. In the field of psychopathology, this phenomenon is often called "lack of insight" (Alenius, Hammarlund-Udenaes, Hartvig, & Lindström, 2010; Cuesta, Peralta, & Zarzuela, 2000). For example, patients who are hallucinating, or who express delusional beliefs, seldom understand that there is something wrong with their minds. Although lack of insight is not one of the diagnostic criteria for schizophrenia listed in the official diagnostic manual (*Diagnostic and Statistical Manual of Mental Disorders*, or DSM-IV; American Psychiatric Association, 1994), it was found to be the most discriminating symptom of schizophrenia in a large, multinational study of the course of that disorder (Sartorius, Shapiro, & Jablonsky, 1974). Dozens of subsequent studies have expanded this body of evidence and point to the conclusion that patients who demonstrate lack of insight show poor response to treatment and worse outcomes (Arango & Amador, 2011; Saravanan et al., 2010).

Detailed consideration of lack of insight for psychotic symptoms indicates that it is actually a rather complex, multidimensional phenomenon (Mintz, Dobson, & Romney, 2003). Consider, for example, the assessment of delusional beliefs. Imagine that a particular patient believes that the FBI has bugged his home and office and that federal agents are following him around with cameras and other recording devices. One dimension of insight would be the extent to which the patient is convinced that this belief is accurate. Some patients might claim that they are absolutely certain of the authenticity of the plot. Others might suspect that it is true, while also acknowledging some chance that they might be mistaken. In other words, conviction is not an all-or-nothing phenomenon. Willingness to consider the possibility that this belief might be mistaken represents one aspect of insight. Another related consideration involves the person's ability to understand someone else's perspective on this belief. Regardless of the patient's own certainty about the belief, what does he imagine other people think about the alleged plot? Some patients might say (particularly during a phase of recovery), "I am still convinced that the plot exists, but my wife does not. I understand that we have different points of view on this issue." A comprehensive understanding of self-knowledge regarding delusional beliefs would require, at the least, judgments regarding both of these considerations. Conviction and perspective are related aspects of self-knowledge regarding delusional beliefs, but they are not identical (Harrow, Rattenbury, & Stoll, 1988; see also Carlson & Kenny, Chapter 15, this volume).

Lack of insight is also an important characteristic of people who are suffering from various kinds of substance use disorders. In the literature concerned with alcoholism, this phenomenon is frequently referred to as "denial of illness" (Dare & Derigne, 2010; Sher & Epler, 2004). People with severe drinking problems are often the last to recognize the nature of their problems. They usually insist that they do not drink too much, and that they can stop anytime they want (as indicated by the large number of times that they have quit, only to return to heavy drinking). Here the various elements associated with self-knowledge expand to include more than simply the recognition that the person is drinking too much. Denial is often assumed to include the person's failure to admit that he or she needs to change the drinking behavior (cut down or abstain), which includes the ability to recognize that heavy drinking has a negative impact on social and occupational adjustment. The assessment of denial may also hinge on consideration of the person's judgment about the *potential* and motivation for change (e.g., the argument "I could stop if I wanted to stop").

In the case of alcoholism, the construct represented by denial of illness is defined by issues that extend beyond the ability to report precisely the number of drinks consumed in a particular period of time. Alcoholics can do that with some accuracy, even though self-report scales leave room for errors (Anthony, Neumark, & Van Etten, 2000). They are much more impaired in being able to recognize and acknowledge the impact of drinking on their lives, and they do not agree with other people's suggestion that they need to change. Sher and Epler (2004) have argued that it will be more useful to focus therapeutic and research efforts on understanding mechanisms involved in *problem recognition*, thus avoiding the ambiguous and somewhat pejorative term *denial*. Their thoughtful review discusses several social-cognitive processes related to problem recognition, as well as the impact of alcohol on self-awareness. They recommend a variety of therapeutic approaches that might be employed with individual patients, depending on the context and the patient's motivation.

Most patients suffering from anorexia nervosa experience a similar inability to recognize the presence and impact of their problems surrounding eating and nutrition (Vandereycken, 2006a, 2006b). Like alcoholics, they are able to record accurately the amount of food that they eat and how much they weigh. In fact, people with eating disorders can be excruciatingly accurate self-observers in that respect. Their lack of insight is evident when they insist that they do not have a problem with their body weight, in spite of the obvious fact that they are severely malnourished. Most patients with anorexia are quite proud of their ability to restrict their intake of food, and resent the efforts of family members and mental health professionals to intervene. Positive outcomes for the treatment of patients with anorexia are typically associated with a meaningful increase in their ability to recognize the nature of their own eating problems (Greenfeld, Anyan, Hobart, Quinlan, & Plantes, 1991).

Obsessive–compulsive disorder (OCD) is another severe form of psychopathology that is often accompanied by a lack of insight. The traditional definition of OCD required that the person recognize that ritualistic behaviors are senseless. For example, a woman who engages in compulsive counting rituals intended to protect the health of her children would have to acknowledge that these behaviors do not really have any influence ("I know that it's silly to do these things, but it makes me feel less anxious"). In other words, the person would have to demonstrate insight in order to meet the diagnostic criteria for OCD. That part of the definition changed with the publication of DSM-IV in 1994. DSM-IV (American Psychiatric Association, 1994) holds that "*at some point* during the course of the disorder, the person has recognized that the obsessions or compulsions are excessive or unreasonable" (p. 423, emphasis added). Several studies support the conclusion that patients with OCD who have poor insight into their condition are less likely to respond positively to treatment and have a poorer long-term course of disorder (Alonso et al., 2008; Catapano et al., 2010; Türksoy, Tükel, Ozdemir, & Karali, 2002).

Different terms are often used to describe self-knowledge as it applies to personality disorders. Here, the formal terminology shifts to the consideration of personal characteristics that are either *ego-dystonic* (thoughts, feelings, or behaviors that are in conflict with the person's image of his or her ideal self) or *ego-syntonic* (consistent with the person's image of him- or herself). Many forms of mental disorder, such as anxiety disorders and mood disorders, are ego-dystonic; that is, people with these disorders are distressed by their symptoms and would prefer to change that aspect of themselves. Personality disorders are usually ego-syntonic. The characteristic behaviors and feelings that define the disorder are acceptable to the person. People with personality disorders frequently do not see themselves as being disturbed. Many forms of personality disorder are defined primarily in terms of the problems that these people create for others rather than in terms of their own subjective distress.

Is the expected level of self-knowledge different for personality disorders than it is for other mental health problems? Clinical folklore in psychiatry has held that people with personality disorders are actually more impaired in this regard than are people suffering from clinical disorders, such as psychosis, alcoholism, and anorexia. In fact, Krueger (2005) reviewed this literature and concluded that clinical disorders and personality disorders cannot be distinguished in this regard (any more than they can be distinguished on the basis of other important dimensions, such as stability of symptoms, age of onset, or response to treatment). He went on to suggest that the study of insight may become important in elucidating the challenging distinction between personality traits and personality disorders; extreme variations on personality traits (e.g., angry hostility, excitement seeking, mistrust) may only rise to the level of becoming a mental *disorder* when accompanied by disturbance in the ability to view one's own behavior from the perspective of others or to recognize the impact of one's behavior on interpersonal relationships.

Most research studies concerned with self-knowledge in personality disorders have focused almost exclusively on one relatively narrow (but important) aspect of insight (i.e., accuracy of self-report; Oltmanns & Turkheimer, 2006). *Accuracy* has been defined in terms of the extent to which people's descriptions of their own personality characteristics agree with descriptions of them provided by people who know them well. This is not a new approach in personality research (see Funder, 1995). In fact, this method for considering insight was initially employed by Flyer, Barron, and Bigbee (1953), who compared the ways target participants described their own personality characteristics to the ways in which they were described by informants. Greater insight was assumed to be present when there was little or no discrepancy between the self-description of an individual and his or her evaluation by well-acquainted judges. Perhaps most interesting is the fact that Flyer and his colleagues were also concerned with *social perception* (i.e., the extent to which the participants were aware of how they were perceived by others). This aspect of their work anticipated by many years the development of studies concerned with metaperception for personality traits (Kenny & DePaulo, 1993; Carlson & Kenny, Chapter 15, this volume).

Research on self-knowledge and personality pathology has focused primarily on the accuracy of self-perceptions, and to a certain extent on the accuracy of metaperceptions. Studies of personality disorders have not attempted, however, to measure the extent to which people with personality disorders recognize the social consequences of their behavior. For example, one study examined convergence between self and informant reports for psychopathic traits and found substantial agreement between self and informants across three separate measures tapping features such as aggressive interpersonal styles and impulsive risk taking (Miller, Jones, & Lynam, 2011). On the basis of this evidence, the investigators commented on the relatively common assumption that psychopaths have poor insight. "Perhaps lack of concern for consequences of these traits has been mistaken for lack of insight into them" (p. 758). The investigators' findings are important, but their interpretation reflects a limited definition of *insight*. Lack of concern for consequences is, in fact, among the most important aspects of insight with regard to any form of psychopathology, including personality disorders.

People who exhibit features of narcissistic personality disorder do seem to be aware of their own reputations (Carlson, Vazire, & Oltmanns, 2011). Narcissists hold exaggerated positive views of their own personality characteristics, but they also recognize that other people view them less favorably than they view themselves. Furthermore, they understand that other people begin to see them in a less favorable light as they get to know them better. It remains to be determined whether narcissists and people with other forms of personality pathology are more specifically aware of the significant interpersonal costs that they pay for their arrogant and entitled approach to interacting with others. Studies aimed at these issues will provide an important addition to the literature regarding self-knowledge and personality disorders.

In relation to some forms of disease and disability, it may actually be adaptive to ignore or deny the impact of a condition. Druss and Douglas (1988) have referred to this phenomenon as "healthy denial," which must be distinguished from lack of insight in mental disorders. People who remain optimistic in the face of fatal cancer, for example, are obviously an inspiration to all of us. But these individuals are not unaware of the medical facts regarding their condition. Their ability to focus on positive aspects of their lives does not preclude participation in active forms of treatment aimed at the disorder from which they are suffering. In the case of mental disorders, lack of insight and denial refer specifically to the failure to recognize problem behaviors and the negative consequences of these behaviors. It is hard to imagine that failure to acknowledge the consequences of delusional thinking or excessive consumption of alcohol or self-imposed starvation can serve an adaptive purpose.

Much could be gained by the development of a broad conception of lack of insight as it applies to many forms of mental disorder. Isolated literatures have developed in each of several fields, and interesting issues have been raised with regard to several specific disorders. A complete definition of self-knowledge regarding specific forms of psychopathology should include the consideration of at least the following related domains:

1. Does the person acknowledge the presence of descriptive features of the disorder? Does the person's self-report of symptoms agree with other ways of measuring diagnostic signs?
2. Can the person recognize how other people view these same descriptive features? Does the person appreciate the perspective of others who have observed his or her behavior?
3. Is the person aware of harmful consequences (both social and biological) that follow as a result of specific problem behaviors? If the person recognizes the presence of symptoms of disorder, does he or she recognize that they are leading to significant problems?
4. Does the person recognize a need for change, regardless of the mode or mechanism that might be used to accomplish it?

Methodological Challenges

Several important methodological issues must be considered in the design of studies regarding self-knowledge for mental disorders in general, or personality pathology in particular. None are more important than those concerned with the identification of participants who exhibit features of the disorder in question. From what source will they be recruited? Should investigators employ a clinical sample or a community sample? Many find their participants by approaching people who are receiving treatment for personality disorders at a clinic or hospital. An alternative strategy is to recruit a sample of community residents, regardless of whether they are in treatment for a specific type of problem. In either method, careful assessments must identify the presence of psychopathology. Clinical samples and community samples both offer advantages and disadvantages.

Many investigators prefer to focus on people receiving treatment because they are clearly disturbed, but seeking treatment for mental health services is influenced by a number of factors other than the presence of psychopathology. Epidemiological studies have demonstrated that most people who qualify for the diagnosis of a mental disorder do not receive treatment (Kessler, Merikangas, & Wang, 2007). In that sense, people identified through hospitals and clinics may not be representative of those people who qualify for a particular diagnosis.

The high rate of comorbidity is another problem associated with clinical samples, particularly when it is used to study personality disorders. It has been shown repeatedly that personality disorders are highly comorbid with major depression and substance use disorders, particularly among patients who are in treatment. When people with personality disorders do seek treatment, it is typically because of concern about these other issues. It therefore seems possible that, by selecting a clinical sample, investigators who are studying self-knowledge of personality disorders might learn more about the impact of depression and substance use disorders, rather than personality problems themselves. For example, people who are in the midst of an episode of depression do not seem to be particularly accurate judges of their own personality characteristics (Klein, Kotov, & Bufferd, 2011). Reliance on clinical samples makes the interpretation of data much more complicated.

Community samples also present important limitations. One is that they do not typically include a concentrated selection of people who exhibit prototypical combinations of a particular disorder. Another issue involves the distinction between normal and abnormal behavior, regardless of the disorder in question. The official diagnostic manual relies on judgments regarding social and occupational impairment in order to justify a formal diagnosis. People in community samples may answer enough questions on a highly structured diagnostic interview to resemble people who are depressed or anxious, or who have other forms of psychopathology. But they also must demonstrate "harm." A clinical sample necessarily includes individuals with symptoms that have caused interference in their lives. In community samples, many people who exhibit features of disorders would not qualify for a diagnosis if clinical significance were taken into consideration (Narrow, Rae, Robins, & Regier, 2002; Paris, 2010). In the end, progress toward understanding psychopathology will depend on the use of both clinical and community samples. Investigators must keep in mind, and try to minimize the impact of, the limitations associated with each approach.

The second important methodological issue involves choice of measurement instruments. Most studies in this field have used two kinds of tools: clinical rating scales based on interviews and self-report questionnaires. Scales that have been developed for the measurement of insight in mental disorders include a variety of considerations (Sanz, Constable, Lopez-Ibor, Kemp, & David, 1998). They often extend well beyond the person's willingness or ability to acknowledge the presence of behaviors or experiences that are considered signs of psychopathology. The Scale to Assess Unawareness of Mental Disorder (SUMD) is a semistructured interview that was developed to measure insight into mental disorders (Amador et al., 1994). The SUMD has probably been the most popular research instrument for measuring lack of insight. This scale includes items that focus on the person's awareness of both the fundamental problem (presence of symptoms) and the social consequences of these symptoms. These are obviously important aspects of self-knowledge. On the other hand, the SUMD also asks the interviewer to rate the extent to which the patient agrees with the clinician's formal diagnosis and recognizes the need to take medication to treat the problem. The latter issues are more concerned with the person's willingness to acquiesce to the clinician's judgment than with the person's ability to know things about him- or herself. The research literature certainly leaves considerable room for disagreement about the most effective and least harmful forms of treatment for disorders such as schizophrenia, alcoholism, anorexia, and personality disorders. There is also room for honest disagreement among trained professionals regarding a specific person's diagnosis. Disagreement between the patient and the clinician on these issues is not necessarily an unambiguous reflection of lack of self-knowledge.

The Brown Assessment of Beliefs Scale (BABS) is also based on a clinical interview and has been used extensively as an index of self-knowledge related to various forms of mental disorder (Eisen et al., 1998). It was developed for use in rating patients' degree of conviction and insight regarding particular beliefs, especially those that might be considered obsessions or delusions. The BABS is based on the premise that insight should be viewed in terms of several related dimensions, including conviction, perception of others' views or beliefs, explanation of differing views, fixity of ideas, attempt to disprove beliefs, and *insight* (defined as the person's ability to assign a psychiatric or psychological cause for the belief that is being examined). These dimensions provide a comprehensive view of many important aspects of pathological beliefs and an interesting perspective on pathological beliefs related to OCD (Eisen et al., 2001), schizophrenia (Kaplan et al., 2006), and eating disorders (Steinglass, Eisen, Attia, Mayer, & Walsh, 2007). However, it does not include a scale concerned with recognizing the social consequences of aberrant beliefs, and it was not designed for use with regard to features of mental disorders that do not revolve around specific beliefs. For these reasons, this important instrument would not be particularly useful for studying self-knowledge regarding personality pathology.

The Beck Cognitive Insight Scale (BCIS) is a 15-item questionnaire that provides a very different perspective on self-knowledge regarding mental disorders (Beck, Baruch, Balter, Steer, & Warman, 2004). The BCIS is focused broadly on attributions, including the person's interpretation of specific events, as well as the recognition of other people's perspectives. Items include the following: "Some of my experiences that have seemed very real may have been due to my imagination," "Some of the ideas I was certain were true turned out to be false," and "There is often more than one possible explanation for why people act the way they do." This instrument is concerned with the person's willingness to consider the possibility that he or she might make errors in interpreting events in the environment. The convergent and discriminant validity of the BCIS has not been evaluated with regard to more general measures of normal and abnormal personality traits (e.g., many items seem to be closely related to constructs such as agreeableness and openness to experience). Like the SUMD, it strays away from a specific focus on the ability to recognize the presence of specific features of psychopathology, and it does not address self-knowledge regarding the consequences of symptoms of mental disorder. For all of these reasons, it should be used cautiously as an index of insight in psychopathology.

The third methodological issue to be considered in studying self-knowledge and psychopathology involves the generation of a valid index of accuracy. Assessment of insight or self-knowledge necessarily requires selection of a standard against which the person's own opinion can be measured. The contrast between two sources obviously lies at the heart of the notion of insight. Disagreement between the person's own perspective and that offered by another source is typically taken to reflect a deficit in knowledge about the self. In most research on mental disorders, the patients' views are compared to those expressed by their therapists. It is important to recognize that judgments made by the latter may also be subject to bias (e.g., Garb, 1998) and should not always be considered to be entirely objective.

In the realm of personality and personality disorders, another option is to use as the criterion the judgments of other people who know the person well. This is an especially attractive alternative when it is possible to collect ratings from a variety of informants (Hofstee, 1994). Averaged across several sources, these ratings have increased reliability and presumably increased validity. They also include a built-in correction for the biases of individual judges, as well as gaps in their knowledge of the person's behavior.

When only one informant is available, the investigator is faced with a serious dilemma. Whom should one choose? Parents, siblings, spouses, friends, coworkers, and neighbors all might provide useful information (Achenbach, Krukowski, Dumenci, & Ivanova, 2005; Klonsky, Oltmanns, & Turkheimer, 2002; Oltmanns & Turkheimer, 2006). On the other hand, any specific person could also provide biased or incomplete information. It is important to consider the level of acquaintance and the situations in which the target and informant have known each other. Parents are obviously likely to have blind spots, and mothers may have different information than fathers. People who are chosen by the participant almost certainly like that person and therefore provide a different perspective than would be given by an informant who does not like the participant (Leising, Erbs, & Fritz, 2010). For all of these reasons, it is important to select informants who are not only available but also able to provide meaningful information about the personality characteristics that are in question.

What Do People Know and What Are the Limits?

The next section of this chapter provides a brief review of current evidence regarding self-knowledge and personality pathology. Of course, this literature is grounded in methods and concepts focused more broadly on normal personality traits. Self–other agreement for personality traits ranges from .40 to .60 (Vazire & Carlson, 2010). As might be expected, agreement increases with the level of acquaintance. Agreement also depends on the types of traits measured, with positive personality traits seemingly agreed upon more easily. Neuroticism, a personality trait characterized by negative affect and associated with many forms of psychopathology, including personality disorders, often shows the lowest self–other agreement (Miller, Pilkonis, & Clifton, 2005).

A few studies have examined levels of self–other agreement for features associated with personality disorders. Two of those studies were conducted by our research group. The Peer Nomination Study was concerned with interpersonal perception for symptoms that define the 10 DSM-IV personality disorders (Oltmanns & Turkheimer, 2006, 2009). It included approximately 2,000 military recruits who were identified and tested in groups of between 27 and 53 recruits. Each group comprised previously unacquainted young adults who had many opportunities to observe each other's behavior after living together in close proximity for a period of 6 weeks. Although this was not a clinical sample of patients being treated for mental disorders, it did include people with significant personality problems. Diagnostic interviews indicated that, consistent with data from other community samples, approximately 10% of the participants qualified for a diagnosis of at least one personality disorder. All participants in each group completed self-report questionnaires, and they also nominated members of their group who exhibited specific features of personality disorders. Everyone served as both a judge and a target. Exactly the same items were included in both the self-report and peer nomination scales. All were lay translations of specific diagnostic features used to define personality disorders in the official psychiatric classification system. Examples include "Is stuck up or 'high and mighty'" (narcissistic personality disorder), "Needs to do such a perfect job that nothing ever gets finished" (obsessive–compulsive personality disorder [OCPD]), and "Has no close friends, other than family members" (schizoid personality disorder).

We compared the self-report scores that recruits provided to describe themselves with the nominations about them provided by their peers. Our results shed light on two central issues related to insight: recognition of symptoms and *metaperception* (i.e., the ability to understand the perceptions of others). Correlations for self–other agreement in the Peer Nomination Study were modest at best, typically in the range between .21 and .30 (Thomas, Turkheimer, & Oltmanns, 2003). Studies in other laboratories have reported similar results (Furr, Dougherty, Marsh, & Mathias, 2007; Klonsky et al., 2002), suggesting that self-reports provide only a limited view of personality pathology.

In spite of differing from others in how they view themselves, can individuals with personality pathology more accurately report how others view them? Perhaps it is easier to admit to negative impressions others have about one than it is to admit to such truths about one's own personality. When assessing normal personality traits, research shows that metaperception is quite good (Vazire, & Carlson, 2010). Relatively few studies have explored this with personality pathology. The Peer Nomination Study did assess "expected peer scores" and asked how participants thought *most* group members would describe them. Although expected peer scores were highly correlated with original self-reports of personality (Carlson, Vazire, & Furr, 2011), the scores were predictive of variability in peer reported personality disorder symptoms above and beyond self-reports, showing that individuals with personality problems may be at least partly aware of negative views that others have, even if they do not agree with them (Oltmanns, Gleason, Klonsky, & Turkheimer, 2005). When self–other agreement was assessed after researchers controlled for expected peer scores, correlations between self and peer reports significantly decreased or disappeared. The expected peer report appeared to be driving the connection between self and other views, again suggesting that key differences exist between how individuals with personality pathology view themselves and how others see them.

Does the difference between how people see themselves and how others see them matter? Data regarding the prediction of consequential life outcomes suggest that it does. Use of informant reports in personality research has allowed us to identify when sources other than the self may be beneficial. Informant report seems to augment information obtained through self-report, providing independent and relevant details that can be helpful in predicting negative life outcomes, such as job success (Oltmanns & Turkheimer, 2009). Our data on military recruits illustrated that for all disorders except OCPD, higher personality disorder scores were associated with greater risk for early discharge among military recruits (Fiedler, Oltmanns, & Turkheimer, 2004). In general, peer reports of personality disorders were better predictors of negative outcomes than self-reports, especially for Cluster B disorders (the "dramatic/erratic" cluster including narcissistic, histrionic, antisocial, and borderline personality disorders). Both self- and informant reports may be useful in identifying meaningful connections between personality problems and adjustment. Although self-reports appear most useful in understanding internalizing problems (e.g., subjective distress, anxiety) informant reports are useful for externalizing problems (e.g., aggression, impulsivity) and more general predictions about occupational outcomes. This finding fits nicely with evidence in the normal personality domain that self-reports are often more helpful when trying to understand internal traits but less effective with highly evaluative traits (Vazire, 2010).

The benefits of informant report have also been documented in relation to physical and mental health outcomes. Research by Smith and his colleagues (2008) showed that among healthy older adults, informant reports of certain personality traits (i.e., anxiety and anger) were a better predictor of coronary artery calcification (an important indicator of coronary artery disease) than self-reports alone. In this case, self-reports would have *underestimated* the health risk associated with a personality trait like angry hostility because an individual was unable to portray this trait as accurately as his or her spouse. Other longitudinal research on functional outcomes among depressed patients by Klein (2003) similarly showed the importance of informant reports, particularly in predicting future social adjustment.

We are currently exploring these issues in a longitudinal study of personality, health, and transitions in later life. The participants constitute a representative sample of adults (ages 55–64) living in the St. Louis metropolitan area. Details about the SPAN Study (St. Louis Personality and Aging Network) are provided by Oltmanns and Gleason (2011). This project focused on personality pathology in later adulthood will shed further light on ways in which self- and informant report operate in relation to personality pathology. Although data collection is still in progress, we have examined self–other agreement in the participants who have been tested up to the present time ($N \sim 900$). One unique benefit of this study is that we have personality data from three sources: the participant, the participant's informant (most often a spouse, child, or sibling), and a trained interviewer familiar with personality disorder symptomatology. Therefore, we are able to explore overlap among all three sources and, in particular, compare evidence obtained from the interviewers and the informants.

Consistent with our previous findings (Oltmanns et al., 2005), self–other agreement for personality disorder symptoms appeared modest at best (ranging from .14 for narcissistic personality disorder to .29 for schizoid personality disorder). Informant–interviewer agreement was similar (ranging from .14 for schizotypal personality disorder to .28 for borderline personality disorder). Self-interviewer agreement was slightly higher (ranging from .23 for antisocial personality disorder to .49 for avoidant personality disorder). Overlap between self-reports and interviewer ratings may be higher because the interviewer must depend on information provided by the participant and must make judgments about personality disorder criteria based on those reports. Again, these results show the value of information obtained in informant reports because it is least tied to an individual's self-report.

Self–other correlations are higher (.41 for borderline personality disorder to .53 for avoidant personality disorder) when the NEO Personality Inventory is used to construct personality disorder prototype scores (Lawton, Shields, & Oltmanns, 2011). The construction of these personality disorder prototypes is based on strong relations between the five-factor model of personality and the structure of DSM-IV personality disorder types (Lynam & Widiger, 2001; Miller et al., 2005). The fact that self–other correlations are stronger using this assessment method may indicate that the negative wording of self-report personality disorder criteria makes it less likely that individuals will endorse items (thus lowering agreement with informants) and that a measure like the NEO, which uses less extreme wording, may capture more accurate personality reports. Perhaps metaperception among individuals high in personality pathology would also improve if the wording on personality disorder inventories were altered.

The limit for self–other agreement is about .50, even for people married for 30 years. Based on the research described earlier, it appears that individuals with personality problems agree even less with their peers about who they are (with a limit closer to .30). Nevertheless, individuals scoring high on personality disorder symptoms do acknowledge that they exhibit some features of personality pathology (especially internal states less easily observed by others). They also seem to be able to provide additional information if they are asked *how they think others see them* (Oltmanns et al., 2005). Informants, on the other hand, appear to offer a unique view that can provide a perspective more helpful in predicting negative life outcomes. Paying attention to both sources of information may be essential as we try to understand personality pathology and its negative consequences better.

Implications of Lack of Self-Knowledge for Personality Disorders

Personality disorders are characterized by their stable and long-lasting negative impact on individuals' lives. Part of the difficulty with personality disorders is reflected in treatment-resistant patterns of thinking and behaving that interfere with treatment. The need to target personality problems has been shown repeatedly in clinical trials with a variety of disorders. Personality disorders have a negative impact on the occurrence, duration, and outcome of depression, substance use disorders, and eating disorders, to name only a few (Alnaes & Torgersen, 1997; Fournier et al., 2008; Zimmerman, Rothschild, & Chelminski, 2005). Research through the Collaborative Longitudinal Personality Disorders Study (CLPS; Skodol et al., 2005) showed that among treatment-seeking adults, individuals with major depressive disorder and a comorbid personality disorder had significantly worse emotional and social functioning over time compared with individuals suffering from major depression alone. The patients with personality disorders were also much more likely to overuse medical resources (compared to patients with major depressive disorder) despite showing lower functioning later (Bender et al., 2006).

Not only is the presence of personality pathology detrimental to treatment outcomes, but also the prevalence of personality disorders in treatment-seeking adults is sometimes as high as 50% (Zimmerman et al., 2005), making the need to address personality pathology in mental health assessment and treatment particularly salient. Assessment of personality disorders in both clinical and research settings most often focuses on self-reports. As previous research has shown (Miller et al., 2005; Oltmanns & Turkheimer, 2009), informant reports, which add unique information about personality pathology not captured through self-reports, help in predicting consequential outcomes. Because personality pathology puts individuals at risk for not improving in treatment, having a broader assessment of personality that includes multiple sources could facilitate the diagnosis and treatment of personality pathology.

People with personality problems see themselves quite differently than do their peers. In that respect, they do appear to have limited insight into their pathology. When these individuals are asked how they think others see them, however, their responses move closer to actual peer reports, showing that they have at least some knowledge of the negative personality traits. A large part of being able to navigate interpersonal situations successfully relates to being able to understand how people perceive one's actions and what implications may emerge. If individuals with personality disorders could become better equipped with metaperception skills, they might also gain increased awareness about their personality problems and the difficulties that result. Treatment focused on increasing awareness of peer perceptions could be a start in educating individuals about their personality pathology (without aggressively attacking these aspects of the self that feel like core elements of who they are). Such awareness would also help us get closer to the information being captured in informant reports, which are tied to functional outcomes predicted less well by self-reports.

Conclusions

Lack of insight and denial of illness have been important topics in the study and treatment of various kinds of mental disorders, ranging from psychosis to alcoholism, eating disorders, and personality pathology. Each of these areas of research has developed its own terminology and assessment instruments. Further progress would be stimulated by the adoption of a standard terminology, as well as more specific measurement tools that address several related dimensions of self-knowledge.

A complete assessment of self-knowledge regarding various forms of pathology necessarily involves four related issues:

1. Does the person recognize specific features of his or her behavior?
2. Is the person able to recognize the perspective that other people have on this same behavior?
3. Does the person appreciate the consequences of these behaviors?
4. Does the person acknowledge the need to change these behaviors?

Each of these topics represents an important aspect of self-knowledge for psychopathology.

In the realm of personality disorder, evidence collected to date is mostly concerned with the first issue and has focused on self–other agreement for features of personality disorders. Findings from several different investigations support the conclusion that people who exhibit increased levels of personality pathology frequently fail to recognize the presence of these symptoms (though they do produce modest agreement with other people who know them well). Furthermore, some evidence suggests that people with personality disorders may appreciate the fact that others see them as showing more features of personality disorder than they see in themselves. Future studies should expand the focus of this line of investigation and explore self-knowledge regarding the social consequences of pathological personality traits and the need to change these problem behaviors.

Pursuit of these basic issues would create a base of knowledge that might stimulate important developments in the treatment of mental disorders (Gabbard & Horowitz, 2009; Ness & Ende, 1994; Sher & Epler, 2004; Vitousek, Watson, & Wilson, 1998). Various dimensions of lack of insight clearly play an important role in the maintenance of many forms of psychopathology. How can we best help people recognize the link between their own behavior and interpersonal problems? How can we improve their willingness to seek treatment for these problems when it is appropriate and effective? Answers to these questions will follow progress in basic research on self-knowledge for psychopathology.

REFERENCES

Achenbach, T. M., Krukowski, R. A., Dumenci, L., & Ivanova, M. Y. (2005). Assessment of adult psychopathology: Meta-analyses and implications of cross-informant correlations. *Psychological Bulletin, 131*, 361–382.

Alenius, M., Hammarlund-Udenaes, M., Hartvig, P., & Lindström, L. (2010). Knowledge and insight in relation to functional remission in patients with long-term psychotic disorders. *Social Psychiatry and Psychiatric Epidemiology, 45*, 523–529.

Alnaes, R., & Torgersen, S. (1997). Personality and personality disorders predict development and relapses of major depression. *Acta Psychiatrica Scandinavica, 95*, 336–342.

Alonso, P., Menchón, J. M., Segalàs, C., Jaurrieta, N., Jiménez-Murcia, S., Cardoner, N., et al. (2008). Clinical implications of insight assessment in obsessive–compulsive disorder. *Comprehensive Psychiatry, 49*, 305–312.

Amador, X. F., Flaum, M., Andreasen, J. C., Strauss, D. H., Yale, S. A., Clark, S. C., et al. (1994). Awareness of illness in schizophrenia and schizoaffective and mood disorder. *Archives of General Psychiatry, 51*, 826–836.

American Psychiatric Association. (1994). *Diagnostic and statistical manual of mental disorders* (4th ed.). Washington, DC: Author.

Anthony, J. C., Neumark, Y. D., & Van Etten, M. L. (2000). Do I do what I say?: A perspective on self-report methods in drug dependence epidemiology. In A. A. Stone, J. S. Turkhan, C. A. Bachrach, J. B. Jobe, H. S. Kurtzman, & V. S. Cain (Eds.), *The science of self-report: Implications for research and practice* (pp. 175–198). Mahwah, NJ: Erlbaum.

Arango, C., & Amador, X. (2011). Lessons learned about poor insight. *Schizophrenia Bulletin, 37*, 27–28.

Beck, A. T., Baruch, E., Balter, J. M., Steer, R. A., & Warman, D. M. (2004). A new instrument for measuring insight: the Beck Cognitive Insight Scale. *Schizophrenia Research, 68*, 319–329.

Bender, D. S., Skodol, A. E., Pagano, M. E., Dyck, I. R., Grilo, C. M., Shea, M. T., et al.

(2006). Prospective assessment of treatment use by patients with personality disorders. *Psychiatric Services, 57,* 254–257.

Carlson, E. N., Vazire, S., & Furr, R. (2011). Meta-insight: Do people really know how others see them? *Journal of Personality and Social Psychology, 101,* 831–846.

Carlson, E. N., Vazire, S., & Oltmanns, T. F. (2011). You probably think this paper's about you: Narcissists' perceptions of their personality and reputation. *Journal of Personality and Social Psychology, 101,* 185–201.

Catapano, F., Perris, F., Fabrazzo, M., Cioffi, V., Giacco, D., De Santis, V., et al. (2010). Obsessive–compulsive disorder with poor insight: A three-year prospective study. *Progress in Neuro-Psychopharmacology and Biological Psychiatry, 34,* 323–330.

Cuesta, M. J., Peralta, V., & Zarzuela, A. (2000). Reappraising insight in psychosis: Multiscale longitudinal study. *British Journal of Psychiatry, 177,* 233–240.

Dare, P. A. S., & Derigne, L. (2010). Denial in alcohol and other drug use disorders: A critique of theory. *Addiction Research and Theory, 18,* 181–193.

Druss, R. G., & Douglas, C. J. (1988). Adaptive responses to illness and disability: Healthy denial. *General Hospital Psychiatry, 10,* 163–168.

Eisen, J. L., Phillips, K. A., Baer, L., Beer, D. A., Atala, K. D., & Rasmussen, S. A. (1998). The Brown Assessment of Beliefs Scale: Reliability and validity. *American Journal of Psychiatry, 155,* 102–108.

Eisen, J. L., Rasmussen, S. A., Phillips, K. A., Price, L. H., Davidson, J., Lydiard, R. B., et al. (2001). Insight and treatment outcome in obsessive–compulsive disorder. *Comprehensive Psychiatry, 42,* 494–497.

Fiedler, E. R., Oltmanns, T. F., & Turkheimer, E. (2004). Traits associated with personality disorders and adjustment to military life: Predictive validity of self and peer reports. *Military Medicine, 169,* 207–211.

Flyer, E. S., Barron, E., & Bigbee, L. (1953). Discrepancies between self-descriptions and group ratings as measures of lack of insight. *USAF Human Resources Research Center Research Bulletin,* No. 53–55.

Fournier, J. C., DeRubeis, R. J., Shelton, R. C., Gallop, R., Amsterdam, J. D., & Hollon, S. D. (2008). Antidepressant medications v. cognitive therapy in people with depression with or without personality disorder. *British Journal of Psychiatry, 192,* 124–129.

Funder, D. C. (1995). On the accuracy of personality judgment: A realistic approach. *Psychological Review, 102,* 652–670.

Furr, R. M., Doughtery, D. M., Marsh, D. M., & Mathias, C. W. (2007). Personality judgment and personality pathology: Self–other agreement in adolescents with conduct disorder. *Journal of Personality 75*(3), 629–662.

Gabbard, G. O., & Horowitz, M. J. (2009). Insight, transference interpretation, and therapeutic change in the dynamic psychotherapy of borderline personality disorder. *American Journal of Psychiatry, 166,* 517–521.

Garb, H. N. (1998). *Studying the clinician: Judgment research and psychological assessment.* Washington, DC: American Psychological Association.

Greenfeld, D. G., Anyan, W. R., Hobart, M., Quinlan, D. M., & Plantes, M. (1991). Insight into illness and outcome in anorexia nervosa. *International Journal of Eating Disorders, 10,* 101–109.

Harrow, M., Rattenbury, F., & Stoll, F. (1988). Schizophrenic delusions: An analysis of their persistence, of related premorbid ideas, and of three major dimensions. In T. F. Oltmanns & B. A. Maher (Eds.), *Delusional beliefs* (pp. 184–211). New York: Wiley.

Hofstee, W. K. B. (1994). Who should own the definition of personality? *European Journal of Personality, 8,* 149–162.

Kaplan, G. B., Phillips, K. A., Vaccaro, A., Eisen, J. L., Posternak, M. A., & MacAskill, H.

S. (2006). Assessment of insight into delusional beliefs in schizophrenia using the Brown Assessment of Beliefs Scale. *Schizophrenia Research, 82*, 279–281.

Kenny, D. A., & DePaulo, B. M. (1993). Do people know how others view them?: An empirical and theoretical account. *Psychological Bulletin, 114*, 145–161.

Kessler, R. C., Merikangas, K. R., & Wang, P. S. (2007). Prevalence, comorbidity, and service utilization for mood disorders in the United States at the beginning of the twenty-first century. *Annual Review of Clinical Psychology, 3*, 137–158.

Klein, D. N. (2003). Patients' versus informants' reports of personality disorders in predicting 7½-year outcome in outpatients with depressive disorders. *Psychological Assessment, 15*, 216–222.

Klein, D. N., Kotov, R., & Bufferd, S. J. (2011). Personality and depression: Explanatory models and review of the evidence. *Annual Review of Clinical Psychology, 7*, 269–296.

Klonsky, E. D., Oltmanns, T. F., & Turkheimer, E. (2002). Informant-reports of personality disorder: Relation to self-reports and future research directions. *Clinical Psychology: Science and Practice, 9*, 300–311.

Krueger, R. F. (2005). Continuity of Axes I and II: Toward a unified model of personality and clinical disorders. *Journal of Personality Disorders, 19*, 233–261.

Lawton, E. M., Shields, A. J., & Oltmanns, T. F. (2011). Five-factor model personality disorder prototypes in a community sample: Self- and informant-reports predicting interview-based DSM-IV diagnoses. *Personality Disorders: Theory, Research, and Treatment, 12*, 279–292.

Leising, D., Erbs, J., & Fritz, U. (2010). The letter of recommendation effect in informant ratings of personality. *Journal of Personality and Social Psychology, 98*, 668–682.

Lynam, D. R., & Widiger, T. A. (2001). Using the five-factor model to represent the DSM-IV personality disorders: An expert consensus approach. *Journal of Abnormal Psychology, 11*, 401–412.

Miller, J. D., Jones, S. E., & Lynam, D. R. (2011). Psychopathic traits from the perspective of self and informant reports: Is there evidence for a lack of insight? *Journal of Abnormal Psychology, 120*(3), 758–764.

Miller, J. D., Pilkonis, P. A., & Clifton, A. (2005). Self and other-reports of traits from the five-factor model: Relations to personality disorders. *Journal of Personality Disorders, 19*(4), 400–419.

Mintz, A. R., Dobson, K. S., & Romney, D. M. (2003). Insight in schizophrenia: A meta-analysis. *Schizophrenia Research, 61*, 75–88.

Narrow, W. E., Rae, D. S., Robins, L. N., & Regier, D. A. (2002). Revised prevalence estimates of mental disorders in the United States. *Archives of General Psychiatry, 59*, 115–123.

Ness, D. E., & Ende, J. (1994). Denial in the medical interview: Recognition and management. *Journal of the American Medical Association, 272*, 1777–1781.

Oltmanns, T. F., & Gleason, M. E. (2011). Personality, health, and social adjustment in later life. In L.B. Cottler (Ed.), *Mental health in public health: The next 100 years*. New York: Oxford University Press.

Oltmanns, T. F., Gleason, M. E., Klonsky, E. D., & Turkheimer, E. (2005). Metaperception for pathological personality traits: Do we know when others think that we are difficult? *Consciousness and Cogntion, 14*, 739–751.

Oltmanns, T. F., & Turkheimer, E. (2006). Perceptions of self and others regarding pathological personality traits. In R. F. Krueger & J. L. Tackett (Eds.), *Personality and psychopathology* (pp. 71–111). New York: Guilford Press.

Oltmanns, T. F., & Turkheimer, E. (2009). Person perception and personality pathology. *Current Directions in Psychological Science, 18*(1), 32–36.

Paris, J. (2010). Estimating the prevalence of personality disorders in the community. *Journal of Personality Disorders, 24*, 405–411.

Sanz, M., Constable, G., Lopez-Ibor, I., Kemp, R., & David, A. S. (1998). A comparative study of insight scales and their relationship to psychopathological and clinical variables. *Psychological Medicine, 28,* 437–446.

Saravanan, B., Jacob, K. S., Johnson, S., Prince, M., Bhugra, D., & David, A. S. (2010). Outcome of first-episode schizophrenia in India: Longitudinal study of effect of insight and psychopathology. *British Journal of Psychiatry, 196,* 454–459.

Sartorius, N., Shapiro, R., & Jablonsky, A. (1974). The International Pilot Study of Schizophrenia. *Schizophrenia Bulletin, 1,* 21–35.

Sher, K. J., & Epler, A. J. (2004). Alcoholic denial: Self-awareness and beyond. In B. D. Beitman & J. Nair (Eds.), *Self-awareness deficits in psychiatric patients: Neurobiology, assessment, and treatment* (pp. 184–212). New York: Norton.

Skodol, A. E., Grilo, C. M., Pagano, M. E., Bender, D. S., Gunderson, J. G., Shea, M. T., et al. (2005). Effects of personality disorders on functioning and well-being in major depressive disorder. *Journal of Psychiatric Practice, 11*(6), 363–368.

Smith, T. W., Uchino, B. N., Berg, C. A., Florsheim, P., Pearce, G., Hawkins, M. (2008). Associations of self-reports versus spouse ratings of negative affectivity, dominance, and affiliation with coronary artery disease: Where should we look and who should we ask when studying personality and health? *Health Psychology, 27,* 676–684.

Steinglass, J. E., Eisen, J. L., Attia, E., Mayer, L., & Walsh, B. (2007). Is anorexia nervosa a delusional disorder?: An assessment of eating beliefs in anorexia nervosa. *Journal of Psychiatric Practice, 13,* 65–71.

Thomas, C., Turkheimer, E., & Oltmanns, T. F. (2003). Factorial structure of pathological personality traits as evaluated by peers. *Journal of Abnormal Psychology, 112,* 1–12.

Türksoy, N., Tükel, R., Ozdemir, O., & Karali, A. (2002). Comparison of clinical characteristics in good and poor insight obsessive–compulsive disorder. *Journal of Anxiety Disorders, 16,* 413–423.

Vandereycken, W. (2006a). Denial of illness in anorexia nervosa—a conceptual review: Part 1. Diagnostic significance and assessment. *European Eating Disorders Review, 14,* 341–351.

Vandereycken, W. (2006b). Denial of illness in anorexia nervosa—a conceptual review: Part 2. Different forms and meanings. *European Eating Disorders Review, 14,* 352–368.

Vazire, S. (2010). Who knows what about a person?: The Self-Other Knowledge Asymmetry (SOKA) model. *Journal of Personality and Social Psychology, 98,* 281–300.

Vazire, S., & Carlson, E. (2010). Self-knowledge of personality: Do people know themselves? *Social and Personality Psychology Compass, 4/8,* 605–620.

Vitousek, K., Watson, S., & Wilson, G. T. (1998). Enhancing motivation for change in treatment-resistant eating disorders. *Clinical Psychology Review, 18,* 391–420.

Zimmerman, M., Rothschild, L., & Chelminski, I. (2005). The prevalence of personality disorders in psychiatric outpatients. *American Journal of Psychiatry, 162,* 1991, 1911–1918.

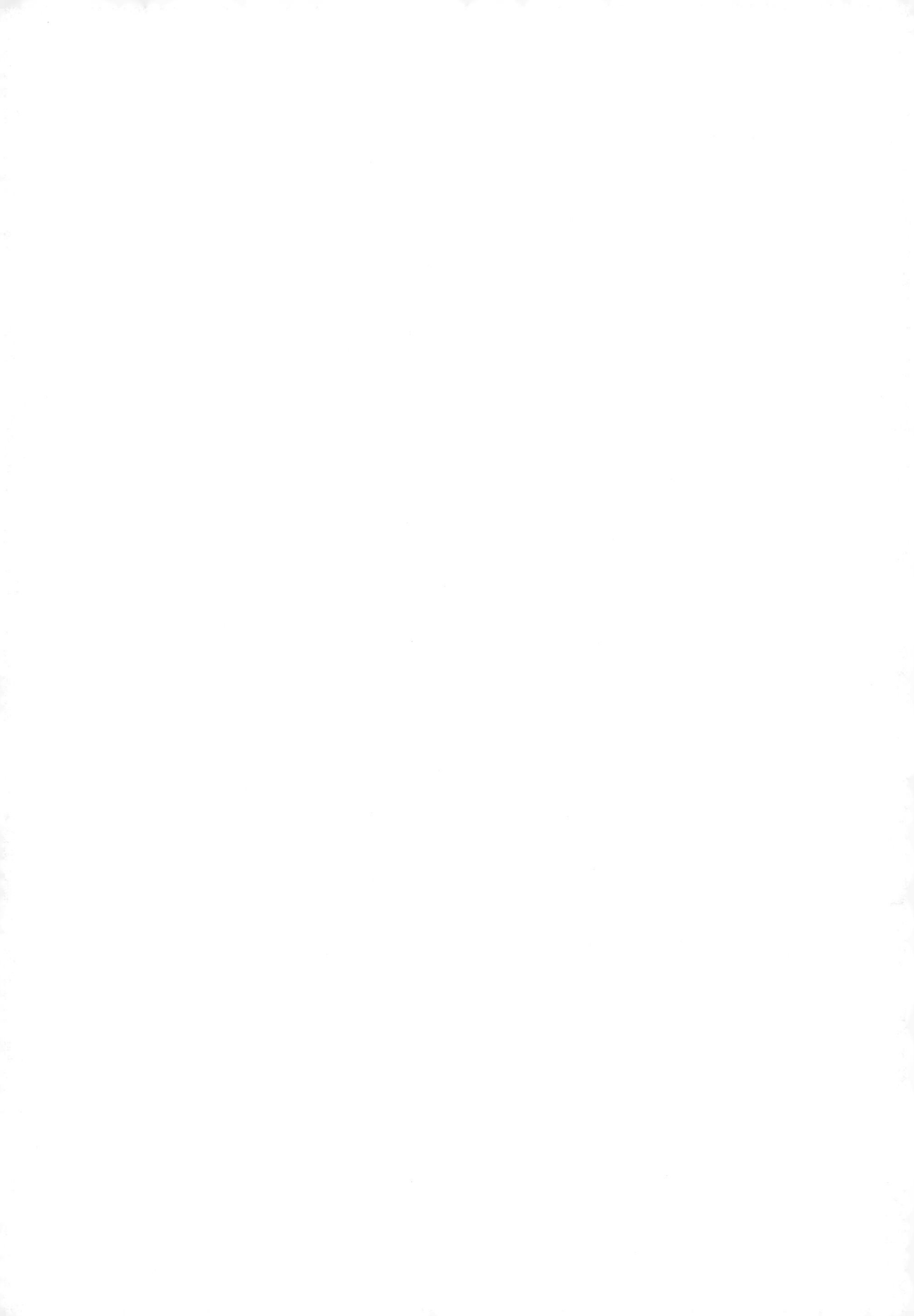

PART III
KNOWING OUR PAST AND FUTURE SELVES

CHAPTER 17

Affective Forecasting
Knowing How We Will Feel in the Future

KOSTADIN KUSHLEV
ELIZABETH W. DUNN

Imagine coming across a vending machine stocked with various forms of self-knowledge. Press one button and out comes an understanding of your own personality; press another and you've got a fistful of knowledge about your own motives or attitudes. Faced with this enticing array of self-knowledge, the wisest choice might lie in selecting an accurate understanding of your own future feelings.

As we show in this chapter, predicting one's own future feelings—making *affective forecasts*—isn't easy. People often make small but systematic errors in forecasting their own emotional responses, and occasionally make more dramatic mistakes. These failures of self-knowledge stem from a variety of sources and carry costs for both individual happiness and societal well-being. Thus, researchers have begun to identify ways to improve this form of self-knowledge. Studying this topic requires methodological care and ingenuity, but doing so can potentially provide important stepping stones in the pursuit of happiness.

What Do People Know—and Not Know—about Their Future Feelings?

Because other reviews of the literature offer excellent typologies of affective forecasting errors (e.g., Hsee & Hastie, 2006; Wilson & Gilbert, 2003), here we present only a brief discussion of the most common types of affective forecasting errors. While researchers have focused on identifying the flaws in affective forecasting, it is important to recognize that these flaws in the foreground stand out against a background of reasonably accurate self-knowledge.

Forecasting Errors

One of the most well-known and widely occurring affective forecasting errors is the *impact bias*—the tendency to overestimate the intensity and duration of emotional responses to future events. Exhibiting the impact bias, people overestimate how happy they will feel at Christmas (Buehler & McFarland, 2001) and how miserable they will feel after failing a driver's test (Ayton, Pott, & Elwakili, 2007) or seeing their preferred candidate lose an election (Gilbert, Pinel, Wilson, Blumberg, & Wheatley, 1998). The impact bias is usually stronger for negative events, with the effects for positive events often significant but smaller (e.g., Buehler & McFarland, 2001; Gilbert et al., 1998).

Although the impact bias may be the most ubiquitous form of forecasting error, people sometimes exhibit just the opposite mistake, underestimating the power of their future affective states (e.g., Dunn, Biesanz, Human, & Finn, 2007). This can occur when people fail to appreciate the potency of their own visceral states (e.g., hunger, thirst) in shaping future decisions and preferences. Such intrapersonal *empathy gaps* have been demonstrated for visceral states ranging from hunger (Read & van Leeuwen, 1998) and sexual arousal (Loewenstein, Nagin, & Paternoster, 1997) to the craving for drugs (Sayette, Loewenstein, Griffin, & Black, 2008).

Occasionally, people exhibit even more dramatic forecasting errors, mistaking sources of misery for sources of joy. Affective forecasts that are this far out of whack typically stem from *inaccurate theories* about the determinants of happiness. For example, most of us believe that having choice is beneficial for our happiness. Yet restricting our ability to choose can sometimes buttress our contentment with what we've got. In one study, people were asked to choose a piece of art to take home, and some of them were told that they would have the option to exchange this piece for a different one. Individuals who were provided with this option experienced less appreciation for their chosen piece of artwork than people who had no such option to exchange. Yet participants failed to anticipate this detrimental effect of choice, relying instead on the assumption that more choice is better (Gilbert & Ebert, 2002).

Forecasting Accuracy

Although we sometimes make dramatic affective forecasting errors, the most common form of forecasting error—the impact bias—tends to be small to medium. In Gilbert and colleagues' (1998) seminal paper, for example, participants consistently overestimated their future affective reactions to positive events (e.g., getting tenure), but the size of this misprediction effect (r) ranged from only .02 to .12 across three different studies. While the effect sizes for mean differences between people's forecasts and experiences were larger for negative events (e.g., romantic breakups) across the same three studies (r's = .38–.41), it is worth recognizing that this affective forecasting bias is not overwhelmingly large.

Indeed, even if people overestimate the absolute intensity of their future affect, they can still exhibit accuracy in predicting the intensity of their feelings relative to other individuals (Mathieu & Gosling, in press). To illustrate, imagine that Paul, Clif, and Ian all make predictions about how they would feel if they got promoted at their jobs, with their predicted happiness scores being 10, 9, and 8, and their actual happiness 8, 7, and 6, respectively. Although Paul overestimates his happiness, he accurately predicts that he will be happier than Clif and Ian. Indeed, a recent meta-analysis of 16 studies documenting mean differences between people's forecasted and actual affect showed that people's affective forecasts on average were correlated ($r = .28$) with their actual affective experiences (Mathieu & Gosling, 2012). Thus, despite systematic biases when people predict how they might feel in the future, individuals show some accuracy in predicting their future feelings relative to others. As we see later in this chapter, affective forecasting errors can have an impact on a variety of important outcomes in the real world (see Rosnow & Rosenthal, 1989, for a discussion of the consequential impact of small effects), but it is important to recognize that people are not entirely without insight into their own emotional futures.

Why Is Self-Knowledge in This Area Limited?

When we make affective forecasts, our capacity for self-knowledge is limited in part because the system we're trying to predict is very different from the system we use to do the predicting. Our basic ability to experience emotions is an ancient capacity that we share with other animals, whereas our ability to *predict* our emotions appears to be uniquely human—a cool new gadget on the timescale of evolution (Gilbert & Wilson, 2007). According to Epstein's (1998) cognitive–experiential self-theory (CEST), emotions are a signature product of the evolutionarily ancient "experiential system," which rapidly and holistically processes information in a concrete, associative fashion. In contrast, the human ability to forecast emotions seems to rely heavily on the newer "rational system," which processes information in a slower and more analytical and abstract manner. Trying to use the rational system to predict the outputs of the experiential system is a little like asking a robot to analyze a poem, and a diverse array of affective forecasting errors arise from this fundamental mismatch (for a more detailed discussion of this perspective, see Dunn, Forrin, & Ashton-James, 2009). As Gilbert and Wilson (2007) argue, "The cortex attempts to trick the rest of the brain by impersonating a sensory system . . . but try as it might, the cortex cannot generate simulations that have all the richness and reality of genuine perceptions" (p. 1354). Building on this argument, we use CEST to provide a broad framework for understanding *why* simulations and actual perceptions systematically diverge.

Holistic versus Analytic

According to CEST, one of the key differences between the rational and experiential systems is that the former processes information more analytically. Drawing on the rational system, forecasters zoom in on a target event, imagining the event largely in isolation from its broader context.[1] This approach can lead forecasters to neglect the temporal context, such that a plate of spaghetti smothered in meat sauce is expected to be nearly as appealing whether it is served for breakfast or dinner (Gilbert, Gill, & Wilson, 2002). This style of thinking also results in *focalism*, whereby people envision a target emotional event while disregarding the important contextual factors that may mitigate its emotional impact (Schkade & Kahneman, 1998; Wilson, Wheatley, Meyers, Gilbert, & Axsom, 2000). When Daniel, for example, is predicting how unhappy he will be if his boyfriend Billy leaves him, he is likely to focus exclusively on how hurtful the breakup will be. The week that Daniel gets dumped, however, may also be filled with abundant sunshine, visits from caring friends, and schoolwork—all of which may contribute to making Daniel's reaction to the breakup less potent than he expected. Finally, because thinking analytically promotes a focus on the differences between the available options, forecasters tend to overlook important similarities across options (Dunn, Wilson, & Gilbert, 2003; Hodges, 1997; Hsee & Zhang, 2004). In contemplating a vacation to Bali versus Belize, forecasters might focus on the fact that Bali has better surfing, while neglecting the fact that both destinations offer interesting wildlife and beautiful weather—leading to an exaggerated belief that Bali will be more fun than Belize.

Hot versus Cold

As well as processing information analytically, the rational system operates in a relatively "cold" manner, processing information dispassionately, whereas the "hot" experiential system is oriented toward pleasure and pain, promoting a more motivated interpretation of information. The rational system is like a judge, balancing the available evidence, while the lawyer of the experiential system builds a story, fitting the evidence to support a desired perspective. Thus, drawing on the rational system, forecasters may go astray by being too fair and balanced. This tendency results in *immune neglect*, whereby forecasters overlook how experiencers will twist the interpretation of an event after it occurs in order to mitigate negative feelings (Gilbert et al., 1998). For example, after being dumped by Billy, Daniel is likely to focus on Billy's annoying habits, making him feel better about the breakup in a way that he would not have anticipated ahead of time. The coldness of the rational system also undermines its capacity to appreciate the power of hot, visceral states, resulting in cold-to-hot empathy gaps (Loewenstein & Schkade, 1999). For example, prior to childbirth, many women make the calculated decision to avoid the use of anesthesia during labor—only to reverse this choice in the heat of the moment (Christensen-Szalanski, 1984).[2]

Associative versus Logical

Whereas the rational system processes information slowly on the basis of abstract logic and conscious appraisal, the experiential system works more quickly by relying on associative thought, interpreting the present though concrete connections to past experiences. This suggests that our emotional experiences may be shaped in part by our implicit associations—which we may overlook if we rely on the rational system in making affective forecasts. Support for this idea comes from a study in which participants were asked to eat a piece of a Red Delicious apple and a piece of Hershey's Bliss chocolate (McConnell, Dunn, Austin, & Rawn, 2011). They were asked to predict how much they would enjoy each food and to rate their actual enjoyment, as well as to complete measures of their implicit and explicit attitudes toward apples and chocolate. Over and above their explicit attitudes, participants' implicit attitudes toward apples and chocolate shaped their actual enjoyment of these foods, but not their expected enjoyment. As a result, participants' implicit attitudes predicted their forecasting errors; individuals with strong positive implicit associations toward chocolate (vs. apples) underestimated how much they would enjoy eating Hershey's Bliss. This suggests that forecasters go astray in part by relying on logic and conscious appraisals, while overlooking the implicit associations that shape actual emotional experiences.

Beyond our associations with individual objects such as apples and chocolate, we have a rich network of "if–then" associations that underlie our personalities (e.g., Mischel, Shoda, & Mendoza-Denton, 2002), which forecasters may also overlook. Shortly after the election of Barack Obama, for example, the joy experienced by his supporters was dampened for neurotic individuals, perhaps because his victory triggered worries about the potential for assassination or the challenges posed by hostile Republicans (Quoidbach & Dunn, 2010). Yet, just prior to the election, participants overlooked their own neuroticism when forecasting how happy they would be if Obama won, thereby exhibiting *personality neglect*.

In short, we have argued that people's simulations of the future are often constructed by the rational system, which operates in a fundamentally different manner than the experiential system. As a result, people may be deprived of accurate self-knowledge because their imaginations are too rational.

Implications of Affective Forecasting Errors

Affective forecasting errors are more than academic curiosities. These errors can impair the pursuit of happiness and health, as well as exacerbate social and economic problems.

Personal Happiness

As noted at the beginning of this chapter, people occasionally mispredict their future affective reactions completely. Because affective forecasts play an important role in decision making (Falk, Dunn, & Norenzayan, 2010), such grave mispredictions could reduce our future happiness by leading us to choose exactly the course of action that would make us less happy. Many of us seem to believe, for instance, that revenge would feel good, which may explain the central place of revenge in both human law and literature. Revenge, however, might be less sweet than we think. In one study, participants were given the chance to exact revenge and punish another player who tried to cheat them out of winning money. Those players who punished the cheater felt worse than players who did not have the chance to exact revenge (Carlsmith, Wilson, & Gilbert, 2008). Yet another group of participants in this study predicted that they would feel better if they had the opportunity to punish the cheater. These findings illustrate how our inaccurate affective forecasts could potentially lead us to choose exactly the thing that would make us less happy.

Subtler forms of affective forecasting errors, however, could potentially boost happiness. In one study, participants who were in negative mood—as compared to participants in a neutral mood—predicted that they would experience stronger positive feelings as a result of desirable future events such as having a nice meal or watching their favorite TV show (Buehler, McFarland, Spyropoulos, & Lam, 2007). Furthermore, the stronger people expected their positive affect to be in the future, the happier and more satisfied they felt in the present. Although the researchers did not examine whether these forecasts were biased, integrating this research with previous work on the impact bias suggests that this bias may not be so bad when it comes to positive events. That is, even if a vacation to the Caribbean isn't as fabulous as we imagine, *expecting* it to be wonderful may provide months of pleasurable anticipation (Loewenstein, 1987).

Personal Health

In addition to influencing personal happiness, affective forecasting errors have been shown to play a role in health decisions. A wide variety of health problems stem from a lack of exercise, and new research suggests that people significantly underestimate how much they would enjoy exercising (Ruby, Dunn, Perrino, Gillis, & Viel, 2011). Furthermore, the less people expect to enjoy exercise, the less they report intending to engage in it. With obesity poised to overtake smoking as the leading cause of death in the United States (Mokdad, Marks, Stroup, & Gerberding, 2004), this research suggests that affective forecasting errors may pose a critical obstacle for public health.

Affective forecasting errors may also prevent people from getting tested for serious health problems. In one study, people overestimated how much distress they would experience if they tested positive for HIV (Sieff, Dawes, & Loewenstein, 1999). Given that people are motivated to avoid negative experiences, expecting to suffer great distress after testing could drive people to postpone being tested, thus potentially endangering their own life and the lives of others.

We are often so motivated to avoid suffering that we will do anything to make ourselves feel better, including taking all kinds of "feel-good" substances, rather than simply relying on the power of the psychological immune system. When participants were asked to imagine being rejected in a dating game, they overestimated how upset they would feel and were more likely to want a mood-enhancing pill, compared to people who actually experienced the rejection (Wilson, Wheatley, Kurtz, Dunn, & Gilbert, 2004). This finding tentatively suggests that people may sometimes overestimate their need for drugs and alcohol in coping with life's setbacks.

Intergroup Relations

Affective forecasting errors may play a role in perpetuating stereotyping and prejudice. In one study, white participants overestimated how much negative emotion they would experience during an interaction with a black person, which they erroneously expected to be more unpleasant than an interaction with a white person (Mallett, Wilson, & Gilbert, 2008). This suggests that affective forecasting errors may lead people to avoid intergroup contact, thereby foregoing experiences that could reduce racism. Indeed, new evidence demonstrates that helping individuals overcome their overly negative expectations regarding intergroup contact can help to promote the development of friendships across groups (Mallett & Wilson, 2010).

Racism may also be perpetuated because people do not react to it as negatively as they themselves would expect. In one study, college students predicted that they would be very distressed if they saw a white person use a racial slur about a black person, but other students who actually witnessed this situation were emotionally unruffled (Kawakami, Dunn, Karmali, & Dovidio, 2009). Forecasters also predicted that they would choose to work with the black victim rather than the white racist on a subsequent task, but experiencers exhibited the opposite preference. These results suggest that, contrary to our expectations, racist acts might have little emotional impact on majority group members and go unpunished.

The findings of these two studies, then, help to explain why racism persists despite apparent changes in explicit attitudes over the past several decades. If I am avoiding interacting with Jamal because I believe that the interaction will be awkward, then this might prevent me from challenging my own stereotypical views of him (and black people in general). At the same time, if I do not challenge my white friends Jeff and Rose when I hear them derogating Jamal because he is black, Jeff and Rose's negative attitudes toward blacks will also go unchallenged.

Economic Implications

Mispredicting our own emotions can also create economic problems. In particular, recent research suggests that the impact bias may lead to loss aversion. Demonstrating classic loss aversion, participants predicted that losing $4 would decrease their current level of happiness more than gaining $4 would increase their level of happiness (Kermer, Driver-Linn, Wilson, & Gilbert, 2006). A different group that actually experienced either a gain or a loss of $4, however, did not show the same aversion toward the loss—the $4 gain and the $4 loss had a similar emotional impact (in opposite directions, of course). Loss aversion creates significant problems for people's economic behavior in the real world, from investing in the stock market to deciding whether to switch retirement plans (Camerer, 2000). For example, because people value what they have (i.e., what they could *lose*) more than what they could acquire (i.e., what they could *gain*), some people willingly forgo the opportunity to choose the many benefits of a new health plan just to preserve the few benefits of their current health plan (Samuelson & Zeckhauser, 1988).

Like loss aversion, the endowment effect can lead to economic problems, from slashing profits to impairing the fluidity of markets. Due to the endowment effect, people value commodities more when they are selling them than when they are buying them. When buyers' agents were asked to make an offer to buy coffee mugs from their owners, the agents consistently made unacceptably low offers to the owners, resulting in few sells (only 19% successful transactions) and low earnings for the agents (only one-third of the amount agents would have earned had they been able to accurately evaluate the value owners placed on their mug; Van Boven, Dunning, & Loewenstein, 2000). Importantly, agents' inability to predict the value placed on the mug by the owner was at least partially due to the agents' inability to predict how *much* they themselves would value the mug if they were owners (an affective forecasting error). In fact, more recent research has shown that when buyers already own an identical mug, they are willing to pay just as much for it as sellers demand (Morewedge, Shu, Gilbert, & Wilson, 2009), presumably because they already know how it feels to be a mug owner, thus eliminating the source of this forecasting error. In short, people's inability to imagine how they would feel about a commodity if they owned it may reduce financial gains and impair the fluidity and profitability of markets by reducing the number of successful transactions.

How Can This Form of Self-Knowledge Be Improved?

By identifying the mechanisms that underlie affective forecasting errors, researchers have been able to develop simple interventions that directly target these specific mechanisms, thereby improving affective forecasts. Of course, like a flu vaccine that only works against specific viral strains, these immunizations are helpful primarily when they are matched with the corresponding strain of forecasting error. Therefore, researchers have also identified skills and interventions that can reduce forecasting errors across a wide variety of situations, akin to vitamins that improve overall health.

Mechanism-Specific Remedies
Reducing Focalism

Focalism and related problems can be combated by encouraging people to adopt a broader perspective (e.g., Dunn et al., 2003; Hoerger, Quirk, Lucas, & Carr, 2009; Wilson et al., 2000). For example, simply asking students to consider how much they enjoy their regular daily activities, from visiting friends to doing homework, reduced their tendency to overestimate how much school football games would influence their happiness (Hoerger et al., 2009). A less direct but perhaps longer-lasting way of reducing focalism among Westerners might lie in living abroad in a more interdependent culture (e.g., Japan). People from interdependent cultures tend to consider contextual factors to a greater extent than do people from independent cultures. It is not surprising, then, that Asians are less prone to focalism than Westerners (Lam, Buehler, McFarland, Ross, & Cheung, 2005). Given that living abroad can produce measurable changes in psychological phenomena such as creativity (Maddux & Galinsky, 2009), spending a year in Japan, for example, might reduce focalism (although no research has directly explored this hypothesis).

Reducing Immune Neglect

Another strategy for reducing affective forecasting errors is to tackle our tendency to ignore our remarkable ability to adapt and make sense of new circumstances. In one study, before making predictions about their quality of life after becoming paraplegic, jurors in the Philadelphia County Courthouse were asked to reflect on their ability to adapt to negative circumstances (Ubel, Loewenstein, & Jepson, 2005). This reflection increased the quality-of-life predictions of the jurors (as compared to the predictions of jurors who did not engage in this reflection). Thus, a simple reflection on adaptation may help us make more balanced affective forecasts.

General "Cures"
Learning from Past Experiences

In addition to targeting specific mechanisms responsible for our affective forecasting errors, we can make better affective forecasts by using some general "cures." One such intuitive strategy lies in learning from past experiences. Learning from the past, however, is more difficult than we might think (Wilson, Meyers, & Gilbert, 2001). This is true in part because the most unusual past events—those events that are least likely to happen again in the future—are often the most memorable (Fredrickson & Kahneman, 1993; Kahneman & Tversky, 1973). When passengers at a train station were prompted to remember a past instance when they missed their train, they typically recalled rather atypical experiences, in which missing the train was especially problematic (Morewedge, Gilbert, & Wilson, 2005). As a result, they expected to be quite unhappy if they missed the train they were currently hoping to catch. This forecasting problem was ameliorated when passengers were instructed to remember *multiple* past instances of missed trains, as opposed to just one. Thus, thinking about a broad array of relevant past experiences may be a productive route to improving affective forecasts.

Increasing Emotional Intelligence

Another general "cure" for our affective forecasting errors is to increase our overall emotional intelligence (EI; i.e., our ability to observe, understand and regulate our emotions). Because some aspects of EI have been shown to improve with training (Nelis, Quoidbach, Mikolajczak, & Hansenne, 2009) and higher EI has been associated with making more accurate affective forecasts (Dunn, Brackett, Ashton-James, Schneiderman, & Salovey, 2007), we might be able to improve the accuracy of our affective forecasts with EI training. Of course, increasing EI would take more time than simply considering nonfocal future events or relevant past experiences. This method of improving affective forecasts, however, is also likely to have more long-lasting and pervasive effect on our ability to predict our emotions. In this sense, then, EI training might be a worthwhile endeavor as a way of reducing the negative personal, societal, and economic consequences of affective forecasting errors.

Learning from Others

In order to increase our own self-knowledge, we may benefit from looking to others. When predicting how much they would enjoy a speed date with a male undergraduate, female undergraduates made smaller affective forecasting errors if they learned how much another woman had enjoyed the date (Gilbert, Killingsworth, Eyre, & Wilson, 2009). Indeed, compared to women who had plentiful information about the young man, women who knew nothing *except* how much this other woman had enjoyed her date with him made better affective forecasts.

Methodological Issues

While most published affective forecasting studies use rigorous methods, many more potentially interesting studies never make it into the journals because of methodological problems. Thus, we offer several basic recommendations for conducting studies of affective forecasting. Although these principles seem fairly obvious, we can confirm from our reviewing experience that they are often violated.

Give Forecasters a Fair Chance

Because researchers in this area often set out to show that forecasters make mistakes, it is essential to give forecasters a fair chance to be right. In particular, it is important to ensure that the situation forecasters are asked to imagine matches the situation experiencers actually encounter. This is harder than it sounds. For example, Kawakami and colleagues (2009) engineered a complex social situation in which experiencers witnessed a white student utter a racial slur about a black student. If forecasters had simply been asked to imagine how they would feel after seeing a white student use this racial slur, they might have envisioned a very different situation than what actually transpired. For this reason, in an initial study, the researchers provided forecasters with a detailed description of the situation that experiencers witnessed. Still, because it is impossible for a written description to convey every important detail of a complex social situation, forecasters in a second study were shown a video of the event that experiencers witnessed, from the experiencers' visual perspective. Of course, this use of video would not be practical in many affective forecasting studies, but regardless of the design used, it is critical for researchers to ensure that the situations forecasters are asked to imagine corresponds as tightly as possible to the situation that experiencers face.

Forecasters and Experiencers Should Be Similar to Each Other

As well as equating the *situations* that forecasters and experiencers confront, researchers should ensure that the *individuals* doing the forecasting and experiencing are as similar to each other as possible. Of course, this goal can be accomplished by randomly assigning participants to the role of forecaster or experiencer. But an important strength of the affective forecasting literature is that researchers often examine people's expected and actual reactions to consequential, real-life events, typically precluding the use of random assignment. For example, we have been interested in examining the predicted and actual emotional benefits of prosocial behavior, and we have considered surveying people who have just participated in charitable activities, such as the Breast Cancer Walk. On that same day, we could ask other people in the same city to predict how they would feel if they had participated in the walk. Comparing walkers' actual feelings with nonwalkers' predicted feelings would, however, be highly problematic. Walkers and nonwalkers might differ in myriad ways—from their athleticism and prosocial orientation to their familiarity with cancer—and any discrepancy between experiences and forecasts might stem from these differences rather than reflect a true error on the part of forecasters. One way to minimize this problem is to survey forecasters and experiencers who are drawn from the same relevant population (e.g., people who have signed up for the Breast Cancer Walk).

Alternatively, researchers can circumvent this problem by using a within-subjects design, in which all participants predict how they will feel after an event, experience the event, then report their actual feelings. But, using a within-subjects design introduces a different problem: The act of making affective forecasts can sometimes alter people's later emotional experiences (or at least their reports of those experiences). For example, the week before an important soccer match, Dolan and Metcalfe (2010) asked fans in one group to predict how they would feel if their team lost the match, whereas other fans were not asked to make any affective forecasts. When surveyed a week after their team lost the match, the fans who had been asked to make the forecast prior to the game rated themselves a whole point lower on a 10-point happiness scale than the fans who had not been asked to make affective forecasts. In other words, the act of making affective forecasts before the event altered participants' emotional ratings after the event. Of course, making affective forecasts does not *always* pollute later emotional reports (e.g., Ruby et al., 2011), and the advantages of within-subject designs sometimes outweigh this potential problem.

Given that both within- and between-subjects designs have limitations, an ideal approach is to use a hybrid design (Loewenstein & Schkade, 1999), in which half the participants make affective predictions but all participants report their actual experiences (for an example of this approach, see Ruby et al., 2011, Study 1). Alternatively, researchers can accomplish the same goal by conducting multiple studies and demonstrating that consistent effects emerge using a combination of between- and within-subjects designs (for an example of this approach, see Gilbert et al., 1998).

Distinguish between Forecasting Extremity, Bias, and Accuracy

In part because of the challenges associated with equating forecasts and experiences, researchers sometimes measure only affective forecasts. This can be a reasonable strategy, but if this methodological approach is used, then researchers should not make any strong claims about forecasting bias or accuracy on the basis of their data. Imagine, for example, asking competitive horseback riders to predict how they would feel after winning a blue ribbon. If riders who predicted the highest levels of joy also reported spending the greatest number of hours at the stable, one might infer that positively biased affective forecasts serve a motivational function (by propelling people to devote more effort to achieving their goal). This conclusion would be inappropriate—extreme affective forecasts do not necessarily reflect bias; that is, individuals who predict relatively extreme emotional reactions may actually *experience* relatively extreme emotions. Thus, forecasting extremity should not be treated as a proxy for forecasting bias.

It is also important to distinguish between bias and overall accuracy (for an excellent illustration of this issue, see Epley & Dunning, 2006). Most studies have examined forecasting biases—directional errors whereby, for example, people significantly overestimate how good they will feel after a positive event. But it is also possible to examine overall accuracy by testing the magnitude of affective forecasting errors rather than their direction. Interestingly, compared to Westerners, East Asians are less susceptible to the impact bias, but they show no advantage in terms of accuracy (measured as the absolute value of the difference between forecasts and experiences or the correlation between forecasts and experiences; Lam et al., 2005). Conversely, individuals who are higher in EI make affective forecasts that are more accurate but no less biased (Dunn et al., 2007). Thus, researchers should first consider whether they expect effects on forecasting bias or overall accuracy, then select methodological and analytical strategies accordingly.

Examine Multiple Situations

In order to show that people make systematic affective forecasting errors, it is valuable to demonstrate that the same pattern emerges across diverse types of situations. For example, Gilbert and colleagues (1998) showed that, due to immune neglect, people overestimated how bad they would feel following romantic breakups, professional failures, upsetting stories, negative feedback, and political defeats. Demonstrating consistency across different situations is particularly essential for research on individual differences in forecasting accuracy and bias. For example, Dunn and colleagues (2007) showed that EI predicted how accurately people forecasted their emotional responses in the domains of academics, politics, and sports. In one of these studies, the same participants were asked to report their predicted and actual emotional responses regarding a graded term paper and a presidential election. Forecasting accuracy was significantly—but only moderately—correlated ($r = .28$, $p < .01$) across these two events. This suggests that individual differences influencing accuracy in one situation may fail to influence accuracy in another. Thus, studies that examine the relationship between individual differences (e.g., gender, personality) and forecasting accuracy in one situation may overestimate the importance of those individual differences for forecasting accuracy more broadly.

While it is important to examine affective forecasting errors across multiple situations, it is less essential to use measures of affect that include multiple items. In an early review paper, Wilson and Gilbert (2003) argued that single-item measures are often adequate for comparing predicted and actual affect, and subsequent studies have supported this perspective by showing that the same affective forecasting biases emerge regardless of whether single or multi-item measures of affect are used (Dunn & Ashton-James, 2008; Ruby et al., 2011). To provide support for the convergent validity of single-item forecasting measures, Quoidbach and Dunn (2010) asked participants to report their predicted and actual feelings on both a single-item measure of happiness and the 20-item Positive and Negative Affect Schedule (PANAS; Watson, Clark, & Tellegen, 1988); they found that the single-item measure was highly correlated with PANAS scores for both forecasts ($r = .70$) and experiences ($r = .73$). Demonstrating the predictive validity of single-item forecasting measures, Ruby and colleagues (2011) showed that participants' intentions to engage in exercise were significantly predicted by their anticipated enjoyment of exercise, regardless of whether anticipated enjoyment was assessed with a single-item or multi-item measure of enjoyment.

In an article titled, "We Have to Break Up," Robert Cialdini (2009) expressed his disillusionment with the state of modern psychology, arguing that demand for methodologically pristine experiments has made publishing field studies very difficult. In light of this important critique of our field by one of its most distinguished practitioners, we would encourage affective forecasting researchers to continue their study of consequential, real-world events, even if this means relying on brief or single-item measure of affect. Whether conducting studies in the field or the laboratory, researchers should strive to minimize differences in (1) the situations faced by forecasters and experiencers, and (2) the types of people doing the forecasting and experiencing. In addition, researchers should clearly distinguish between forecasting extremity, bias, and overall accuracy, while seeking to uncover similar patterns across diverse situations.

Conclusion

Returning to our self-knowledge vending machine, we have seen that a number of errors arise when we try to predict our future emotions—metaphorically speaking, when we're expecting Coke, we very often get Pepsi, and occasionally end up with a totally unexpected pack of peanuts. Many of these errors arise because of differences in the mental machinery that underlies our ability to experience emotions and our ability to anticipate them. Although such errors are sometimes harmless, they can pose obstacles to the well-being of both individuals and societies. By using clever, rigorous methods, however, researchers have successfully identified ways to overcome these obstacles, thereby helping people get what they expect, or at least expect what they're getting.

NOTES

1. For a more thorough discussion of the role of contextual factors in affective forecasting errors, see Gilbert and Wilson (2007).
2. The most effective way to combat cold-to-hot empathy gaps seems to lie in giving forecasters a taste of the hot state they will later experience (e.g., Loewenstein et al., 1997). Of course, if forecasters are placed in a hot state and experiences later occur in a cold state, this can result in the converse error, termed hot-to-cold empathy gaps (see Loewenstein, 2005, for a review).

REFERENCES

Ayton, P., Pott, A., & Elwakili, N. (2007). Affective forecasting: Why can't people predict their emotions? *Thinking and Reasoning, 13*, 62–80.

Buehler, R., & McFarland, C. (2001). Intensity bias in affective forecasting: The role of temporal focus. *Personality and Social Psychology Bulletin, 27*, 1480–1493.

Buehler, R., McFarland, C., Spyropoulos, V., & Lam, K. C. H. (2007). Motivated prediction of future feelings: Effects of negative mood and mood orientation on affective forecasts. *Personality and Social Psychology Bulletin, 33*, 1265–1278.

Camerer, C. (2000). Prospect theory in the wild: Evidence from the field. In D. Kahneman & A. Tversky (Eds.), *Choices, values and frames* (pp. 288–300). Cambridge, UK: Cambridge University Press.

Carlsmith, K. M., Wilson, T. D., & Gilbert, D. T. (2008). The paradoxical consequences of revenge. *Journal of Personality and Social Psychology, 95*, 1316–1324.

Christensen-Szalanski, J. J. (1984). Discount functions and the measurement of patients' values: Women's decisions during childbirth. *Medical Decision Making, 4*, 47–58.

Cialdini, R. B. (2009). We have to break up. *Perspectives on Psychological Science, 4*, 5–6.

Dolan, P., & Metcalfe, R. (2010). "Oops . . . I did it again": Repeated focusing effects in reports of happiness. *Journal of Economic Psychology, 31*, 732–737.

Dunn, E. W., & Ashton-James, C. (2008). On emotional innumeracy: Predicted and actual affective responses to grand-scale tragedies. *Journal of Experimental Social Psychology, 44*, 692–698.

Dunn, E. W., Biesanz, J. C., Human, L. J., & Finn, S. (2007). Misunderstanding the affective consequences of everyday social interactions: The hidden benefits of putting one's best face forward. *Journal of Personality and Social Psychology, 92*, 990–1005.

Dunn, E. W., Brackett, M. A., Ashton-James, C., Schneiderman, E., & Salovey, P. (2007). On emotionally intelligent time travel: Individual differences in affective forecasting ability. *Personality and Social Psychology Bulletin, 33*, 85–93.

Dunn, E. W., Forrin, N., & Ashton-James, C. E. (2009). On the excessive rationality of the emotional imagination: A two-systems account of affective forecasts and experiences. In K. D. Markman, W. M. P. Klein, & J. A. Suhr (Eds.), *The handbook of imagination and mental simulation* (pp. 331–346). New York: Psychology Press.

Dunn, E. W., Wilson, T. D., & Gilbert, D. T. (2003). Location, location, location: The misprediction of satisfaction in housing lotteries. *Personality and Social Psychology Bulletin, 29*, 1421–1432.

Epley, N., & Dunning, D. (2006). The mixed blessings of self-knowledge in behavioral prediction: Enhanced discrimination but exacerbated bias. *Personality and Social Psychology Bulletin, 32*, 641–655.

Epstein, S. (1998). Cognitive–experiential self-theory. In D. F. Barone, M. Hersen, & V. B. Van Hasselt (Eds.), *Advanced personality* (pp. 211–238). New York: Plenum Press.

Falk, C. F., Dunn, E. W., & Norenzayan, A. (2010). Cultural variation in the importance of expected enjoyment for decision making. *Social Cognition, 28*, 609–629.

Fredrickson, B. L., & Kahneman, D. (1993). Duration neglect in retrospective evaluations of affective episodes. *Journal of Personality and Social Psychology, 65*, 45–55.

Gilbert, D. T., & Ebert, J. E. J. (2002). Decisions and revisions: The affective forecasting of changeable outcomes. *Journal of Personality and Social Psychology, 82*, 503–514.

Gilbert, D. T., Gill, M. J., & Wilson, T. D. (2002). The future is now: Temporal correction in affective forecasting. *Organizational Behavior and Human Decision Processes, 88*, 430–444.

Gilbert, D. T., Killingsworth, M. A., Eyre, R. N., & Wilson, T. D. (2009). The surprising power of neighborly advice. *Science, 323*, 1617–1619.

Gilbert, D. T., Pinel, E. C., Wilson, T. D., Blumberg, S. J., & Wheatley, T. P. (1998). Immune neglect: A source of durability bias in affective forecasting. *Journal of Personality and Social Psychology, 75*, 617–638.

Gilbert, D. T., & Wilson, T. D. (2007). Prospection: Experiencing the future. *Science, 317*, 1351–1354.

Hodges, S. D. (1997). When matching up features messes up decisions: The role of feature matching in successive choices. *Journal of Personality and Social Psychology, 72*, 1310–1321.

Hoerger, M., Quirk, S. W., Lucas, R. E., & Carr, T. H. (2009). Immune neglect in affective forecasting. *Journal of Research in Personality, 43*, 91–94.

Hsee, C. K., & Hastie, R. (2006). Decision and experience: Why don't we choose what makes us happy? *Trends in Cognitive Sciences, 10*, 31–37.

Hsee, C. K., & Zhang, J. (2004). Distinction bias: Misprediction and mischoice due to joint evaluation. *Journal of Personality and Social Psychology, 86*, 680–695.

Kahneman, D., & Tversky, A. (1973). On the psychology of prediction. *Psychological Review, 80*, 649–744.

Kawakami, K., Dunn, E., Karmali, F., & Dovidio, J. F. (2009). Mispredicting affective and behavioral responses to racism. *Science, 323*, 276–278.

Kermer, D. A., Driver-Linn, E., Wilson, T. D., & Gilbert, D. T. (2006). Loss aversion is an affective forecasting error. *Psychological Science, 17*, 649–653.

Lam, K. C. H., Buehler, R., McFarland, C., Ross, M., & Cheung, I. (2005). Cultural differences in affective forecasting: The role of focalism. *Personality and Social Psychology Bulletin, 31*, 1296–1309.

Loewenstein, G. (1987). Anticipation and the valuation of delayed consumption. *Economic Journal, 97*, 666–684.

Loewenstein, G. (2005). Hot–cold empathy gaps and medical decision making. *Health Psychology, 24,* 49–56.

Loewenstein, G., Nagin, D., & Paternoster, R. (1997). The effect of sexual arousal on predictions of sexual forcefulness. *Journal of Crime and Delinquency, 32,* 443–473.

Loewenstein, G., & Schkade, D. A. (1999). Wouldn't it be nice?: Predicting future feelings. In D. Kahneman, E. Diener, & N. Schwartz (Eds.), *Well being: The foundations of hedonic psychology* (pp. 85–105). New York: Russell Sage Foundation.

Maddux, W. W., & Galinsky, A. D. (2009). Cultural borders and mental barriers: The relationship between living abroad and creativity. *Journal of Personality and Social Psychology, 96,* 1047–1061.

Mallett, R. K., & Wilson, T. D. (2010). Increasing positive intergroup contact. *Journal of Experimental Social Psychology, 46,* 382–387.

Mallett, R. K., Wilson, T. D., & Gilbert, D. T. (2008). Expect the unexpected: Failure to anticipate similarities leads to an intergroup forecasting error. *Journal of Personality and Social Psychology, 94,* 265–277.

Mathieu, M. T., & Gosling, S. D. (2012). The accuracy or inaccuracy of affective forecasts depends on how the question is framed: A meta-analysis of past studies. *Psychological Science, 23,* 161–162.

McConnell, A. R., Dunn, E. W., Austin, S. N., & Rawn, C. D. (2011). Blind spots in the search for happiness: Implicit attitudes and nonverbal leakage predict affective forecasting errors. *Journal of Experimental Social Psychology, 47,* 628–634.

Mischel, W., Shoda, Y., & Mendoza-Denton, R. (2002). Situation-behavior profiles as a locus of consistency in personality. *Current Directions in Psychological Science, 11,* 50–54.

Mokdad, A. H., Marks, J. S., Stroup, D. F., & Gerberding, J. L. (2004). Actual causes of death in the United States, 2000. *Journal of the American Medical Association, 291,* 1238–1245.

Morewedge, C. K., Gilbert, D. T., & Wilson, T. D. (2005). The least likely of times: How remembering the past biases forecasts of the future. *Psychological Science, 16,* 626–630.

Morewedge, C. K., Shu, L. L., Gilbert, D. T., & Wilson, T. D. (2009). Bad riddance or good rubbish?: Ownership and not loss aversion causes the endowment effect. *Journal of Experimental Social Psychology, 45,* 947–951.

Nelis, D., Quoidbach, J., Mikolajczak, M., & Hansenne, M. (2009). Increasing emotional intelligence: (How) is it possible? *Personality and Individual Differences, 47,* 36–41.

Quoidbach, J., & Dunn, E. W. (2010). Personality neglect: The unforeseen impact of personal dispositions on emotional life. *Psychological Science, 21,* 1783–1789.

Read, D., & van Leeuwen, B. (1998). Predicting hunger: The effects of appetite and delay on choice. *Organizational Behavior and Human Decision Processes, 76,* 189–205.

Rosnow, R. L., & Rosenthal, R. (1989). Statistical procedures and the justification of knowledge in psychological science. *American Psychologist, 44,* 1276–1284.

Ruby, M. B., Dunn, E. W., Perrino, A. L., Gillis, R., & Viel, S. C. (2011). The invisible benefits of exercise. *Health Psychology, 30,* 67–74.

Samuelson, W., & Zeckhauser, R. (1988). Status quo bias in decision making. *Journal of Risk and Uncertainty, 1,* 7–59.

Sayette, M. A., Loewenstein, G., Griffin, K. M., & Black, J. J. (2008). Exploring the cold-to-hot empathy gap in smokers. *Psychological Science, 19,* 926–932.

Schkade, D. A., & Kahneman, D. (1998). Does living in California make people happy?: A focusing illusion in judgments of life satisfaction. *Psychological Science, 9,* 340–346.

Sieff, E. M., Dawes, R. M., & Loewenstein, G. (1999). Anticipated versus actual reaction to HIV test results. *American Journal of Psychology, 112,* 297–311.

Ubel, P. A., Loewenstein, G., & Jepson, C. (2005). Disability and sunshine: Can hedonic predictions be improved by drawing attention to focusing illusions or emotional adaptation? *Journal of Experimental Psychology: Applied, 11,* 111–123.

Van Boven, L., Dunning, D., & Loewenstein, G. (2000). Egocentric empathy gaps between owners and buyers: Misperceptions of the endowment effect. *Journal of Personality and Social Psychology, 79,* 66–76.

Watson, D., Clark, L. A., & Tellegen, A. (1988). Development and validation of brief measures of positive and negative affect: The PANAS scales. *Journal of Personality and Social Psychology, 54*(6), 1063–1070.

Wilson, T. D., & Gilbert, D. T. (2003). Affective forecasting. *Advances in Experimental Social Psychology, 35,* 345–411.

Wilson, T. D., Meyers, J., & Gilbert, D. T. (2001). Lessons from the past: Do people learn from experience that emotional reactions are shortlived? *Personality and Social Psychology Bulletin, 27,* 1648–1661.

Wilson, T. D., Wheatley, T., Kurtz, J., Dunn, E., & Gilbert, D. T. (2004). When to fire: Anticipatory versus postevent reconstrual of uncontrollable events. *Personality and Social Psychology Bulletin, 30,* 1–12.

Wilson, T. D., Wheatley, T., Meyers, J. M., Gilbert, D. T., & Axsom, D. (2000). Focalism: A source of durability bias in affective forecasting. *Journal of Personality and Social Psychology, 78,* 821–836.

CHAPTER 18

Past Selves and Autobiographical Memory

COLLEEN M. KELLEY
LARRY L. JACOBY

"Knowing who we were" presupposes a relatively long life marked by change, including straightforward developmental progressions from childhood to adulthood, as well as more dramatic reinventions, resurrections, or extreme makeovers. A sense of self that evolves over time is a relatively recent invention. In fact, Baumeister (1987) argued that the modern conception of self formed partially as a result of the change from living inside one's medieval village, where everyone knew everyone else and roles were fixed, toward living among strangers in new locations and the consequent need to establish one's value for economic and social transactions. "Knowing who we were" might be important in creating a narrative story of one's self that sustains a feeling of continuity and fulfillment (McAdams, 2001). So, for example, one might take pride in having grown up in a small town with few options but making one's way toward a role in a larger society with some minor fame, or perhaps greater wealth. However, sustaining such a narrative wouldn't require much in the way of detailed knowledge and memories of prior self, and in fact the narrative might be relatively unconstrained by past reality (see also Adler, Chapter 20, this volume).

Memory for past selves includes memory for knowledge about one's past: abstractions such as roles and traits, tendency toward particular emotional expressions and moods, mental and physical health, patterns of behavior in relation to significant others, where we've lived, our jobs, our relationships. One might say "I was very shy in high school, but now I've learned to interact easily with strangers." However, as in the case of our current selves, our past selves are also constructed and reconstructed out of specific events we have experienced. Retrieving one event (a childhood memory of not answering the phone because one didn't want to talk with strangers) versus another event (giving an impromptu hula hoop performance for strangers) support contradictory views of whether one was shy or not in the past. Processes of selective retrieval produce selective views of our past selves.

The focus of our own research has been on memory for particular prior episodes rather than on autobiographical memory but, as we will show, the two topics are closely related. Of particular interest to us is a distinction between recollection, a consciously controlled use of memory, and more automatic influences of memory along with attribution processes. Recollection is consciously controlled in that attention is required to constrain retrieval processes to memory for a particular prior experience. Automatic influences of memory, in contrast, are less constrained, and reflect memory of the same form as revealed by indirect tests of memory. Even very dense amnesics show preserved memory measured by means of indirect tests. This form of memory, commonly called *implicit* memory, is akin to implicit attitudes (e.g., Greenwald & Banaji, 1995), in that it is measured indirectly and its effects occur without knowledge of their source. Just as implicit attitudes can bias interpretation of a current event, so can implicit or automatic influences of memory bias interpretation of memory for the past. Such effects can result in ideas coming immediately to mind with the force of truth in response to memory queries, which we term *memory fluency* or an *accessibility bias*. Using the fluency with which an idea is perceived or retrieved as a basis for memory may play a particularly large role in memory for past selves from the more distant past. However, fluency is a less reliable basis for memory than is recollection.

First we review the role of autobiographical memory in self-functions. We then discuss the role of memory accuracy in autobiographical memory, and do so by distinguishing between recollection and automatic influences of memory. Our emphasis on memory for prior episodes highlights the importance of cues for retrieval provided by context, with the result being multiple selves, dependent upon the particular aspect of the self that is activated by the environment. The presence of multiple selves is most dramatic for those with multiple personalities (e.g., Eich, 1989). However, we argue that effects of context on retrieval processes produce similar variability in those supposedly having a single personality. Largely because of automatic influences of memory, along with processes involved in the reconstruction of memory, there is the potential for false memories ranging from the mundane to the self-defining. Finally, we discuss determinants of whether memories will be accessed or forgotten, and speculate about how accessing and forgetting contribute to changes in the self over time.

Autobiographical Memory and Self-Knowledge

Autobiographical memory refers to memories of one's personal past, and differs from memory as it is typically studied in the laboratory in that the timescales are much longer, the events are more complex, and of course, the events are self-relevant and sometimes emotion-laden (Rubin, 2006). Autobiographical memory helps establish a sense of continuity of the self over time (Brewer, 1986; Conway, 1996). People also use autobiographical memory to establish and maintain social connections, to present themselves to new acquaintances or love interests through stories that illustrate the self. Autobiographical memory also serves an essential function in problem solving, as current dilemmas lead people to search memory for prior experiences that could hold the key to a solution. The problem can be relatively mundane, or it can be a concern that lies at the heart of self-knowledge.

Bluck, Alea, Habermas, and Rubin (2005) explored the functions of autobiographical memory by having people rate how often they attempted to remember past experiences for particular purposes, using a measure they developed called Thinking about Life Experiences, or TALE. Self-continuity emerged as a factor tapped by questions such as remembering "when I want to understand who I am now" or "when I am concerned about whether I am still the same type of person I was earlier." The social relationship function was tapped by items such as "when I want to strengthen a friendship by sharing old memories with friends" and "when I want to develop a closer relationship with someone." Surprisingly, the broadest factor was retrieving autobiographical memory in a directive way, aimed at solving problems. This problem-solving factor included items related to emotional regulation (e.g., "when I feel down and want to make myself feel better" and "when I am facing a challenge and I want to give myself confidence"). The problem-solving factor also included items such as "when I am searching for a solution to a problem"; "when I want to learn from my past mistakes"; "when something happens to me and I want to look back to see what caused it"; or "when I want to reinterpret old events in the light of things that have happened since." These latter items point to the fact that autobiographical memory is used deliberately to create changes in self-knowledge, as well as to establish self-continuity over time.

Autobiographical memories are also used to define one's identity (Singer & Salovey, 1993), by supporting the emergence of new self-images, namely, roles such as professor and parent, and traits such as adventurous or confident. Researchers have explored particular self-images by asking participants to complete statements repeatedly beginning with "I am." Rathbone, Moulin, and Conway (2008) asked participants to use their self-images as cues to retrieve autobiographical memories from a time when that self-image was a significant part of their identity. The memories that were most accessible using a particular self-image as a cue were memories that formed around the time the person reported that the self-image emerged. So, for example, a person who says "I am adventurous" may then use that as a cue to generate memories of a time when being adventurous was a particularly key part of his or her identity and report a memory of a solo trip in late adolescence that instigated the emergence of the self-image of adventurousness. The events themselves create changes in self-images, and the corresponding autobiographical memories are linked to and provide ready evidence for the self-images.

Autobiographical Memory in Models of the Self

Mischel's (2004) theory of personality argues for consistency not on the level of traits across all situations but at the level of patterns for a particular person across different situations. We would extend that position to suggest that effects of the situation are sufficiently powerful to produce multiple selves, with differences among selves being less dramatic but akin to those shown by people suffering from dissociative identity disorder. Retrieval of specific autobiographical memories contributes to variability in perception and behavior rather than the invariance that would come from abstractions such as traits. A model in the spirit of such variability is McConnell's (2011) multiple self-aspects framework, which proposes that the self-concept is a collection of many context-dependent selves. McConnell illustrates his framework with an example of a woman, Rachel, whose sense of self includes "Mike's girlfriend," "sorority sister," "Jewish," "daughter," and "student." Each self-aspect is associated with certain traits, some of which crop up in several self-aspects, and others of which are unique to particular aspects. Particular self-aspects are activated by the environment (entering a classroom vs. going on a date), and so direct context-appropriate interaction.

A layer of autobiographical memories could be added to self-models such as that of McConnell, creating a more specific underpinning to self-aspects. The resulting model would have similarities with Conway and Pleydell-Pierce's (2000; Conway, 2005) self-memory system, which emphasizes the hierarchical organization of autobiographical memory and knowledge, and a control system called the working self. As Rathbone and colleagues (2008) note, new experiences support the emergence of new aspects of the self. Memories of dates and conversations with a new partner would be the basis for the origination of new self-aspects, such as "Mike's girlfriend." Being reminded of autobiographical memories related to an aspect of self would affect behavior by activating that self-aspect. A student whose mind wanders to last night's date during a lecture would have her girlfriend aspect activated, which would change percepts and behavior temporarily. In addition to such effects mediated by activation of a self-aspect, remembering a certain event should also directly affect behavior and perception, by biasing interpretations of a situation or person, and providing ready access to different behavioral options (Benjamin & Ross, 2010).

Accuracy of Memory and Self-Knowledge

If autobiographical memories play a role in shaping current self-knowledge, then there must be a relationship between the fidelity of autobiographical memories and the fidelity of self-knowledge. Although there is seldom a record of events against which researchers can evaluate the accuracy of autobiographical memory, cases where people are remembering verifiable information, such as what grade they obtained in a high school course, or what party they voted for in an election years before, reveal that memory is often biased by general knowledge and later changes, as we discuss later. However, there are hints that even the recollection of vivid details is no guarantee that the event in the memory really occurred.

One case where we know that people have inaccurate autobiographical memories is when twins dispute ownership of a memory. Sheen, Kemp, and Rubin (2001) cued same-sex twins to come up with autobiographical memories from when they were 8 to 12 years old and found that most twins had memories where at least one twin must have been wrong about which twin was the protagonist in the remembered event. Many of these events were not routine but were rather distinctive, often emotional events one might expect to be recallable a decade later when the twins were interviewed. For example, in one disputed memory, both twins said it was the other who stole candy from a shop; both said they danced all night with X at a school dance;

and both said the other ran away from home and "Mum and I searched frantically for her." The memories disputed by the twins included important events that might shape one's self-knowledge, yet one twin is wrong.

False memories are not confined to twins. People reportedly appropriate ownership of memories that come from movies or television, as in the case of Ronald Reagan telling a story about something he witnessed in the war, when actually it was an incident from one of his movies. Whole autobiographical memories can also be created with laboratory techniques, leading to false memories of episodes such as being lost in a mall as a child (Loftus & Pickrell, 1995), tipping over a punch bowl at a wedding (Hyman & Pentland, 1996), or playing a childhood prank (Lindsay et al., 2004). These experimenters convince people that an event happened by using a parental report or doctored photograph, and ask them to try to remember the event via imagery and retrieval of related memories (for a recent review, see Newman & Lindsay, 2009). For example, photographs of each participant's grade school class were used as memory aids for retrieval of the suggested event of putting toy slime in the teacher's desk (Lindsay, Hagen, Read, Wade, & Garry, 2004). Rather than increasing veridical recall, the photograph vastly increased the likelihood of false recall, perhaps by helping participants gain access to childhood events that could serve as building blocks for the suggested events.

People vary in suggestibility to false memories in life and in the laboratory. To understand such individual differences, Clancy, McNally, Schacter, Lenzenweger, and Pitman (2002) recruited people who had recovered memories of a likely false traumatic event, that of being abducted by aliens, then tested their memory in a simple paradigm that often creates errors in memory. In the DRM paradigm, participants study a list of words that are associated with a particular critical word (e.g., the *sleep* list includes *bed*, *night*, *rest*, *pillow*) but not the critical word itself (*sleep*). When memory for the list is later tested, there is a high likelihood of mistakenly recalling or recognizing the unpresented critical word, partly because people have a hard time distinguishing words they actually heard on the list from words they merely thought about while studying the list (for a review, see Gallo, 2010). People who had recovered a "memory" of being abducted by aliens, or who believe they were abducted but have not yet recovered the memory, were more likely to recall and recognize falsely the critical words in the DRM paradigm than participants who denied ever being abducted by aliens. A similar propensity toward false memories in the DRM paradigm was found in people who believe they have experienced past lives (Meyersburg, Bogdan, Gallo, & McNally, 2009). The propensity toward false memory in the laboratory and in real life may partially reflect a deficit in *source monitoring*, the process of distinguishing between memories of imagined events or events that were read about, compared to events that were actually experienced (Johnson, Hashtroudi, & Lindsay, 1993).

Source monitoring is compromised when the evidence that distinguishes memories from different sources is lacking. So, for example, people normally can tell that an event was only imagined rather than actually perceived because there are more perceptual details in an actual event. People with particularly vivid imaginations are more prone to mistake memories of imagined events for perceived memories. If someone's memory is generally lacking in specific perceptual details, he or she might also have a difficult time telling memory for perceived events from memory for imagined events. Sorting out the source of a memory is also compromised if people do not spontaneously attempt to monitor memory, as in the case of older adults (Dywan & Jacoby, 1990; see also Rhodes & Kelley, 2005).

The false memory studies were inspired by reports of therapists working with patients to retrieve memories of past physical or sexual abuse that the therapist assumed must exist. Best-selling self-help books concocted symptom checklists, "diagnosed" people as having being abused as children, then provided a manual for retrieving those memories. The manuals (see, e.g., Frederickson, 1992) recommended techniques such as hypnosis, free association journal writing, massage, and art therapy. Early chapters depicted horrific acts of abuse, which could provide a source of involuntary images during people's later attempts to retrieve a memory of their own abuse. Retrieval suggestions in the self-help manuals were to imagine freely events such as being abused in childhood, and "letting yourself see whatever pops into your head" (Frederickson, 1992, p. 109). The manuals directed help seekers to suspend normal processes of source monitoring, telling them that the long-repressed memories of abuse would not be like normal memories. Subsequent research by Loftus, Hyman, Lindsay, and colleagues increased the suspicion that such techniques hold the possibility of creating self-defining memories that are false (Newman & Lindsay, 2009). An added risk with such suggestive therapeutic techniques is that people who expect to enter psychotherapy in the future tend to be more likely to believe that they have experienced, but forgotten, childhood experiences of abuse and trauma (Rubin & Boals, 2010). Believing in the plausibility that an event occurred in the past makes one particularly vulnerable to the creation of false memories.

Without conditions such as suggestion from an authority and repeated attempts to imagine the suggested event, false memories for most of the people most of the time may be minor variations on experienced events that would not impair self-knowledge. In a study of true and false memories among people who had turned over extensive diaries, the researchers made up a recognition test of descriptions of events recorded in the diary, and plausible foils that differed from a true event in one, two, or three attributes of activity, location, and other persons involved. On the recognition test, with no suggestions from the experimenter, false events that were entirely new combinations of familiar activities, locations, and participants were "remembered" only 7% of the time (Burt, Kemp, & Conway, 2004).

A more widespread source of inaccuracies in memory for past selves stems from cases where we attempt to retrieve simple facts about our prior selves, rather than detailed false memory of events. We often reconstruct the past by drawing on knowledge. Ross (1989) has shown that our implicit theories about who we are now, and whether we think a dimension should be stable or vary over time, shape our reconstruction of our personal past. The particularly remarkable cases are the distortions that can be induced when theories are incorrect. We apparently have a fairly generous capacity to fill in "memories" so that they are congruent with who we are now when we have a mistaken theory of stability. Older people who currently are in the Republican Party but had actually registered as Democrats when they were younger misremembered being lifelong Republicans, perhaps because they believe that political affiliation represents a set of core values that do not change across the lifespan. We also have a capacity to rewrite history to fit change we think must have occurred, even when it did not. So, for example, students who took (sadly) an ineffectual study skills course that did not bring up their grades nonetheless felt they had improved because they now misremembered their earlier grades as worse (Conway & Ross, 1984; Ross, 1989; Ross & Wilson, 2003).

When Recollection Succeeds: Limits on False Memory

Bahrick, Hall, and Berger (1996) assessed college students' memory for their high school grades, a memory that could be checked against transcripts. Recall accuracy was far better for grades of A (89%) than for grades of D (29%). The better recall for higher grades might be due to their pleasantness, and perhaps a lack of rehearsal of negative events. However, a second factor that contributed to grade inflation in memory was reconstructive inference. "A" students were great at remembering their A's (93% recalled), but much less successful at remembering their C's (50%). If students were unable to remember their grade in a particular course, the most reasonable guess would be the grade they normally earned.

An important question is whether reconstructive processes can run roughshod over memories that are otherwise available, making recollection of the actual earned mark impossible, or whether such distortion primarily happens when memories are forgotten. Bahrick and colleagues (1996) originally proposed that distortion could block access to recall, such that distortion produced forgetting. However, their findings supported the less dramatic conclusion that distortions do not displace memories, but, rather, reconstructive processes that use generic knowledge ("I was an 'A' student") fill in when recollection fails. The degree of distortion in memory was measured as a bias to move actual B, C, or D grades up or down (although most grades were moved up); A's and F's were not included because they could only be misremembered in one direction. If it were the case that reconstructive processes blocked access to memories that would otherwise be available, the distortion bias ought to correlate with the accuracy of recall such that those who showed the most distortion bias produced less correct recall. Such a correlation was not found, which led Bahrick and colleagues to conclude that the distortions fill in gaps when specific memories are forgotten.

We (Jacoby, Woloshyn & Kelley, 1989) employed a "false fame" paradigm to gain more direct evidence that bias effects occur only when recollection fails. In the first phase of those experiments, a list of names (e.g., Sebastian Weisdorf) was presented and participants were correctly informed that the names were those of people who were not famous. Those old nonfamous names were then intermixed with new nonfamous names and new famous names on a test of fame judgments. This procedure places recollection in opposition to the fame-biasing effects of having previously read the old nonfamous names. On the fame test, recollection of reading the name on the earlier list of nonfamous names allows one to know that the name should be judged "nonfamous." But if recollection fails, having read the nonfamous name earlier increases its familiarity and produces a bias toward judging it as "famous." Similarly, in the Bahrick and colleagues (1996) study of memory for grades, if recollection of a particular grade failed, the familiarity of "A" due to receiving A's in other classes led people to mistakenly think they had received an A in the course.

We predicted that divided attention, compared to full attention, while reading the nonfamous names in the first phase of the fame experiments would reduce the probability of recollection but leave automatic influences of memory unchanged. In line with this prediction, dividing attention in the first phase increased the probability of mistakenly calling old nonfamous names "famous" but did not influence responding to new nonfamous names. A similar increase in false fame occurred when we delayed the fame judgment test by 24 hours, producing a "sleeper effect" (Jacoby, Kelley, Brown, & Jasechko, 1989). Recollection of reading the names in the list of nonfamous names fell off, but the familiarity of the nonfamous names that had been read 24 hours earlier held up. Nonfamous names became famous overnight.

The false fame experiments support the distinction between recollection and automatic influences of memory, as well as the role of attribution processes. False fame reflects a misattribution of the familiarity of a name to its fame when the familiarity actually arose from presentation of the name in an earlier phase of the experiment. Later, we describe other misattributions of this sort, and their importance. In the false fame experiments, we gained evidence supporting the distinction between recollection and automatic influences by placing the two forms of memory in opposition. Subsequent experiments expanded on the opposition procedure to produce a process dissociation procedure that allows one to separately measure effects of manipulations on recollection and automatic influences of memory. Jacoby, Bishara, Hessels, and Hughes (2007) used the process dissociation procedure to examine probabilistic retroactive interference in a situation that was meant to mimic the recall of high school grades (Bahrick et al., 1996). Those experiments also found that the biasing effects of the recent past on memory for the more distant past occur only when recollection fails.

The accessibility bias that is responsible for false fame and for the false recall of high school grades is very similar to the accessibility of ideas that come to mind in response to cues in tests of implicit memory. Even people who are profoundly amnesic and show little or no recollection of events following brain injury can nonetheless be affected in very specific ways by past experience on a test of implicit memory. A typical indirect or implicit test is stem-cued completion, such as giving the first word that comes to mind that starts with *ch*. If someone has recently encountered a word that fits, such as *cheese*, there is a bias to complete the stem with that word. In the case of the accessibility bias, a particular word might come to mind on a cued recall test because it was read several times in an interference phase.

Experiments by Jacoby and colleagues (2007) supported these two independent processes of recollection and accessibility bias. The argument for two independent memory processes was supported by finding dissociations. There are variables that affect recollection, such as study time and attention at encoding, that have no effect on the accessibility bias. There are also variables that affect the accessibility bias that have no affect on the probability of recollection. Parallel studies show that an accessibility bias can be established before the list that is to be memorized (Hay & Jacoby, 1999; Jacoby, Debner, & Hay, 2001) and thereby produce proactive interference.

Older adults may be particularly prone to false memory that results from an accessibility bias. The independence of the accessibility bias in Jacoby and colleagues (2007) and Bahrick and colleagues' (1996) studies means that the accessbility bias does not override the likelihood of correct recollection but merely fills in when recollection fails. However, in those experiments, young adults are instructed to engage in conscious recollection. In some populations, such as older adults, people may not engage in such constrained retrieval, so the accessibility of prior habits may dominate behavior. An example is the case of action slips. An aging professor who typically flew to conferences was chagrined when he could not find his return ticket at the end of the conference, so he bought a new ticket and flew home. When his flight arrived in his hometown, he called his wife to come pick him up. His wife informed him that she would be pleased to do so but could not because he had driven their only car to the conference! Here, the professor's failure to recollect having driven to the conference provided an opening for the prior habit to be accessed and serve as the basis for an action slip—going to the airport to fly home. Recollection is often achieved by a deliberate process of elaborating on a retrieval cue to allow people to tightly constrain what ideas come to mind, such as thinking back to a particular time and place. In contrast, the accessibility bias is a less effortful, more automatic basis for responding that reflects global factors, such as experience in the form of habits. In terms of implications for self-knowledge, we can certainly gain access to memories of our past selves by engaging in controlled retrieval, even if our current self is quite different, but once memory fails, we may end up reporting whatever comes to mind simply because it is very accessible due to more recent experiences.

Older adults' lessened ability to recollect makes them particularly vulnerable to scam artists. One version is that the scam artist appears at the house of an older adult and offers to reseal her driveway for $100. When the job is done, the older adult prepares to pay the $100, when the scam artist says "No, I told you, it's $100 per bucket of sealer!" These statements may be so compelling that the older adults make no further attempt to recollect what was actually said.

Older adults are more likely than young adults to find highly accessible ideas so compelling that they bypass any attempt at constrained retrieval. The result is that older adults can be "captured" by a false memory in ways similar to the scam artist's ploy described earlier. For example, Jacoby, Bishara, Hessels, and Toth (2005) had older and younger adults study lists of word pairs (e.g., *knee bone*). At the time of the memory test, a prime word that was either misleading (*bend*) or correct (*bone*), or a control set of ampersands (&&&&&&) was presented for half a second just prior to presenting the cue for recall (*knee–b__n__*). Older adults were much more likely to produce the misleading prime as a response than were younger adults. Details of the results suggested that older adults were often captured by the prime, and they did not even attempt recollection when a prime was presented. Crucially, Jacoby and his colleagues asked for subjective reports of whether participants remembered the target word (*bone* or *bend*) or it just seemed familiar, or whether it was a guess. Older adults showed dramatic levels of false remembering, with a .43 probability of reporting they "remembered" the misleading prime, compared to .04 for young adults. This extraordinary level of false memory occurred even though the memory performance of older and younger adults had been equated in the baseline condition by allowing more time for older adults to study the words.

We suspect that there are situations in which even young adults could be captured by ideas that come to mind quickly and forcefully, and accept them as memories, without attempting recollection. Controlled recollection is attention-demanding and time-consuming. Individual differences such as impulsivity and low motivation for accuracy, and states such as alcohol intoxication or sleep deprivation may change the probability with which people rely on the first thing that comes to mind as a basis for remembering, rather than invest in more controlled retrieval.

Memory and the Fluency Heuristic

Memory for past selves takes place over time spans that are measured in decades rather than the minutes we typically use in laboratory studies, and retrieval after a long delay is increasingly reconstructive rather than reproductive (Bartlett, 1932) as recollection drops off sharply. People may be particularly likely to use the fluency heuristic as a basis for remembering events in the distant past. The fluency heuristic is activated when the ease of perceiving a person, place, or event, or the ease with which an idea comes to mind, is interpreted as familiarity. It parallels Tversky and Kahneman's (1973) notion of the availability heuristic, whereby the ease of generating instances of an event is interpreted as an indication of high frequency. In experiments demonstrating the fluency heuristic, Jacoby and Whitehouse (1989) manipulated the ease of perceiving words on a recognition test by brief presentation of words that either matched or mismatched a subsequently presented recognition test word. The argument was that prior presentation of a matching word would give people a start on perceiving the word, such that when the word came up on the computer screen for the recognition test, it would be felt to be fluently perceived, and so judged as familiar. That indeed occurred, with both hits and false alarms increasing as a function of being preceded by the matching prime word, but only in a condition where the presentation was sufficiently short that participants did not see the prime, and so did not attribute the ease of processing the recognition test item to the matching prime. A key aspect of the fluency effect is that people cannot readily pin the fluent processing on some obvious manipulation or source, such as word frequency, and so attribute their fluent processing to having seen the test item in the past (for a review, see Kelley & Rhodes, 2002). A parallel effect occurs in *cued recall*, when the ease of generating a word in response to cue is subtly manipulated (Lindsay & Kelley, 1996), and people report what they generate as a memory.

    An inspiration for the Jacoby and Whitehouse demonstration that fluent processing can be interpreted as familiarity was Titchener's speculation about the experience of déjà vu. Titchener used the example of a person about to cross a busy street in a new city, who glances at the shops across the street, but then quickly turns his attention back to his own side of the street to check for traffic before crossing. Upon arriving at the other side, the person might experience very fluent perception of the shops, and so feel a sense of familiarity that would be experienced as déjà vu if he were unable to recollect his first glance. Jacoby and colleagues have since determined that recollection is greatly reduced by divided attention during encoding, but processing that produces later fluency is more robust and requires minimal perceptual processing during encoding. If we hear or see reports of events happening to others while our attention is divided, we may not recollect the event later, but we may find it strangely fluent, and so suspect that it was something that happened to us. Recent experiences can also serve as sources of fluent processing while attempting to recognize a person or event from the more distant past. These multiple sources of fluency make it a far less diagnostic basis for remembering our past selves than the recollection of specific details.

Fluency of perception and thought is a primary component of subjective experience. Depending on the situation, fluency may be taken as an indicator not of familiarity, but of truth, beauty, certainty, or simplicity (for a review, see Kelley & Rhodes, 2002). For example, people interpret ease of problem solving as reflecting the objective difficulty of the problem (Kelley & Jacoby, 1996). Fluency serves as a basis for a variety of metacognitive judgments, including confidence (Kelley & Lindsay, 1993; Koriat, Ma'ayan, & Nussinson, 2006) and judgments of learning (Rhodes & Castel, 2008). Fluency may well be the basis for judgments about the current self or about a past self, giving easily generated ideas about the self a ring of truth, or leading one to hold those ideas with greater confidence.

Memory Retrieval: Remembering versus Forgetting Past Selves

What determines our ability to access past selves, and what leads to our forgetting them? Memory retrieval is cue-driven. As described in our discussion of multiple selves, details of the current circumstance, including physical context, serve as powerful cues for retrieval. Evidence of the power of such context effects is provided by Godden and Baddeley's (1975) finding that divers who studied words underwater or on the dock retrieved them better in the matching context than in the mismatching context. Similarly, psychoactive states such as alcohol or marijuana intoxication can serve as the context of an event that can later cue memories. Cues encountered in the environment or produced by an ongoing train of thought drive retrieval of memories. The cues can produce spontaneous remindings (Hintzman, 2011) or involuntary memories (Berntsen, 2010). People also engage in deliberate retrieval, cueing themselves recursively in an attempt to remember.

A major theory of forgetting is that context changes slowly over time, or drifts, and the loss of contextual cues leads older memories to be less and less accessible. Complex contextual change can create a boundary between events and so reduce access to memories of prior events (Isarida & Isarida, 2010). Students head off to college, changing location, roles, friends, and tasks compared to those in their adolescent lives. New jobs often require another change of location, role, friends and tasks, and so on. The changes accompanied by combined cues of place, roles, other people, and habitual emotions may help define cut points between past selves, with an accompanying reduction in spontaneous access to autobiographical memories from that time.

The diminished access to autobiographical memories over time and self-changes is illustrated in an unpublished diary study recounted by Lindsay and Read (2006). Participants were each given eight of their diary entries recorded 7 to 60 years earlier. For 30–40% of the diary entries queried, people were surprised by their memory of long-forgotten events. One woman had forgotten an earlier serious romantic relationship when she was 17, until she read about it in the diary; two participants had forgotten that their parents had been injured in car crashes. These instances of "recovered memories" highlight the importance of cues for access to past selves or self-aspects, and furthermore, indicate that the past self can differ so much from the current self that the past becomes nearly inaccessible. It might take more cues, such as returning to a childhood home, reentering an old role, or visiting a long-out-of-touch friend, to plunge one back into access with a prior self.

In addition to spontaneous reminding due to the presence of external cues, such as other people, places, and situations, people engage in deliberate reinstatement of cues in their imagination as a means of gaining access to memories. Smith (1979) illustrated the power of reinstatement of physical cues in a paradigm involving environmental context change between learning a list of words in one room and being tested on memory for the words in a second, very different room. The change of context produced worse memory for the words, but telling people to imagine themselves back in the original room where they learned the list enhanced memory. As Tulving (1985) noted, memory allows us to travel through time as well as space.

Acts of memory create interconnections among current and past selves, little wormholes across space and time. People who engage in more autobiographical remembering ought to end up with more of a sense of continuity among their past selves, whereas people who rarely look back (or go back) to earlier contexts might feel that their past selves are almost as different from them as other people.

Just as we can mentally reinstate cues to *enhance* remembering of a past self or self-aspect, we can shift cues mentally to *reduce* remembering of a past self. Directed forgetting is a laboratory paradigm whereby people typically memorize a list of words and then are told by the experimenter to forget those words, as they were simply for practice, and then a second list of word is presented for memorization. At test, participants are surprised with a recall test for the to-be-forgotten list. Remarkably, people remember fewer words after being told to forget than in the control condition in which the first list was followed by instructions to remember those words.

A major mechanism of directed forgetting is that people who are told to forget attempt to "clear their heads" by thinking of something outside the experiment. For example, a young woman reported that when she was told to forget the list of words she had just studied, she started thinking about her sister's upcoming wedding, and the dress fitting that was going to happen that weekend in Miami. Sahakyan and Kelley (2002) hypothesized that this is a case of the person mentally effecting a context change, which would lower access to memories from the prior list. We tested the mental context change theory of directed forgetting by having participants study a list of words; then, rather than asking them to forget the words, we told them to think for a minute about what they would do if they were invisible (Experiment 1), or to imagine their parents' house (Experiment 2). We thought that both of those manipulations would induce imagined contexts that were dissimilar from the participants' original context at the beginning of the experiment. Then we presented the second list of words, followed by a test of the first list. Both of these imaginary changes of context led to worse memory for the first list of words because of the mismatch of the encoding context and the context available at testing.

We assume contexts vary in similarity, and the more context is changed between encoding and retrieval, the greater the disruption in access to memories encoded before the change. To sharpen the measurement of degree of context change, Delaney, Sahakyan, Kelley, and Zimmerman (2010) used distance and time as proxies for context similarity, and found that a mental context shift instantiated by thinking of a place one hadn't been for some time (imagining one's parent's house) had a larger disruptive effect on access to memory for the just-studied list than thinking of a place one may have been a few hours ago (imagining one's current apartment). In fact, the longer one had not been to one's parent's house, the more disruptive the effect of thinking about it on memory for the list just studied. Similarly, being prompted to remember a foreign vacation had a larger disruptive effect on access to memory for the just-studied list than remembering a domestic vacation.

To return to the idea of multiple-contextualized selves, people have a greater or lesser degree of overlap in the attributes associated with different selves (daughter, student, girlfriend). A student in a lecture whose mind wanders to a date from the night before may have greater trouble remembering the threads of the lecture when he or she tunes back if the reverie activates a self-aspect that has no overlapping attributes with the student self. Aspects of current self and past selves also differ in degree of overlap, with more change happening on some dimensions (relationship in college vs. relationship with husband) than others (daughter, Jewish). The degree of change should have important implications for memory of past selves, with less access along dimensions of greater change.

An important dimension of self-knowledge is knowledge of one's mental and physical health, both current and over the life course, and it is a dimension where people experience major changes. It is thus a test case for dramatic instances of forgetting prior self-aspects that are no longer part of the current self. A recent study found that about half of the people who experience an episode of a clinical mental disorder such as depression, anxiety, or alcohol or drug abuse forget about it. Moffitt and her colleagues (2010) compared the lifetime incidence of depression, anxiety, or alcohol or drug abuse between the ages of 18 and 32, as measured with retrospective reports from participants, versus the lifetime incidence of those disorders in participants in a different study that computed incidence rates using four clinical assessments at ages 18, 21, 26, and 32. The mean age of participants was equal between the two studies, but those assessed with retrospective reports could report even childhood episodes, whereas those assessed contemporaneously via clinical interviews could only report current episodes and those that occurred in the past year. Nonetheless, the lifetime estimates were half as high when based on retrospective reports compared to contemporaneous assessments, indicating that people forget even life-altering experiences.

Moffit and her colleagues (2010) proposed that forgetting happened for the people who experienced a single episode of a disorder, rather than for those who had recurrent episodes. Moving on to a period of improved mental health would mean that the current self does not match the formerly depressed or anxious self, and so the current self is not a good retrieval cue for the past self. In the diary study cited earlier (Lindsay & Read, 2006), people failed to recognize 30% of tested events, including events extended over time. One participant reported, "I can't believe I suffered from and apparently was treated for depression—at that age! If I had been asked whether I have ever been depressed, I would have said *no*." Another said, "I was 14 when I wrote these entries . . . I was a monarchist. I'm not now, and it's embarrassing. I never thought I was." Change can indeed reduce access to past selves.

Summary and Conclusions

Our life story, in the form of autobiographical memory, likely reflects editing by a second-rate novelist, enhancing the main character but omitting much of the complexity and contradiction that comprise the life we have actually lived. Our past selves are less consistent across situations and with our current self than is generally believed. Our current, strongly held beliefs, those that are important for our definition of self sometimes unknowingly contradict earlier-held beliefs (e.g., Ross, 1989). Access to past selves is driven by cues, such that dramatic changes between current and past selves lead to little or no access to past selves. Due to the powerful effects of context, both external context and internal context produced by our own thoughts, we have multiple selves rather than the single self that is featured in the narrative of our autobiographical memory (McConnell, 2011). Memory for prior events plays a key role in the generation of selves, and we speculate that retrieval of specific memories also directs behavior and affects perception, contributing to the contextualized and multifaceted nature of the self. If variety is the spice of life, most of us have a life that is less bland than we imagine.

Autobiographical memory is a mix of true recollections and convenient fictions. When listening to a parent or grandparent reminisce, their lives can seem remarkably interesting. However, we can gain comfort in knowing that our own life story will likely become more interesting with time. The multiple forms of memory include automatic influences of memory as well as recollection. Reliance on automatic influences, along with attribution and reconstruction processes, can result in inaccuracies of memory. Retellings, as well as other forms of repetition, increase the fluency with which ideas come to mind. Reliance on the fluency heuristic or accessibility bias can produce memory inaccuracies that range from the inconvenient action slip (flying back from a conference to which one drove) to the catastrophic (believing one was the victim of sexual abuse when one was not). Our parents and grandparents may unknowingly include memory inaccuracies that make their stories more interesting and reflect automatic influence from their prior tellings in combination with forgetting.

One might become so impressed by memory inaccuracies as to conclude that memory is generally untrustworthy. However, accessibility bias plays a role only when recollection fails. Recollection is a more accurate basis for memory judgments than are automatic influences of memory. We also suspect that memory is more accurate outside the laboratory than is suggested by the recent boom of experiments showing false memory. Memory illusions, like perceptual illusions, are useful, in that both reveal the processes that underlie performance but reflect systems that are generally accurate. Memory for where we have been is subject to illusions, just as is perception of where we are going, but both are generally sufficiently well adapted to support survival.

REFERENCES

Bahrick, H. P., Hall, L. K., & Berger, S. A. (1996). Accuracy and distortion in memory for high school grades. *Psychological Science, 7*, 265–271.

Bartlett, F. C. (1932). *Remembering: A study in experimental and social psychology.* New York: Cambridge University Press.

Baumeister, R. F. (1987). How the self became a problem: A psychological review of historical research. *Journal of Personality and Social Psychology, 52,* 163–176.

Benjamin, A. S., & Ross, B. H. (2010). The causes and consequences of reminding. In A. S. Benjamin (Ed.), *Successful remembering and successful forgetting: A Festschrift in honor of Robert A. Bjork* (pp. 71–88). New York: Psychology Press.

Berntsen, D. (2010). The unbidden past: Involuntary autobiographical memories as a basic mode of remembering. *Current Directions in Psychological Science, 19,* 138–142.

Bluck, S., Alea, N., Habermas, T., & Rubin, D. C. (2005). A tale of three functions: The self-reported uses of autobiographical memory. *Social Cognition, 23,* 91–117.

Brewer, W. F. (1986). What is autobiographical memory? In D.C. Rubin (Ed.), *Autobiographical memory* (pp. 25–49). Cambridge, UK: Cambridge University Press.

Burt, C., Kemp, S., & Conway, M. (2004). Memory for true and false autobiographical event descriptions. *Memory, 12,* 545–552.

Clancy, S. A., McNally, R. J., Schacter, D. L., Lenzenweger, M. F., & Pitman, R. K. (2002). Memory distortion in people reporting abduction by aliens. *Journal of Abnormal Psychology, 111,* 455–461.

Conway, M. A. (1996). Autobiographical knowledge and autobiographical memory. In D. C. Rubin (Ed.), *Remembering our past: Studies in autobiographical memory* (pp. 67–93). Cambridge, UK: Cambridge University Press.

Conway, M. A. (2005) Memory and the self. *Journal of Memory and Language, 53,* 594–628.

Conway, M. A., & Pleydell-Pearce, C. W. (2000). The construction of autobiographical memories in the self-memory system. *Psychological Review, 107,* 261–288.

Conway, M., & Ross, M. (1984). Getting what you want by revising what you had. *Journal of Personality and Social Psychology, 47,* 738–748.

Delaney, P. F., Sahakyan, L., Kelley, C., & Zimmerman, C. A. (2010). Remembering to forget: The amnesic effect of daydreaming. *Psychological Science, 21,* 1036–1042.

Dywan, J., & Jacoby, L. L. (1990). Effects of aging on source monitoring: Differences in susceptibility to false fame. *Psychology and Aging, 5,* 379–387.

Eich, E. (1989). Theoretical issues in state dependent memory. In H. L. Roediger III & F. I. M. Craik (Eds.), *Varieties of memory and consciousness: Essays in honour of Endel Tulving* (pp. 331–354). New York: Erlbaum.

Fredrickson, R. (1992). *Repressed memories: A journey to recovery from sexual abuse.* New York: Simon & Schuster.

Gallo, D. A. (2010). False memories and fantastic beliefs: 15 years of the DRM illusion. *Memory and Cognition, 38,* 833–848.

Godden, D. R., & Baddeley, A. (1975). Context-dependent memory in two natural environments: On land and underwater. *British Journal of Psychology, 66,* 325–331.

Greenwald, A. G., & Banaji, M. R. (1995). Implicit social cognition—attitudes, self-esteem, and stereotypes. *Psychogical Review, 102,* 4–27.

Hay, J. F., & Jacoby, L. L. (1999). Separating habit and recollection in young and elderly adults: Effect of elaborative processing and distinctiveness. *Psychology and Aging, 14,* 122–134.

Hintzman, D. L. (2011). Research strategy in the study of memory: Fads, fallacies, and the search for the "coordinates of truth." *Perspectives on Psychological Science, 6,* 253–271.

Hyman, I. E., Jr., & Pentland, J. (1996). The role of mental imagery in the creation of false childhood memories. *Journal of Memory and Language, 35,* 101–117.

Isarida, T., & Isarida, T. K. (2010). Effects of simple- and complex-place contexts in the multiple context paradigm. *Quarterly Journal of Experimental Psychology, 63*, 2399–2412.

Jacoby, L. L., Bishara, A. J., Hessels, S., & Hughes, A. (2007). Probabilistic retroactive interference: The role of accessibility bias in interference effects. *Journal of Experimental Psychology: General, 136*, 200–216.

Jacoby, L. L., Bishara, A. J., Hessels, S., & Toth, J. P. (2005). Aging, subjective experience, and cognitive control: Dramatic false remembering by older adults. *Journal of Experimental Psychology: General, 134*, 131–148.

Jacoby, L. L., Debner, J. A., & Hay, J. F. (2001). Proactive interference, accessibility bias, and process dissociations: Valid subjective reports of memory. *Journal of Experimental Psychology: Learning, Memory, and Cognition, 27*, 686–700.

Jacoby, L. L., Kelley, C. M., Brown, J., & Jasechko, J. (1989). Becoming famous overnight: Limits on the ability to avoid unconscious influences of the past. *Journal of Personality and Social Psychology, 56*, 326–338.

Jacoby, L. L., & Whitehouse, K. (1989). An illusion of memory: False recognition influenced by unconscious perception. *Journal of Experimental Psychology: General, 118*, 126–135.

Jacoby, L. L., Woloshyn, V., & Kelley, C. M. (1989). Becoming famous without being recognized: Unconscious influences of memory produced by dividing attention. *Journal of Experimental Psychology: General, 118*, 115–125.

Johnson, M. K., Hashtroudi, S., & Lindsay, D. S. (1993). Source monitoring. *Psychological Bulletin, 114*, 3–28.

Kelley, C. M., & Jacoby, L. L. (1996). Adult egocentrism: Subjective experience versus analytic bases for judgment. *Journal of Memory and Language, 35*, 157–175.

Kelley, C. M., & Lindsay, D. S. (1993). Remembering mistaken for knowing: Ease of retrieval as a basis for confidence in answers to general knowledge questions. *Journal of Memory and Language, 32*, 1–24.

Kelley, C. M., & Rhodes, M. G. (2002). Making sense and nonsense of experience: Attributions in memory and judgment. *Psychology of Learning and Motivation, 41*, 293–319.

Koriat, A., Ma'ayan, H., & Nussinson, R. (2006). The intricate relationships between monitoring and control in metacognition: Lessons for the cause-and-effect relation between subjective experience and behavior. *Journal of Experimental Psychology: General, 135*, 36–69.

Lindsay, D. S., Hagen, L., Read, J. D., Wade, K. A., & Garry, M. (2004). True photographs and false memories. *Psychological Science, 15*, 149–154.

Lindsay, D. S., & Kelley, C. M. (1996). Creating illusions of familiarity in a cued recall remember/know paradigm. *Journal of Memory and Language, 35*, 197–211.

Lindsay, D. S., & Read, J. D. (2006). Adults' memories of long-past events. In. G.-G. Nilson & N. Ohta (Eds.), *Memory and society: Psychological perspectives* (pp. 51–72). Hove, UK: Psychology Press.

Loftus, E. F., & Pickrell, J. E. (1995). The formation of false memories *Psychiatric Annals, 25*, 720–725.

McAdams, D. P. (2001). The psychology of life stories. *Review of General Psychology, 5*, 100–122.

McConnell, A. R. (2011). The multiple self-aspects framework: Self-concept representation and its implications. *Personality and Social Psychology Review, 15*, 3–27.

Meyersburg, C. A., Bogdan, R., Gallo, D. A., & McNally, R. J. (2009). False memory propensity in people reporting recovered memories of past lives. *Journal of Abnormal Psychology, 118*, 399–404.

Mischel, W. (2004). Toward an integrative science of the person. *Annual Review of Psychology, 55*, 1–22.

Moffitt, T. E., Caspi, A., Taylor, A., Kokaua, J., Milne, B. J., Polanczyk, G., et al. (2010). How common are common mental disorders. Evidence that lifetime prevalence rates are doubled by prospective versus retrospective ascertainment. *Psychological Medicine, 40,* 899–909.

Newman, E. J., & Lindsay, D. S. (2009). False memories: What the hell are they for? *Applied Cognitive Psychology, 23,* 1105–1121.

Rathbone, C. J., Moulin, C. J. A., & Conway, M. A. (2008). Self-centered memories: The reminiscence bump and the self. *Memory and Cognition, 36,* 1403–1414.

Rhodes, M. G., & Castel, A. D. (2008). Memory predictions are influenced by perceptual information: Evidence for metacognitive illusions. *Journal of Experimental Psychology: General, 137,* 615–625.

Rhodes, M. G., & Kelley, C. M. (2005). Executive processes, memory accuracy, and memory monitoring: An aging and individual difference analysis. *Journal of Memory and Language, 52,* 578–594.

Ross, M. (1989). Relation of implicit theories to the construction of personal histories. *Psychological Review, 96,* 341–437.

Ross, M., & Wilson, A. E. (2003). Auobiographical memory and conceptions of the self: Getting better all the time. *Current Directions in Psychological Science, 12,* 66–69.

Rubin, D. C. (2006). The basic-systems model of episodic memory. *Perspectives on Psychological Science, 1,* 277–311.

Rubin, D. C., & Boals, A. (2010). People who expect to enter psychotherapy are prone to believing that they have forgotten memories of childhood trauma and abuse. *Memory, 18,* 556–562.

Sahakyan, L., & Kelley, C. M. (2002). A contextual change account of the directed forgetting effect. *Journal of Experimental Psychology: Learning, Memory, and Cognition, 28,* 1064–1072.

Sheen, M., Kemp, S., & Rubin, D. (2001). Twins dispute memory ownership: A new false memory phenomenon. *Memory and Cognition, 29,* 779–788.

Singer, J. A., & Salovey, A. P. (1993). *The remembered self.* New York: Free Press.

Smith, S. M. (1979). Remembering in and out of context. *Journal of Experimental Psychology: Human Memory and Learning, 5,* 460–471.

Tulving, E. (1985). Memory and consciousness. *Canadian Psychology, 26,* 1–12.

Tversky, A., & Kahneman, D. (1973). Availability: A heuristic for judging frequency and probability. *Cognitive Psychology, 5,* 207–232.

CHAPTER 19

Self-Conceptualization, Self-Knowledge, and Regulatory Scope

A Construal-Level View

CHERYL J. WAKSLAK
YAACOV TROPE
NIRA LIBERMAN

Decades of research in social psychology highlight the impact the situation exerts on people's attitudes, judgments, and behaviors. From the opinions of other people (Asch, 1956) to the instructions of an authority (Milgram, 1965), to previously unscrambled sentences (Srull & Wyer, 1979) and the race of an experimenter (Lowery, Hardin, & Sinclair, 2001), research has illustrated the incredible power of the situation to influence the self-concept and behavior. At the same time, people do show consistent patterns of behavior that differ reliably from one person to another (Digman, 1990), and people intuitively believe that the self exists (Bem & Allen, 1974). Given that the self is characterized by both variety and consistency, how do we best think of self-knowledge? Does knowing the self mean being able to predict accurately how the self will act in a given context, or can one know the self as it exists in general, even if the self in any one given context might act quite differently?

In this chapter, we distinguish between two modes of self-representation, and argue that these different types of self-representations can be accurate (and inaccurate) in different ways. In particular, we suggest that self-representations act as self-guides, regulating the self across different contexts, and that the nature of a self-guide varies according to the proximity of the self-regulation context, something we term *regulatory scope*. Guides for dealing with proximal issues (e.g., issues to occur in the near future or a nearby location) will be concrete and contextualized, coinciding with a representation of the self that heavily considers the context in which the self will be enacted. Guides for regulating across distance (regarding, e.g., issues delayed in time or to occur in a distant location) will be more abstract and generalized, incorporating a representation of the self that is generalized beyond any one immediate context. Concrete self-representations, which incorporate the situational impact that will likely influence the self's expression in a given context, may thereby lead to precise predictions about the self's operations within that context. This type of self-representation is thus useful for regulating the self in proximal contexts, where one typically has a large degree of relevant knowledge about oneself and the surrounding situation. Abstract self-representations, which are schematic reflections of information that is true of the self in general, are also, for this reason, inherently imprecise. Because they do not take into account the dramatic effect the situation in fact does have on behavior, these self-representations may appear inaccurate, in that they do not allow precise predictions about the manner of self-expression in any one particular context. At the same time, this form of self-representation is, on some level, a mirror to the "true" self, the aspect of oneself that is consistent and generalizable, reflecting how one is different from others and uniquely oneself. Indeed, we believe it is for this reason that abstract self-guides are used to regulate across distance, to bridge mentally between the self as it exists in the here and now and the self as it will exist in a distant context.

In this chapter we more fully develop this distinction between abstract and concrete self-guides and the way in which these self-guides can be especially useful in regulating the self in different contexts. Supporting this distinction and its association with distance, we describe research suggesting that self-representation changes as a function of psychological distance, with representations of a distant self reflecting more superordinate qualities and exhibiting more schematicity and consistency. Building on this, we review accumulating evidence that (1) general self-characteristics (including personality traits, values, ideology, general attitudes, etc.) are more predictive of the evaluations, goals, plans, and preferences people have for distant than near situations, and that (2) people view their behavior in distant situations as having more implications for the self. Finally, we end by returning to the issue of accuracy, and discuss this important issue as it relates to our construal account of self-conceptualization.

Abstract and Concrete Self-Guides

Research on psychological distance points to the many ways in which objects and events can be psychologically close or distant from us (see Trope & Liberman, 2010, for a recent review). They may be geographically nearby or remote, occur in the near or distant future, be probable or improbable, and involve others who are socially close to us or distant. For successful functioning, individuals must be able to regulate their behavior not only for the here and now but also for the there and then; likewise, they must be able to navigate both probable and improbable situations, and effectively relate with both socially close and distant people. In other words, self-regulation at times concerns proximal objects and at other times, more distal ones. We refer to the extent to which one's goals and interactions involve objects that are distant on spatial, temporal, social, and hypotheticality dimensions as *degree of regulatory scope*.

Viewing the self as a representation that is called to mind to guide one's interactions with the world (cf. Higgins, 1996), and bearing in mind long-standing research suggesting that individuals maintain a variety of self-representations (cf. Markus & Wurf, 1987), our central argument in this chapter is that degree of regulatory scope—the extent to which self-regulation involves proximal or distal objects—influences the type of self that is activated to guide self-regulation and the type of self-characteristics that will ultimately be reflected in one's decisions, attitudes, and behaviors. The self that is called to mind for interacting with the world in distant contexts will consist of abstract and general self-conceptions that reflect the self's perceived essence or gist; this self will therefore act as a general self-guide. In contrast, the self that is called to mind to guide self-regulation in proximal contexts will be more concrete and specific, taking into account the situational context in which self-regulation will occur and thereby acting as a more contextualized self-guide. This distinction is related to one we have made more generally between high-level construals, abstract and general representations that distill an item's gist, and low-level construals, concrete and contextualized representations that fail to distinguish between defining and less defining item features (see Trope & Liberman, 2010, for a more thorough discussion of this distinction).

Why might there be this association between regulatory scope and the degree to which self-representations used to guide self-regulation are more abstract or concrete? We contend that abstract, decontextualized representations of the self are useful guides for self-regulation in distal contexts because high-level construals are more likely than low-level construals to remain unchanged across distance. When regulating the self in a distant context it is necessary to transcend mentally the currently experienced self; adopting an abstract self-guide that highlights aspects of the self that remain invariant across situations allows one to do this and is therefore the most appropriate guide for such self-regulation. That is, if we regulate behavior from a proximal perspective as we travel through time, it makes sense to call to mind a contextualized self in each moment to guide that regulation. But, if we would like our self as it exists in the moment to regulate the self in the future, we need to connect those two selves, to think of the self in a way that serves to bridge (but not deny) a current self-conceptualization with a future, contextualized self. Aspects of the self that allow this connection are high-level construal in nature, since these reflect our overall, general self-properties that are invariant across individual context-dependent selves, which may be viewed as more specific contextualizations of one's underlying general self.

Importantly, the tendency to activate an abstract self-guide when regulatory scope is high should exist even when details are not likely to change across distance. We assume that, in general, effects of distance on construal are overgeneralized, making them persist even if the initial reasons that gave rise to the association are no longer present. Accordingly, people should adopt high-level self-representations when they consider themselves in distant contexts, even if they are thinking of the self within a particular context for which specific information is readily available, or if the particular future context is unlikely to be dramatically different from the current one. For example, individuals might consider how they will act within a given role about which they have precise information and that they currently occupy; nevertheless, we would expect behaviors and choices made within that context to more closely relate to general self-conceptions when regulatory scope is high than when it is low (i.e., when there is increased distance in time, space, social dimensions, or hypotheticality). Put differently, although it is possible that distance may sometimes be related to the availability of information, or may at times influence the accessibility of low-level versus high-level aspects, we would expect to find distance-related shifts in representation even when specific, concrete information is available and readily accessible; indeed, our premise is that because of a generally functional relationship between distance and abstraction, such concrete information will be construed differently when considered from a near versus distant vantage point.

The Effect of Distance on Self-Representation

An initial implication of the association we propose between regulatory scope and the type of self-guide that is activated is that distance should have a direct influence on people's self-representations. Adopting a high-level construal on the self would involve extracting the essence or gist of the self, imposing an order or structure on self-representation, and using more abstract and superordinate self-identifications. This perspective on the self, which should be adopted when considering a future self, emphasizes the unity rather than the variety that characterizes the self, and is similar to the self-concept that many personality researchers explicitly seek to capture by asking for reports of general personality traits and typical self-characteristics, as opposed to personality traits and characteristics expressed within a given context (e.g., Goldberg, 1999; however, see Mischel & Shoda, 1995, for one general critique of this approach).

Exploring this association, we examined people's near and distant future self-representations (Wakslak, Nussbaum, Liberman, & Trope, 2008). In an initial study, for example, we looked at the level of abstraction and inclusiveness individuals displayed when describing themselves using social categories. Participants described themselves in the near or distant future on a questionnaire that consisted of 14 groups of social categories, organized in hierarchies of two to five levels. For example, one hierarchy was as follows: a person; a man–woman; a young man–woman; a man–woman in his or her early–late 20s; a man–woman age ____ (a five-level hierarchy, ordered from the broadest, high-level category to the narrowest, low-level category). Participants chose the characteristic from each group that seemed to describe themselves most appropriately. As expected, participants chose more broad and superordinate descriptions when describing themselves in the near versus distant future.

Follow-up studies extended beyond social identities to self-descriptions more generally. For example, using the Linville (1985) measure of self-complexity, participants describing themselves as they would be in the distant future exhibited more simple, less complex self-representations than those describing themselves in the near future. Similar results emerged using the self-structure measure of self-concept differentiation (Donahue, Robins, Roberts, & John, 1993), which examines the degree to which individuals see themselves similarly across social contexts. If people think about themselves in more general terms in the distant future, even when considering a self that is situated within a particular context, their self-descriptions across different contexts should exhibit greater consistency when thinking about one's distant rather than near future self. Indeed, participants were more consistent in indicating their personality in five different social roles (student, son–daughter, friend, employee, romantic partner) when they made judgments about themselves a year from now versus tomorrow.

If people think about the distant future self in a general, decontextualized manner, an intriguing implication is that it should be easier for them to make general trait judgments about the distant rather than the near future self. Using a classic me–not-me reaction time paradigm (e.g., Kuiper, 1981; Markus, 1977), participants viewed a series of adjectives and quickly indicated whether each trait was or was not self-descriptive. As expected, participants were faster to make such general trait judgments when thinking about themselves in the distant future than when thinking about themselves in the near future; on some level, then, participants had an easier time making a general statement about who they were for a remote rather than proximal self. Moreover, the effect was consistent across adjectives of different valence, suggesting it was not due to a mere case of people exhibiting a more positive outlook on a distant future self.

This analysis has implications for the predictions and inferences people will make about their future behavior. Traditional measures of the general self-concept (without time specification) assess decontextualized and stable attributes (e.g., the type of person one typically is). We expected that the general self, thus assessed, is more likely to be reflected in predictions people make about their behavior in the more distant future than the near future because, when thinking about the distant future, one will call to mind a general self-representation to guide behavioral predictions. In contrast, when considering the near future, one will call to mind a contextualized self-representation to inform these expectations, and one's predictions are therefore less likely to correlate with a general sense of self. Supporting this argument, we found that general assessments people made about themselves on traits related to the Big Five trait dimensions were better predictors of their later reports of how they would act in terms of these traits in three different situations (having an argument with someone, meeting with unfamiliar people, and attending a birthday party) when the situations were to occur in the distant future than when they were to occur in the near future. Furthermore, expectations for distant behaviors showed a higher degree of cross-situational consistency than expected near future behaviors.

We view this effect as related to a more widespread phenomenon: If the self-guide called upon to regulate distant contexts is general, whereas that called upon to regulate near contexts is specific and contextualized, then it is the choices, attitudes, and behaviors relevant to distant contexts that will be more strongly in line with general self-characteristics. We turn now to review a range of findings that are consistent with this perspective.

Self-Regulation of Distant and Near Contexts

The idea that abstract and general self-guides will regulate behavior in distant contexts, whereas concrete and contextualized self-guides will regulate behavior in proximal contexts has implications for a range of issues related to self-regulation, including the role of values in guiding behavior, the effects of one's ideology on attitude expression, social judgment, performance expectations, bargaining behavior, and self-control.

Values as Behavioral Guides

Values are abstract, schematic mental constructs that should be invoked as part of an individual's general self-concept. If a general self-representation is used to guide behavior in distant contexts, we would expect one's values to be more readily applied to psychologically distal than to proximal situations. For example, one's general achievement values should better predict signing up for a challenging course to be offered in the distant future than the near future. (Note, however, that we are not suggesting values will never predict proximal behavior; if the situational context is not especially strong, we might expect values to predict proximal behavior, albeit more weakly than distant behavior.) Recent research by Eyal, Sagristano, Trope, Liberman, and Chaiken (2009; see also Torelli & Kaikati, 2009) examined this suggestion. For example, in one study, participants indicated the importance of a range of values using Schwartz's 1992 value questionnaire. They then imagined 30 behaviors (e.g., "rest as much as I can") and indicated the likelihood of performing each behavior in either the near or distant future. Correlations between the rated importance of the values and the likelihood of performing behaviors corresponding to that value were higher for behaviors planned for the distant (average correlation = .40) rather the near future (average correlation = .25), in line with our general contention that broad and general self-aspects invoked as part of an abstract self-guide exert a greater influence on self-regulation when regulatory scope is high. Interestingly, Eyal and colleagues (2009) also found that while values predicted participants' intentions for the distant future, situational constraints were more predictive of their near future intentions. For example, whereas the number of distant future hours participants were willing to volunteer was predicted by their benevolence values, it was the convenience of the timing that predicted the number of hours participants volunteered for the near future. A concrete self-representation that considers the self within a particular situational context was thus more relevant for guiding proximal behaviors than distant ones.

Also supporting an association between one's distant self and one's values is research by Kivetz and Tyler (2007), who argue that the content of distant future self-representations tends to be idealistic, whereas the content of near future self-representations tends to be pragmatic. Participants choosing characteristics that would best describe themselves in the distant (vs. near) future, for example, increasingly selected characteristics that reflected an idealistic self-activation and its concomitant value system (e.g., "putting my values and principles above all other considerations," "fulfilling my inner potential"), as opposed to characteristics that reflected a pragmatic self-activation (e.g., "mostly guided by practical considerations"). This differential self-activation then guided identity versus instrumental preferences, with distal condition participants preferring to select a bank with superior identity attributes (e.g., treating customers with respect) over a bank with superior instrumental attributes (e.g., having low fees). Intriguingly, while these authors suggest that the content of distant selves tends to be identity-related and that distant future preferences therefore tend to focus on identity concerns, they also find that when individuals' general guiding principle in life is in fact to prefer instrumental over identity attributes their distant, abstract self guides them to instrumental choices.

Extending this work on values to the domain of morally offensive behavior, Eyal, Liberman, and Trope (2008) argued that people judge generally immoral acts as more offensive and generally moral acts as more virtuous when the acts are psychologically distant rather than near. Thus, transgressions against core values that are deemed harmless due to extenuating circumstances (e.g., eating one's dead dog) are judged more severely when imagined from a more distant temporal or social perspective. Conversely, moral acts which might have had ulterior motives (e.g., adopting a disabled child when a government pays high adoption pensions) are judged more positively from a distance. The findings suggest that one's general views toward a moral activity are likely to guide judgments of distant acts, whereas contextual aspects related to that activity will have an impact on proximal judgments. In a similar vein, Agerström and Björklund (2009) find that people act more in line with altruistic moral principles over selfish hedonistic motives with increased temporal distance. Moreover, they find that this is moderated by the degree to which people generally value the altruistic and hedonistic motives implicated in a moral dilemma: Distance only influences moral expression when participants more strongly value altruistic than hedonistic values at a general level. This is consistent with our general contention that increased regulatory scope activates an abstract self-guide that emphasizes the self's central qualities and general values, leading decisions about distant contexts to be increasingly in line with these characteristics.

An intriguing corollary of this demonstrated association between regulatory scope and the impact of one's important values is findings that suggest invoking a high-level construal of the self by focusing on one's important values creates a general tendency to focus on the "big picture." Recent research, for example, demonstrates that self-affirmation procedures in which people describe their most (vs. least) important values lead people to adopt a widespread high-level construal orientation that transfers to subsequent tasks, even when such tasks are unrelated to protecting self-integrity (Wakslak & Trope, 2009; see also Schmeichel & Vohs, 2009). For example, after affirming (vs. disaffirming) the self, people perform better at tasks associated with abstract, gestalt thinking and less well at tasks associated with concrete, detail-oriented thinking. This suggests that focusing on one's important values is one way to activate directly an abstract self-guide, which will then guide information processing and self-regulation.

Effects of Ideology on Attitudes and Behavior

Like values, *ideologies* are broad constructs that can be conceptualized as aspects of one's general self-concept. These ideologies may inform individual attitudes about specific issues expressed in specific contexts to a greater or lesser degree. Research widely demonstrates, for example, that our attitudes shift, often outside of our awareness, in response to other people in our local social context, including communication partners, significant others, and even total strangers (Baldwin & Holmes, 1987; Davis & Rusbult, 2001; Higgins & Rholes, 1978; Kawakami, Dovidio, & Dijksterhuis, 2003; Lowery et al., 2001). We might expect to see such social tuning (and correspondingly less ideological behavior) more in proximal than in distal situations. When an attitude object is psychologically near, the self-guide called to mind to regulate self-expression will be contextualized and sensitive to the context. Attitudes expressed will therefore be attuned to the particular social context and likely be affected by incidental attitudes of others in the social situation rather than by one's ideology. Conversely, when the attitude object is distant, a general self should guide self-regulation. Evaluation will therefore be less affected by the incidental attitudes of salient others and, instead, reflect one's ideology.

A series of studies by Ledgerwood, Trope, and Chaiken (2010) tested the hypothesis that attitudes align more with those of another person in the local social context when psychological distance is low (vs. high). Using an anticipated interaction paradigm, participants read about a policy that would increase the deportation of illegal immigrants starting either next week (near future) or next year (distant future), and learned that their discussion partner was either in favor of or against deporting illegal immigrants. They then privately reported how likely they would be to vote in favor of the policy. Participants' voting intentions shifted toward the interaction partner's attitude when the policy was set to be implemented in the near future, but not when it was to be implemented in the distant future. However, voting intentions more strongly reflected participants' previously assessed ideological values when the policy was to be implemented in the distant (vs. near) future. Specifically, the more participants valued preserving the societal status quo, the more they supported a distant future policy that would enforce the deportation of illegal immigrants (for an extensive discussion of the way in which these findings and general conceptualization qualify and extend Fishbein and Ajzen's (1974, 1975) influential work on the compatibility principle, see Ledgerwood, Trope, & Liberman, 2010, pp. 266–268).

Social Judgment

General attitudes should predict not only attitudes toward issues but also judgments about other social targets. Exploring the nature of near and distant social judgment, Henderson and Wakslak (2010) recently examined the way that social judgments about a proximal and a distal target are differentially influenced by situational cues and general attitudes about a target's behavior. In one study, for example, participants were first exposed to a semantic prime activating the concept of either recklessness or adventurousness and then asked to make judgments about a person skydiving (an ambiguously reckless activity) in either a near or a distant spatial location. They also provided general ratings of how they felt about skydiving. Evaluations of the proximal, but not distal, target assimilated toward the semantic primes (i.e., individuals primed with the concept of recklessness evaluated the proximal skydiver more negatively then those primed with adventurousness). In contrast, participants' ratings of how they generally felt about skydiving were associated with evaluations of the distal skydiver but not the proximal one. This latter point was underscored in a follow-up study in which participants were first asked to generate characteristics that generally describe someone who would ride a high-speed motorbike, and then to evaluate a target person engaging in this same ambiguous behavior in a physically close or far away location. Participants' general attitude toward the activity was positively related to their evaluation of the target for those in the physically distant condition, but completely unrelated for those in the physically near condition. This is in line with our contention that an abstract self-guide regulates interactions in the distant future and that, therefore, general self-characteristics such as one's general opinions will influence judgments when regulatory scope is high.

Ability versus Task Characteristics

Like judgments of others, expectations of oneself should be increasingly based on general self-characteristics with increased distance. One example in which this is relevant is when people predict their own performance outcomes. If an abstract, general self-guide is called to mind when a context is distal, general perceptions of one's ability should guide predictions about distant performance outcomes. In contrast, a more contextualized representation of one's abilities would take into account specifics of the task itself; such factors should thus guide predictions of proximal performance outcomes. Testing this hypothesis, Nussbaum, Liberman, and Trope (2006) examined participants' predictions of their performance on a general knowledge quiz expected to take place either on the same day or 2 months later. The questions were the same but in either a relatively multiple-choice (easy) or open-ended (hard) format. In another study, the quiz consisted of questions with either two response alternatives (relatively easy) or four response alternatives (relatively hard). The researchers also assessed participants' perceived ability in each knowledge domain (e.g., how generally knowledgeable they were in geography, history, etc.). As expected, the results showed that as the temporal distance from the performance increased, participants were increasingly likely to base their performance predictions on their perceived ability in each knowledge domain, and less likely to base those predictions on the specific format of the questions in the quiz. High perceived ability led participants to expect better performance on the distant future quiz, whereas a relatively easy task format led participants to expect better performance on the near future quiz.

Cooperative versus Competitive Bargaining

Another area in which people often have general views of themselves relates to their social value orientation, whether people are oriented toward cooperation (have a prosocial orientation) or competition (have a pro-self orientation). An abstract self-guide that is called to mind to regulate distant contexts should highlight one's general motivational orientation, which should then guide behavior in bargaining and negotiation contexts. In line with this, Giacomantonio, De Dreu, and Mannetti (2010) found that an individual's general social value orientation was related to ultimatum bargaining behavior when psychological distance was high, but not when it was low. When psychological distance was high, individuals with a general prosocial orientation made higher offers to their partner than did individuals with a general pro-self orientation; when psychological distance was low, individuals' general social value orientation did not influence offers. These findings present an important caveat to other findings that suggest a more general effect by which distance influences cooperative behavior (e.g., Sanna, Chang, Parks, & Kennedy, 2009), and support our general argument that whereas an abstract, general self-guide regulates behavior in distant contexts, a concrete, contextualized self-guide regulates behavior in proximal contexts.

Self-Control

A key aspect of self-regulation is *self-control*, the ability to withhold immediate pleasure in anticipation of more long-term gain. Consistent with the process of a more abstract self-guide regulating behavior when regulatory scope is high, Rogers and

Bazerman (2008) conceptualize self-control as a struggle between a "should-self," which encourages control of the self, and a "want-self," which encourages immediate gratification, and argue that the should-self is more abstract in nature and increasingly dominant with increased distance. Supporting this argument, they find that (1) the should-shelf operates at a higher level of construal (i.e., it is more abstract and superordinate) than the want-self, and (2) people are correspondingly increasingly likely to select should-choices when the choices will be implemented in the distant future rather than the near future; that is, people are more likely to make binding choices that they see as should-choices (e.g., choosing to donate to charity, supporting an increase in the price of fossil fuel to reduce consumption, engaging in physical exercise) when they are committing now to a choice whose consequences will be felt in the distant (vs. near) future.

This work dovetails well with that of Fujita, Trope, Liberman, and Levin-Sagi (2006), who find that self-control is heightened when a high-level (vs. low-level) construal orientation is directly activated, as well as research by Freitas, Salovey, and Liberman (2001) showing that self-control is heightened in the context of obtaining negative but useful feedback when the feedback is delayed rather than imminent. It is also consistent with research on children's delay of gratification, which has demonstrated that greater temporal and spatial distance from a tempting object enhances self-control (Metcalfe & Mischel, 1999; Mischel, Shoda, & Rodriguez, 1989). As a whole, then, findings from the self-control literature are strongly in line with our argument that enhanced regulatory scope activates an abstract self to guide behavior, leading distant decisions to be increasingly in line with individuals' superordinate and defining concerns.

Altogether, the research reviewed in this section suggests that regulatory scope changes the degree to which our values, ideologies, general attitudes, and core superordinate concerns influence our judgments, decisions, and behaviors. Although people may have less information on average about distant situations, activation of an abstract self-guide in such contexts leads to self-regulation that is in line with our important, defining self-attributes. In a somewhat ironic way, then, people may often act in ways that are better reflections of who they are as a whole when they are removed from a situation on some dimension. In the next section we explore an intriguing corollary of this: If an abstract, general self guides distant behavior such that general self-characteristics are expressed to a greater degree in distant contexts, then individuals may see behaviors performed in distant contexts as stronger reflections of their general selves.

Distant Behavior as Expressions of Oneself

Research we reviewed earlier suggests that the distant self is represented in a more abstract, general way, and that general self-characteristics more strongly influence distant judgments and behavior. It is possible, then, that individuals will be more willing to draw conclusions about the self from their distant behavior; that is, given that distant behaviors are more strongly guided by an abstract, general self, and more linked with general self-characteristics than are near behaviors, individuals should be more likely to think that distant behaviors communicate something about the general self.

Future Behaviors as Reflections of the General Self

Drawing on earlier studies that suggested individuals more closely link their distant future actions to their general self than they do their near future actions, which are increasingly expected to be influenced by the situational context, Wakslak and colleagues (2008) examined whether people would identify distant future behaviors, more than near future behaviors, as "saying something" about who they are in general. Participants were presented with a list of 25 activities that represent extracurricular behaviors in which students frequently engage (e.g., "adopting a kitten," "organizing a surprise party for a friend"), imagined themselves doing each activity either sometime in the present week (near future condition) or in a week 1 year later (distant future condition), and indicated the extent to which doing this activity would say something about them ("If you behave in the described way, how much will it express who you are; that is, how much will it say something about you, your character and your preferences?"). As expected, activities imagined in the distant future were perceived as more self-expressive than activities imagined in the near future, an effect that occurred for positive and also for neutral and negative behaviors.

These findings concerned a case where participants considered the degree to which a series of random behaviors would be self-expressive if they chose to pursue them. What if, in contrast, individuals first thought about their general self-characteristics and then considered activities that went against these general traits? If a distant context calls to mind an abstract, general self, they should expect behaviors consistent with that general self, and should therefore judge situations in which they did not act in a trait-consistent manner as not being reflective of the self. In other words, whereas behaviors in general should be seen as more self-expressive when performed in the distant future, this should not be the case for countertrait behaviors. Examining this idea, we had people first describe their typical self-characteristics by rating themselves on a series of positive and negative traits and then imagine themselves engaging in a series of activities in either the near or distant future, each of which was designed to contradict one of the aforementioned traits (e.g., the scenario "you arrive half an hour late to a job interview" was inconsistent with the trait "punctual"). Participants then indicated the extent to which each scenario would be congruent with their underlying, general self ("If you find yourself in this situation . . . how much will it reflect your "real" self, be consistent with what you really are?"). As expected, negative correlations between the degree to which people endorsed a general trait and the degree to which they reported that a countertrait behavior would be a reflection of their "real" self were stronger when they imagined doing the behaviors in a distant as opposed to a near context. This effect was consistent across the valence of the traits. Individuals thus seem to expect their distant behavior, more than their near behavior, to match up with their self-characteristics; consequently, they more strongly rejected situations in which their behavior would be inconsistent with their general traits.

Self-Perception Effects

An interesting implication of this analysis is for self-perception phenomena (Bem, 1972). If individuals judge distant behavior to be more self-expressive than near behavior, it is possible that inducing a behavior related to the distant future (vs.

the near future) will lead individuals to draw conclusions more strongly about their general attitudes from that behavior. In line with this idea, Libby, Shaeffer, Eibach, and Slemmer (2007) illustrated that when people visualize themselves performing a behavior from a distant, third-person perspective (as opposed to a proximal, first-person perspective) they adopt general attitudes that are more strongly in line with the imagined behavior, and then are actually more likely to carry out the behavior in question. Specifically, on the evening before the 2004 U.S. presidential election, their participants (all registered voters) pictured themselves voting in the upcoming election from either a third-person perspective (which induces people to think about the self more abstractly, in terms of general dispositions) or from a first-person perspective (which induces people to think about the self more concretely). They then indicated their attitudes toward and opinions about voting (how good or bad it was to vote, how important it was to vote, etc.), and, in a follow-up measure after the election, whether they had actually voted. In line with predictions, to picture voting from the third-person perspective caused subjects to adopt a stronger pro-voting mindset, which consequently led participants in this group to actually vote in greater numbers.

Reporting behaviors that one did in a distant (rather than proximal) context has a similar impact on self-perception. For example, in a modified version of a classic self-perception task developed by Salancik and Conway (1975), participants completed a behavioral checklist for a class they had taken during the past semester (a proximal time point) or during a semester a year prior (a distal time point). The checklist was constructed so that some participants were induced to report a greater balance of positive to negative behaviors than others (accomplished by pairing the positive behaviors with the word *occasionally* and negative behaviors with the word *frequently*, which makes it relatively easy to agree to having done the positive behaviors and relatively hard to agree to having done the negative behaviors, or reversing the word pairing in a different condition). Classic work suggests a self-perception effect of this word-pairing manipulation on course attitudes: When induced to report a greater balance of positive to negative behaviors, participants are more favorable in their evaluations of the course (inferring that they must have liked the course from the relatively positive behaviors they report having done during it; Salancik & Conway, 1975). This pattern, however, was moderated by the distance manipulation. When the course was taken at a distant time point, results showed the classic self-perception effect; when the course was taken at a more proximal time point, there was no self-perception effect of reported behaviors on course evaluation, a pattern that remained when controlling for self-reported memory of the time points (Wakslak, 2012). This finding is in line with our argument that people consider their behavior in distant contexts as a reflection of their general attitudes and opinions, whereas they see proximal behavior as less tied to who they are.

Distance and Self-Knowledge

Given that the self can be both contextualized and generalizable, what does it mean to have knowledge of the self? Is knowing the self synonymous with being able to predict aspects of the self accurately within a specific, concrete context, or can one know oneself more generally? If a person's self-reports of his or her general attitudes, personality, values, and so forth, fail to predict his or her behavior within a given situation but still predict her or his plans for distal situations, would we characterize such self-views as inaccurate? According to our framework, important parts of a person's self-concept, his or her values, attitudes, and general beliefs, oftentimes fail to predict actual behavior. Describing this pattern as reflecting inaccurate self-views, however, might be a harsh characterization given that such self-views predict a person's plans for the distant future and ideas of how he or she should behave. Moreover, such high-level self-aspects are general ways of knowing the self whose accuracy relates to the self as it exists across disparate contexts, rather than the self as it exists at any single moment.

More generally, a construal-level framework is useful for distinguishing between different types of inaccuracy. For example, one type of inaccuracy occurs when a person uses an abstract self-guide to predict behavior that is ultimately guided by a concrete self-guide. This type of inaccuracy arises because prediction is based on one type of self-representation (a general self), but actual behavior is based on a different self-representation (a contextualized self); an example is when we predict an evaluation that we will have within some distant future situation but this is not the evaluation we arrive at when we actually encounter that situation. This is a common error, and one that has been widely described within the robust literature on affective forecasting (see Gibert & Wilson, 2007, for a review). This type of error in prediction is particularly interesting when the distant context was known and could have been taken into account during prediction, but was not taken into account because of the overgeneralized tendency (discussed earlier) to rely on high-level self-guides to deal with distal situations. The same basic error is less interesting from a psychological perspective when people really do not know the details that will ultimately guide their behavior (e.g., they do not know that at the time of the rally they will have a bad cold and therefore not attend it). In such cases it is indeed reasonable to make predictions based on an abstract self-representation, even if there is imprecision inherent in the resulting predictions, as this is likely to lead to a more accurate prediction than relying on an incorrectly specified contextualized self, such as the self that is relevant to the currently experienced context.

A second kind of inaccuracy occurs when people's behavior is in fact guided by principles (e.g., because people precommitted to a choice or because the behavior in question is generalized, in the sense of being summed over many situational instances) but a concrete self-guide is used to make predictions (as would be the case when predictions are made from a proximal perspective). This type of prediction error, however, may be less common than the former because predictions are more typically made from a distant point in time and concern a specific behavior that is not precommitted. In addition, predictions that are based on low-level, more concrete constructs tend to be less confident (see Nussbaum et al., 2006); because lower-level construals distinguish less clearly between essential and inessential aspects, they typically offer less clear predictions than do high-level construals. Thus, even when people make predictions based on low-level construals, they are relatively less likely to rely on them.

In summary, then, we see levels of construal as involving a tradeoff between reliability and precision: high-level self-construals comprise (subjectively) core aspects that are invariant and therefore afford reliable predictors but sacrifice precision. Often, high-level construal self-representations will be relatively inaccurate reflections of actual self-expression, which occurs within a particular context and is influenced by that context; incorporating contextual information about the distant context into predictions made about that context should increase precision and therefore accuracy. However, representing the self in a high-level fashion offers a reliable way of thinking about the self across contexts, of finding the commonality that links oneself in the here and now to oneself as it will exist in different, distal situations. Low-level construal self-representations, in contrast, specify particular and concrete self-aspects and therefore afford more precision; these representations, however, are less reliable because they reflect secondary aspects that are therefore variable (i.e., not always associated with the self). It is therefore functional to negotiate self-representation by progressively incorporating contextualized self-aspects as one gets closer to a given context because with increasing proximity, reliability of such self-aspects increases. The evidence presented earlier suggests that this is what people in fact tend to do: call to mind abstract self-guides when considering a distant context and concrete self-guides when considering a proximal one. Although this tendency is generally functional, it leads to particular biases and cases where accuracy may be improved by considering aspects of the self that are different than those emphasized in the self-guide cued by the situation's proximity or distance.

A set of related issues concerns the possibility of people having metaknowledge about this effect of distance on self-representation. If people are aware of these differences, they may strategically use them to nudge themselves into making decisions that are consistent with their high-level, general self, much as the precommitment literature has shown that people are often willing to take proactive action such as cancellation of alternatives, self-imposed penalties, and so forth, in order to nudge themselves into self-control behavior (e.g. Ariely & Wertenbroch, 2002; Trope & Fishbach, 2000). Although undoubtedly multidetermined, people certainly at times establish delayed starting dates when making consequential decisions about controversial issues; as just one example, consider the tendency of government bodies to debate bills that would go into effect at a significantly later time point. Although extant research has not examined this, it would be intriguing for people to have a meta-awareness that decisions they make for near and distant contexts are different. Moreover, even if people do not have this knowledge, it would be intriguing to examine whether being taught about this relationship would make people willing to make decisions earlier or to delay outcomes so as to benefit from the perspective offered by distance.

Conclusion

We have argued in this chapter that the type of self-guide that is activated varies according to regulatory scope, the degree of distance inherent in a self-regulation context. Guides for dealing with proximal contexts will reflect a contextualized self that takes into account concrete aspects of the situation; guides for dealing with distal contexts will be abstract reflections of one's general self-characteristics. Evidence suggests that the nature of near and distant self-representations differ along these lines, that general self-characteristics are stronger predictions of decisions, evaluations, and behavior relevant to distant (vs. near) contexts, and that people view behavior in distant contexts as having more implications for the self. Abstract and concrete self-representations are accurate and inaccurate in different ways, though we believe that the link between self-representation and regulatory scope is rooted in a functional tradeoff between reliability and precision. The connection between self-representation and distance, while leading to particular patterns of behavior and particular inaccuracies, enables people to effectively cognize, emote, and act on what is present, as well is what is not present, within their current environment. It is thus an extremely useful mechanism through which people are able to regulate behavior across situations that differ markedly in the degree to which they require transcendence of current experience and engagement in mental travel.

REFERENCES

Agerström, J., & Björklund, F. (2009). Moral concerns are greater for temporally distant events and are moderated by value strength. *Social Cognition, 27,* 261–282.

Ariely, D., & Wertenbroch, K. (2002). Procrastination, deadlines, and performance: Self-control by precommitment. *Psychological Science, 13*(3), 219–224.

Asch, S. E. (1956). Studies of independence and conformity: A minority of one against a unanimous majority. *Psychological Monographs, 70.*

Baldwin, M. W., & Holmes, J. G. (1987). Salient private audiences and awareness of the self. *Journal of Personality and Social Psychology, 52,* 1087–1098.

Bem, D. J. (1972). Self-perception theory. In L. Berkowitz (Ed.), *Advances in experimental social psychology* (Vol. 6, pp. 1–62). New York: Academic Press.

Bem, D. J., & Allen, A. (1974). On predicting some of the people some of the time: The search for cross-situational consistencies in behavior. *Psychological Review, 81,* 506–520.

Davis, J. L., & Rusbult, C. E. (2001). Attitude alignment in close relationships. *Journal of Personality and Social Psychology, 81,* 65–84.

Digman, J. M. (1990). Personality structure: Emergence of the five-factor model. *Annual Review of Psychology, 41,* 417–440.

Donahue, E. M., Robins, R. W., Roberts, B. W., & John, O. P. (1993). The divided self: Concurrent and longitudinal effects of psychological adjustment and social roles on self-concept differentiation. *Journal of Personality and Social Psychology, 64,* 834–846.

Eyal, T., Liberman, N., & Trope, Y. (2008). Judging near and distant virtue and vice. *Journal of Experimental Social Psychology, 44,* 1204–1209.

Eyal, T., Sagristano, M. D., Trope, Y., Liberman, N., & Chaiken, S. (2009). When values matter: Expressing values in behavioral intentions for the near vs. distant future. *Journal of Experimental Social Psychology, 45,* 35–43.

Fishbein, M., & Ajzen, I. (1974). Attitudes toward objects as predictors of single and multiple behavioral criteria. *Psychological Review, 81,* 59–74.

Fishbein, M., & Ajzen, I. (1975). *Belief, attitude, intention, and behavior: An introduction to theory and research.* Reading, MA: Addison-Wesley.

Freitas, A. L., Salovey, P. & Liberman, N. (2001). Abstract and concrete self-evaluative goals. *Journal of Personality and Social Psychology, 80,* 410–424.

Fujita, K., Trope, Y., Liberman, N., & Levin-Sagi, M. (2006). Construal levels and self-control. *Journal of Personality and Social Psychology, 90,* 351–367.

Giacomantonio, M., De Dreu, C. K., & Mannetti, L. (2010). Now you see it, now you don't: Interests, issues, and psychological distance in integrative negotiation. *Journal of Personality and Social Psychology, 98*(5), 761–774.

Gilbert, D. T., & Wilson, T. D. (2007). Prospection: Experiencing the future. *Science, 317*, 1351–1354.

Goldberg, L. R. (1999). A broad-bandwidth, public-domain, personality inventory measuring the lower-level facets of several five-factor models. In I. Mervielde, I. Deary, F. De Fruyt, & F. Ostendorf (Eds.), *Personality psychology in Europe* (Vol. 7, pp. 7–28). Tilburg, The Netherlands: Tilburg University Press.

Henderson, M. D., & Wakslak, C. J. (2010). Psychological distance and priming: When do semantic primes impact social evaluations? *Personality and Social Psychology Bulletin, 36*, 975–985.

Higgins, E. T. (1996). The "self digest": Self-knowledge serving self-regulatory functions. *Journal of Personality and Social Psychology, 71*, 1062–1083.

Higgins, E. T., & Rholes, W. S. (1978). "Saying is believing": Effects of message modification on memory and liking for the person. *Journal of Experimental Social Psychology, 14*, 363–378.

Kawakami, K., Dovidio, J. F., & Dijksterhuis, A. (2003). Effect of social category priming on personal attitudes. *Psychological Science, 14*, 315–319.

Kivetz, Y., & Tyler, T. R. (2007). Tomorrow I'll be me: The effect of time perspective on the activation of idealistic versus pragmatic selves. *Organizational Behavior and Human Decision Processes, 102*, 193–211.

Kuiper, N. A. (1981). Convergent evidence for the self as a prototype: The "inverted-U RT effect" for self and other judgments. *Personality and Social Psychology Bulletin, 7*, 438–443.

Ledgerwood, A., Trope, Y., & Chaiken, S. (2010). Flexibility now, consistency later: Psychological distance and construal shape evaluative responding. *Journal of Personality and Social Psychology, 99*, 32–51.

Ledgerwood, A., Trope, Y., & Liberman, N. (2010). Flexibility and consistency in evaluative responding: The function of construal level. In M. P. Zanna & J. M. Olson (Eds.), *Advances in experimental social psychology* (Vol. 43, pp. 257–295). San Diego, CA: Academic Press.

Libby, L. K., Shaeffer, E. M., Eibach, R. P., & Slemmer, J. A. (2007). Picture yourself at the polls: Visual perspective in mental imagery affects self-perception and behavior. *Psychological Science, 18*, 199–203.

Linville, P. W. (1985). Self-complexity and affective extremity: Don't put all of your eggs in one cognitive basket. *Social Cognition, 3*, 94–120.

Lowery, B. S., Hardin, C. D., & Sinclair, S. (2001). Social influence effects on automatic racial prejudice. *Journal of Personality and Social Psychology, 81*, 842–855.

Markus, H. (1977). Self-schemata and processing information about the self. *Journal of Personality and Social Psychology, 35*, 63–78.

Markus, H., & Wurf, E. (1987). The dynamic self-concept: A social psychological perspective. *Annual Review in Psychology, 38*, 299–337.

Metcalfe, J., & Mischel, W. (1999). A hot/cool-system analysis of delay of gratification: Dynamics of willpower. *Psychological Review, 106*, 3–19.

Milgram, S. (1965). Some conditions of obedience and disobedience to authority. *Human Relations, 18*, 57–76.

Mischel, W., & Shoda, Y. (1995). A cognitive–affective system theory of personality: Reconceptualizing situations, dispositions, dynamics, and invariance in personality structure. *Psychological Review, 102*, 246–268.

Mischel, W., Shoda, Y., & Rodriguez, M. L. (1989). Delay of gratification in children. *Science, 244*, 933–938.

Nussbaum, S., Liberman, N., & Trope, Y. (2006). Predicting the near and distant future. *Journal of Experimental Psychology: General, 135*, 152–161.

Rogers, T., & Bazerman, M. H. (2008). Future lock-in: Future implementation increases selection of "should" choices. *Organizational Behavior and Human Decision Processes, 106,* 1–20.

Salancik, G. R., & Conway, M. (1975). Attitude inferences from salient and relevant cognitive content about behavior. *Journal of Personality and Social Psychology, 32,* 829–840.

Sanna, L. J., Chang, E. C., Parks, C. D., & Kennedy, L. A. (2009). Construing collective concerns: Increasing cooperation by broadening construals in social dilemmas. *Psychological Science, 20,* 1319–1321.

Schmeichel, B. J., & Vohs, K. D. (2009). Self-affirmation and self-control: Affirming core values counteracts ego depletion. *Journal of Personality and Social Psychology, 96,* 770–782.

Schwartz, S. H. (1992). Universals in the content and structure of values: Theoretical advances and empirical tests in 20 countries. In M. P. Zanna (Ed.), *Advances in experimental social psychology* (Vol. 25, pp. 1–65). New York: Academic Press.

Srull, T. K., & Wyer, R. S. (1979). The role of category accessibility in the interpretation of information about persons: Some determinants and implications. *Journal of Personality and Social Psychology, 37,* 1660–1672.

Torelli, C. J., & Kaikati, A. M. (2009). Values as predictors of judgments and behaviors: The role of abstract and concrete mindsets. *Journal of Personality and Social Psychology, 96,* 231–247.

Trope, Y., & Fishbach, A. (2000). Counteractive self-control in overcoming temptation. *Journal of Personality and Social Psychology, 79,* 493–506.

Trope, Y., & Liberman, N. (2010). Construal level theory of psychological distance. *Psychological Review, 117,* 440–463.

Wakslak, C. J. (2012). *The effect of timing on self-perception.* Manuscript in preparation, City University of New York.

Wakslak, C. J., Nussbaum, S., Trope, Y., & Liberman, N. (2008). Representations of the self in the near and distant future. *Journal of Personality and Social Psychology, 95,* 757–773.

Wakslak, C. J., & Trope, Y. (2009). Cognitive consequences of affirming the self: The relationship between self affirmation and object construal. *Journal of Experimental Social Psychology, 45,* 927–932.

CHAPTER 20

Sitting at the Nexus of Epistemological Traditions
Narrative Psychological Perspectives on Self-Knowledge

JONATHAN M. ADLER

To inquire about self-knowledge implicitly suggests that there is a self that can be known in a verifiable way. Several psychological disciplines have developed creative and innovative methods for identifying and overcoming barriers to assessing the self in an objective manner. Yet from the perspectives adopted by the growing field of narrative psychology, the very mission of identifying objective self-knowledge is fraught. One of the most exciting elements of the field of narrative psychology is its location at the nexus of two epistemological traditions. On the one hand, narrative psychologists share many of the same concerns with validity, reliability, and prediction that are at the heart of most scientific psychological inquiry. On the other hand, narrative perspectives embrace the fundamental subjectivity of stories. Rather than regarding personal narratives as veridical accounts of what took place in an individual's life, stories are construed as revealing important psychological data about the individual's approach to making meaning out of those experiences. This meaning is idiosyncratic, dynamic, and deeply subjective; but it also turns out to be relatively stable, reliably assessed, and highly predictive of important psychological outcomes. By virtue of straddling this epistemological line, narrative perspectives offer an incredibly generative theoretical orientation toward the matter of self-knowledge. In this chapter I discuss narrative psychology's elegant, if sometimes uncomfortable, blending of epistemological traditions as they apply to the topic of self-knowledge. In doing so, I hope to shed light on the contributions and limitations of different approaches, and to illuminate the potential of continuing to walk this epistemological line.

Two Epistemological Approaches

The Paradigmatic Mode

Jerome Bruner, a pioneer in the field of narrative psychology, has written extensively about two complementary modes of thought that are brought to bear in approaching human psychology. Bruner (1986) terms one of these *the paradigmatic mode*, which, he suggests, "attempts to fulfill the ideal of a formal, mathematical system of description and explanation. It employs categorization or conceptualization and the operations by which categories are established, instantiated, idealized, and related to one another to form a system" (p. 12). Indeed, the paradigmatic mode is the mode of science and is therefore concerned with logical argument, classification, and prediction. "Good" paradigmatic explanations are those that conform to a coherent and rational accounting of reality. They are typically grounded in specific, falsifiable, and unambiguously phrased hypothetical assertions that can be evaluated using the scientific method in the service of describing, explaining, and predicting phenomena. Not simply focused on the accuracy of their methods, paradigmatic approaches prescribe a framework for the task of conducting scholarship. Indeed, paradigmatic arguments are immensely powerful and occupy a position of supreme authority in modern industrialized societies (e.g., McLeod, 1997). The vast majority of modern psychological science embraces a fundamentally paradigmatic approach, and the other chapters in this volume are likely to do so as well, although few are likely to explicitly state as much.

The Narrative Mode

The other epistemological paradigm that Bruner identified is labeled *the narrative mode*. This mode of thought is concerned with how people make sense of their experiences through telling stories about them. These stories are about "human or humanlike intention and action and the vicissitudes and consequences that mark their course" (Bruner, 1986, p. 13). They capture people's own explanations about what they want and how they go about achieving it. In contrast to scientific explanations, narratives do not aspire to be generalized, impersonal, or decontextualized. Narrative approaches reject the notion of the scientific method, instead embracing hermeneutic perspectives. From this standpoint, narratives are regarded as being deeply rooted in the specific, interpreted history of the individual. Far from mere literary productions, the stories people weave about their experiences serve as a foundational element of identity, what McAdams (1993) called "the stories we live by." Indeed, the collection of stories that individuals craft about their lives can be understood as their "narrative identity" (McAdams, 2001).

The question of what makes a "good" narrative is much less straightforward than identifying the criteria for a "good" paradigmatic argument. While the criteria for evaluating scientific explanations enjoy such widespread consensus as to be implicit in most scientific discourse (though still discussed among philosophers of science), scholars working in the narrative mode continue to debate vigorously the nature of a good story. Offering a comprehensive account of that debate is well beyond the scope of this chapter, but one of the primary criteria by which personal narratives are evaluated within narrative psychology, and one that makes for an especially relevant example for the domain of self-knowledge, is their coherence (e.g., Habermas & Bluck, 2000; Hyvärinen, Hydén, Saarenheimo, & Tamboukou, 2010; McAdams, 2006).

At the most basic level, stories must be understandable to their audience if they are to convey their meaning adequately, no matter how simple the message (e.g., Labov, 1972). Indeed, the story "is a basic building block of human communication" (McLeod, 1997, p. 32); stories are the vehicles by which meaning is encapsulated for the individual and then transmitted to others. Stories serve a "binding" function that holds together a sequence of moments, focused on preventing "the utter dispersion of experience, its evaporation into nothingness" (Freeman, 2010, p. 171). A certain degree of coherence is simply necessary for this goal to be adequately fulfilled. But the standards of coherence against which stories may be assessed far exceed the grammatical and syntactic levels. In striving to organize the vicissitudes of human intention, personal narratives serve to unite temporally the present self with the selves of the past and of the future (e.g., McAdams, 2001). This diachronic integration, or *temporal coherence*, provides the through-line through which the moment of the story is connected to the moment of the storytelling (e.g., Adler & McAdams, 2007b). Although stories may be told with scenes that do not fall within a linear chronological order, such as flashbacks or imagined future scenarios, the audience must be able to sequence the events into a temporally coherent arc (e.g., Mandler, 1984). Indeed, Bruner (1990) argued that narrative's "principle property is its inherent sequentiality" (p. 43). According to Bruner, temporal coherence is not simply a criterion by which narratives may be evaluated; it is a definitional standard for the form.

Habermas and Bluck (2000) suggest that good narratives espouse other types of coherence beyond the temporal dimension. First, personal stories ought to contain *causal coherence*, instructive points that explain the connections between different sets of actions or account for apparent discontinuities. Causal coherence shows up in narratives when the narrator describes the ways in which he or she views different elements of the story as being linked. This can be as simple as a cause-and-effect account of an experience, or it can be as sophisticated as joining specific historical events to one's developing sense of self. Such instances of causal connection are a key way experiences are connected to the narrator's identity (Pals, 2006). For example, when difficult experiences happen in adulthood, the individual is faced with the challenge of narrating these difficulties in a way that is either consonant with his or her existing life narrative or revising that narrative to accommodate the new circumstances (Pals, 2006). Second, personal narratives express *thematic coherence*, the repetition of often implicit judgments about the narrator or main character that, when assessed holistically, reveal a consistency in the nature of that character (Habermas & Bluck, 2000). For example, a story about a man's life may contain several anecdotes about volunteering, working as a teacher, and the joys of being a parent, thus adding up to a coherent thematic assessment of the man as an especially generative person. Third, Habermas and Bluck assert that personal narratives ought to adhere to a *cultural concept of biography*. Personal narratives are adapted from templates available to the individual within his or her cultural context, "master narratives," or outlines for how lives are supposed to unfold (e.g., Hammack, 2008). This assertion is supported by Bruner's (1990) suggestion that personal stories "[make] comprehensible a deviation from a canonical cultural pattern" (pp. 49–50). When people tell stories that deviate too widely from these social scripts, they can be hard to interpret; thus, cultural fluency can be considered a criterion for narrative coherence. These four elements of narrative coherence are far from the only ones that have been proposed and debated, but they capture the ways in which scholars working from a narrative perspective evaluate good stories from a narrative approach.

It is tempting to regard coherence as a linear concept when it comes to evaluating narratives, with higher degrees of coherence being better. There is certainly empirical evidence documenting the significant detrimental consequences of low levels of coherence for the narrator. For example, people suffering from psychopathology have been shown to have low levels of coherence in their stories (e.g., Adler, Chin, Kolisetty, & Oltmanns, in press; Lysaker & Lysaker, 2006). In the adult attachment literature, the criteria for secure attachment are highly aligned with the coherence of participants' responses on the Adult Attachment Interview (e.g., Bouchard et al., 2008). Low levels of narrative coherence have also been associated with more simplistic worldviews, low psychological maturity, and low trait Openness to experience (e.g., Adler, Wagner, & McAdams, 2007). Certainly low narrative coherence impedes the believability of a story, which is associated with poor outcomes for the narrator.

Yet, as Freeman (2010) pointed out, "Some people become imprisoned by too-coherent narratives" (p. 168). High levels of narrative coherence can be bad for the narrator as well. Life is messy, and embracing the complexity of lived experience is vital if one is to have a believable narrative. This may be especially important in the wake of difficult life experiences. In an example drawn from an empirical study of personal narratives, Pals (2006) described two dimensions along which stories may be assessed. One was labeled *coherent positive resolution*, or a sense that the story of an episode is adequately wrapped up at the end with a sense of closure. This dimension, which bears strong relationship to the types of coherence discussed earlier, was associated with positive subjective well-being. The other dimension was labeled *exploratory processing*, or a sense that the narrator was actively engaged in reflecting upon and analyzing challenges and changes in his or her life. This exploratory dimension was uniquely associated with psychological maturity (as assessed by Loevinger's [1976] construct of ego development). Pals's data indicated that narratives espousing a combination of coherent positive resolution and exploratory processing were those that best supported positive self-transformation for the narrator after difficult life experiences. This suggests that a glossing over of potentially incongruous details, or a rigid adherence to a tight story line, may be detrimental to the narrator, much as low levels of coherence may be.

It is worth noting that within the tradition of narrative approaches there are disagreements concerning the privileged status of coherence. The editors of a recent volume titled *Beyond Narrative Coherence* wrote that their book

> challenges [the centrality of narrative coherence] *theoretically* (positioning it historically; indicating its problems), *methodologically* (in showing its often problematic consequences, finding new methods with which to approach broken narratives), and *ethically* (by showing how the coherence paradigm privileges middle-class conventionality and marginalizes the experiences of artistically creative as well as politically traumatized people). (Hyvärinen et al., 2010, p. 2, original emphasis)

The very assertion that coherence ought to be the standard by which narratives are evaluated is contentious among some scholars operating from a hermeneutic approach. Yet in the afterword to the volume, after concurring with the spirit of the preceding chapters and many of their conclusions, Freeman (2010) adroitly points out that "this 'anti-coherence'—or even anti-narrativism—bespeaks a coherence of its own, that it is the inverted image of, and is thus parasitic upon, the very coherence it rejects and replaces" (pp. 167–168). In other words, there is an implicit coherence in the rallying cry against coherence put forth by many of the authors in this volume. Coherence, it seems, is inescapable to a certain degree. Within the narrative tradition the debate about the role of coherence in evaluating the quality of narratives is likely to continue for some time, but for the moment, it convincingly remains central.

The Two Approaches

The paradigmatic mode and the narrative mode of thought are distinct epistemological traditions. These represent two fundamentally different ways of organizing knowledge; one approach is not reducible to the other, nor is one approach an emergent property of the other. The two approaches are not arranged hierarchically but stand beside each other with unique contributions and unique limitations.

Perhaps not surprisingly, there are internal tensions among psychologists studying personal narratives that are grounded in the seeming incompatibility of these two epistemological approaches (e.g., Bakan, 1966; Craik, 1996; Josselson & Lieblich, 1993). On the one hand, positivists studying narratives from the paradigmatic mode can be dismissive of narrative epistemological approaches, suggesting that because the insights they provide are not necessarily grounded in the scientific method and therefore do not obviously generalize, they are not valid sources for the study of truth. On the other hand, hermeneutic researchers working in the narrative mode criticize paradigmatic approaches as overly reductionist, as failing to capture adequately the vibrant diversity of individual human experience and violating the beauty of narratives as data. Both positions are fair, sound, and appropriate, yet both are also wholly informed by their particular epistemological traditions. In the remainder of this chapter I hope to offer insights about self-knowledge gleaned from both paradigmatic and narrative perspectives, and to consider the potential for a pluralistic approach.

Accuracy in Self-Knowledge from Two Approaches[1]

A fundamental issue facing the emerging field of research on self-knowledge is the accuracy of the knowledge under question. Embedded in the central proposition *What do people know about themselves?* is the assumption that certain knowledge is to be considered more accurate than other knowledge. For example, Vazire (2010) has recently developed a model of self-knowledge that capitalizes on the documented asymmetries in accuracy of self-reports compared to other-reports to assess when the individual is a better or worse informant about him- or herself than others. The matter of accuracy in self-knowledge is approached quite differently by paradigmatic and narrative epistemological traditions.

Vazire and Mehl (2008) provide a nice review of the scholarly research on accuracy of self-knowledge from a paradigmatic perspective. They highlight the importance of identifying criterion measures for evaluating the accuracy of various perspectives (traditional self-report and other-report). Some social-psychological traditions, such as the study of naive realism (e.g., Pronin, Lin, & Ross, 2002) and attributional theory (e.g., Sweeny, Anderson, & Bailey, 1986) focus on the scientific assessment of people's explanations for the world and their role in it. Studies in this vein often identify a disconnect between participants' perceptions and an externally validated measure of reality. Elegant research designs have produced criterion measures separate from either self- or other-report, such as ratings of behavior in the laboratory by trained and reliable experts, or by using ecological criterion measures that attempt to assess a representative sample of the target's behavior (Vazire & Mehl, 2008). In the typical paradigmatic approach to studying accuracy of self-knowledge, the individual's ability to predict his or her behavior is pitted against the perspective of someone else (typically a close friend or family member) and the established criterion measure, and stronger associations between the prediction and the behavior are taken as most accurate. The underlying assumption of research in this mold is that individuals' conscious construal of themselves may or may not align with an objective, externally assessed measure of them, and that the external criterion is to be privileged. In such research the typical scientific concerns are of utmost importance: the reliability and validity of the measures used, the rigor of the study design, and so forth. The array of creative approaches to studying self-knowledge from across the paradigmatic spectrum is on display in the other chapters in this volume.

Perhaps somewhat surprisingly, narrative approaches to self-knowledge also value accuracy, but the definition of *accuracy* is different than that embraced by paradigmatic approaches. Narrative perspectives challenge the privileged status of external criterion measures, asserting instead that the self is a fundamentally internal and subjective phenomenon, not subject to external validation. From a narrative epistemological approach, the story one tells may include both conscious and unconscious elements, but the story itself is to be regarded as the privileged focus of inquiry. To say that a story is accurate from a narrative perspective therefore implies that it is *believable* (e.g., McAdams, 2006). While paradigmatic approaches seek to identify objective accuracy criteria, narrative approaches regard accuracy as fundamentally relational—there is always an audience that is evaluating the story. Indeed, if narrative accuracy is to be understood as believability, one must always question, "Believable by whom?"

What then makes for a believable story? Once again, coherence is a major standard by which narrative believability can be assessed. Stories that deviate widely from the types of coherence described earlier—temporal, causal, thematic, and cultural–biographical—are less believable. Consider a hypothetical story wherein the temporal sequencing of events is dramatically inconsistent: The protagonist gets married, then learns to walk, then raises her granddaughter, and then is born. The temporal incoherence leads the audience simply to dismiss the story (and potentially the narrator) as unbelievable.[2] Yet, in addition to these types of coherence, McAdams (2006) advances an additional component by which we ought to evaluate stories. He suggests that personal narratives must reflect the actual lived experience of the narrator. Indeed, stories may be highly coherent in their temporal sequencing, causal connections, thematic elements, and adherence to cultural standards for biography, but may be complete confabulation. Without a doubt, narratives themselves are fundamentally interpretative in nature and cannot be taken as accurate accounts of one's experience. Spence (1982) distinguished between "historical truth and narrative truth," the distinction between what actually happened and the individual's interpretation of what happened (pp. 27–28). Given that all narratives are the products of reconstructed and biased perceptions, it simply does not make sense to assess personal stories primarily by their veracity. Yet despite the interpretive leap, for stories to be believable they must conceivably adhere to the historical events of a person's life.

There may be an inherent tension between the coherence of a narrative and its believability. Narratives that are not sufficiently coherent are, at worst, not interpretable by the audience and, at best, evidence of disruptions in psychological well-being and maturity. Yet narratives that are overly coherent may be exaggeratedly divorced from the nuances of lived experience. At this point, whether believability ought to be considered an additional criterion by which narratives are to be evaluated is far from settled, and the vast majority of research on the topic has focused on the primary dimensions of coherence.

I would like to suggest that beyond the dominance of coherence in evaluating narratives and the additional suggestion that "good" narratives are those that are believable, narratives may also be judged by their ability to support the psychological well-being of their narrator. As I describe in more detail below, there has been significant scholarship on narratives that strives to identify those components of personal stories that are associated with various features of mental health. I assert that this emphasis reveals a deeper belief that narratives are created and told in the service of supporting the well-being of the narrator. Coherence may be thought of as a definitional criterion for narratives; a collection of statements cannot be properly labeled as a "narrative" without an internal coherence. Believability may be understood as fundamental to narratives as they are communicated to others; the success of a story is grounded in its believability. Yet supporting the well-being of the narrator undergirds the psychological function of narratives for the storyteller. Wilson (2002) refers to this as the "peace-of-mind" criterion (p. 221). He suggests that effective narratives recede into the background of the individual's consciousness rather than dominating his or her daily thoughts, and that narratives that are successful in doing so provide a sense of peace with themselves. Thus, rather than focusing on accuracy, narratives ought to be evaluated by their coherence, believability, and ability to support the psychological well-being of the narrator.

Walking the Epistemological Line

Thus far, I have described some of the differences between paradigmatic approaches and narrative approaches to self-knowledge and highlighted the divergence in their grappling with the accuracy of self-knowledge. I now turn to ways in which scholars have worked to bring together the strengths of these epistemological traditions.

While the range of scholarship broadly subsumed under the label *the narrative study of lives* (e.g., Josselson & Lieblich, 1993) spans the epistemological spectrum, a growing body of work within this tradition has embraced methods that incorporate both narrative and paradigmatic approaches. It is first important to clarify the distinction between epistemology and methodology: *Epistemology* provides the broader philosophical approach to knowledge that grounds a particular inquiry, while *methodology* is the set of techniques a scholar uses in pursuing a particular question (e.g., Grecco, 1999). It is not appropriate to reduce the paradigmatic tradition to quantitative methods and the narrative tradition to qualitative methods, although in practice this is the most common distinction in their approach. Research that attempts to walk the epistemological line between paradigmatic and narrative traditions often draws on mixed methodological designs, incorporating both qualitative and quantitative elements.

The primary way such epistemologically blended studies are accomplished is by collecting personal stories as a vehicle for conducting scientific research. In a typical study, extensive narratives are collected from a group of participants, and other variables of interest, such as mental health or psychological maturity, are also assessed. The narratives are coded using reliable and valid systems by raters who have demonstrated statistical reliability in using the coding system with a subset of narratives drawn from the dataset. This coding process is the method by which rich individual stories are digested, such that they can be empirically compared with each other, and such that themes across participants' narratives may be assessed with respect to other variables (see King, 2004, for a more in-depth overview of typical research methods). I provide some examples of research using this approach in the next section.

Whether this method succeeds in walking the epistemological line between narrative and paradigmatic approaches is up for debate. Certainly within mainstream personality and social psychology, research conducted in this manner often takes the guise of paradigmatic science when it is published. Reports of such studies often include descriptive and inferential statistics alongside lengthy narrative excerpts. In doing so, research in this vein runs the risk of satisfying no one. Paradigmatic scholars sometimes find such research deficient, as it is still grounded in personal stories that cannot aspire to present veridical accounts of what actually took place. Paradigmatic accuracy is nowhere to be found in such data. Narratives are fundamentally subjective and, while they can be an excellent source for investigating meaning-making processes, mainstream paradigmatic researchers still have somewhat mixed feelings about their value. On the other hand, hermeneutic scholars working in the narrative mode are also sometimes put off by research that seeks to blend an emphasis on personal stories with quantitative approaches to data analysis. Such endeavors can be seen as an affront to the narrative epistemology, disregarding or underprivileging the value of the contributions qualitative narratives can make. Scholarship that blends approaches is surely restricted in its ability both to fulfill narrative aspirations of capturing the idiosyncratic and the personal in rich and nuanced ways, and to achieve the experimental control privileged by paradigmatic traditions.

In spite of these legitimate mutual objections, there is much to be gained for research on self-knowledge from attempting to walk the epistemological line. Scholarship in this vein manages to provide research participants with a phenomenological experience that embraces the ethos of narrative research, treating the individual as the expert on his or her own life. Research practices that include the collection of personal narratives strive to cultivate a feeling of empowerment and authority in participants (e.g., Fivush & Marin, 2007; Riessman, 2008). Doing so alleviates some of the skepticism and fear that permeate the subjective experience of potential participants in psychological research studies (e.g., Marshall et al., 2001). For example, one widely used instrument for collecting narratives within the field of personality psychology, the Life Story Interview (McAdams, 2008) directs the researcher to say to participants: "Please know that my purpose in doing this interview is not to figure out what is wrong with you or to do some kind of deep clinical analysis . . . [my] main goal is simply to hear your story." Such instructions put the participant at ease and suggest that the specifics of his or her own story will be most privileged. In my own experience conducting this type of research, participants often find the act of participating to be rewarding in and of itself. For example, a participant in one of my studies of psychotherapy noted, "Just describing these feelings now makes me feel better and more enthusiastic about therapy. This step in the research I think actually helps my therapy. Thank you." At the same time, epistemologically pluralistic studies are able to obtain data that may be analyzed in the service of identifying generalities across participants, the primary goal of paradigmatic social science. Thus, such approaches can foster the collection of empirical data, while preserving the open and welcoming research experience for participants that is deeply and justly prized by narrative researchers.

Self-Knowledge on the Epistemological Line

What follows are several examples of research on the self that strives to blend narrative and paradigmatic approaches. In each case, personal narratives were collected alongside other data. The aim of this research was to illustrate the relationship between meaning-making processes best captured in the stories of individuals and outcomes or correlates that generalize across a group of participants. The research described below provides a few examples of work that embraces personal narratives as a unique and vital vehicle for assessing self-knowledge, while operating in a fundamentally paradigmatic mode of inquiry. They demonstrate how the individual meaning instantiated in personal narratives can be stable, reliably assessed, and predictive of important outcomes.

A pair of longitudinal studies offers insight on how people view their own personality development during the often tumultuous college years. In one study, McAdams and colleagues (2006) collected personal narratives and other data concerning personality traits from two groups of college students, half freshmen and half seniors. The participants were asked to reflect on 10 key moments in their lives and to provide rich narrative accounts of these experiences. Narratives were collected 3 months after the initial time point and again 3 years after that. The authors found that the thematic continuity of the narratives was high—equivalent to that of personality traits—especially in terms of their emotional tone and overall complexity. This study established that the thematic ways in which college students made sense of their lives remained relatively stable, despite the developmental challenges associated with this period of emerging adulthood. In doing so, it suggests that the process of constructing a self-story engages particular narrative styles that remain fairly consistent over time.

In another study, Lodi-Smith, Geise, Roberts, and Robins (2009) collected personality trait data from college students during their freshman year of college and again in their senior year. At the second time point, the researchers also asked participants to provide detailed narratives reflecting on the ways in which their own personality had changed over the course of college. The results of the study indicated that two aspects of the narratives—affective processes that involved positive valence, and exploratory processes that involved coherent causal explanations for change—were associated with increases in emotional health over the 4 years, independent of changes in personality traits. This study suggests that narrative processes have unique predictive value above and beyond the contribution of other, non-narrative constructs, such as personality traits.

Each of these two studies demonstrates the distinct benefits of blending narrative and paradigmatic approaches. The particular constellation of findings indicate that subjective, idiosyncratic meaning-making processes stand alongside objective, generalizable measures of personality in understanding students' development over the college years. In each case, the narratives provide rich, detailed accounts that could not be adequately assessed by answers on Likert-type scale items. For example, in reflecting on her time in college, one of the participants in the study by Lodi-Smith and colleagues (2009, p. 686) stated, "My personality has not changed much, but my perception of life has changed." This brief excerpt demonstrates the disconnect between actual personality change as assessed by trait measures given at several time points and the individual's insight into her own development. While the questionnaire data can tell researchers whether this individual's trait profile evolved during 4 years, this young woman has her own take on her growth. By virtue of its design, such research implicitly values both paradigmatic and narrative perspectives on the self. Research such as that represented by these longitudinal studies demonstrates how the study of self-knowledge may benefit from perspectives that blend paradigmatic and narrative approaches in investigating identity development.

In another set of studies, researchers have employed paradigmatic and narrative approaches to assess the relationship between meaning-making processes and mental health. As mentioned earlier, narrative researchers have been particularly interested in determining the distinct features of personal stories that differentially relate to high levels of subjective well-being versus psychological maturity, or the complexity and nuance of meaning-making processes (typically measured via Loevinger's [1976] concept of ego development). The ways in which these two dimensions of psychological functioning are associated with narrative strategies of self-making have been explored in a variety of ways. For example, a series of studies by King and colleagues investigating people's adaptations to significant life transitions (King & Raspin, 2004; King, Scollon, Ramsey, & Williams, 2000; King & Smith, 2004) reveals that different approaches to storytelling relate differently to subjective well-being and psychological maturity. When individuals undergo a significant transition, they are faced with the psychological task of grappling with the self that they will no longer become, what King calls "lost possible selves" (e.g., King & Raspin, 2004; King & Smith, 2004). For instance, when people get divorced, they must make sense of the married self they can no longer be (King & Raspin, 2004). In studies focused on transitions ranging from divorce, to the coming-out process in gay men and lesbians, to the discovery that the child one is about to have will be born with Down's syndrome, King and her colleagues have found that the salience of the lost possible self—how often participants thought about it—was negatively related to subjective well-being. In contrast, the elaboration of the lost possible self—the amount of vivid detail in people's narratives about this self—was related to psychological maturity, both concurrently at the time of the narrative and years down the road. In this work, the rich, ideographic meaning instantiated in personal stories is blended with widely accepted scientific measures of subjective well-being and psychological maturity, leading to a mixed-methods window into the importance of narratives.

In a different example, Bauer, McAdams, and Sakaeda (2005) found that individuals high in subjective well-being tended to frame their stories of personal growth in terms of intrinsic concerns dealing with humanistic interests, such as fostering meaningful relationships and contributing to society. In contrast, individuals high in psychological maturity framed their stories of personal growth in terms of integrative concerns fostering social-cognitive development, such as the desire for new perspectives or learning to understand one's life in terms of even greater richness of meaning. Both relationships between the personal memories and the mental health outcomes remained significant when the impact of personality traits was statistically controlled. As in the program of research by King and colleagues, this study by Bauer and colleagues demonstrates the ways in which different perspectives on self-knowledge differentially relate to aspects of psychological health.

Finally, in some of my own research I have investigated the ways in which different approaches to narrating one's experience in psychotherapy relate to uneven outcomes among clients. In a pair of studies, one qualitative (Adler & McAdams, 2007a) and one quantitative (Adler, Skalina, & McAdams, 2008), the characteristics of clients' therapy stories were differentially related to subjective well-being and psychological maturity following treatment. In both studies, participants who described their experiences in therapy by heavily incorporating the theme of *personal agency*—a sense that one is in control of his or her circumstances—were more likely to have high levels of subjective well-being. In contrast, participants high in psychological maturity framed the experience as a coherent story of personal growth. In a third longitudinal investigation (Adler, 2012), increases in the theme of agency were observed over the course of treatment and these increases temporally preceded improvements in participants' mental health. This relationship between changes in the narratives and subsequent changes in mental health remained consistent across a variety of demographic differences in participants and their therapists, as well as when dispositional personality traits were statistically controlled. In addition to the quantitative results, Adler (2012) also featured an in-depth case study of one participant's story as it unfolded over time. These studies further illustrate the contribution of mixed-methods narrative research to the understanding of self-knowledge as it relates to psychological health.

In each of these examples, the researchers have sought to blend the benefits afforded by obtaining rich qualitative narratives from participants as they describe some of the major impacts on their sense of self, from divorce to periods of significant personal growth, to psychotherapy, with the strengths of comparative paradigmatic science. There is no question that the methodological pluralism each study espoused represents an innovative approach to tapping the personal experience of the individual participant, while simultaneously deriving rigorous scientific conclusions that generalize beyond the specific samples under investigation. Whether these studies and others like them are equally successful in embracing two truly distinct epistemological traditions is less clear. Each of the specific studies described earlier certainly conforms to the standards of paradigmatic inquiry. I contend that, at least in terms of the phenomenological experience the study provided to the research participants, one that elicited mostly unconstrained accounts of personal experiences, scholarship in this vein does achieve at least some of the goals of narrative epistemological approaches. As such, study designs that incorporate personal narratives but ultimately use these data to answer scientific questions about the nature of self-knowledge can be understood as walking the epistemological line.

Conclusion: The Case of "Tim" and Epistemological Pluralism

In conceptualizing a topic as multifaceted and important as self-knowledge, one epistemological approach cannot be considered sufficient. The emerging tradition of scientific research on self-knowledge, elegantly brought together for the first time in this handbook, provides an excellent foundation for paradigmatic perspectives on who we are and how we come to know ourselves. This tradition of research aspires to answer some of the most vital questions concerning self-knowledge; to explore the limits of self-knowledge, the methodological challenges in evaluating self-knowledge, and the implications for different ways of knowing the self. At the same time, a distinct epistemological approach, one that embraces the personal, idiosyncratic, and fundamentally subjective nature of the storied self, stands as a valuable counterpoint. Indeed, scientifically documenting "glaring inaccuracies in self-perception" (Vazire & Mehl, 2008, p. 1202) is absolutely vital to combating reliable misperceptions. But the meaning that individuals ascribe to their experiences and instantiate in personal narratives, however flawed or inaccurate, ought to be treated with care.

Much of this handbook focuses on the distinction between *what is true* about self-knowledge and *what people believe is true* based on their privileged status as interpreters of their sense of self. From the perspective of certain philosophers of science, this distinction can be conceptualized as one between causal and meaningful explanations (e.g., Brendel, 2000). *Causal explanations* seek to explain the true underlying connections between phenomena. In contrast, *meaningful explanations* seek to describe the relationship between phenomena in terms of the ways humans make sense of them, whether these ways are accurate or not. Causal explanations, operating in the paradigmatic mode of thought, are evaluated by their validity, reliability, and precision. In contrast, meaningful explanations, operating in the narrative mode of thought, are evaluated by their ability to capture coherently and believably the shifting motivations of their characters and to support the narrator's well-being.

It may appear self-evident that causal explanations are to be privileged over meaningful explanations; if we are able to determine what was really going on, why would we choose to value someone's potentially flawed and certainly biased stories about what happened? Yet Brendel (2000) provides an elegant example of these two approaches that illustrates their surprising interdependence. This example does as much to affirm the contribution of both paradigmatic and narrative perspectives as it does to further complicate the picture, thus demonstrating the benefits of adopting both approaches.

Brendel (2000) presents a brief case study of a man named "Tim" who suffered from the delusion that he was put on this planet to atone for Adolf Hitler's sins. This belief led to intense suffering for Tim, and his days were spent in anguish. Yet, despite the unremitting agony, Tim refrained from committing suicide out of the conviction that his continued existence was responsible for sparing humanity from the otherwise imminent consequences of Hitler's havoc. Brendel makes clear that a causal explanation of Tim's condition would refer to the evident disruptions in his neurophysiology. Nevertheless, the idiosyncratic explanation that Tim ascribes to his condition "cannot be understood in causal terms. It can be made intelligible only in terms of Tim's life story and the meaningful connections that constituted his subjectivity" (p. 188). Tim's meaningful explanation had itself become causal—the individual and subjective narrative he wove about his experience was responsible for keeping him alive. From any paradigmatic perspective, Tim's explanation cannot be considered accurate. But from the perspective of his personal narrative, the story was a matter of life and death. Writing specifically about the context of psychiatric treatment, Spence (1982) suggested, "Once a given construction has acquired narrative truth, it becomes just as real as any other kind of truth; this new reality becomes a significant part of the [psychotherapeutic] cure" (p. 31). Once fully articulated, the narrative can impact and shape experience in a way that can be validly and reliably assessed using paradigmatic science. Tim's story might conform to the standards of coherence but would certainly fail to achieve the criterion of believability. At the same time, it served a vital purpose (in the full sense of the word *vital*). Tim's case reveals the limits of valuing accuracy in self-knowledge above all else, and it also suggests there is more to good stories than their believability. As for supporting his well-being, Tim's case is highly nuanced. On the one hand, his day-to-day existence was quite painful. On the other hand, he found some existential peace in the notion that he was fulfilling his ultimate purpose. From a narrative perspective, Tim's story was successful in achieving the coherence and well-being criteria of good narratives, but it failed to be believable and could not be considered accurate from a paradigmatic perspective. This case study illustrates how both paradigmatic and narrative perspectives have their flaws, and it suggests that bringing them together offers many benefits to the study of self-knowledge.

As the field of scholars working on self-knowledge continues to coalesce, it is vital that they adopt epistemologically pluralistic approaches to their pursuit. One of the great philosophers of science, Karl Popper (1963), wrote, "It is imperative that we give up the idea of ultimate sources of knowledge, and admit that all knowledge is human; that it is mixed with our errors, our prejudices, our dreams, and our hopes; that all we can do is grope for truth even though it is beyond our reach. There is no authority beyond the reach of criticism" (p. 39). This perspective of humility is most likely to promote a vibrant and prolific emerging field focused on explaining self-knowledge.

NOTES

1. It is worth noting that in regard to the study of the self, the word *knowledge* often connotes beliefs that have been externally validated (e.g., Vazire, 2010). In light of the epistemological conflict about the centrality of such externally verifiable truths within the field of research on personal stories, I will continue to use the term *self-knowledge*. I recognize that positivists may regard the work I am going to review as more accurately characterized as being focused on "self-views," whereas hermeneutic scholars may regard the conflation of "knowledge" and "truth" as meaningless.

2. Note that it is *possible* to impose a temporal coherence even to this seemingly incoherent sequence of events: Perhaps the protagonist is wheelchair-bound until after her wedding, at which point she learns to walk, which leads her to embrace this new phase of her life by having children and ultimately a granddaughter whom she raises, after which she feels like such a completely new person that she considers herself "born" as a new person. This illustration reveals the seductive pull of temporal coherence—the reader *wants* to impose some logic to the sequence of events. It also demonstrates the standard of causal coherence: Without offering *explanatory* connections between the events in the life, the story cannot be considered coherent and therefore believable.

REFERENCES

Adler, J. M. (2012). Living into the story: Agency and coherence in a longitudinal study of narrative identity development and mental health over the course of psychotherapy. *Journal of Personality and Social Psychology, 102*(2), 367–389.

Adler, J. M., & McAdams, D. P. (2007a). The narrative reconstruction of psychotherapy. *Narrative Inquiry, 17*(2), 179–202.

Adler, J. M., & McAdams, D. P. (2007b). Time, culture, and stories of the self. *Psychological Inquiry, 18*(2), 97–99.

Adler, J. M., Chin, E. D., Kolisetty, A. P., & Oltmanns, T. F. (in press). The distinguishing characteristics of narrative identity in adults with features of Borderline Personality Disorder: An empirical investigation. *Journal of Personality Disorders*.

Adler, J. M., Skalina, L. M., & McAdams, D. P. (2008). The narrative reconstruction of psychotherapy and psychological health. *Psychotherapy Research, 18*(6), 719–734.

Adler, J. M., Wagner, J. W., McAdams, D. P. (2007). Personality and the coherence of psychotherapy narratives. *Journal of Research in Personality, 41*(6), 1179–1198.

Bakan, D. (1966). *The duality of human existence*. Boston: Beacon.

Bauer, J. J., McAdams, D. P., & Sakaeda, A. R. (2005). Interpreting the good life: Growth memories in the lives of mature, happy people. *Journal of Personality and Social Psychology, 88*(1), 203–217.

Bouchard, M., Target, M., Lecours, S., Fonagay, P., Tremblay, L., Schacter, A., et al. (2008). Mentalization in adult attachment narratives: Reflective functioning, mental states, and affect elaboration compared. *Psychoanalytic Psychology, 25*, 47–66.

Brendel, D. H. (2000). Philosophy of mind in the clinic: The relation between causal and meaningful explanation in psychiatry. *Harvard Review of Psychiatry, 8*, 184–191.

Bruner, J. (1986). *Actual minds, possible worlds*. Cambridge, MA: Harvard University Press.

Bruner, J. (1990). *Acts of meaning*. Cambridge, MA: Harvard University Press.

Craik, K. H. (1996). The objectivity of persons and their lives: A noble dream for personality psychology? *Psychological Inquiry, 7*(4), 326–330.

Fivush, R., & Marin, K. A. (2007). Place and power: A feminist perspective on self-event connections. *Human Development, 50,* 111–118.

Freeman, M. (2010). "Even amidst": Rethinking narrative coherence. In M. Hyvärinen, L. C. Hydén, M. Saarenheimo, & M. Tamboukou (Eds.), *Beyond narrative coherence* (pp. 167–186). Philadelphia: Benjamins.

Greco, J. (1999). What is epistemology? In J. Greco & E. Sosa (Eds.), *The Blackwell guide to epistemology* (pp. 1–32). New York: Blackwell.

Habermas, T., & Bluck, S. (2000). Getting a life: The emergence of the life story in adolescence. *Psychological Bulletin, 126*(5), 748–769.

Hammack, P. L. (2008). Narrative and the cultural psychology of identity. *Personality and Social Psychology Review, 12*(3), 222–247.

Hyvärinen, M., Hydén, L. C., Saarenheimo, M., & Tamboukou, M. (2010). *Beyond narrative coherence.* Philadelphia: Benjamins.

Josselson, R., & Lieblich, A. (Eds.). (1993). *The narrative study of lives* (Vol. 1). Newbury Park, CA: Sage.

King, L. A. (2004). Measures and meaning: The use of qualitative data in social and personality psychology. In C. Sansone, C. C. Morf, & A. T. Panter (Eds.), *The Sage handbook of methods in social psychology* (pp. 173–194). New York: Sage.

King, L. A., & Raspin, C. (2004). Lost and found possible selves, subjective well-being, and ego development in divorced women. *Journal of Personality, 72,* 603–632.

King, L. A., Scollon, C. K., Ramsey, C., & Williams, T. (2000). Stories of life transition: Subjective well-being and ego development in parents of children with Down syndrome. *Journal of Research in Personality, 34,* 509–536.

King, L. A., & Smith, N. G. (2004). Gay and straight possible selves: Goals, identity, subjective well-being, and personality development. *Journal of Personality, 72,* 967–994.

Labov, W. (1972). *Language in the inner city.* Philadelphia: University of Pennsylvania Press.

Lodi-Smith, J., Geise, A. C., Roberts, B. W., & Robins, R. W. (2009). Narrating personality change. *Journal of Personality and Social Psychology, 96*(3), 679–689.

Loevinger, J. (1976). *Ego development.* San Francisco: Jossey-Bass.

Lysaker, P. H., & Lysaker, J. T. (2006). A typology of narrative impoverishment in schizophrenia: Implications for understanding the processes of establishing and sustaining dialogue in individual psychotherapy. *Counseling Psychology Quarterly, 19*(1), 57–68.

Mandler, J. M. (1984). *Stories, scripts, and scenes: Aspects of schema theory.* Hillsdale, NJ: Erlbaum.

Marshall, R. D., Spitzer, R. L., Vaughn, R., Mellman, L. A., MacKinnon, R. A., & Roose, S. P. (2001). Assessing the subjective experience of being a participant in psychiatric research. *American Journal of Psychiatry, 158*(2), 319–321.

McAdams, D. P. (1993). *The stories we live by: Personal myths and the making of the self.* New York: Guilford Press.

McAdams, D. P. (2001). The psychology of life stories. *Review of General Psychology, 5*(2), 100–122.

McAdams, D. P. (2006). The problem of narrative coherence. *Journal of Constructivist Psychology, 19,* 109–125.

McAdams, D. P. (2008). *Interviewer guide for the life story interview.* Unpublished manuscript, Northwestern University, Chicago. Available at *www.sesp.northwestern.edu/foley/instruments/interview.*

McAdams, D. P., Bauer, J. J., Sakaeda, A., Anyidoho, N. A., Machado, M., Magrino, K., et al. (2006). Continuity and change in the life story: A longitudinal study of autobiographical memories in emerging adulthood. *Journal of Personality, 74*(5), 1371–1400.

McLeod, J. (1997). *Narrative and psychotherapy*. London: Sage.

Pals, J. L. (2006). Narrative identity processing of difficult life experiences: Pathways of personality development and positive self-transformation in adulthood. *Journal of Personality, 74*(4), 1079–1110.

Popper, K. (1963). *Conjectures and refutations*. New York: Routledge.

Pronin, E., Lin, D. Y., & Ross, L. (2002). The bias blind spot: Perceptions of bias in self versus others. *Personality and Social Psychology Bulletin, 28*(3), 369–381.

Riessman, C. K. (2008). *Narrative methods for the human sciences*. Los Angeles: Sage.

Spence, D. P. (1982). *Narrative truth and historical truth: Meaning and interpretation in psychoanalysis*. New York: Norton.

Sweeny, P. D., Anderson, K., & Bailey, S. (1986). Attributional style in depression: A meta-analytic review. *Journal of Personality and Social Psychology, 50*(5), 974–991.

Vazire, S. (2010). Who knows what about a person?: The self–other knowledge asymmetry (SOKA) model. *Journal of Personality and Social Psychology, 98*(2), 281–300.

Vazire, S., & Mehl, M. R. (2008). Knowing me, knowing you: The accuracy and unique predictive validity of self-ratings and other-ratings of daily behavior. *Journal of Personality and Social Psychology, 95*(5), 1202–1216.

Wilson, T. D. (2002). *Strangers to ourselves: Discovering the adaptive unconscious*. Cambridge, MA: Harvard University Press.

PART IV
MOTIVES AND BIASES IN SELF-KNOWLEDGE

CHAPTER 21
Illusions of Self-Knowledge

KATHERINE E. HANSEN
EMILY PRONIN

The valley of Delphi, on the slopes of Mount Parnassus in central Greece, is famous for more than its awe-inspiring beauty. It is there that ancient Greeks trekked in the hopes of obtaining prophecies about themselves from the god Apollo. The path to self-knowledge was not easy. Coming from Athens, the typical prophecy seeker had to endure a nearly 200 km hike in the Mediterranean heat (prophecies were not offered in the wintertime). The answer to one's question ultimately came, via an Oracle channeling Apollo, in the form of mysterious, bordering on uninterpretable, riddles.

Harnessing the wisdom of Apollo was a tough way to attain self-knowledge. It seems easier to sit down in a comfortable chair, rest our chin in our hand, and take a moment for self-reflection. Unfortunately, looking inward to attain self-knowledge is more difficult than it seems. The lenses through which we look are far from objective, and they can distort, cloud, and color what we see in ways that, for example, sometimes present us with overly positive self-views and other times present us with overly negative ones (Alicke, 1985; Dunning, Meyerowitz, & Holzberg, 1989; Kruger, 1999). The problem goes deeper than such distortions: Self-reflection only reveals those things—memories, emotions, beliefs, motives—that occupy our current conscious experience. By focusing on what we find when we look inward, we blind ourselves to those things that are inaccessible via introspection (Nisbett & Ross, 1980; Nisbett & Wilson, 1977; Wilson, 2002). For example, we may misread the cause of our current happy mood because we cannot consciously perceive the source (or activity) of the neurochemical processes that have recently triggered our dopaminergic system, so we instead rely on what we can perceive, even if it is not truly diagnostic.

This chapter focuses on illusions of self-knowledge. Those illusions can involve erroneous beliefs about what we are like, such as the illusion that we are smarter or prettier than we really are. Illusions of self-knowledge go deeper than that, though. They also involve erroneous beliefs about how self-knowledge is itself obtained. A fundamental illusion of self-knowledge is the illusion that it derives primarily from introspection, or looking inward (e.g., Pronin, 2009; Pronin & Kugler, 2007). At the entrance to the Oracle of Delphi, visitors were greeted with the famous command "Know Thyself." It may seem ironic that this command was put forth in a location where people went to learn about themselves from an external source. Perhaps, though, the command had a different purpose—to remind people that self-knowledge can sometimes best be obtained by looking outward to the opinions of others, especially those wiser than ourselves and with more detached perspectives, rather than by sitting and reflecting, chin in hand.

In the discussion that follows, we first explore various illusions of self-knowledge and the role of inappropriate reliance on introspection in fostering these illusions. We begin by looking at the ways in which people misperceive things about themselves, such as traits and abilities, as a result of their systematic focus on internal information. These misperceptions commonly involve self-aggrandizing distortions that stem from people placing too much weight on things such as positive intentions as opposed to actual behavior. We then turn more directly to people's inappropriate faith in what they can learn about themselves by "looking inward," suggesting that a major illusion about self-knowledge is that self-knowledge itself derives from the unique ability to access one's own mental processes. After reviewing these major pitfalls in self-knowledge, the chapter examines their implications for social interaction—with a focus on consequences for interpersonal intimacy and social conflict. Finally, we describe a number of ways, rooted in the theoretical underpinnings of this chapter, in which illusions of self-knowledge may be overcome.

The Introspection Illusion: A Guiding Framework

People are constantly immersed in a world of their own desires, thoughts, and feelings; as a result, people tend to use that "inner world" as their primary source of information about themselves, even when other avenues of information could lead to a more accurate understanding. Research has documented people's overreliance on information gained by introspection. We have referred to this tendency as an *introspection illusion*—a disproportionate weighting of introspective information when assessing oneself, but not others (e.g., Pronin, 2008, 2009; Pronin, Berger, & Molouki, 2007; Pronin & Kugler, 2007).

The problem with looking inward for self-understanding is multifold. For one, people do not have conscious access to much of the information that they would require to gain self-understanding. For example, if a person wants to know why he sometimes gets sad during the holidays or why he loves baroque music but not country music, he may not have access to those reasons. At the heart of this problem is people's lack of appreciation for that fact about themselves. People introspect to gain self-knowledge because they do not recognize the limits of introspection. As Wilson, Hodges, and LaFleur (1995, p. 17) put it: "People are often unaware of their own unawareness." Reliance on introspection comes at the cost of not paying attention to another important source of information: behavior. People sometimes are sufficiently immersed in their inner lives that they disregard what they do outwardly. As this chapter explores, these tendencies are at the core of many of people's illusions of self-knowledge.

Things We Think We Know about Ourselves That Are *Not True*

People are confident that they know themselves (Dunning, 2005). This section reviews research suggesting that we know ourselves less well than we think we do, in part because we think ourselves better than we really are. In reviewing this research we begin to make the case for how people's reliance on introspection produces illusory self-knowledge.

Enhancement Illusions

When people are asked about what they are like, they can readily report on their traits and abilities ("I'm funny, a night owl, and a great salsa dancer"). Perhaps unsurprisingly, people's reports are often biased in a self-aggrandizing way. Despite the fact that it is a statistical impossibility, most people believe they are friendlier, smarter, more honest, and more persistent than the average person, a bias known as the "better-than-average effect" (Alicke, 1985). Academics like us are likely no exception: In a 1977 study, Cross reported that 94% of professors claimed to do better work than their peers.

The correlation between self-perception and reality can thus be weak. Mabe and West (1982) conducted a meta-analysis on the relationship between self-assessment and objective performance across a variety of domains, finding a correlation of .29 in performance accounted for by people's self-perceptions. Correlations tended to be weak for assessments involving complex social skills (e.g., managerial competence) and stronger for assessments in which objective feedback was readily available. However, even when objective measures are readily available, people's self-assessments often disregard the information provided by those measures. For example, the correlation between people's perceptions of their own intelligence and their performance on various measures of intelligence is about .2 to .3 (Hansford & Hattie, 1982). Ironically, most people insist that they are less susceptible than most other people to the better-than-average effect (Friedrich, 1996; Pronin, Lin, & Ross, 2002).

Part of the reason for the better-than-average effect involves people's reliance on internal information. For instance, in assessing the impressiveness of her vocabulary, Jane may focus on all the arcane words that she knows but rarely ever uses, whereas her friend John can only observe the commonplace words that Jane uses in everyday speech. People's overreliance on introspection also prevents their considering others' abilities, even when they are explicitly assessing their own performance relative to those others (Kruger, 1999). When assessing their own relative competence at something like riding a bicycle, people focus on how capable they are (e.g., rarely falling off the bicycle) and fail to note others' similar competence. This error can lead people to exaggerate their inabilities as well. For example, when thinking about how one cannot juggle, one may fail to consider that most other people cannot juggle either, a failure that can lead to the perception that one is less capable than average (e.g.,

Kruger, 1999; Moore & Small, 2007; Weinstein & Lachendro, 1982). Thus, apparent self-enhancement illusions may have less to do with a motivation to self-enhance than with the information that people use in making self assessments—information that can lead not only to self-enhancing views but also to self-deprecating ones.

Unrealistic Optimism and Control Illusions

People can be unrealistically optimistic about their personal outcomes. These illusions about the self can have benefits for mental and physical health, for example, by providing a buffer against random failures or facilitating psychological coping with grave medical conditions (e.g., Taylor & Brown, 1988; Taylor, Lerner, Sherman, Sage, & McDowell, 2003). Unrealistic optimism also can foster harmful beliefs and behaviors, such as when it seems to render unnecessary the sort of wise behaviors that could promote future health or economic security (e.g., Robins & Beer, 2001; Weinstein, 1980). Although unrealistic optimism has a self-aggrandizing flavor to it (fostering people's impression that their futures are uniquely rosy), the mechanisms underlying it go beyond a motivation to self-enhance. The effect is at least partially rooted in the weight that people place on a critical type of introspective information: their intentions. For example, in situations in which people think they can impact their outcomes (like driving), the bias toward unrealistic optimism is especially pronounced (Klein & Helweg-Larson, 2002). Pronin (2009) examined roots of unrealistic optimism in an experiment in which people rated their likelihood of attaining various positive and negative outcomes (e.g., living past 80, getting fired from a job). Those participants also rated how much their attainment of these outcomes would be a reflection of their own personal intentions and of general population base rates. A second group of participants made these same three sets of ratings about a fellow student. The results showed that not only were participants unrealistically optimistic about their own (but not a fellow student's) future, but also this unrealistic optimism was rooted in the greater weight they placed on their own intentions. Essentially, students felt that they would be successful and healthy in the future because they focused on that *intention*, whereas they assessed a fellow student's outcomes by focusing on population base rates.

A related type of overoptimism involves people's undue confidence in their likelihood of personal success when it comes to chance events, an effect known as the *illusion of control* (Langer, 1975). In cases where people are specifically trying to attain an outcome, they assume that attainment of the desired outcome is brought about by their own behavior, even in instances when the outcome would have occurred regardless. For example, Matute (1996) found that, under naturalistic conditions, people aiming to extinguish an aversive noise mistakenly perceived that pressing the space bar on a keyboard had an effect on terminating the noise when in reality it had no such effect.

Such illusions of control have been traced to the inappropriate weight that people place on their own internal thoughts (e.g., Wegner, 2004). Instances of *magical thinking* provide a striking illustration (Pronin, Wegner, McCarthy, & Rodriguez, 2006). Magical thinking occurs when people believe they have caused outcomes for which there is no known scientific account for such causation, such as when people believe that they caused their favorite baseball player to hit a home run by sitting on the sofa and visualizing that outcome. Pronin and her colleagues (2006) conducted a series of experiments demonstrating the origins of such magical thinking in the weight people place on their thoughts. In one experiment, participants were asked to place a voodoo hex on another person (a confederate posing as another participant). Those participants who first were induced to privately think ill of the person on whom they placed the hex felt responsible when that person later claimed to have contracted a headache; those participants who entertained no ill thoughts before placing the hex (which involved sticking pins in a voodoo doll) did not feel responsible.

Prediction Illusions

People are overconfident about the accuracy of the predictions they make about their futures (Dunning, Heath, & Suls, 2004). In fact, people sometimes are more accurate at predicting the behavior of other people than of themselves. For example, in a study by Epley and Dunning (2000), 83% of surveyed undergraduates predicted they would buy flowers in a campus charity drive, but only 43% actually did. The students were far more accurate at predicting their peers' behavior—they predicted that 56% of other students would buy a flower. One root of such overoptimistic predictions for oneself can be found in the introspection illusion. For instance, when we are thinking about whether or not we will donate money to a charity in the future, we are mostly aware of our feelings of goodwill and our desire to help. We are not thinking about our poor track record when it comes to donating, our upcoming credit card bill, or the various situational barriers that will keep us from giving.

Our overvaluation of introspection also leads us astray in predicting our affective reactions to future events. People sometimes assume that such events will impact them for longer than they actually do—known as an *error in affective forecasting* (Wilson & Gilbert, 2003). In these cases, people become so caught up in the information that is prominent to them introspectively (i.e., information about what a future emotion will *feel* like) that they fail to introspect about all of the aspects of their lives that will not change. If we focus on how horrid it will be if the political candidate we most fear becomes President, while we ignore the fact that our lives involve more than just politics, we may overestimate how long the devastating effects of this event will last (Gilbert, Pinel, Wilson, Blumberg, & Wheatley, 1998).

Our inaccuracy in predicting our future emotions extends to how we perceive our future desires. When predicting what we will want in the future, we have difficulty separating ourselves from our current internal state; we are so wrapped up in what we want right now that we fail to account for the fact that we may not always feel this way. Since we only have introspective access in the moment and lack such access into our future selves, we make our predictions using the wrong information. For example, researchers found that when asking workers right after lunch what late-afternoon snack they would want 1 week later, the workers predicted a preference for something light and healthy (an apple) as opposed to something more filling (a candy bar), despite the fact that they were regularly hungry in the late afternoon (Read & van Leeuwen, 1998). They relied on their current feeling of satiety rather than looking, for example, to their past behavior at snacktime.

Things We Think We Know about Ourselves That We *Cannot Know*

The previous section explored a number of illusions of self-knowledge arising from our overweighting of information available in introspection. These illusions produce erroneous conclusions about what we are like, what we can achieve, and what our futures hold. In these cases, there is informational value to be found in introspection; the problem is that we rely on introspective information at the expense of taking into account other diagnostic sources of information. It is helpful to know about one's intentions in order to predict one's behavior, as long as we do not overweight these intentions at the expense of other information—but there also are cases when introspection holds little informational value. Those cases involve trying to access processes that operate nonconsciously and therefore leave no introspective traces. The following section explores three such examples from our research.

Unconscious Bias

People possess a bias blind spot when it comes to recognizing their own biases (e.g., Pronin, Gilovich, & Ross, 2004; Pronin et al., 2002, 2007). While people readily recognize others' commissions of cognitive and motivational biases ranging from the fundamental attribution error to better-than-average effect, they tend not to recognize those same biases in themselves. This illusion of objectivity presents a profound barrier to self-knowledge. None of us are capable of true "objectivity"—of seeing things apart from the lenses of our own perceptual processes. While we sometimes are aware in the abstract of our susceptibility to bias, the fact that bias typically operates unconsciously prevents our having knowledge of it when its impact is actually occurring (Ehrlinger, Gilovich, & Ross, 2005; Pronin, 2009). This lack of self-knowledge about our own susceptibility to bias has meaningful consequences. It can lead us unwittingly to make decisions based on biased judgments that affect our health, achievement, and well-being.

Roots In Introspection

This bias blind spot is rooted in the undue weight that people place on introspection. In a series of experiments, Pronin and Kugler (2007) demonstrated this underlying mechanism. In one study, participants took a purported test of their social intelligence. Previously, that test had been shown to elicit a classic self-serving bias—those told they did poorly viewed it as invalid, whereas those told they did well viewed it as valid (Pronin et al., 2002); the test also had been shown to elicit a bias blind spot—those who took it denied being biased in evaluating it even while they imputed that bias to a fellow test taker. Pronin and Kugler (2007) examined what information test takers (vs. observers) relied on when assessing bias. In their experiment, test takers received negative feedback about their performance. They then offered their thoughts about the test's validity (those thoughts were tape-recorded) and assessed that validity on a scale. Finally, they evaluated whether their assessment was biased by their test score. Test takers showed the usual bias blind spot in seeing their assessments as relatively objective (and more objective than how observers saw them). Moreover, whereas observers imputed more bias to test takers who were more critical of the test, test takers ignored that behavioral indicator of bias and instead claimed objectivity based on introspection. When they looked inward for signs of bias, they found none (as indicated by their thought reports), and it was this absence of internal information that led them to deny bias. Notably, observers who had seen test takers' thought reports did not similarly conclude that those actors had been free of bias (indeed, they ignored those reports entirely in favor of attending to the actors' behavior).

Claiming Objectivity

People's reliance on internal information for assessing bias can blind them to biased decisions even when they know that they have used a biased decision-making strategy. In a series of recent experiments, we (Hansen, Pronin, Gerbasi, & Todorov, 2011) have been exploring this tendency. Our studies investigate instances in which people *know* that they have used a biased decision-making strategy but nevertheless are *still* inclined to view their resulting decisions as objective (even when those decisions are, in fact, biased).

In one experiment, participants were asked to evaluate a series of paintings for artistic merit either in an explicitly biased way—by always looking to see who painted it prior to seeing the painting, or in an explicitly objective way—by always shielding oneself from the name (and fame) of the painter before judging the painting. Half of the paintings were attributed to names from the phone book rather than to famous artists such as Picasso or Monet. Prior to rating the paintings, participants who were about to use the explicitly biased strategy rated it as biased and those who were about to use the explicitly objective strategy rated it as objective. Those who were about to use the biased strategy, therefore, correctly recognized it as biased. But this knowledge did not extend to how they saw themselves. Analyses showed that those using the biased strategy were in fact biased in their ratings of the paintings (they rated the paintings attributed to famous artists as having more artistic merit than those attributed to nonfamous artists). However, those participants claimed that their ratings were objective. Indeed, they saw their ratings as no less objective than those in the objective condition saw their own ratings (see Figure 21.1). The introspection illusion provides a key to understanding this result. When people attempted to judge their own objectivity, they introspected to find the answer. In so doing, they saw no signs of the bias (because it operated unconsciously), and they therefore concluded that they had been objective in spite of the biased nature of their decision process.

Bias Protection Procedures

The implications of this blind spot are meaningful. If people do not recognize their biases, they cannot try to correct or prevent them. Fortunately, a foolproof solution exists: We can institute procedures that prevent people from being biased in the first place by "protecting" them from potentially biasing influences, a practice referred to as *exposure control* (Gilbert, 1993; Wilson & Brekke, 1994). For example, doctors do not need to recognize their personal susceptibility to the biasing effects of gifts from pharmaceutical representatives in order to institute a policy that prevents that bias by prohibiting such gifts. Similarly orchestra members do not need to believe

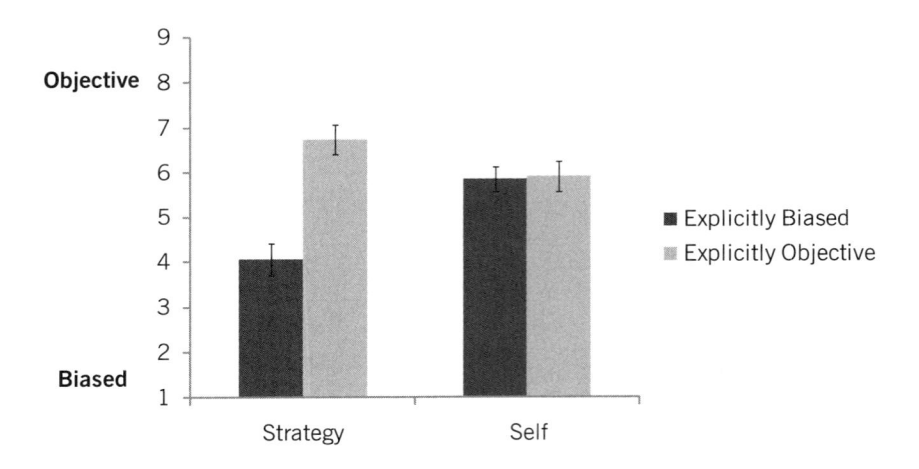

FIGURE 21.1. People's ratings of bias in their judgmental strategy and in their subsequent self-judgment.

that they personally are susceptible to bias in order to institute a policy that puts auditioners behind a curtain that conceals their gender and ethnicity. A related case, closer to the authors' own experience, involves the idea of "blind review" for journal article submissions. Indeed, each of these policies is sometimes formally instituted.

However, in a recent study, Mueller and Pronin (2012) demonstrated people's opposition to antibiasing procedures that would be imposed on them personally. High school teachers and members of college singing groups were asked about various antibiasing procedures that involved "blinding" individuals to potentially biasing information. Those procedures involved, for example, blind auditioning for orchestras, blind treatment in drug trials, and—critically—blind auditioning for singing groups and blind grading for teachers. The result was that participants supported antibiasing procedures the least when those procedures addressed their own potential bias. Singing group members and high school teachers both claimed that blinding procedures were less necessary for them personally than for others in their situation (i.e., other singing group members, other teachers). They also claimed that those procedures were less necessary in their situation than in others. Indeed, teachers endorsed blinding procedures more for singing groups than for teachers, whereas singing-group members endorsed blinding procedures more for teachers than for singing-group members.

Prejudice

The example of blinding procedures brings to light an important source of bias: implicit group-based prejudice. A wealth of research has documented people's capacity to hold implicit prejudices based on race, gender, age, and other group-based variables. These prejudiced attitudes are often not in line with people's conscious reports about how they perceive members of those groups (e.g., Devine, 1989; Greenwald & Banaji, 1995). Given the unconscious nature of these attitudes, introspection can lead one astray in inferring their presence.

In one study, Dovidio, Kawakami, and Gaertner (2002) found that, following an interaction with a black participant, white participants looked to their introspective evidence (i.e., their consciously accessible attitudes) to evaluate the interaction—and thereby concluded that they had been friendly. The black participants, however, saw the interaction differently. White participants' nonverbal behavior revealed their negative *implicit* attitudes, leading to an uncomfortable interaction for black participants. In instances such as these, people's reliance on introspection blinds them to group-based distinctions in their behavior that stem from implicit attitudes.

Implicit Social Influence

Studies in social psychology have demonstrated people's nonconscious conformity to those around them, from failing to intervene as a bystander (Darley & Latane, 1968) to mimicking the physical gestures of one's conversation partners (Chartrand & Bargh, 1999). Such cases of conformity represent another blind spot in people's self-knowledge. In domains ranging from political beliefs to clothing purchases, people deny the impact of social influence (Pronin et al., 2007). Reliance on introspection contributes to this mistaken self-assessment. In one experiment by Pronin and colleagues (2007), college students in California read descriptions of various political initiatives allegedly up for vote in that state. Each initiative had no partisan bent but allegedly was backed by either the Democrats or the Republicans. After reading each initiative, participants listed their thoughts about it and indicated how they would vote. They also indicated their party affiliation. Another group of participants served as observers. Each observer read about the various initiatives and saw one randomly selected voter's thoughts about those initiatives, as well as that voter's indication of how he or she would vote and his or her party affiliation. Voters were heavily swayed by their political party in choosing their positions. At the same time, voters thought that they were less influenced than did observers. Why? Voters and observers relied on different information. Voters paid more attention to their thoughts, whereas observers focused more on the alignment of the voter's party with his or her votes.

The Reasons for Our Preferences

Sometimes we know our preferences without knowing the reasons why we prefer them. Charles might know that he prefers Doris over Evelyn to be his girlfriend, without having access to the true source of that preference (e.g., Nisbett & Ross, 1980; Nisbett & Wilson, 1977). In cases like this, people's reliance on introspection can lead them astray in inferring their true preferences (Wilson et al., 1993, 1995).

In one experiment, Wilson and colleagues (1993) asked college students to choose among several posters that they could keep. Some students were instructed that before making their choice they should introspect about that choice and about the reasons for it. In the end, those participants were not as happy with their choice as were their peers who did not analyze the reasons for their preference. The former group placed too much weight on the introspective content that they happened to generate, and this blinded them to their more enduring attitudes. More generally, this research on the effects of analyzing reasons demonstrates how people can get into trouble by trying to access something (the reasons for their feelings) to which they do not have access, but think they do. The result is ironic: People can find themselves unhappy with their decisions not because they failed to think about them but because they thought about them too much (and in the wrong way).

Free Will

It is highly unlikely that we will see the debate over the existence of free will resolved anytime soon. The debate has raged for eons, and smart people just disagree about whether humans have free will. In the case of most of the complex actions we take and decisions we make, it is probably impossible to assess whether they were the product of free will.

One potential reason why the free-will debate continues to rage is that people have dueling intuitions about whether free will exists, and those depend on whether it is their *own* free will or *others'* free will being considered (Pronin & Kugler, 2011). When we think about ourselves, we have an internal sense of free will. We feel as though our desires and intentions precede and influence our actions, and that when critical decision points arise we choose what path to take. However, when we think about others, we often feel that their decisions were predictable in advance, by their personality traits, their background, and so forth. In a series of experiments, Pronin and Kugler (2011) explored this self–other asymmetry. In one study, college students saw their own futures and pasts as less predictable a priori than those of their peers. This self–other difference was associated with students' viewing their own futures as best predicted by looking to their ongoing intentions and preferences, while viewing others' futures as best predicted by preexisting personality traits.

Illusions of Self-Knowledge in Social Interaction

Thus far in this chapter we have looked at how the introspection illusion influences people's thoughts about their traits, abilities, decisions, and behavior. We now turn to the realm of social interaction, and to how illusions of self-knowledge resulting from introspection affect the ways in which people see themselves and others in social settings. We look at illusions of self-knowledge as they pertain to how "knowable" people think they appear to others (and vice versa), and as they pertain to how people think their disclosures are perceived and interpreted by others.

Perceiving Others' Knowledge of Us

People think that their self-knowledge is superior to others' self-knowledge. Indeed, they sometimes are so skeptical of others' self-knowledge that they think they know others better than those others know themselves (although they rarely have the reverse belief involving others' knowledge of them exceeding their own self-knowledge). This phenomenon was demonstrated in a series of experiments by Pronin, Kruger, Savitsky, and Ross (2001). For example, in one experiment, college roommates reported on their own and their roommate's self-knowledge, as well as their own and their roommate's knowledge of each other. The roommates generally reported that they knew themselves better than their roommate knew *themselves*—and that, for some dimensions (e.g., messiness), their knowledge of their roommate exceeded that roommate's self-knowledge.

In a series of follow-up studies, Pronin and colleagues (2001) explored the source of these effects. It involved individuals' tendency to define themselves in terms of unobservable characteristics at the same time that they defined others in terms of observable characteristics. For example, individuals thought that what defined them was more like the part of the iceberg that lies "below the surface," in comparison to others, whose defining characteristics they saw as more above the surface. Also, when asked to write descriptions of when they were most like themselves, or when their close friend was most like him- or herself, their descriptions again differed on this dimension. Coders rated the self-descriptions as more likely to involve private and unobservable features (e.g., personal thoughts and musings) than the other-descriptions. Individuals tend to assume that in their own case self-knowledge derives from looking inward but that others may best gain self-knowledge by looking at observable behavior—notably, the same behavior to which an outsider with sufficient opportunities could be privy.

While we often see ourselves as uniquely hidden, there also are times when we feel the complete opposite—when we think that our inner selves are *transparent* to those around us. This apparently opposing phenomenon can be reconciled by considering the heavy weight that people place on introspective information. In particular, people experience so-called "illusions of transparency" in cases where they are acutely aware of their internal experiences and that awareness causes them to lose sight of others' ignorance (Gilovich, Savitsky, & Medvec, 1998). When we experience strong emotions, for example, we may feel so aware of our internal emotional state that we believe it is being externally projected to those around us. It seems reasonable to us that if we feel something incredibly strongly, everyone around us must notice. It turns out, however, that even in times of extreme embarrassment, we do not garner nearly as much attention as our internal lives insist we merit.

Illusions and Thwarted Intimacy

A fundamental way in which people come to know each other is through self-disclosure. However, people do not seem to accurately understand the impact of their own self-disclosures. That lack of understanding constitutes a type of illusion of self-knowledge, as actors think they know how their revelations come across when in fact they do not. As a consequence, when people self-disclose they may ironically create distance while seeking intimacy.

A common disclosure when seeking intimacy with another person involves talking about what one *values*. People cherish their most important values—whether those be maintaining close family relationships, pursuing a satisfying career, staying healthy and fit, or keeping one's faith—and the intensity with which people hold those values may lead them to assume that "opening up" about them is an intimate and personally revealing thing to do. Pronin, Fleming, and Steffel (2008) found that people indeed view their value disclosures as revealing, but that recipients of those disclosures instead view them as banal and uninformative. For example, in one experiment, pairs of college students were instructed to open up to each other about their most important values. After doing so, the students felt that they had opened up to their partner but that their partner had revealed little to them. This asymmetry was found to be rooted in weight given to introspection: When individuals disclosed to another, they saw their disclosure as revealing because they heavily weighted the intense internal feelings that they associated with their most important values; when individuals were the recipient of another's disclosure, by contrast, they instead judged the disclosure by the overt behavior it entailed. That overt behavior generally involved a brief and commonplace disclosure about a value shared by most people.

While people are quick to disclose their values, they often shudder to open up about their more negative qualities, such as their fears and insecurities. This poses a problem for establishing intimacy, as people are likely to feel that others cannot truly know or love them if those others only know the good things. Research by Gromet and Pronin (2009) suggests that people are incorrect in assessing how others will react to their revelations of fears and insecurities. In a series of experiments, Gromet and Pronin asked college students to reveal personal fears and insecurities (or more positive qualities) to a peer and then to rate how much that peer would like them after hearing the negative (or positive) disclosure. Other students in each experiment served as recipients rather than as disclosers, and they heard a peer's disclosure (negative or positive) and then rated how much they liked that peer. The experiments showed that disclosers of personal fears and insecurities assumed that recipients would like them far less than those recipients actually did following the disclosure. The roots of this asymmetry rested in disclosers' inability to escape from their own introspective awareness. Specifically, disclosers assessed how their revelations would be perceived by focusing on the negativity they associated with their fears and insecurities. By doing so, they failed to recognize that, from the perspective of recipients, those disclosures indicated the positive and intimacy-building qualities of openness, genuineness, and honesty. Recipients were more affected by the honesty and genuineness that they associated with the "negative" disclosures than by the negative content of the disclosures themselves.

Taken together, the research by Pronin, Fleming, and Steffel (2008) and by Gromet and Pronin (2009) conveys an important message about self-disclosures. People misperceive what is conveyed by their own self-disclosures and, as a result, their attempts at intimacy can be thwarted. They may think they are opening up when they reveal their values, but those on the other side may instead feel rebuffed by the banality of those disclosures. In contrast, people may shy away from opening up about fears and insecurities even though they crave such disclosures for establishing intimacy, when in fact those disclosures would be perceived in a positive light.

Illusions and Social Conflict

Imagine how an argument between two people would be affected by both individuals' ignorance of their own biases. This ignorance, or "bias blind spot," is a profound illusion of self-knowledge that has important consequences for social conflict. First, it generally leads people to view their adversaries' positions as biased. If two people disagree and each is convinced that he or she sees things "as they are," then each is likely to conclude that it must be the *other* person whose views are clouded by the distorting lenses of self-interest, ideology, and so forth (Pronin, Gilovich, & Ross, 2004; Ross

& Ward, 1995). Where does this leave the disagreeing parties? A second consequence issuing from the bias blind spot involves the escalating conflict that typically results from people's perception that their adversary is biased (Kennedy & Pronin, 2008, 2012; Pronin, Kennedy, & Butsch, 2006).

In a series of experiments, Kennedy and Pronin (2008) found that the tendency to see others as biased, while preserving faith in one's own objectivity, is especially prominent in cases of disagreement. Additionally, they found that people react to such bias perceptions with conflict-escalating approaches. For example, in one experiment, undergraduate students were confronted with an adversary who disagreed with them regarding an (allegedly) impending grading policy change at their school. Those who were experimentally induced to see that adversary as biased rather than objective, by virtue of that person's written comments about the policy issue, behaved more aggressively toward that person (according to coders of participants' written responses, and according to participants' own reported intentions). It is not hard to see how this process could elicit a downward spiral of conflict. Indeed, Kennedy and Pronin found that seeing one's adversary as biased leads to more conflictual responding, which in turn leads one's adversary to see one as yet more biased and therefore as deserving aggressive rather than cooperative treatment.

The bias blind spot offers but one example of how illusions of self-knowledge can promote and perpetuate social conflict. Another instance involves the sort of self-enhancement illusions reviewed earlier. In that instance, conflict may arise as people discover (or anticipate; e.g., Carlson, Vazire, & Oltmanns, 2011) the gulf between how they see themselves and how others see them. That gulf is likely to make self-perceivers feel disrespected and underestimated by those around them, while making those others feel frustrated by the apparent arrogance and self-delusion of those with whom they are dealing.

Overcoming the Illusions

Our overreliance on introspection clearly produces illusions of self-knowledge that can have negative consequences. In our concluding section, we explore a number of ways in which people may be able to "overcome" their problematic overreliance on introspection.

Education and Experience

Experience

We sometimes can get beyond our overoptimistic illusions about the self through life experience. For example, Kulik and Mahler (1987) found that students who were already suffering from an acute illness, compared to healthy students, were more realistic about their risk for future health problems. Unfortunately, they remained as overoptimistic as their peers in non-health domains. Another study found that students who had recently survived an earthquake became more realistic about the possibility of being in other natural disasters (Burger & Palmer, 1992). This return to realism was again, however, situation-specific and was found to have dissipated 3 months later.

Introspective Education

Pronin and Kugler (2007) tested a form of education that directly targeted people's reliance on introspection. The prediction was that educating people about the limits of introspection would lessen a classic effect linked to introspective overweighting (i.e., people's blindness to their own biases). In one experiment, half of the participants read an article detailing a number of social-psychological phenomena that occur nonconsciously, such as implicit prejudice effects. The article was titled "Unaware of Our Unawareness" after the classic article by Nisbett and Wilson (1977) and the related quotation in Wilson, Hodges, and LaFleur (1995, p. 17). By focusing on the importance of nonconscious processes, it offered a heavy dose of evidence regarding the perils of relying on introspection. The other half of the participants read an unrelated article and served as a control condition. Participants then completed a standard bias blind spot measure, in which they rated their susceptibility relative to their peers to a number of common biases.

Pronin and Kugler (2007) found that while those in the control condition showed the usual bias blind spot, those who received introspective education did not display a bias blind spot (and the two conditions differed significantly from each other). This finding suggests that *introspective education*—education about nonconscious processes, the limits of introspection, and the perils of overweighting introspective information—is a promising tool for helping individuals to attain more accurate self-knowledge.

Ignoring Introspection

If introspection misleads us, then it seems logical that one way to correct for this would be to pay less attention to introspection and more to behavior. In one experiment, researchers instructed people to ignore their subjective, internal experiences when making a decision for which they would normally show extreme temporal discounting (Pronin, Olivola, & Kennedy, 2008). People were asked to decide whether or not they would defer a more proximal monetary reward in favor of a larger monetary reward further in the future. They were asked to make this decision either for themselves now (i.e., choose between $50 now vs. $65 in a couple of months), for a fellow student now, or for a future self (i.e., choose between $50 in a couple of months vs. $65 a couple of months after that). Without any special instructions, most people displayed temporal discounting when choosing for the present self (i.e., preferring $50 now) but did not show that discounting for a future self or other. A fourth experimental condition tested whether the discounting effect for present selves would be eliminated if participants were given instructions to ignore current introspective experience. When participants were instructed to make a decision for the present self, while diverting their attention from their ongoing emotions, the discounting effect diminished powerfully—that is, participants chose the larger more distal reward as often as they had for future selves or others (see Figure 21.2).

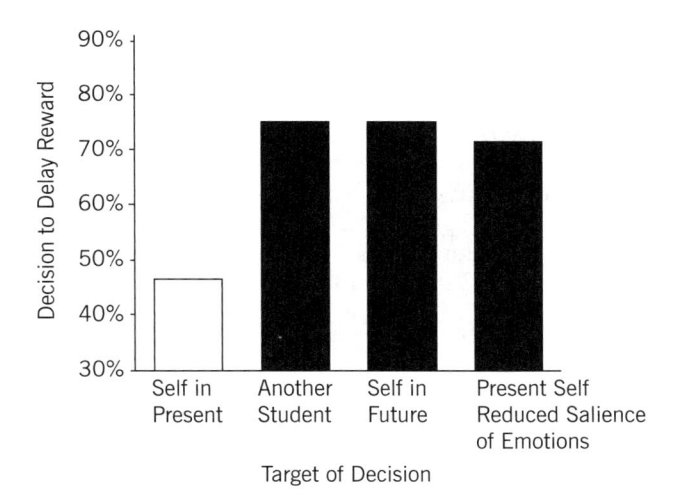

FIGURE 21.2. Decisions to defer a lottery reward on behalf of the present self, the future self, a fellow student, or the present self with that self's attention diverted from ongoing emotions. From Pronin, Olivola, and Kennedy (2008). Copyright 2008 by Sage Publications. Reprinted by permission.

Returning to Delphi: Self-Knowledge from Others' Knowledge

Time and again, research has shown that others sometimes know us better than we know ourselves. Our peers and even complete strangers can sometimes predict our behavior better than we can (e.g., Epley & Dunning, 2000; Vazire & Mehl, 2008). One explanation for this surprising effect is that others take our behavior into account—a source of information that we too often disregard in favor of introspection. For example, this review has described how others are more likely than ourselves to recognize our bias, and our conformity, because of those others' attention to behavioral information that we disregard.

There is a larger message here, and one implied in this chapter's introduction: The perspectives of others have much to offer us in the pursuit of self-knowledge. Indeed, in cases where illusions of self-knowledge are common, we may be better off adopting others' perspectives on us than attending to our own. Of course, this message is likely to be hard for most of us to accept, as the ultimate illusion of self-knowledge may be our blindness to the very illusions that distort our self-knowledge. Trekking to the Oracle of Delphi may not have provided the answer to all quests for self-knowledge, but the arduousness of that path does tell us something quite true about the difficulty of the quest for self-knowledge.

ACKNOWLEDGMENT

This material is based on work supported by the National Science Foundation (Grant No. 0742394).

REFERENCES

Alicke, M. D. (1985). Global self-evaluation as determined by the desirability and controllability of trait adjectives. *Journal of Personality and Social Psychology, 49,* 1621–1630.

Burger, J. M., & Palmer, M. (1992). Changes in and generalization of unrealistic optimism following experiences from stressful events: Reactions to the 1989 California earthquake. *Personality and Social Psychology Bulletin, 18,* 39–43.

Carlson, E. N., Vazire, S., & Oltmanns, T. F. (2011). You probably think this paper's about you: Narcissists' perceptions of their personality and reputation. *Journal of Personality and Social Psychology, 101*(1), 185–201.

Chartrand, T. L., & Bargh, J. A. (1999). The chameleon effect: The perception–behavior link and social interaction. *Journal of Personality and Social Psychology, 76,* 893–910.

Cross, P. (1977). Not can but *will* college teaching be improved? *New Directions for Higher Education, 17,* 1–15.

Darley, J. M., & Latane, B. (1968). Bystander intervention in emergencies: Diffusion of responsibility. *Journal of Personality and Social Psychology, 8,* 377–383.

Devine, P. G. (1989). Stereotypes and prejudice: Their automatic and controlled components. *Journal of Personality and Social Psychology, 56,* 5–18.

Dovidio, J. F., Kawakami, K., & Gaertner, S. L. (2002). Implicit and explicit prejudice and interracial interaction. *Journal of Personality and Social Psychology, 82,* 62–68.

Dunning, D. (2005). *Self-insight: Roadblocks and detours on the path to knowing thyself.* New York: Psychology Press.

Dunning, D., Heath, C., & Suls, J. M. (2004). Flawed self-assessment: Implications for health, education, and the workplace. *Psychological Science in the Public Interest, 5,* 69–100.

Dunning, D., Meyerowitz, J. A., & Holzberg, A. D. (1989). Ambiguity and self-evaluation: The role of idiosyncratic trait definitions in self-serving assessments of ability. *Journal of Personality and Social Psychology, 57,* 1082–1090.

Ehrlinger, J., Gilovich, T., & Ross, L. (2005). Peering into the bias blind spot: People's assessments of bias in themselves and others. *Personality and Social Psychology Bulletin, 31,* 680–692.

Epley, N., & Dunning, D. (2000). Feeling "holier than thou": Are self-serving assessments produced by errors in self or social prediction? *Journal of Personality and Social Psychology, 79,* 861–875.

Friedrich, J. (1996). On seeing oneself as less self-serving than others: The ultimate self-serving bias? *Teaching of Psychology, 23,* 107–109.

Gilbert, D. T. (1993). The assent of man: Mental representation and the control of belief. In D. M. Wegner & J. W. Pennebaker (Eds.), *The handbook of mental control* (pp. 57–87). Englewood Cliffs, NJ: Prentice-Hall.

Gilbert, D. T., Pinel, E. C., Wilson, T. D., Blumberg, S. J., & Wheatley, T. P. (1998). Immune neglect: A source of durability bias in affective forecasting. *Journal of Personality and Social Psychology, 75,* 617–638.

Gilovich, T., Savitsky, K., & Medvec, V. H. (1998). The illusion of transparency: Biased assessments of others' ability to read one's emotional states. *Journal of Personality and Social Psychology, 75,* 332–346.

Greenwald, A. G., & Banaji, M. R., (1995). Implicit social cognition: Attitudes, self-esteem, and stereotypes. *Psychological Review, 102,* 4–27.

Gromet, D. M., & Pronin, E. (2009). What were you worried about?: Actors' concerns about revealing fears and insecurities relative to observers' reactions. *Self and Identity, 8,* 342–364.

Hansen, K. E., Pronin, E., Gerbasi, M., & Todorov, A. (2011). *Unaffected by bias: The effects of knowingly utilizing a biased strategy.* Unpublished manuscript.

Hansford, B. C., & Hattie, J. A. (1982). The relationship between self and achievement/performance measures. *Review of Educational Research, 52*, 123–142.

Kennedy, K. A., & Pronin, E. (2008). When disagreement gets ugly: Perceptions of bias and the escalation of conflict. *Personality and Social Psychology Bulletin, 34*, 833–848.

Kennedy, K. A., & Pronin, E. (2012). Bias perception and the spiral of conflict. In J. Hanson (Ed.), *Ideology, psychology, and law* (pp. 410–446). New York: Oxford University Press.

Klein, C., & Helweg-Larson, M. (2002). Perceived control and the optimistic bias: A meta-analytic review. *Psychology and Health, 17*, 437–446.

Kruger, J. (1999). Lake Wobegon be gone!: The "below-average effect" and the egocentric nature of comparative ability judgments. *Journal of Personality and Social Psychology, 77*, 221–232.

Kulik, J., & Mahler, H. (1987). Health status, perceptions of risk and prevention interest for health and nonhealth problems. *Health Psychology, 6*, 15–27.

Langer, E. J. (1975). The illusion of control. *Journal of Personality and Social Psychology, 32*, 311–328.

Mabe, P. A., III, & West, S. G. (1982). Validity of self-evaluation of ability: A review and meta-analysis. *Journal of Applied Psychology, 67*, 280–286.

Matute, H. (1996). Illusion of control: Detecting response-outcome independence in analytic but not in naturalistic conditions. *Psychological Science, 7*, 289–293.

Moore, D. A., & Small, D. A. (2007). Error and bias in comparative judgment: On being both better and worse than we think we are. *Journal of Personality and Social Psychology, 92*, 972–989.

Mueller, P., & Pronin, E. (2012). [Blinding procedures as evaluated by the self and others]. Unpublished raw data.

Nisbett, R. E., & Ross, L. (1980). *Human inference: Strategies and shortcomings of social judgment.* Englewood Cliffs, NJ: Prentice-Hall.

Nisbett, R. E., & Wilson, T. D. (1977). Telling more than we can know: Verbal reports on mental processes. *Psychological Review, 84*, 231–259.

Pronin, E. (2008). How we see ourselves and how we see others. *Science, 320*, 1177–1180.

Pronin, E. (2009). The introspection illusion. *Advances in Experimental Social Psychology, 41*, 1–66.

Pronin, E., Berger, J. A., & Molouki, S. (2007). Alone in a crowd of sheep: Asymmetric perceptions of conformity and their roots in an introspection illusion. *Journal of Personality and Social Psychology, 92*, 585–595.

Pronin, E., Fleming, J. J., & Steffel, M. (2008). Value revelations: Disclosure is in the eye of the beholder. *Journal of Personality and Social Psychology, 95*, 795–809.

Pronin, E., Gilovich, T., & Ross, L. (2004). Objectivity in the eye of the beholder: Divergent perceptions of bias in self versus others. *Psychological Review, 111*, 781–799.

Pronin, E., Kennedy, K., & Butsch, S. (2006). Bombing versus negotiating: How preferences for combating terrorism are affected by perceived terrorist rationality. *Basic and Applied Social Psychology, 28*, 385–392.

Pronin, E., Kruger, J., Savitsky, K., & Ross, L. (2001). You don't know me, but I know you: The illusion of asymmetric insight. *Journal of Personality and Social Psychology, 81*, 639–656.

Pronin, E., & Kugler, M. B. (2007). Valuing thoughts, ignoring behavior: The introspection illusion as a source of the bias blind spot. *Journal of Experimental Social Psychology, 43*, 565–578.

Pronin, E., & Kugler, M. B. (2011). People believe they have more free will than others. *Proceedings of the National Academy of Sciences USA, 107*, 22469–22474.

Pronin, E., Lin, D. Y., & Ross, L. (2002). The bias blind spot: Perceptions of bias in self versus others. *Personality and Social Psychology Bulletin, 28,* 369–381.

Pronin, E., Olivola, C. Y., & Kennedy, K. A. (2008). Doing unto future selves as you would do unto others: Psychological distance and decision making. *Personality and Social Psychology Bulletin, 34,* 224–236.

Pronin, E., Wegner, D. M., McCarthy, K., & Rodriguez, S. (2006). Everyday magical powers: The role of apparent mental causation in the overestimation of personal influence. *Journal of Personality and Social Psychology, 91,* 218–231.

Read, D., & van Leeuwen, B. (1998). Time and desire: The effects of anticipated and experienced hunger and delay to consumption on the choice between healthy and unhealthy snack food. *Organizational Behavior and Human Decision Processes, 76,* 189–205.

Robins, R. W., & Beer, J. S. (2001). Positive illusions about the self: Short-term benefits and long-term costs. *Journal of Personality and Social Psychology, 80,* 340–352.

Ross, L., & Ward, A. (1995). Psychological barriers to dispute resolution. *Advances in Experimental Social Psychology, 27,* 255–304.

Taylor, S. E., & Brown, J. D. (1988). Illusion and well-being: A social psychological perspective on mental health. *Psychological Bulletin, 103,* 193–210.

Taylor, S. E., Lerner, J. S., Sherman, D. K., Sage, R. M., & McDowell, N. K. (2003). Are self-enhancing cognitions associated with healthy or unhealthy biological profiles? *Journal of Personality and Social Psychology, 85,* 605–615.

Vazire, S., & Mehl, M. R. (2008). Knowing me, knowing you: The accuracy and unique predictive validity of self-rating and other-ratings of daily behavior. *Journal of Personality and Social Psychology, 95,* 1202–1216.

Wegner, D. M. (2004). Précis of *The illusion of conscious will*. *Behavioral and Brain Sciences, 27,* 649–692.

Weinstein, N. D. (1980). Unrealistic optimism about future life events. *Journal of Personality and Social Psychology, 58,* 806–820.

Weinstein, N. D., & Lachendro, E. (1982). Egocentrism as a source of unrealistic optimism. *Personality and Social Psychology Bulletin, 8,* 195–200.

Wilson, T. D. (2002). *Strangers to ourselves: Discovering the adaptive unconscious*. Cambridge, MA: Belknap/Harvard University Press.

Wilson, T. D., & Brekke, N. (1994). Mental contamination and mental correction: Unwanted influences on judgments and evaluations. *Psychological Bulletin, 116,* 117–142.

Wilson, T. D., & Gilbert, D. T. (2003). Affective forecasting. *Advances in Experimental Social Psychology, 35,* 345–411.

Wilson, T. D., Hodges, S. D., & LaFleur, S. J. (1995). Effects of introspecting about reasons: Inferring attitudes from accessible thoughts. *Journal of Personality and Social Psychology, 69,* 16–28.

Wilson, T. D., Lisle, D. J., Schooler, J. W., Hodges, S. D., Klaaren, K. J., & LaFleur, S. J. (1993). Introspecting about reasons can reduce post-choice satisfaction. *Personality and Social Psychology Bulletin, 19,* 331–339.

CHAPTER 22
Classic Self-Deception Revisited

DELROY L. PAULHUS
ERIN BUCKELS

In common parlance, *self-deception* is the act of lying to oneself. When more rigorous definitions are attempted, this straightforward notion quickly becomes complex, if not impossibly paradoxical. Especially problematic is the assumption that self-deception is analogous to deceiving others. These difficulties have undermined the feasibility of operationalizing the concept and conducting research. Despite this checkered history, the possibility of confirming the existence self-deception remains so seductive that we enter the fray one more time.

Rather than clarifying the concept, the theoretical literature on self-deception has become more abstruse and unwieldy. Recent treatises and responses thereto confirm the lack of consensus (e.g.,McKay & Dennett, 2009; Mele, 1997). Instead, we see a diversity of competing but overlapping and intertwining concepts. Blatant challenges include recommendations to replace self-deception with concepts such as bad faith (Sartre, 1943/1982), disavowal of engagement (Fingarette, 1969), wishful thinking (Szabados, 1985), akrasia (Pears, 1984), positive illusions (Taylor & Brown, 1988), and the adaptive unconscious (Wilson, 2002).

The advent of psychology's cognitive revolution encouraged the study of more empirically tractable concepts such as confirmation bias (Kunda, 1990), self-signaling (Mijovic-Prelec & Prelec, 2010), dynamic complexity (Paulhus & Suedfeld, 1988), ethical fading (Tenbrunsel & Messick, 2004), cognitive avoidance (Greenwald, 1997), self-serving processing (von Hippel, Lakin, & Shakarchi, 2005), and time discounting (Ainslie, 1997). As he had done with other psychological conundra, Zajonc (1980) opened the door with evidence that affect and cognition follow independent routes to awareness. Thus, the information-processing approach easily incorporates the dual processing implicit in self-deception.

Serious consideration of this plethora of conceptual competitors is beyond the mandate of this chapter. Instead, a brief summary of the key issues will have to suffice (the first section of the chapter). We then turn to several influential operationalizations that have led most directly to empirical investigation. Ultimately, we single out one of these—the Quattrone–Tversky paradigm—to generate and explain new data on the curious phenomenon of cheating on practice tests (the second section). Finally, we summarize and critique the individual-difference literature (the third section).

Overview of the Issues

Everyday Self-Deception

We begin by pointing to a common but puzzling observation: People sometimes appear to believe something that they must know is false. As observers, we conclude that such behavior is self-deceptive because the contradictory evidence should be obvious to all—especially the perpetrator. This phenomenon goes well beyond exaggeration, faking, or simple lying: In those cases, the individual is aware of uttering a falsehood. Instead, self-deception seems to be something deeper and more complicated—even paradoxical.

Consider some anecdotal examples. An otherwise pleasant young man is clearly an alcoholic but bridles at others saying so. He refuses to acknowledge the truth even though the evidence is obvious: There are empty bottles hidden throughout his apartment, and his boss has often sent him home for drinking on the job. Again, it doesn't count as self-deception if he knows he's an alcoholic but is simply lying about it.

Consider another case, where a young woman has a deep-seated hatred of her mother but cannot admit it to herself. The signs of this hatred are abundant: She angers quickly at any mention of her mother and makes a face when forced to discuss her. Perhaps the young woman cannot admit her feelings because much guilt and shame would surely ensue. What kind of horrible person hates her mother—the one who brought her into this world and sacrificed to raise her?

Consider the father who cannot believe that his only son, his pride and joy, is actually guilty of the heinous crimes alleged by the police. Because his reason for living would be shattered, the father cannot allow himself to believe the accusations. But he winces at every ring of the phone, fearing that it is the police calling (once again) about his son's latest misdeed.

The more carefully one analyzes such cases, the fuzzier the notion of self-deception becomes. The apparent duality of thought seems to implicate some process equivalent to the psychoanalytic unconscious: That traditional framework easily accommodates cases where an emotional conflict influences an individual's behavior while remaining inaccessible. At a conscious level, details about the conflict are unavailable or, at least, obscure. The unconscious, however, "knows" the truth. This terminology has proved so useful in framing complex behavior that it is now part of everyday lay conversations (Westen, 1998).

Unfortunately, such anecdotes—whether from personal experience or insights from clinicians—constitute the bulk of the evidence for the existence of self-deception. Before we describe the limited empirical literature, two other sources of evidence warrant mention.

Soft Versions of Self-Deception

People are often inaccurate about aspects of their lives. But few of these self-inaccuracies implicate a self-deceptive process. Some follow from systematic limitations in our self-knowledge (Kihlstrom, 2001; Wilson, 1985). Others result from simple misinformation. For example, you may not have been told that you were adopted: In that case, you may have been purposely deceived by others. Or you may believe that you have a genius-level IQ because you accidently misscored a take-home IQ test. Your recall of the fact that you hated your parents at age 10 may have faded along with other early memories. None of these cases qualifies as self-deception.

Other everyday phenomena seem to smack of self-deception but are less dramatic. They might be labeled as "soft" self-deception. You might set your watch 10 minutes ahead to ensure that you get to an appointment on time. How can that possibly work? You know very well your watch is 10 minutes fast. Yet people say it helps them to be on time—perhaps because the initial conclusion that they are late shocks them into action. Or take procrastination: Although the strategy has never paid off before, we again put off making that unpleasant phone call. Our intellectual powers allow us to devise impressive rationalizations for staying longer in bed or waiting until the last minute to write a paper.

It is a stretch to label such cases as self-deception. They are better placed into the category of crude coping mechanisms. When confronted, perpetrators immediately acknowledge the facts. The term *self-deception* should be reserved for cases where strong psychological forces prevent us from acknowledging a threatening truth about ourselves.

Evolutionary Basis

But isn't truth distortion inherently maladaptive? Not so, according to a growing number of writers taking an evolutionary perspective. They argue that human beings engage in self-deception because it is built into the genes of our species (Lockard & Paulhus, 1988; Trivers, 1985). According to evolutionary theory, such psychological tendencies were gradually insinuated into our genetic makeup. The genes of individuals lacking this mechanism suffered a reproductive disadvantage (Krebs & Denton, 1997; Krebs, Denton, & Higgins, 1988).

But how could such irrationality be adaptive? One argument is that complete awareness of our motives would interfere with effectively satisfying them (Trivers, 1985). Believing that something is true facilitates its coming to fruition (Starek & Keating, 1991; von Hippel & Trivers, 2011). For example, confidence in making the Olympic team is a necessary (but not sufficient) condition for making the dream come true. Fending off an attacker is facilitated by exaggerated confidence. In both cases, however, there are negative consequences to inaccuracy: In the first case, one may delay reproduction with 4 years of futile workouts; in the second case, one may unnecessarily put life at risk. Overall, however, there is good reason to believe that a modicum of self-deception is adaptive (Baumeister, 1993).

Such arguments set the stage for debates over the existence of self-deception. If evolutionarily coherent, then self-deception does not have to be viewed as a human aberration (Lockard & Paulhus, 1988).

Theoretical History and Background

Self-deception is often discussed in the context of psychoanalytic theory. Rather than one of many defense mechanisms, self-deception is thought to be a necessary component of all psychoanalytic defenses (Sackeim, 1988). Each one entails the paradoxical element noted earlier: There must be at least one moment of self-deception for the successful operation of a defense mechanism. Readers familiar with defenses such as projection, intellectualization, and repression will understand the argument that, in each case, a person has to be both unaware and hyperaware of the disturbing information (Lockie, 2003; Westen, 1998).

Cases where the biased belief is maintained under continual confrontation might be labeled *deep self-deception*. As in the psychoanalytic notion of repression, some conflicts may quickly be resolved in favor of the psychologically comfortable option: Subsequently, an anxiety signal triggers an avoidance process that helps maintain the contradictory state with no further confrontation.

As a result, psychoanalytic theory has always been pessimistic about the possibility of people recognizing their own self-deceptions. However, clinicians and nonclinicians alike believe that insight is possible at some point down the line ("I must have been self-deceived about that relationship"). Such insight may not be possible until strong affect has subsided and a more objective analysis is possible. This psychoanalytic perspective continues to have broad appeal (see Paulhus, Fridhandler, & Hayes, 1997).

Skepticism

Over 70 years ago, Freud's ideas about self-deception were attacked by the celebrated philosopher, Jean-Paul Sartre. Along with many nonphilosophers, Sartre (1943/1982) dismissed the idea of self-deception as impossible. How can one know something and not know it at the same time?

This criticism continues to resonate with some contemporary commentators (Gergen, 1997; Kihlstrom, 2001; Szabados, 1985). They remain dubious about the very existence of deep self-deception. Some of this criticism smacks of residual antipathy toward psychoanalysis. Other writers seem concerned that the label of self-deception lets perpetrators off the moral hook (Fingarette, 1969). Other critics are simply skeptical about a processing system that requires monitoring and management of potentially upsetting self-knowledge. Continuous monitoring would require significant cognitive resources. Such cases, they argue, are better described as suppression, mental control, self-regulation, or repetitive coping (for a variety of sources, see Wegner & Pennebaker, 1993). Again, this suppression task would seem downright impossible without some awareness of the threatening thought.

Information Processing

Surprising to some early critics was the fact that the feasibility of self-deception has been supported by some of the most rigorous research in cognitive psychology. There is no longer any debate about the fact that many processes operate without awareness.

Moreover, we now know that the human cognitive apparatus allows for multiple representations of the same stimulus: Indeed, the modular nature of the brain allows for contradictory information to be stored in two different parts of the brain (Fodor, 1983). Finally, we also know that emotional aspects of a stimulus are processed more quickly than is the content. For example, it has been shown that, with a polygraph, the emotional impact of a word can be detected before the word is understood consciously (Zajonc, 1980).

Given the solid evidence for these cognitive processes, the possibility of self-deception becomes quite feasible. Several of these dual-process theories have been reviewed by Chaiken and Trope (1999; see also Gawronski & Bodenhausen, Chapter 3, this volume). In all these theories, one process deals with the informational content of the stimulus; the other with the emotional content. Moreover, the emotional system operates more quickly, thereby allowing the mind to set up preemptive roadblocks for the unacceptable. Greenwald's (1997) "junk-mail" analogy nicely explains how disturbing evidence can be overlooked indefinitely by responding with avoidance tactics to prevent any prospect of it surfacing.

Beyond Motivated Cognition

With this body of research in mind, Mele (1997) attempted to "deflate" the language of self-deception by arguing that all such phenomena can be reduced to various types of motivated cognition (Kunda, 1990). Others (including yours truly) disagree. A satisfactory explanation of self-deception requires not only motivated cognition but also the additional feature of discrepant representations. Its uniqueness may follow from the direct involvement of the self. To aid in their decision, readers should explore the review of motivated cognition by Helzer and Dunning (Chapter 23, this volume).

Experimental Inductions

So far we have established that (1) clinicians are confident that certain of their patients have deceived themselves, (2) self-deception is compatible with evolutionary psychology, and (3) the human information-processing system allows for self-deception.

On the empirical side, small advances have been made using a variety of operationalizations. For example, researchers have concluded that self-deception is easier in the future than in the present (Robinson & Ryff, 1999) and more likely in private than in public conditions (Smith & Whitehead, 1993). It appears only when a credible excuse is available (Ditto & Lopez, 1992) and when feedback about accuracy is vague (Sloman, Fernbach, & Hagmayer, 2010).

Nonetheless, direct experimental evidence for the existence of self-deception is hard to come by. Of course, it takes just one valid demonstration to confirm the possibility. But such demonstrations have proved to be challenging even in tightly controlled laboratory studies. In fact, only a handful of studies (described below) claim to have confirmed an instance of self-deception. We leave it to the reader to decide whether these studies are convincing or not.

Gur and Sackeim

Harold Sackeim and Ruben Gur are credited with developing systematic criteria for self-deception (Sackeim & Gur, 1978), as well as laying out experimental evidence for its existence (Gur & Sackeim, 1979). Their criteria for demonstrating self-deception included (1) evidence for simultaneous but contradictory beliefs, only one of which is conscious, and (2) evidence that this discrepancy is motivated.

Their experimental paradigm built on the fact that people typically find the sound of their own voices to be aversive. Subjects were asked to distinguish their own from a series of voices and indicate so by saying "me" or "not me." Under certain conditions, subjects failed to acknowledge hearing their own voices.

At the same time subjects were hooked up to a polygraph that measured emotional responses to the voices. In short, the experimental setup provided two sources of information about whether the subjects recognized their own voices—an oral response, and an emotional response measured by polygraph.

Although the polygraph invariably showed a blip in reaction to the subject's own voice, the oral response was often inaccurate. In particular, *false denials were common*: Subjects said "not me" even though the polygraph invariably detected their voices. Such false denials suggested a bifurcation of awareness: The individual knows something and does not know it at the same time.

The researchers also predicted systematic changes in false denials depending on the need to avoid self-confrontation. This need was induced in some subjects by threatening their self-esteem using a standard failure induction. Indeed, after subjects' self-esteem was threatened, the frequency of false denials increased.

According to Sackeim and Gur (1978), false denials indicate that subjects believe X and do not believe X at the same time. Moreover, this lack of awareness is motivated by intrapsychic concerns (maintaining self-esteem). Together, the experiments appear to demonstrate an instance of self-deception. Of course, they do not address how widespread the phenomenon is. Instead, they point out that a single instance is all that is required to confirm that self-deception is possible.

The need for such elaborate laboratory orchestration is not without its critics. The artificiality and complexity of the Sackeim–Gur paradigm does little to convince many observers that self-deception is at large in everyday life.

Quattrone and Tversky

The second study claiming to demonstrate self-deception was conducted by psychologists George Quattrone and Amos Tversky (1984). Their theoretical rationale was based on the common belief that changing one's score on any correlated variable can change a significant outcome. For example, assume for the moment that intellectuals tend to smoke pipes. The individual who believes that smoking a pipe will make him into an intellectual is being self-deceptive. Given that doctors are typically the source of bad news about one's health, some individuals choose to avoid doctors. They, too, are engaging in self-deception. Put another way, people often believe that correlation guarantees causation.

Although such beliefs are common, they are more likely (or more irrational) under motivated conditions. As such, Quattrone and Tversky attempted to demonstrate that the experience of pain, which was self-evident under control conditions, could be minimized if its long-term implications were sufficiently serious.

The Pain Paradigm

The experimenters exploited a cold pressor test, where participants are asked to immerse one hand in very cold water and keep it there "as long as you can stand it." Before taking the test, some of the participants were threatened with information about an unfortunate correlate of the pain experience: "People who feel a lot of pain from the cold water have a weakness in their cardiovascular system. This defect leads to early heart attacks and a short lifespan."

Results showed that participants receiving this information rated the task as less painful than did a control group. They even held their hand in the cold water longer. They seemed to be trying to convince themselves that they didn't have the life-threatening cardiovascular defect. They were engaging in self-deception, according to Quattrone and Tversky, because they wouldn't acknowledge—even to themselves—the pain that they surely were experiencing.

A potential concern that participants were simply engaging in impression management. Specifically, they may have minimized their pain reports in the health threat condition to avoid the public embarrassment. The researchers went to great lengths to minimize this possibility. For example, they used two experimenters: one to provide information about health consequences, and another to collect pain reports. See Quattrone and Tversky (1984) for other arguments to counter accusations of impression management.

Another concern was that actual pain, not just its perception, was being modified by such manipulations. This concern was overcome in a conceptual replication recently conducted by Sloman and colleagues (2010). Instead of modifying pain reports, the researchers showed that dot-tracking speed could be increased or decreased by telling participants that tracking speed was associated with higher or lower intelligence. The fact that control over tracking speed is immediate and conscious was used to argue that this motivated behavior was a form of self-deception.

Reflection on the Key Experiments

At this point, readers may or may not be convinced that these studies demonstrate self-deception. What they should be convinced of is that confirmation of self-deception is incredibly difficult. Remember that a convincing experiment has to show that an individual believes something and disbelieves it at the same moment. The Sackeim-Gur (1978) study appears to have accomplished this goal directly; the Quattrone-Tversky (1984) study provides only indirect evidence of contradictory beliefs. On the other hand, the latter paradigm better captures everyday self-deception and permits any number of follow-up studies to explore the theoretical issues.

Cheating On Practice Tests

The most recent research exploiting the Quattrone-Tversky paradigm comes from our own laboratory. We have conducted a series of studies on the phenomenon of cheating on practice tests (Buckels & Paulhus, 2011; Paulhus, Nathanson, & Lau, 2005). Although common, this paradoxical behavior seems to meet the Quattrone–Tversky (1984) criteria for self-deception.

To prepare for an important test, it is common for students to take practice versions of the actual test. Preparation courses and handbooks for the SAT, GRE, MCAT, and so forth, do a thriving business and all include practice tests. On the surface, the purpose of practice tests is to diagnose one's current capability in this domain: They are designed to give test takers a realistic sense of where they stand and how much effort remains to reach their desired level of competence.

My discussions with Kaplan employees indicate that clients frequently cheat on the practice tests. In our pretests, we found that more than one-third of students take more than the allotted time on a practice test for the GRE. But if the purpose is realistic self-assessment, then why would anyone cheat on a practice test?

The answer appears to be self-deception for the sake of maintaining a positive self-evaluation. This positivity can be assured with a high score on the practice test. As Quattrone and Tversky (1984) argued, people believe that any change to a predictor will change the outcome: They have confused diagnostic contingencies with causal contingencies.[1] In this case, people seem to believe that even an underhanded way of improving practice test scores will improve their ability to perform better on ability tests in the future. By implication, such improvements will lead to greater scholastic success.

Our Studies

Our laboratory has recently generated several studies designed to confirm this form of self-deception. Following the Quattrone–Tversky (1984) model, we stepped up the motivation for subjects to perform well on (what were described as) GRE practice tests. We also provided them with an opportunity to cheat by taking extra time. As far as participants could tell, such cheating would go undetected. At the same time, the ambiguity of taking a test online would permit subjects to believe the altered results.

Study 1

Participants were randomly assigned to complete a vocabulary test under one of three conditions: (1) a self-enhancement condition, where the test was described as predicting future life success; (2) a reward condition, where a prize of $200 was awarded for a top score; or (3) a control condition. They were advised that the time limit was 8 minutes: This countdown time appeared on the screen in full view at all times. However, the experimenter did not stop participants after 8 minutes.

Despite the fact that participants were well aware of the time limit and of the elapsed time, 37% of participants cheated by taking longer than the allotted time. As expected, participants in the self-enhancement condition displayed the greatest amount of cheating, that is, significantly longer test times than those in the reward and control conditions. Those who cheated were thereby unable to score higher on the test.

Directly after completing the task, participants were asked, "Why did you take extra time?" Those who had taken extra time justified their behavior with comments such as "I was compensating for being distracted" or "Otherwise my score would not represent my true ability." Overall, their message was that the cheated score was more accurate.[2] In short, the motivated subjects had come to believe in their obviously fudged scores.

Study 2

To confirm that a behavior is motivated, the researcher must show that its direction can be reversed (Martin & Tesser, 2009; Sackeim & Gur, 1978). Otherwise, the motivation condition may have induced some other effect (e.g., arousal or distraction) that could explain the extra time taken. Hence, we needed to establish that the effect could be reversed. But is it possible to motivate student participants to perform worse than normal?[3]

To this end, we added a self-handicapping condition to Study 2. This induction was not easily effected: We had to convince educated subjects that doing well on an ability test was indicative of a negative outcome. Eventually, we found one that had some credibility. Drawing on the stereotype that genius and insanity often go hand in hand, we informed subjects about research linking high test scores to the style of creativity often found in people with schizophrenia.

Once again, participants in the self-enhancement condition cheated most (and achieved the highest scores). Participants in the self-handicapping condition cheated least (and scored lowest).

Apparently, self-handicappers found ways to sabotage their own performance! We investigated this apparent sabotage in several ways. First we examined the pattern of work times. Compared to the control condition, the self-handicapping group spent significantly less time working on the items. In fact, their median duration was actually less than the allotted 8 minutes. Not only their overall score but also the proportion of correct answers was lower. Perhaps their effort was reduced; perhaps they purposely put down wrong answers.

See the summary of conditions and results in Table 22.1. Together, these results indicate the self-deceptive nature of cheating on practice tests. Subjects can be motivated to excel or fail on a test that is supposed to inform them about their current ability level. The design and outcomes of our studies are consistent with the Quattrone–Tversky paradigm in indicating that such behavior is part of a more general (and apparently nonconscious) tendency purposely to bias predictors in the direction of desired outcomes.

Bottom Line

Arguably, the key controversy over self-deception centers on whether individuals can ever hold two thoughts that are both simultaneous and contradictory. The consciously proclaimed belief (e.g., "My future is secure") should defer to overwhelming evidence that contradicts it. In the studies reviewed here, subjects' proclaimed beliefs were challenged by direct experience of their pain (Quattrone & Tversky, 1984), by

TABLE 22.1. Summary of Inductions and Outcomes in Our Cheating Research

Induction	Instructions	Test time taken	Test score outcome
Study 1			
1. Enhancement	Good performers go on to successful lives.	8.5 minutes	Highest
2. Monetary reward	Reward of $200 for best performance.	8.3 minutes	Intermediate
3. Control group	No instructions.	8.1 minutes	Lowest
Study 2			
1. Enhancement	Good performers go on to successful lives.	8.5 minutes	Highest
2. Handicapping	People who do well are prone to schizophrenia.	7.9 minutes	Lowest
3. Control group	No instructions.	8.1 minutes	Intermediate

Note. Participants were instructed that the allotted time was 8 minutes but were not prevented from continuing.

observing their contradictory behavior (Sloman et al., 2010), or by observing their own cheating (Paulhus et al., 2005). In all three cases, perpetrators "should" have been aware of the contradictory evidence. Ultimately, this criterion may rest on moral as well as factual grounds (Paulhus, Fridhandler, & Hayes, 1997).

Individual Differences In Self-Deception

The research cited so far has focused on situational inducements/opportunities to engage in self-deception. As early as Frenkel-Brunswik (1939), other writers have focused on individual differences in self-deception. As in the conceptual debates, the focal measurement contrast is self-deception versus other-deception. In other words, the positive bias observed in self-descriptions may be aimed at the self or at others. Cronbach (1945), for example, made this distinction while discussing biases in questionnaire responses. The K scale developed for the Minnesota Multiphasic Personality Inventory (MMPI) was specifically targeted at self-deception. However, the first instrument specifically distinguishing self-deception and other-deception did not arrive until Sackeim and Gur (1978). That measure exhibited a coherent pattern of correlations with the MMPI validity scales.

Later, Paulhus (1984) refined the Gur–Sackeim scales while confirming their distinctiveness. To avoid the connotation of outright lying, the label *other-deception* was replaced with *impression management*. Later psychometric analyses of the Self-Deception Scale prompted the separation of two subscales: Self-Deceptive Enhancement (SDE) and Self-Deceptive Denial (SDD) (Paulhus & Reid, 1991). A further distinction was needed to acknowledge the difference between agentic and communal forms of self-deception (Paulhus, 2002; Paulhus & John, 1998).

The SDE scale taps a form of narcissistic exaggeration and outperforms impression management scales in predicting ego-relevant outcomes. Its correlates include tendencies toward overclaiming (Paulhus, Harms, Bruce, & Lysy, 2003), hindsight bias (Paulhus, 1998b), and other self-favoring biases (Hoorens, 1995). High-SDE individuals also exhibit a discordance with reality, as indicated by a discrepancy in self-ratings of agency relative to ratings by group consensus (Paulhus, 1998a). Nonetheless, SDE correlations with concrete performance are invariably positive (Johnson, 1995; Starek & Keating, 1991). More recently, SDE has also shown utility in moderating the validity of other self-report scales (Otter & Egan, 2007). For example, controlling for SDE served to improve the validity (defined by the correlation with observer ratings) of self-report neuroticism (Berry, Page, & Sackett, 2007).

Indirect operationalizations of individual differences have also been used. One example is the tendency to engage in self-serving bias (SSB) (Ditto & Lopez, 1992; von Hippel et al., 2005). Ditto and Lopez established its cross-situational consistency and showed that the SSB could predict a behavioral index of cheating[4] (von Hippel et al., 2005). Not surprisingly, such indexes are less commonly used than questionnaire measures.

How many types of self-deceptive tendencies are there? Paulhus and John (1998) addressed this question by factoring a set of 60 self-criterion discrepancies calculated from a broad range of personality and ability variables. They isolated two large factors, namely, agentic and communal enhancement. This two-factor model has been replicated by others (Honkaniemi & Feldt, 2008; Lönnqvist, Verkasalo, & Bezmenova, 2007; Vecchione & Alessandri, in press).

Limitations

From the beginning, difficulties in interpretation have dogged social desirability scales (Paulhus, 2002). For the most part, however, the critiques have been directed at impression management scales, based primarily on their overlap with actual positive traits (e.g., Uziel, 2010). To date, we are unaware of any critiques leveled at individual-difference measures of self-deception.

Unfortunately, only modest headway has been achieved in linking the individual-difference research with the definitional criteria for self-deception addressed in the prominent experimental paradigms. The task of diagnosing contradictory beliefs within the same questionnaire has proved especially daunting. Instead, self-deceptive tendencies have been investigated as predictable aspects of established traits (e.g., narcissism) and cultural styles (Lalwani, Shavitt, & Johnson, 2006).

We can point to several research programs that do capture the spirit of dual representation. Instead of the label *self-deception*, those programs have applied terms such as *repression* and *defensiveness* (see Paulhus et al., 1997). The work on repressive style exemplifies the contrast between behavior collected at different levels of awareness (e.g., Bonanno & Singer, 1990; Coifman, Bonanno, Ray, & Gross, 2007; Weinberger, 1990). The extensive body of work on the dynamics of narcissism includes demonstrations of distinctive reactions of narcissists under threat and no-threat conditions (for a review, see Morf & Rhodewalt, 2001). Finally, the dualism model is evident in work contrasting implicit and explicit self-esteem (Jordan, Spencer, Zanna, Hoshino-Browne, & Correll, 2003): Of the four combinations, most fragile is the individual with high explicit and low implicit self-esteem.

Such individuals tend to overreact to criticism by exhibiting extreme negative affect (Kernis & Goldman, 2006). All of these empirically based approaches have supported the conclusion that some individuals more than others manage to maintain multiple representations of the same information—and that one of those representations induces sufficient distress to minimize its full availability to conscious awareness.

Conclusions

Clinicians are certain about the operation of self-deception in some of their patients. Given its complexity, it is not surprising that only a handful of empirical studies claim to have confirmed the phenomenon. Instead, the bulk of writing on self-deception has been published by philosophers who—unlike psychologists—do not have to collect data to support their claims. Based on the work reviewed here, our position is that self-deception research has advanced sufficiently to confirm its existence as a genuine human phenomenon.

Most convincing to us is the research based on the Quattrone–Tversky paradigm, which provides a simple but powerful framework for pursuing the otherwise elusive phenomenon of self-deception. Several laboratories, including our own, have exploited this paradigm and provided conceptual replications of the original operationalization. Using a variety of labels, the search for an effective individual-difference measure continues among personality researchers.

Implications

The notion of self-deception implicates a deep-seated psychological process that eventuates in a distorted self-perception. As in the case of other motivated biases, the victim possesses the information to draw the correct conclusion but, for emotional reasons, does not do so. Self-deception goes further to suggest that both the accurate and inaccurate representations remain active. To regulate dangerous information most effectively, one must, at some level, recognize and manage it. As such, it may be seen as the most extreme version of motivated bias.

The phenomenon of self-deception may play an important, if hidden, role in a variety of human endeavors. Despite its evolutionary roots, the long-term impact of self-deception in the modern world appears to be predominantly toxic (see Leary & Toner, Chapter 25, this volume). It places limitations on the ability of humans to stave off social and political conflict. It impairs any rational approach to financial prosperity. Its psychological mechanism entails an intrapsychic pressure to trade off or, at least, balance two fundamental motivations: People seek accurate information about their world and its complexity; they also need to defend against information that would undermine the values and ideas on which their identities are constructed. It remains to be seen whether our vital intrapsychic lies are best interpreted in moral or factual terms.

NOTES

1. Of course, changing some predictors does benefit future performance: for example, studying the dictionary, reviewing high-school mathematics. These behaviors actually do play a causal role in improving one's abilities, as well as future test scores.

2. Note the contrast with purposeful watch setting: When people are reminded that they purposely set their watch ahead, they immediately acknowledge the real time.

3. Such self-handicapping was successfully induced in recent studies by Sloman et al. (2010).

4. Unfortunately, their self-deception index did not correlate significantly with SDE.

REFERENCES

Ainslie, G. (1997). If belief is a behavior, what controls it? *Behavioral and Brian Sciences, 20*, 102–104.

Baumeister, R. F. (1993). Lying to yourself: The enigma of self-deception. In M. Lewis & C. Saarni (Eds.), *Lying and deception in everyday life* (pp. 166–183). New York: Guilford Press.

Berry, C. M., Page, R. C., & Sackett, P. R. (2007). Effects of self-deceptive enhancement on personality–job performance relationships. *International Journal of Selection and Assessment, 15*, 94–109.

Bonanno, G. A., & Singer, J. L. (1990). Repressive personality style: Theoretical and methodological implications for health and pathology. In J. L. Singer (Ed.), *Repression and dissociation: Implications for personality theory, psychopathology, and health* (pp. 435–470). Chicago: University of Chicago Press.

Buckels, E., & Paulhus, D. L. (2011, June). *Cheating on practice tests: A matter of self-deception?* Paper presented at the annual meeting of the Canadian Psychological Association, Toronto.

Chaiken, S., & Trope, Y. (1999). *Dual-process theories in social psychology.* New York: Guilford Press.

Coifman, K. G., Bonanno, G. A., Ray, R. D., & Gross, J. J. (2007). Does repressive coping promote resilience?: Affective–autonomic response discrepancy during bereavement. *Journal of Personality and Social Psychology, 92*, 745–758.

Cronbach, L. J. (1945). Response sets and test validity. *Educational Psychological Measurement, 6*, 475–494.

Ditto, P. H., & Lopez, D. F. (1992). Motivated skepticism: Use of differential decision criteria for preferred and non-preferred outcomes. *Journal of Personality and Social Psychology, 63*, 568–584.

Fingarette, H. (1969). *Self-deception.* New York: Humanities Press.

Fodor, J. (1983). *The modularity of mind.* Cambridge, MA: MIT Press.

Frenkel-Brunswik, E. (1939). Mechanisms of self-deception. *Journal of Social Psychology, 10*, 409–420.

Gergen, K. J. (1997). Detecting self-deception. *Behavioral and Brain Sciences, 20*, 114–115.

Greenwald, A. G. (1997). Self-knowledge and self-deception: Further consideration. In M.S. Myslobodsky (Ed.), *The mythomanias: The nature of deception and self-deception* (pp. 51–71). Mahwah, NJ: Erlbaum.

Gur, R. C., & Sackeim, H. A. (1979). Self-deception: A concept in search of a phenomenon. *Journal of Personality and Social Psychology, 37*, 147–169.

Honkaniemi, L., & Feldt, T. (2008). Egoistic and moralistic bias in real-life inventory responses. *Personality and Individual Differences, 45,* 397–311.

Hoorens, V. (1995). Self-favoring biases, self-presentation, and the self–other asymmetry in social comparison. *Journal of Personality, 63,* 793–817.

Johnson, E. A. (1995). Self-deceptive responses to threat: Adaptive only in ambiguous circumstances. *Journal of Personality, 63,* 759–791.

Jordan, C. H., Spencer, S. J., Zanna, M. P., Hoshino-Browne, E., & Correll, J. (2003). Secure and defensive high self-esteem. *Journal of Personality and Social Psychology, 85,* 969–978.

Kernis, M. H., & Goldman, B. M. (2006). A multicomponent conceptualization of authenticity: Theory and research. *Advances in Experimental Social Psychology, 38,* 283–357.

Kihlstrom, J. F. (2001). Dissociative disorders. In P. B. Sutker & H. E. Adams (Eds.), *Comprehensive handbook of psychopathology* (3rd ed., pp. 259–276). New York: Plenum Press.

Krebs, D. L., & Denton, K. (1997). Social illusions and self-deception: The evolution of biases in person perception. In J. A. Simpson & D. T. Kenrick (Eds.), *Evolutionary social psychology* (pp. 21–47). Hillsdale, NJ: Erlbaum.

Krebs, D. L., Denton, K., & Higgins, N. (1988). On the evolution of self-knowledge and self-deception. In K. McDonald (Ed.), *Sociobiological perspectives on human behavior* (pp.103–139). New York: Springer-Verlag.

Kunda, Z. (1990). The case for motivated reasoning. *Psychological Bulletin, 108,* 480–498.

Lalwani, A. K., Shavitt, S., & Johnson, T. (2006). What is the relation between cultural orientation and socially desirable responding? *Journal of Personality and Social Psychology, 90,* 165–178.

Lockie, R. (2003). Depth psychology and self-deception. *Philosophical Psychology, 16,* 127–148.

Lockard, J. S., & Paulhus, D. L. (Eds.). (1988). *Self-deception: An adaptive mechanism?* Englewood Cliffs, NJ: Prentice-Hall.

Lönnqvist, J. E., Verkasalo, M., & Bezmenova, I. (2007). Agentic and communal bias in socially desirable responding. *European Journal of Personality, 21,* 853–868.

Martin, L. L., & Tesser, A. (2009). Five markers of motivated behavior. In G. B. Moskowitz & H. Grant (Eds.), *The psychology of goals* (pp. 257–276). New York: Guilford Press.

McKay, R. T., & Dennett, D. C. (2009). The evolution of misbelief. *Behavioral and Brain Sciences, 32,* 493–561.

Mijovic-Prelec, D., & Prelec, D. (2010). Self-deception as self-signaling: A model and experimental evidence. *Philosophical Transactions of the Royal Society B: Biological Sciences, 365,* 227–240.

Mele, A. R. (1997). Real self-deception. *Behavioral and Brain Sciences, 20,* 91–136.

Morf, C. C., & Rhodewalt, F. (2001). Unraveling the paradoxes of narcissism: A dynamic self-regulatory processing model. *Psychological Inquiry, 12,* 177–196.

Otter, Z., & Egan, V. (2007). The evolutionary role of self-deceptive enhancement as a protective factor against antisocial cognitions. *Personality and Individual Differences, 43,* 2258–2269.

Paulhus, D. L. (1984). Two-component models of socially desirable responding. *Journal of Personality and Social Psychology, 46,* 598–609.

Paulhus, D. L. (1986). Self-deception and impression management in test responses. In A. Angleitner & J. S. Wiggins (Eds.), *Personality assessment via questionnaire* (pp. 143–165). New York: Springer-Verlag.

Paulhus, D. L. (1998a). Interpersonal and intrapsychic adaptiveness of trait self-enhancement: A mixed blessing? *Journal of Personality and Social Psychology, 74,* 1197–1208.

Paulhus, D. L. (1998b). *Manual for Balanced Inventory of Desirable Responding* (BIDR-7). Toronto: Multi-Health Systems.
Paulhus, D. L. (2002). Socially desirable responding: The evolution of a construct. In H. Braun, D. N. Jackson, & D. E. Wiley (Eds.), *The role of constructs in psychological and educational measurement* (pp. 67–88). Hillsdale, NJ: Erlbaum.
Paulhus, D. L., Fridhandler, B., & Hayes, S. (1997). Psychological defense: Contemporary theory and research. In J. A. Johnson, R. Hogan, & S. R. Briggs (Eds.), *Handbook of personality psychology* (pp. 543–579). New York: Academic Press.
Paulhus, D. L., Harms, P. D., Bruce, M. N., & Lysy, D. C. (2003). The over-claiming technique: Measuring self-enhancement independent of ability. *Journal of Personality and Social Psychology, 84,* 681–693.
Paulhus, D. L., & John, O. P. (1998). Egoistic and moralistic bias in self-perceptions: The interplay of self-deceptive styles with basic traits and motives. *Journal of Personality, 66,* 1024–1060.
Paulhus, D. L., Nathanson, C., & Lau, K. S.-L. (2005, August). *Cheating on practice tests: A matter of self-deception?* Paper presented at the annual meeting of the American Psychological Society, New York.
Paulhus, D. L., & Reid, D. B. (1991). Enhancement and denial in social desirable responding. *Journal of Personality and Social Psychology, 60,* 307–317.
Paulhus, D. L., & Suedfeld, P. (1988). A dynamic complexity model of self-deception. In J. S. Lockard & D. L. Paulhus (Eds.), *Self-deception: An adaptive mechanism?* (pp. 132–145). Englewood Cliffs, NJ: Prentice-Hall.
Pears, D. (1984). *Motivated irrationality.* Oxford, UK: Clarendon Press.
Quattrone, G. A., & Tversky, A. (1984). Causal versus diagnostic contingencies: On self-deception and the voter's illusion. *Journal of Personality and Social Psychology, 46,* 236–248.
Robinson, M. D., & Ryff, C. D. (1999). The role of self-deception in perceptions of past, present, and future happiness. *Personality and Social Psychology Bulletin, 25,* 595–606.
Sackeim, H. A. (1988). Self deception: A synthesis. In J. S. Lockard & D. L. Paulhus (Eds.), *Self deception: An adaptive mechanism?* (pp. 146–165). Englewood Cliffs. NJ: Prentice-Hall.
Sackeim, H. A., & Gur, R. C. (1978). Self-deception, other-deception and consciousness. In G. E. Schwartz & D. Shapiro (Eds.), *Consciousness and self-regulation: Advances in research* (Vol. 2, pp. 139–197). New York: Plenum Press.
Sartre, J.-P. (1982). *Mauvaise foi* and the unconscious. In R. Wollheim & J. Hopkins (Eds.), *Philosophical essays on Freud.* Cambridge, MA: Cambridge University Press. (Original work published 1943)
Sloman, S. A., Fernbach, P. M., & Hagmayer, Y. (2010). Self-deception requires vagueness. *Cognition, 115,* 268–281.
Smith, S. H., & Whitehead, G. I. (1993). The use of self-deceptive strategies as a function of the manipulation of publicness: The role of audience information. *Contemporary Social Psychology, 17,* 8–13.
Starek, J. E., & Keating, C .F. (1991). Self-deception and its relationship to success in competition. *Basic and Applied Social Psychology, 12,* 145–152.
Szabados, B. (1985). The self, its passions, and self-deception. In M. W. Martin (Ed.), *Self-deception and self-understanding* (pp. 143–168) Lawrence: University Press of Kansas.
Taylor, S. E., & Brown, J. D. (1988). Illusion and well-being: A social psychological perspective on mental health. *Psychological Bulletin, 103,* 193–210.
Tenbrunsel, A. E., & Messick, D. M. (2004). Ethical fading: The role of self-deception in unethical behavior. *Social Justice Research, 17,* 223–236.

Trivers, R. (1985). *Social evolution*. Menlo Park, CA: Benjamin/Cummings.

Uziel, L. (2010). Rethinking social desirability scales: From impression management to interpersonally oriented self-control. *Perspectives on Psychological Science, 5*, 243–262.

Vecchione, M., & Alessandri, G. (in press). Alpha and beta traits and egoistic and moralistic self-enhancement: A point of convergence between two research traditions. *Journal of Personality*.

von Hippel, W., Lakin, J. L., & Shakarchi, R. J. (2005). Individual differences in motivated social cognition: The case of self-serving information processing. *Personality and Social Psychology Bulletin, 31*, 1347–1357.

von Hippel, W., & Trivers, R. (2011). The evolution and psychology of self-deception. *Behavioral and Brain Sciences, 34*, 1–56.

Wegner, D. M., & Pennebaker, J. W. (Eds.). (1993). *Handbook of mental control*. Englewood Cliffs, NJ: Prentice-Hall.

Weinberger, D. A. (1990). The construct validity of the repressive coping style. In J. L. Singer (Ed.), *Repression and dissociation: Implications for personality theory, psychopathology, and health* (pp. 337–386). Chicago: University of Chicago Press.

Westen, D. (1998). The scientific legacy of Sigmund Freud: Towards a psychodynamically informed psychological science. *Psychological Bulletin, 124*, 333–371.

Wilson, T. D. (1985). Self-deception without repression: Limits on access to mental states: In M. W. Martin (Ed.), *Self-deception and self-understanding* (pp. 95–116). Lawrence: University Press of Kansas.

Wilson, T. D. (2002). *Strangers to ourselves: Discovering the adaptive unconscious*. Cambridge, MA: Harvard University Press.

Zajonc, R. B. (1980). Feeling and thinking: Preferences need no inferences. *American Psychologist, 35*, 151–175.

CHAPTER 23

On Motivated Reasoning and Self-Belief

ERIK G. HELZER
DAVID DUNNING

In 2010, a team of political scientists published a study with a curious result. They invited roughly 200 residents of Eastern Iowa to take part in a hypothetical presidential primary election for either the Democratic or Republican Party. Participants read about various candidates, gathered information about each one, and then selected their tentative favorite. The research team then introduced an important wrinkle. For some participants, their favorite candidate continued to express ideologically consistent opinions, presumably opinions the participant liked. For others, the candidates expressed opinions that opposed the participants' stance about 25% of the time. For yet another group, the candidate almost completely reversed—taking positions that disagreed with the participant about 75% of the time (Redlawsk, Civettini, & Emmerson, 2010).

At the end of the study, participants were asked to offer a final decision about which candidate they preferred. Not surprisingly, participants whose candidates stayed uniformly true to participants' own views showed little change from their initial preferences. Also unsurprising, participants confronting candidates who ended up mostly disagreeing with them tended to lower significantly their initially positive impression of the candidate. But what about participants whose preferred candidates showed 25% disagreement? One might expect that participants would like these candidates less than the candidates who showed uniform agreement. But that is not what the research team found. Instead, participants confronting candidates displaying this level of disagreement rated them *more*, not less, favorably than they had when they offered their initial rating (Redlawsk et al., 2010). How could this be? How could disagreement lead to greater liking rather than its opposite?

What this study shows is that a little disagreement never got in the way of potentially vigorous *motivated reasoning*, which refers to thought or analysis that is aimed at supporting some favored conclusion. People like to think, for example, that their future is a bright and benign one, and so may bend, massage, mold, select, or favor arguments and evidence that favor that conclusion over its opposite (Beckman, 1973; Ditto & Lopez, 1992; Kunda, 1990; Pyszczynski, Greenberg, & Holt, 1985; Willis, 1981; Wyer & Frey, 1983). In the Iowa study, one can see how people might engage in motivated reasoning after they had come to prefer a specific candidate. Perturbed by seemingly disagreeable "flaws" in their candidates, people may have reacted by explaining away those flaws or bolstering other aspects of the candidate's politics (Festinger, 1957). Indeed, the research team found presumed evidence of this, in that participants spent more time reading and thinking over disagreements than agreements with their favored candidates (Redlawsk et al., 2010).

Some Introductory Notes about Motivated Reasoning

If people engage in motivated reasoning to defend a hypothetical candidate in some fictional presidential primary in a researcher's laboratory, imagine how strongly they react when thinking about actual people for whom they have real feelings. Take, for example, how much people might engage in motivated reasoning when it is the *self* who is in question. That issue is the focus of this chapter: How does motivated reasoning influence thinking about the self? And to what extent does it enhance or detract from people's understanding of themselves?

However, before beginning our discussion of motivated reasoning and self-knowledge, we must make a few introductory points. First, in a sense, all reasoning is motivated in some way. A mathematician is motivated to prove some theorem, but that is not the sense of motivation on which we focus herein. The motivation spurring on the mathematician is simply the need to know, or curiosity, which has been shown to be an important driver of human thought (Dunning, 2001; Kruglanski, Orehek, Dechesne, & Pierro, 2009). Similarly, people might be motivated by a desire to be accurate in their thinking, but, again, this is not what we specifically mean by motivated reasoning (Dunning, 2001). Furthermore, people might be motivated to reach an impression of the world that is coherent and that contains no puzzling or discomforting contradictions. For several years, from the 1940s to the 1970s, social psychology emphasized this press toward cognitive consistency (for a review, see Abelson et al., 1968), and in fact it lay at the heart of the original formulation of both cognitive dissonance (Festinger, 1957) and balance (Heider, 1946) theories. But this kind of motivation is, again, not the motivated reasoning discussed in this chapter.

What we mean, and what researchers typically mean, when talking about motivated reasoning in contemporary psychological research is thought that is *directional* (i.e., thought that favors some predetermined conclusion that the individual desires to reach; Kunda, 1990). This type of reasoning has many names: *wishful thinking, rationalization, self-affirmation,* and *defensive processing,* just to name a few (Ditto & Lopez, 1992; Festinger, 1957; Steele, 1988; Taylor, 1983; Taylor & Brown, 1988). It can take on two forms. First, there may be some explicit conclusion in conscious deliberation that the individual favors reaching—such as people convincing themselves (as much as the job interviewer) that they are the best person for the job (Ditto & Lopez, 1992; Kunda, 1987, 1990).

Second, there may be some background belief that the individual does not wish to contradict, even if the belief is never made explicit. For example, much work has shown that people judge others in ways that reaffirm that they themselves are lovable and capable human beings. Even when the self is not explicitly mentioned, people are more likely to judge as capable a target who shares their own strengths and weaknesses, while a dissimilar other tends to be seen as less skilled (for reviews, see Dunning, 1999, 2007).

As such, motivated reasoning holds two general implications for self-knowledge. First, motivated reasoning leads to conclusions that contain a good deal of bias. The conclusions that people reach often may lie some distance from objective truth or an impartial reading of the evidence. Second, motivated reasoning leads people to persist in believing conclusions about themselves far more than they should. Even when the evidence suggests that people should revise what they think about themselves, motivated reasoning allows them to cling to favored beliefs and attitudes.

We begin our discussion by describing some primary strategies people use to reason their way toward a desired conclusion. We then turn to current controversies in the literature, focusing, for example, on whether motivated reasoning *actually* leads to inaccuracies in self-knowledge. We conclude with lingering questions about this topic that have yet to be satisfactorily answered and thus require further theoretical and empirical work.

Strategies of Motivated Reasoning

The psychological literature is full of research documenting a wide array of strategies people use to travel closer to conclusions they wish to reach (for reviews, see Baumeister & Newman, 1994; Dunning, 2001; Kunda, 1990). We focus more narrowly on the strategies that have the greatest implications for self-knowledge and -understanding. The conclusions people wish to reach about themselves may influence how they process information about the world in any number of ways—some blatant, some subtle.

Motives Influence the Framing of Information Seeking

One of the most powerful—and subtle—strategies people can use to arrive at desired conclusions is to frame the questions they ask in a biased manner, making confirmation of a desired conclusion more likely than disconfirmation. Imagine people who want to assess their social abilities. They could begin by asking themselves, "Am I extroverted?" or "Am I shy?" These two questions may seem like two sides of the same self-assessment coin, but a long-standing body of work shows that people answer these two questions in very different ways: Ask people if they are extroverted and they primarily search for positive evidence that they are extroverted. After finding it, people tend to believe they are outgoing, gregarious individuals. However, ask the same people if they are shy, and they tend to search for evidence that they are reticent and private people, which can lead them to think that they are more reserved and inhibited (Kunda, Fong, Sanitioso, & Reber, 1993; Snyder & Swann, 1978).

A number of factors can influence the question people initially pose to themselves and thus the conclusion they ultimately reach. The frame of a question can be suggested by an outside source, such as a salesman or therapist, or from a recent experience. Our assertion, though, is that a person's directional motives may possess a similar influence. It is likely that most people favor asking questions that suggest positive conclusions over negative ones. They prefer to ask themselves if they are intelligent rather than stupid, good-looking rather than unattractive, healthy rather than unhealthy, and, outgoing rather than shy. Once these question frames are in place, a confirmatory bias takes over that favors favorable conclusions over alternatives (Mussweiler & Strack, 1999; Pyszczynski & Greenberg, 1987). Indeed, Mussweiler (2003) has argued that such a confirmatory process underlies any number of social comparisons in which people engage to uphold their positive self-views.

Motives Influence the Quantity and Quality of Information Sought

But, sometimes, even if people adopt a congenial question frame, the evidence they gather may not conform to their wishes. Motives likely influence what people do when they encounter favorable versus unfavorable information, altering how much evidence and what quality of evidence people demand before they can cut off an information search and move toward a conclusion.

People show a tendency not to need much evidence in favor of conclusions they like. However, when it comes to conclusions they would rather avoid, they show a marked tendency to demand more evidence and to place whatever uncongenial evidence they have under intense scrutiny. In a phrase, people seem to adopt a "Can I believe?" stance to favorable conclusions: Any evidence permitting them to believe favorable conclusions is taken at face value. For unfavorable conclusions, they adopt a "Must I believe?" stance, asking instead whether they are compelled to believe an unfriendly message (Dawson, Gilovich, & Regan, 2002; Gilovich, 1991).

The different treatment given to favorable versus unfavorable evidence is best illustrated by work on *motivated skepticism* (Ditto & Lopez, 1992), which has shown that people accept congenial information more or less effortlessly, but examine uncongenial information with a fine-toothed comb. In one study, participants were given a kit to test for the (actually fictitious) medical condition thioamine acetylase (TAA) deficiency, which they were told was linked to unfortunate pancreatic disorders later in life. Participants were instructed to spit into a cup, dip a testing strip into the saliva, and wait for it either to change color or stay the same (to indicate the absence or presence of the deficiency).

Ditto and Lopez (1992) covertly observed that participants receiving "good news"—the test result indicating no increased risk for pancreatic problems—accepted the information readily. They waited less time for a color change in the strip and they did not engage in any retesting behaviors (e.g., redipping the strip just to be sure of the result). Those who received the "bad news," on the other hand, waited longer before accepting the results of the test and engaged in retesting behaviors three times more often than their peers.

Skepticism was also observed in participants' explicit responses to the test. Those who received the "bad news" thought the test was less accurate and the conclusions less severe, than did those who received the "good news." In follow-up work, participants proved ready to discount an unfavorable test if there was a reason it might be invalid but did not discount a favorable test if it contained the same flaw (Ditto, Scepansky, Munro, Apanovitch, & Lockhart, 1998).

Motives Guide the Interpretation of Key Social Concepts and Behaviors

Consider a trait that most of us would like to claim: gifted scholarship. Of course, not every academic can rightfully claim the trait, but many do, probably more than are justified. What allows them to make the claim? One possibility stems from the fact that the trait itself is ambiguous. What exactly constitutes *gifted scholarship*? Is it the number of publications one has? Professional accolades? Or perhaps it is a trait revealed by teaching evaluations. In essence, one way people may achieve motivated conclusions about themselves involves how they define the traits and abilities that they wish to possess.

Self-Serving Definitions of Social Concepts

Each scholar probably possesses his or her own idiosyncratic standard or definition of good scholarship, and, for most people, that idiosyncratic definition is probably self-serving in nature. A great deal of research (for reviews, see Critcher, Helzer, & Dunning, 2011; Dunning, 1999) suggests that the definitions people assign to positive traits (e.g., *sophisticated*) just happen to be the very qualities that they themselves possess (Dunning & Cohen, 1992; Dunning & McElwee, 1995; Dunning, Meyerowitz, & Holzberg, 1989; Dunning, Perie, & Story, 1991). A wine expert emphasizes knowledge of fine wines in his or her definition of *sophisticated*. A person who has read many books emphasizes a more bookworm-like variant of the term. In contrast, the qualities people assign to unfavorable traits (e.g., *submissive*) tend to be qualities they fail to see in themselves. Thus, one way people can support desired self-impressions is to form their definition of a particular trait with reference to their own behaviors and qualities.

Note that the key to motivated self-assessment in these examples is *trait ambiguity*—assessing the self on traits that can be defined in any number of ways. As evidence of this, when researchers reign in people's ability to exploit ambiguity in their definitions by assigning them a specific and concrete definition of an otherwise ambiguous trait (e.g., they are presented a definition of *sophisticated* that includes only being able to speak foreign languages and cooking gourmet meals), people offer self-assessments that are significantly less self-enhancing (Dunning et al., 1989).

Self-Serving Labels Applied to Behavior

Another avenue for motivated reasoning in self-understanding lies at the intersection of a concrete instance of behavior and the more abstract label a person assigns to it. Take the act of completing a tedious laboratory task (e.g., writing number words—*one, two, three, four*—continuously for 4 minutes): How might a person make meaning out of that behavior? Jordan and Monin (2008) put participants in such a situation and later asked them to assess their own moral qualities and the moral qualities of another participant in the experiment. Under normal circumstances (i.e., when participants were led to believe that both they and the other participant had been made to complete the exact same task), people did not tend to imbue the act of completing the task with a particular self-serving meaning. They rated their own morality and the morality of the other participant roughly equally. In another condition, participants simply witnessed the other participant (actually a confederate) refuse to do the task before rating the other participant's morality. Here, again, participants assessed themselves and the confederate roughly equally.

However, in the key condition, participants were put in a position that was potentially threatening to their sense of self. Having just spent 4 minutes completing the dreary and tedious task, participants witnessed a confederate refuse to complete the very same task with no adverse consequence. Faced with the uncongenial possibility that they had just played the sucker, participants showed a motivated shift in thought. Participants rated their own morality (but not their intelligence, confidence, or sense of humor) as higher than the morality of the participant who refused to complete the task. In participants' minds, their efforts at the banal task were demonstrative of moral character rather than gullibility. A second study confirmed the motivational nature of this shift in moral self-perceptions, in that it did not arise if participants first engaged in a self-esteem-building exercise.

Keeping Accounts of Behavior

A final way people maintain favorable views of self is to balance the choices they make against one another to ensure that, on balance, they send adequate signals that they are worthy and capable individuals; that is, people at times can indulge in less-than-admirable behavior if they have first built up their "bona fides" as moral and respectable individuals. By building up accounts of desirable behavior, they obscure any chance that their indulgent transgressions can be interpreted as anything significant about their overall character.

Work on *moral licensing* shows this balancing most directly, thus revealing how people can engage in questionably immoral or stigmatized behavior without worrying about the dishonor often associated with that behavior, provided that they feel that have adequately signaled their moral worth elsewhere. For example, when people are feeling particularly moral, they may—paradoxically—give themselves permission to act in morally questionable ways with no consequence for their own self-views. In a well-known demonstration, Monin and Miller (2001) offered participants an opportunity to signal their good moral credentials by disagreeing with a number of sexist views, then observed their responses to a subsequent task in which they chose the best candidate for a job usually linked to men. Relative to control participants, participants who had just established their nonsexist credentials by rejecting blatantly biased statements made *more* biased hiring decisions, in that they were more likely to pick a man over a woman for a stereotypically male job in law enforcement.

In similar set of studies, Sachdeva, Iliev, and Medin (2009) showed that people were *less* charitable than control participants following a reminder of their own positive traits, and *more* charitable than controls following a reminder of their own negative traits. Such a result makes little sense unless one posits the idea that people engage in moral accounting to ensure that they can see themselves as good and moral agents. Thus, if people have already been given the opportunity to signal their moral worth (via a recitation of their positive qualities), they need not repeat costly moral behavior and can instead engage in some questionable actions. However, when this signal has been interrupted or undermined by a reminder of their shortcomings, people are energized to restore a positive self-image via moral behavior.

Current Issues in Motivated Reasoning Theory and Research

Decades of research on motivated reasoning has offered a number of classic demonstrations of its operation in people's day-to-day thinking about themselves. Without a doubt, motivated reasoning exists and serves as a primary line of defense that protects people's self-views from potentially damaging or conflicting information. But the exact implications of motivated reasoning for social thought and life remain somewhat controversial, spurring current research and enduring debates.

Do Congenial Conclusions Necessarily Reflect Motivated Reasoning?

One issue concerns the frequency and scope of motivated reasoning. People come to congenial conclusions all the time, but that does not necessarily mean that those conclusions were inspired by motivated reasoning. A number of flaws in thinking, including everyday heuristics for evaluating information, may give rise to congenial conclusions even without any particular biasing motivation.

Consider one of the most common and visible biases suggesting motivated reasoning in self-perception, the above-average effect, the statistically impossible phenomenon in which the average person rates his or her skill, on average, as way above average (Alicke, 1985; Alicke & Govorun, 2005; Guenther & Alicke, 2010; Dunning, Heath, & Suls, 2004). Although the above-average effect looks like it must be a product of motivated reasoning, this is not necessarily the case. Other nonmotivational quirks of thinking can lead to a good deal of above-average responding.

For example, one could propose that the above-average effect arises because self-serving motivations prompt people to ask questions in such a way that almost guarantees a favorable self-impression (e.g., asking whether they are more intelligent than their peers, rather than whether their peers are more intelligent than them). Such question frames, however, can just as easily be prompted by nonmotivational factors, producing above-average effects in contexts that clearly have nothing to do with motivation. Consider three workshop tools that one might own: a hammer, a screwdriver, and a saw. If someone were to ask you if the hammer is a more useful tool than the other two, you are likely to agree (i.e., it is good for pounding nails, and opening nuts when you cannot find the nutcracker)—making the hammer an above-average tool. But here is the trick. You are likely to do the same for the screwdriver if asked about it (e.g., it's essential for screws, and for opening balky cans) and for the saw (e.g., it cuts wood cleanly, and in an emergency can be used as a musical instrument).

In other words, if one is given a pointed hypothesis by an external agent about one object within the group, one is likely to hunt for information that confirms the hypothesis. Having found confirmatory evidence, one will conclude (perhaps wrongly, but not because of any particular motivation) that the object in question is above average. But here's the rub: Because each tool is useful in its own way, and the ways in which a particular tool is more useful than the others become salient when that tool is the focus of attention, it is easy to slip into claiming that the tool is more useful than others (Giladi & Klar, 2002; Klar & Giladi, 1997); that is, even though the guiding question is a comparative one, people often fail to complete the comparison in their thinking, focusing on the central object and thinking only about how useful that particular object is (Kruger, 1999; Weinstein & Lachendro, 1982).

Does this mean that the above-average effect is really a nonmotivated phenomenon? Not necessarily, since current research suggests that motivational dynamics are often in play in producing the effect. In one illustrative study, participants were asked to rate themselves along 23 different trait dimensions. Four to 8 weeks later, they were handed the exact same set of ratings and were told that the ratings came either from themselves or from some other student at their university. They were then asked to provide the rating that a "typical student" in their university would give. When participants thought that the ratings came from someone else, their ratings for the "typical student" closely mimicked the ratings they were given. However, when participants were reminded that the ratings were actually their own, their assessments of the "typical student" changed, with participants rating the student much more negatively than they did in the other group. Motivated to think of themselves as superior to others, participants now seemed impelled to maintain a gap in perception between self and other that favored the self. Such a motivation was absent when they considered ratings that they thought came from another person (Guenther & Alicke, 2010).

Does Motivated Reasoning Necessarily Lead to Error in Self-Knowledge?

The question of whether motivated reasoning leads to error in self-knowledge is also a topic of disagreement. On first pass, it may seem almost impossible that the sorts of cognitive tricks prompted by motivation would fail to lead to some kind of systematic distortion in self-understanding. Surely, differential treatment of flattering versus unflattering evidence should lead to errors and omissions in a person's global self-evaluation.

Self-Immunization

An argument can be made, however, that people can hold vaulted views of themselves yet still maintain an accurate impression of the world and their place in it. Theorizing by Greve and Wentura (2003) suggests that people can achieve this happy state by simultaneously holding uniformly positive self-evaluations at an abstract (i.e., trait) level and knowing their limitations and weaknesses at a more concrete (i.e., behavioral) level. Greve and Wentura have labeled this possibility *self-immunization*.

As one demonstration of accuracy at the concrete level but self-enhancement at the abstract level, Greve and Wentura (2003) asked participants to tackle a general knowledge test in which they were asked a variety of questions from four different domains of knowledge (e.g., politics, science, history, art). They competed against a confederate, allowing the experimenters to assign participants randomly to perform better than the confederate on two of the four domains and worse on the other two. Later, when participants were asked to offer self-assessments, Greve and Wentura found that participants were able to recall accurately the areas of knowledge in which they excelled and in which they failed—that is, they showed no evidence of distorting the raw data of their concrete experience in a self-serving direction. At the behavioral level, they were largely accurate.

However, at a more abstract or trait level, participants showed no allergy to self-enhancement. When asked which domains were most indicative of overall intelligence, participants tended to choose the domains in which they themselves had purportedly beaten the confederate. Thus, at a more "conceptual" level, participants could exploit ambiguity to think well of themselves, even though they remained accurate at a more concrete level. Studies like these (for a demonstration of self-immunization using implicit measures, see Wentura & Greve, 2004) suggest that people may be able to maintain knowledge of their concrete strengths and weaknesses, but may put a spin on this information as a way of maintaining positive global self-views (for a similar view, see Armor & Taylor, 1998).

In effect, Greve and Wentura (2003) argue that people can reasonably possess rosy self-impressions yet maintain accuracy, too. Note, though, that to maintain this ideal balance, people must stay aware of the often hazy but critically important line between their *knowledge* (i.e., information about concrete behavioral performance) and *inference* (i.e., the more flattering opinions they extract about themselves at the abstract trait level) (see Critcher, Helzer, & Dunning, 2011; Schneider, 2001). To the extent that they are successful at recognizing where actual information ends and more subjective opinion or "spin" begins, they can have positive impressions about the self yet maintain accurate self-insight. For example, Erik can believe in his subjective inference that he is more "sports savvy" than David because he knows (objectively) more about baseball. And David can be just as justified in extolling his own subjective evaluation that his sports savvy is excellent because he knows (objectively) more about soccer than Erik does.

However, if they wish to remain accurate in their self-assessments and not just self-enhancing, Erik must acknowledge that his "sports savvy" is primarily in the domain of baseball; David must acknowledge that his "sports savvy" is primarily in soccer; and both must acknowledge that their "sport savvy" likely would not necessarily translate to expertise in football, basketball, tennis, golf, cricket, polo, rugby, wrestling, boxing, and virtually every other sport. Without this understanding, the happy marriage between (abstract) self-enhancement and (concrete) self-knowledge begins to dissolve.

Put another way, as the line between subjective interpretation and objective knowledge blurs, the potential for accuracy in the realm of self-insight diminishes. In the previous example, if Erik or David infers from his self-perceived sports savvy (rather than a more concrete review of his specific knowledge of baseball or soccer) that he can beat the other in a sport trivia contest, one of them is by definition going to be in error. Or, to the extent that their subjective inferences cause them to distort either online or retrospective accounts of their objective performance, they will again be led to distorted self-views.

Indeed, much empirical work suggests that people have a very difficult time keeping their subjective inference and objective knowledge straight. First, people tend not to think of their inferences as subjective. They create self-serving templates of intelligence, leadership, and so on, and construe them as universal—just as applicable to others as they are to the self (for reviews, see Dunning, 1999, 2002a, 2002b). For example, Erik will use expertise in baseball as a cue to expertise about sports in general; David will do the same with his expertise in soccer. Second, people's subjective self-views prompt them to misremember objective performances. People with high self-impressions of themselves tend to believe they have performed better in the past than they have actually done. People with low self-impressions tend to underestimate how well they have done (McFarland, Ross, & De Courville, 1989; Story, 1998).

In addition, people's abstract notions of themselves also influence how well they think they are achieving on a given concrete task as they complete it. Those who believe they are skilled think they are doing better than those who think they are less skilled, even when equating actual performance. In one demonstration of this phenomenon, Ehrlinger and Dunning (2003, Study 1) asked participants to evaluate their abstract reasoning ability before completing a standardized test of that sort of reasoning. Once they had completed the test, participants evaluated how they had performed relative to their peers on the test. Noting that participants showed the usual self-enhancement bias on their performance estimates (on average, people thought they performed in the 61st percentile), Ehrlinger and Dunning examined the relationship between participants' chronic self-views (measured before the task), their actual performance, and their estimated performance. The results indicated that participants' estimates of their objective performance were predicted by their subjective self-views, but not by their actual performance.

In other words, participants based their performance evaluations on their a priori beliefs about their abilities, and showed little sensitivity to actual performance. To be sure, participants' self-views were not totally divorced from reality (the one-item measure of people's global self-perceptions of ability significantly predicted actual performance), and, as such, stable self-views were not useless bases for self-evaluation. However, the broader point is that participants leaned heavily (indeed, too heavily) on these subjective beliefs when predicting a single instance of performance and showed little insight into their concrete performance on the task at hand (see also Critcher & Dunning, 2009).

Looking across the prediction literature, there are numerous examples of people making poor concrete self-predictions about the future because they base those predictions on subjective self-views (Buehler, Griffin, & Ross, 1994; Epley & Dunning, 2000; Koehler & Poon, 2006). As one striking example, medical students' self-rated ability at the end of medical school correlates strongly ($r > .50$) with their self-rated ability in the first year of medical school, even though the former ratings tend to be unrelated to more objective measures of performance ability, including supervisor ratings and final board exams (Arnold, Willoughby, & Calkins, 1985). Taken together, findings like these raise serious doubts about whether people can distinguish between concrete information about themselves and more abstract (and flattering) self-evaluations. Thus, to our minds, inaccuracies at the abstract level of self-evaluation pose serious threats to self-knowledge, broadly construed. However, Greve and Wentura (2003) make an opposite claim, with other theorists more in the middle (e.g., Schneider, 2001), meaning that more analysis and empirical study on this issue would be worthwhile.

Can Motivated Reasoning Be Corrected?

If motivated reasoning leads to error, how might one overcome it? Two techniques have been proposed: one straightforward and the other trickier. The straightforward way to correct for motivated reasoning applies to many other reasoning problems as well. Because people tend to look for confirming information, and often stop short of considering all the information they should, one simple way to correct for biases—including motivated ones—is explicitly to *consider the opposite*. For example, if one's thoughts are leading one to conclude, with confidence, that one will obtain a well-paying job after college, or a seat at a highly-ranked law or medical school, the best corrective is to consider explicitly why such a conclusion might be wrong. What could go wrong to prevent that job or postgraduate career? What could one have forgotten to do to make those outcomes more assured?

Much work shows that considering the opposite does a good deal to remove biases in people's conclusions, especially those promoted by confirmatory thinking (Lord, Lepper, & Preston, 1984), anchoring (Mussweiler, Strack, & Pfeiffer, 2000), and the hindsight bias (Arkes, Faust, Guilmette, & Hart, 1988). This technique works even better than simple exhortations to be fair and impartial in decision making. Explicitly asking people why a prediction might be wrong causes them to be significantly less overconfident in that prediction (Hoch, 1985; Koriat, Lichtenstein, & Fischhoff, 1980).

A second technique works specifically to alleviate motivated biases and involves asking people to engage in *self-affirmation* by considering an aspect or part of themselves that they hold in high regard and that makes them proud (friends and family, scientific values, artistic values, etc.). They write a short essay about a time they were proud of something related to that self-aspect. The net effect of this exercise is that people are subsequently much more likely to accept threatening information (for reviews, see Sherman & Cohen, 2006; Steele, 1988). For example, doing a self-affirmation exercise makes people more likely to accede to the idea that they are at risk for HIV, and to purchase more condoms as a response (Sherman, Nelson, & Steele, 2000). Such exercises make people more open-minded, that is, more willing to listen to and consider the arguments of people who disagree with their own positions on politics and morality (Cohen, Aronson, & Steele, 2000). To be sure, no one knows exactly why self-affirmation exercises work—they just do, as has been demonstrated in a wide variety of domains of some consequence to the people involved (see Sherman & Cohen, 2006).

Contemporary and Future Questions

Questions about motivated reasoning still exist and are at the center of current (and, we believe, future) empirical research in psychology and related fields. Some of these questions are classic and enduring ones, and methodological and theoretical advances now make them amenable to empirical study. Let us consider three such questions in turn.

The Relation of Motivated Reasoning to Self-Deception

The first question focuses on the relationship between motivated reasoning and self-deception. Traditionally, the two concepts have not been considered the same thing (see Paulhus & Buckels, Chapter 22, this volume, for a discussion of self-deception). People can surely reason their way toward beliefs that are not true, but that is not exactly what is meant by self-deception. As traditionally defined, *self-deception* involves the paradoxical situation in which a person believes X to be true, but convinces him- or herself of not-X. Philosophers have long argued about how, or whether, such a bifurcated belief system could be maintained (see Mele, 1997, 2001).

However, if one relinquishes this strict definition, motivated reasoning emerges as a paradigmatic case of self-deception. Suppose that the quest for self-knowledge involves an inferential race between a correct belief about oneself ("When it comes to relationships, I am only about as caring as the average person") and an incorrect, but flattering one ("I'm probably a better boyfriend than most guys I know"). Now, suppose that a person's capacity for motivated reasoning allows him or her to construct and alter the race course so that one belief (the congenial, but incorrect one) will almost always win out over the other (Mele, 1997)—and will do so without leaving the slightest trace of suspicious play. An interesting question for future research is how people alter the race course without awareness of the effort to do so. We can offer two possibilities for future empirical work.

Motivated Reasoning Can Operate Nonconsciously

One way for motivated reasoning to do its work without leaving a conscious trace is to situate its operations outside of awareness. Many cognitive tasks are completed nonconsciously. Just to speak a sentence, a person needs to choose words, conjugate verbs, and rearrange words into comprehensible phrases, clauses, and sentences—and much of this work takes place before any product of it reaches consciousness (Bargh, 1994).

Recent work suggests that the impact of motivated reasoning extends down into processes that are clearly nonconscious. For example, what the visual system presents to consciousness can be shaped by motivated preferences. In one illustrative study, Balcetis and Dunning (2006) told participants that a computer was about to assign them to one of two fates. The first was pleasant and involved drinking some freshly squeezed orange juice. The second was unpleasant and involved drinking a foul-smelling pink and green concoction euphemistically described as an "organic garden smoothie." Half of the participants would receive the orange juice if the computer showed them a letter of the alphabet; the other half would receive it if the computer showed them a number. The computer then showed them an image that looked like it could be either the letter *B* or the number 13. Participants tended to report seeing the image that assigned them to the orange juice much more often than they did the image that assigned them to the smoothie. Subsequent experiments demonstrated that participants truly did see the image they wanted to see and were not merely lying to the experimenter.

Motivated Reasoning Resides in the Past

Another trick about motivated reasoning is that it need not always be actively motivated; that is, once people have formed a congenial belief (e.g., "I am an excellent driver/student/cook"), that crystallized belief is available for them for the foreseeable future. It merely becomes part of their belief system, and need not be "redistorted" by motivated reasoning. Thus, one can often reach distorted conclusions based on illusory self-beliefs crafted long ago and need no additional motivated reasoning in the present. In this way, the motivated and distorted nature of these beliefs remains hidden, and the person stays blissfully self-deceived.

To date, no research we are aware of shows that motivated beliefs, once crystallized, remain in the person's belief system to distort future conclusions about the self. However, one recent series of studies has shown evidence of at least the first step in the process. Motivated beliefs, once formed, tend to stick—that is, to become functionally autonomous from the circumstances that created them. In its specifics, this work asked whether the timing of self-affirmation exercises mattered (Critcher, Dunning, & Armor, 2010). Would self-affirmation prevent people from acting defensively toward threatening information if the affirmation came after the threat rather than before?

To address this question, Critcher, Dunning, and Armor (2010) asked some participants to complete self-affirmation exercises before they responded to a threat—such as failing a test. Others completed the self-affirmation only after responding to the threat. The researchers found that self-affirmation before the threat tended to stop people from being defensive, the usual self-affirmation result. However, if the self-affirmation came after people had already responded to the threat through defensive self-enhancement, the exercise did nothing to reduce the amount of defensive resistance to the threat that people displayed. That defensive reaction, now completed, had crystallized and was not "undone" by the introduction of self-affirmation; that is, once in place, those defensive conclusions were presumably positioned to distort future conclusions that individuals might reach about themselves and their place in the world.

Relation of Motivated Reasoning to Reality Constraints

In her groundbreaking review article on motivated reasoning, Kunda (1990) asserted that people maintain a nuanced dance between their wishes on the one hand and reality on the other (echoing Heider, 1958, who offered a similar analysis of people's need to balance desired conclusions with conclusions warranted by data). People do tend to reach favorable conclusions, but those conclusions are heavily hemmed in by "reality constraints." Indeed, work in the 1990s showed just how much reality constraints matter. People tended to provide unrealistically positive self-views, for example, only when the traits in question were ambiguous enough for motivated reasoning to have some leeway to provide favorable interpretations. Instead, when the meaning of a trait was clear (e.g., *punctual, neat, mathematically skilled*), researchers saw *no* distortion in self-judgment, despite participants' obvious desire to see themselves as positively as possible (Dunning et al., 1989). Hsee (1995, 1996) also showed that motivated reasoning produced distorted judgments only when the factors justifying conclusions were elastic in their application—that is, there was some play in what factors were relevant versus not relevant. When those factors were more clear-cut in their applicability, no motivated distortion was found.

Recent current events, however, suggest that reality constraints may not be as restrictive as this past work suggests. As of the writing of this chapter, people can be shown to believe ideas that have been patently proved time and again to be false. For example, despite voluminous evidence to the contrary, in February 2011, a full 51% of respondents planning to vote in the 2012 Republican Presidential primaries believed that the current U.S. President, Barack Obama, was not born in the country, and thus ineligible for his office, and another 28% were unsure (Public Policy Polling, 2011). Of Americans, roughly 20% thought that Obama was Muslim, with such perceptions more widespread (34%) among those (conservative Republicans) who presumably oppose his presidency (Pew Forum on Religion and Public Life, 2010).

Thus, it appears that a reexamination of the interplay between motivation and reality constraints may be in order. When are motivated distortions reigned in by factual evidence? And when does motivation triumph despite evidence and constrictions from the real world?

Perception of Motivated Reasoning in Self versus Other

The final question has to do with how well people understand the impact of motivated reasoning in their everyday world and lives. To be sure, one question that seems settled is that people underestimate just how much their own judgments are molded by wishes, preferences, and fears. In study after study, people describe themselves as more unbiased than their peers (Pronin & Kugler, 2007; Pronin, Lin, & Ross, 2002), whether or not the bias involved is motivational.

But how do people calibrate their beliefs about the extent to which their peers' thoughts are guided by motivated wishes and desires? Do people understand, for example, how much other people rationalize? Or do they over- or underestimate it? Given the commonness of motivated reasoning in everyday life, getting its impact right would seem to be an important source of social wisdom.

To date, there are very few investigations of people's understanding of motivated reasoning in the social world. One extant study, for example, finds that people overestimate motivated reasoning—that people are "naive cynics." People expect that their peers will take too much credit for positive contributions to joint projects but deny responsibility for setbacks. It turns out that although the former assumption is correct, the latter is not. People are just as likely to accept their share of blame for failures—even overdoing it—as they are to take credit for successes (Kruger & Gilovich, 1999). Further work, however, is needed to flesh out whether this is a general tendency or just an isolated instance of a social fallacy.

Concluding Remarks

To understand self-understanding, one must study closely the impact of motivations on people's reasoning about the self and their social world. To be sure, people want to achieve an accurate understanding of themselves, but they seem not to mind holding flattering impressions of themselves as well. Thus, to gauge how people come to understand themselves—and, more importantly, how they *mis*understand themselves, one must first grasp the when, how, and why of motivated reasoning. As researchers interested in people's capacity for genuine self-knowledge, we must take seriously not only the pervasiveness of motivated processes in self-understanding but also the nuances that govern the interplay between self-flattery and self-insight. We must further understand that motivated processes present difficult challenges to the Delphic admonition to "Know Thyself."

REFERENCES

Abelson, R. P., Aronson, E., McGuire, W. J., Newcomb, T. M., Rosenberg, M. J., & Tannenbaum R. H. (1968). *Theories of cognitive consistency: A sourcebook.* Chicago: Rand McNally.

Alicke, M. D. (1985). Global self-evaluation as determined by the desirability and controllability of trait adjectives. *Journal of Personality and Social Psychology, 49,* 1621–1630.

Alicke, M. D., & Govorun, O. (2005). The better-than-average effect. In M. D. Alicke, D. A. Dunning, & J. I. Krueger (Eds.), *The self in social judgment* (pp. 85–106). New York: Psychology Press.

Arkes, H. R., Faust, D., Guilmette, T. J., & Hart, K. (1988). Eliminating the hindsight bias. *Journal of Applied Psychology, 73,* 305–307.

Armor, D. A., & Taylor, S. E. (1998). Situated optimism: Specific outcome expectancies and self-regulation. In M. P. Zanna (Ed.), *Advances in experimental social psychology* (Vol. 30, pp. 309–379). New York: Academic Press.

Arnold, L., Willoughby, T. L., & Calkins, E. V. (1985). Self-evaluation in undergraduate medical education: A longitudinal perspective. *Journal of Medical Education, 60,* 21–28.

Balcetis, E., & Dunning, D. (2006). See what you want to see: The impact of motivational states on visual perception. *Journal of Personality and Social Psychology, 91,* 612–625.

Bargh, J. A. (1994). The Four Horsemen of automaticity: Awareness, efficiency, intention, and control in social cognition. In R. S. Wyer, Jr. & T. K. Srull (Eds.), *Handbook of social cognition* (2nd ed., pp. 1–40). Hillsdale, NJ: Erlbaum.

Baumeister, R. F., & Newman, L. S. (1994). Self-regulation of cognitive inference and decision processes. *Personality and Social Psychology Bulletin, 20,* 3–19.

Beckman, L. (1973). Teachers' and observers' perceptions of causality for a child's performance. *Journal of Educational Psychology, 65,* 198–204.

Buehler, R., Griffin, D., & Ross, M. (1994). Exploring the "planning fallacy": Why people underestimate their task completion times. *Journal of Personality and Social Psychology, 67,* 366–381.

Cohen, G. L., Aronson, J., & Steele, C. M. (2000). When beliefs yield to evidence: Reducing biased evaluation by affirming the self. *Personality and Social Psychology Bulletin, 26,* 1151–1164.

Critcher, C. R., & Dunning, D. (2009). How chronic self-views influence (and mislead) self-assessments of performance: Self-views shape bottom-up experiences with the task. *Journal of Personality and Social Psychology, 97,* 931–945.

Critcher, C. R., Dunning, D., & Armor, D. A. (2010). When self-affirmation reduces defensiveness: Timing is key. *Personality and Social Psychology Bulletin, 36,* 947–959.

Critcher, C. R., Helzer, E. G., & Dunning, D. (2011). Self-enhancement via redefinition: Defining social concepts to ensure positive views of self. In M. D. Alicke & C. Sedikides (Eds.), *Handbook of self-enhancement and self-protection* (pp. 69–91). New York: Guilford Press.

Dawson, E., Gilovich, T., & Regan, D. T. (2002). Motivated reasoning and performance on the Wason selection task. *Personality and Social Psychology Bulletin, 28,* 1379–1387.

Ditto, P. H., & Lopez, D. F. (1992). Motivated skepticism: Use of differential decision criteria for preferred and nonpreferred conclusions. *Journal of Personality and Social Psychology, 63,* 568–584.

Ditto, P. H., Scepansky, J. A., Munro, G. D., Apanovitch, A. M., & Lockhart, L. K. (1998). Motivated sensitivity to preference-inconsistent information. *Journal of Personality and Social Psychology, 75,* 53–69.

Dunning, D. (1999). A newer look: Motivated social cognition and the schematic representation of social concepts. *Psychological Inquiry, 10,* 1–11.

Dunning, D. (2001). On the motives underlying social cognition. In N. Schwarz & A. Tesser (Eds.), *Blackwell handbook of social psychology: Vol. 1. Intraindividual processes* (pp. 348–374). New York: Blackwell.

Dunning, D. (2002a). The relation of self to social perception. In M. R. Leary & J. P. Tangney (Eds.), *Handbook of self and identity* (pp. 421–441). New York: Guilford Press.

Dunning, D. (2002b). The zealous self-affirmer: How and why the self lurks so pervasively behind social judgment. In S. Fein & S. Spencer (Eds.), *Motivated social perception: The Ontario Symposium* (Vol. 9, pp. 45–72), Mahwah, NJ: Erlbaum.

Dunning, D. (2007). Self-image motives and consumer behavior: How sacrosanct self-beliefs sway preferences in the marketplace. *Journal of Consumer Psychology, 17,* 237–249.

Dunning, D., & Cohen, G. L. (1992). Egocentric definitions of traits and abilities in social judgment. *Journal of Personality and Social Psychology, 63,* 341–355.

Dunning, D., Heath, C., & Suls, J. (2004). Flawed self-assessment: Implications for health, education, and the workplace. *Psychological Science in the Public Interest, 5,* 69–106.

Dunning, D., & McElwee, R. O. (1995). Idiosyncratic trait definitions: Implications for self-description and social judgment. *Journal of Personality and Social Psychology, 68,* 936–946.

Dunning, D., Meyerowitz, J. A., & Holzberg, A. D. (1989). Ambiguity and self-evaluation: The role of idiosyncratic trait definitions in self-serving assessments of ability. *Journal of Personality and Social Psychology, 57,* 1082–1090.

Dunning, D., Perie, M., & Story, A. L. (1991). Self-serving prototypes of social categories. *Journal of Personality and Social Psychology, 61,* 957–968.

Ehrlinger, J., & Dunning, D. (2003). How chronic self-views influence (and potentially mislead) estimates of performance. *Journal of Personality and Social Psychology, 84,* 5–17.

Epley, N., & Dunning, D. (2000). Feeling "holier than thou": Are self-serving assessments produced by errors in self or social prediction? *Journal of Personality and Social Psychology, 79,* 861–875.

Festinger, L. (1957). *A theory of cognitive dissonance.* Stanford, CA: Stanford University Press.

Giladi, E. E., & Klar, Y. (2002). When standards are wide of the mark: Nonselective superiority and inferiority biases in comparative judgments of objects and concepts. *Journal of Experimental Psychology: General, 131,* 538–551.

Gilovich, T. (1991). *How we know what isn't so: The fallibility of human reason in everyday life.* New York: Free Press.

Greve, W., & Wentura, D. (2003). Immunizing the self: Self-concept stabilization through reality-adaptive self-definitions. *Personality and Social Psychology Bulletin, 29,* 39–50.

Guenther, C. L., & Alicke, M. D. (2010). Deconstructing the better-than-average effect. *Journal of Personality and Social Psychology, 99,* 755–770.

Heider, F. (1946). Attitudes and cognitive organization. *Journal of Psychology, 21,* 107–112.

Heider, F. (1958). *The psychology of interpersonal relations.* New York: Wiley.

Hoch, S. J. (1985). Counterfactual reasoning and accuracy in predicting personal events. *Journal of Experimental Psychology: Learning, Memory, and Cognition, 11,* 719–731.

Hsee, C. K. (1995). Elastic justification: How tempting but task-irrelevant factors influence decisions. *Organizational Behavioral and Human Decision Process, 62,* 330–337.

Hsee, C. K. (1996). Elastic justification: How unjustifiable factors influence judgments. *Organizational Behavior and Human Decision Processes, 66,* 122–129.

Jordan, A. H., & Monin, B. (2008). From sucker to saint: Moralization in response to self-threat. *Psychological Science, 19,* 809–815.

Klar, Y., & Giladi, E. E. (1997). No one in my group can be below average: A robust positivity bias in favor of anonymous peers. *Journal of Personality and Social Psychology, 73,* 885–901.

Koehler, D. J., & Poon, C. S. K. (2006). Self-predictions overweight strength of current intentions. *Journal of Experimental Social Psychology, 42,* 517–524.

Koriat, A., Lichtenstein, S., & Fischhoff, B. (1980). Reasons for confidence. *Journal of Experimental Psychology: Human Learning and Memory, 6,* 107–118.

Kruger, J. (1999). Lake Wobegon be gone!: The "below-average effect" and the egocentric nature of comparative ability judgments. *Journal of Personality and Social Psychology, 77,* 221–232.

Kruger, J., & Gilovich, T. (1999). "Naive cynicism" in everyday theories of responsibility assessment: On biased assumptions of bias. *Journal of Personality and Social Psychology, 76,* 743–753.

Kruglanski, A. W., Orehek, E., Dechesne, M., & Pierro, A. (2009). Three decades of lay epistemics: The why, how and who of knowledge formation. *European Review of Social Psychology, 20,* 146–191.

Kunda, Z. (1987). Motivated inference: Self-serving generation and evaluation of causal theories. *Journal of Personality and Social Psychology, 53,* 37–54.

Kunda, Z. (1990). The case for motivated reasoning. *Psychological Bulletin, 108,* 480–498.

Kunda, Z., Fong, G. T., Sanitioso, R., & Reber, E. (1993). Directional questions direct self-conceptions. *Journal of Experimental Social Psychology, 29,* 63–86.

Lord, C. G., Lepper, M. R., & Preston, E. (1984). Considering the opposite: A corrective strategy for social judgment. *Journal of Personality and Social Psychology, 47,* 1231–1243.

McFarland, C., Ross, M., & De Courville, N. (1989). Women's theories of menstruation and biases in recall of menstrual symptoms. *Journal of Personality and Social Psychology, 57,* 522–531.

Mele, A. (2001). *Self-deception unmasked.* Princeton, NJ: Princeton University Press.

Mele, A. R. (1997). Real self-deception. *Behavioral and Brain Sciences, 20,* 91–136.

Monin, B., & Miller, D. T. (2001). Moral credentials and the expression of prejudice. *Journal of Personality and Social Psychology, 81,* 33–43.

Mussweiler, T. (2003). Comparison processes in social judgment: Mechanisms and consequences. *Psychological Review, 110,* 472–489.

Mussweiler, T., & Strack, F. (1999). Hypothesis-consistent testing and semantic priming in the anchoring paradigm: A selective accessibility model. *Journal of Experimental Social Psychology, 35,* 136–164.

Mussweiler, T., Strack, F., & Pfeiffer, T. (2000). Overcoming the inevitable anchoring effect: Considering the opposite compensates for selective accessibility. *Personality and Social Psychology Bulletin, 26,* 1142–1150.

Pew Forum on Religion and Public Life. (2010). *Growing number of Americans say Obama is a Muslim.* Unpublished manuscript, Washington, DC.

Pronin, E., Lin, D. Y., & Ross, L. (2002). The bias blind spot: Perceptions of bias in self versus others. *Personality and Social Psychology Bulletin, 28,* 369–381.

Pronin, E., & Kugler, M. B. (2007). Valuing thoughts, ignoring behavior: The introspection illusion as a source of the bias blind spot. *Journal of Experimental Social Psychology, 43,* 565–578.

Public Policy Polling. (2011). *Huckabee tops GOP field, 51% are birthers and love Palin.* Unpublished manuscript, Raleigh, NC.

Pyszczynski, T., & Greenberg, J. (1987). Toward an integration of cognitive and motivational perspectives on social inference: A biased hypothesis-testing model. In L. Berkowitz (Ed.), *Advances in experimental social psychology* (Vol. 20, pp. 297–340). New York: Elsevier.

Pyszczynski, T., Greenberg, J., & Holt, K. (1985). Maintaining consistency between self-serving beliefs and available data: A bias in information evaluation following success and failure. *Personality and Social Psychology Bulletin, 11*, 179–190.

Redlawsk, D. P., Civettini, A. J. W., & Emmerson, K. M. (2010). The affective tipping point: Do motivated reasoners ever "get it"? *Political Psychology, 31*, 563–593.

Sachdeva, S., Iliev, R., & Medin, D. L. (2009). Sinning saints and saintly sinners: The paradox of moral self-regulation. *Psychological Science, 20*, 523–528.

Schneider, S. L. (2001). In search of realistic optimism: Meaning, knowledge, and warm fuzziness. *American Psychologist, 56*, 250–263.

Sherman, D. K., & Cohen, G. L. (2006). The psychology of self-defense: Self-affirmation theory. In M. P. Zanna (Ed.) *Advances in experimental social psychology* (Vol. 38, pp. 183–242). San Diego, CA: Academic Press.

Sherman, D. K., Nelson, L. D., & Steele, C. M. (2000). Do messages about health risks threaten the self?: Increasing the acceptance of threatening health messages via self-affirmation. *Personality and Social Psychology Bulletin, 26*, 1046–1058.

Snyder, M., & Swann, W. B. (1978). Hypothesis-testing in social interaction. *Journal of Personality and Social Psychology, 36*, 1202–1212.

Steele, C. M. (1988). The psychology of self-affirmation: Sustaining the integrity of the self. In L. Berkowitz (Ed.), *Advances in experimental social psychology* (Vol. 21, pp. 261–302). San Diego, CA: Academic Press.

Story, A. L. (1998). Self-esteem and memory for favorable and unfavorable personality feedback. *Personality and Social Psychology Bulletin, 24*, 51–64.

Taylor, S. E. (1983). Adjustment to threatening events: A theory of cognitive adaptation. *American Psychologist, 38*, 1161–1173.

Taylor, S. E., & Brown, J. D. (1988). Illusion and well-being: A social psychological perspective on mental health. *Psychological Bulletin, 103*, 193–210.

Weinstein, N. D., & Lachendro, E. (1982). Egocentrism as a source of unrealistic optimism. *Personality and Social Psychology Bulletin, 8*, 195–200.

Wentura, D., & Greve, W. (2004). Who wants to be . . . erudite?: Everyone! Evidence for automatic adaptation of trait definitions. *Social Cognition, 22*, 30–53.

Willis, T. A. (1981). Downward comparison principles in social psychology. *Psychological Bulletin, 90*, 245–271.

Wyer, R. S., & Frey, D. (1983). The effects of feedback about self and others on the recall and judgments of feedback-relevant information. *Journal of Experimental Social Psychology, 19*, 540–559.

CHAPTER 24

From "Out There" to "In Here"
Implications of Self-Evaluation Motives for Self-Knowledge

MICHAEL J STRUBE

Each day we navigate through complex environments, real and imagined, physical and social, that are fraught with the prospects of pleasure and peril. By careful choice and deft reaction, we can negotiate a path that is prosperous, physically and psychologically. Traveling well, however, requires *self-knowledge*—an awareness of who we are, what we can do, and the limitations that we possess. How do we arrive at our self-knowledge, and how well do we know ourselves? In this chapter I focus on the role played by self-evaluation motives in the acquisition of self-knowledge and the implications of these motives for studying the nature of self-knowledge. Along the way I suggest an alternative way to view self-evaluation motives, one that places them in the larger context of how people fit into the environments they inhabit. This person–environment (P-E) fit perspective has important implications for how self-knowledge is conceived and measured.

Let me begin with an assumption that undergirds what I have to say and helps place matters in context. Like others (e.g., Sedikides & Skowronski, 2000; Sedikides, Skowronski, & Gaertner, 2004; Yost, Strube, & Bailey, 1992) I assume that the self evolved as a powerful adaptation to assist coping with the complex social and physical environments of our ancestors—a world inhabited by reproductive adversaries that were also our social and cultural collaborators. Such a world strikes a fragile balance between individual and collective concerns, requiring the ability to represent self and others symbolically. In a very basic sense, then, "survival" is the answer to the question "What is the self *for*?" A major part of the self that helps us survive is the accumulated knowledge of who we are—our self-attributes broadly defined. But how do we know what we know about ourselves? How do we arrive at the self-knowledge that we experience as our own, are able to report to others, use as guides to our behavior, and embrace as *me*?

One answer that has emerged over the past 60 years is that a handful of self-evaluation motives exert powerful influences that guide the transformation of information "out there" to a self "in here." Self-evaluation motives provide systematic and strategic ways of bringing us in contact with, avoiding, constructing, reacting to, and processing the wealth of possible self-relevant information "out there." In doing so, over our lives we construct the self that helps us survive—survive in the very basic Darwinian sense of our evolutionary past and in a broader and more "cultured" sense today. In the discussion that follows, I provide commonly used definitions of the most common self-evaluation motives, briefly trace their history, and summarize the current state of affairs. In this effort, I make no attempt to provide a comprehensive review; even book-length treatments of single motives (e.g., Alicke & Sedikides, 2010) stretch the ability to provide complete coverage. Next, I discuss the implications of common self-evaluation motives for self-knowledge and bias. Last, I suggest that the current way that these motives are conceptualized is deficient for addressing the link to self-knowledge. I offer an alternative perspective that places the self-evaluation motives in a broader context, one that emphasizes the fit of a person's self-attributes to the demands of the environment. This alternative view identifies challenges to the way self-knowledge is defined and assessed.

The Big Four

It has become typical to define self-evaluation as arising from four basic motives—*self-enhancement, self-assessment, self-verification*, and *self-improvement* (Sedikides & Strube, 1997; see also Helzer & Dunning, Chapter 23, this volume).[1] Self-enhancement represents not only striving to place the self in a positive light (sometimes called *positivity strivings*) but also defending or protecting the self from threat (e.g., Alicke & Sedikides, 2009). Self-assessment represents striving to achieve an accurate representation of the self, sometimes at the expense of positive self-regard, but in the service of reducing uncertainty about self-attributes (e.g., Trope, 1983, 1986). Self-verification represents striving to maintain consistency in self-perceptions (often in relation to the views held about us by important others), in the service of producing and maintaining a predictable and controllable world (e.g., Swann, 1990; Swann et al., 2003). Self-improvement (sometimes called *self-expansion*) represents striving to grow and expand the self beyond its current boundaries or limits in the service of identifying new avenues for self-expression (e.g., Taylor, Neter, & Wayment, 1995; Wayment & Taylor, 1995).

Early work on each motive progressed largely in isolation, with few attempts to integrate them in any fashion. The importance of each motive was apparent (see Sedikides & Strube, 1995; 1997) but their relation to each other was largely unknown (though speculations were frequently offered, e.g., Strube, 1990). Claims for supremacy soon followed, as did attempts to determine a "winner" in something akin to cage matches to declare a single victor. The contestants were most often self-enhancement pitted against either self-assessment (e.g., Strube & Roemmele, 1985; Trope & Pomerantz, 1998) or self-verification (e.g., Katz & Beach, 2000). Occasionally all three joined the fray (e.g., Sedikides, 1993). If anything was certain from this early work, it was that matters were hardly simple. Indeed, it often was clear that motive expression depended on other variables (e.g., task diagnosticity, self-attribute centrality, self-attribute uncertainty, uncertainty orientation) and that the motives often worked in concert (e.g., Bosson & Swann, 2001), perhaps even serving a larger purpose.

More recent work has continued to map the moderators, boundary conditions, and relations of the motives to each other (e.g., Chang-Schneider & Swann, 2010; Neff & Karney, 2002), relations to other processes (e.g., Leonardelli & Lakin, 2010) and to extend the research to new samples and situations. It is now clear, for example, that self-motives extend to the groups and collectives that define the self (e.g., Chen, Chen, & Shaw, 2004; Chen, Taylor, & Jeung, 2006; Stets & Harrod, 2004), consistent with the view that selves do not exist in isolation but are embedded in social environments (Sedikides & Brewer, 2001). Researchers have also begun exploring self-evaluation motives over the age span (e.g., Reijntjes, Thomaes, Kamphuis, de Castro, & Telch, 2010; Trzesniewski, Kinal, & Donnellan, 2010) and in a variety of cultures (e.g., Chiu, Wan, Cheng, Kim, & Yang, 2010; Heine & Raineri, 2009; Sedikides, 2007; Spencer-Rodgers, Boucher, Peng, & Wang, 2009). Not surprisingly, the prominence of these motives varies by age in sensible ways and the nature of their expression depends on culture (though the motives themselves appear universal). Individuals also vary in their preferences for particular motives (e.g., Anseel & Lievens, 2007; Hepper, Gramzow, & Sedikides, 2010; Strube & Yost, 1993). Finally, there have been important attempts to demonstrate the applied implications of the self-motives (e.g., Anseel & Lievens, 2006, 2007; Anseel, Lievens, & Levy, 2007; Arndt & Goldenberg, 2010; Dauenheimer, Stahlberg, Spreemann, & Sedikides, 2002; Halliwell & Dittmar, 2005; Neiss, Sedikides, Shahinfar, & Kupersmidt, 2006; Pinel & Swann, 2000; Seyle & Swann, 2007; Swann & Chang-Schneider, 2008).

After decades of research and hundreds of studies, we would seem to be on firm footing in making the link from self-evaluation motives to self-knowledge. At a high level, we might expect that people know what their motives allow them to know, reflecting filters or emphases that particular self-motives impose on the processing of self-relevant information.[2] The self-enhancement motive, for example, predicts that our self-perceptions should be positively biased because we encounter and interpret the world in ways that reveal our positive self-attributes in sharper relief than our limitations. This should especially be true for higher-level self-attributes than for lower-level acts because the former are more easily interpreted in self-serving ways that defy verification by others. The self-assessment motive, in contrast, predicts that we ought to be quite accurate about our self-attributes, especially those that can be verified by others and that are tied to clear and important outcomes or standards. The self-verification motive offers a rather different kind of prediction—whether or not our self-views are accurate in some objective sense, we strive to bring the views of others in line with our own and so there should be substantial self–other correspondence, especially for others who are important to us and whose expectations we care about. Similarly, because understanding the views of others and the impact we have on others plays such a central role in self-verification strivings, *meta-accuracy* (i.e., our knowledge of how others perceive us) should be substantial as well, at least among well-acquainted and vested others. The self-improvement motive is harder to pin down. In part this reflects the fact that among members of the self-motive family, self-improvement is the runt of the litter, having come along much later and so having much less research available to map its boundary conditions and implications. We might venture the prediction that self-improvement requires both accuracy and bias—accuracy so that our self-improvement efforts are strategic and have some hope of success, but also positively biased because improvement likely depends on the promise or hope of success to carry us through the periods of uncertainty that we likely will encounter (cf. Armor, Massey, & Sackett, 2008; Taylor & Brown, 1988).

But, of course, we should not expect a decisive winner here any more than we would get in the larger literature on motive presence and influence. Indeed, at a lower and more nuanced level, we should expect the influence of self-motives on self-knowledge to be guided by moderators. As such, self-knowledge should be fluid and its nature dependent on the self-motives that are active at the time self-knowledge is produced and possibly when it is probed. Immediately, then, we see a potential problem in asking simple questions such as "Do people hold accurate or biased self-views?" or "Do others agree with assessments we have of ourselves?" It depends. Does *this* person, at *this* time, for *this* self-attribute have a good reason to be accurate? Was an important uncertainty about a central trait reduced by seeking diagnostic information from a trusted source? Or is the self-attribute in question of low importance *right now*, to the target and others? The answers to these kinds of questions surely have an impact on whether a particular person is accurate or biased about a particular self-attribute assessed at a particular time. They likely influence as well whether that person's views are shared by others. Indeed, simple questions about accuracy and bias are largely off the mark. Stated differently, most self-knowledge is highly dependent on *context*—context that is highly idiosyncratic to the individual, requiring careful attention to how and why the particular self-knowledge is relevant at particular times and in particular environments.[3] Viewed outside the context of self-evaluation motives, the answers to questions about accuracy or bias are likely to be quite muddled.

What do the data say? We can certainly find evidence to support the influence of most of the self-motives on self-knowledge. Perhaps most prominent are positivity biases in what people know (or claim to know) about themselves. The well-known better-than-average effect (e.g., Guenther & Alicke, 2010), for example, is one of the easiest phenomena to demonstrate and follows naturally from the self-enhancement motive.[4] Likewise, people easily and commonly take advantage of ambiguous concepts (e.g., intelligence, creativity) to construe them in ways that boost the positivity of self-views (Critcher, Helzer, & Dunning, 2010). Indeed, in general, people are wrong in a lot ways when asked to report on themselves, and the errors are hardly random. When the errors are valenced, the overwhelming tendency is to bias matters in the direction of self-enhancement. This might be taken as evidence for the prominence, perhaps even supremacy, of the self-enhancement motive in guiding self-perception, but I think a different interpretation is plausible. In most cases, researchers probe the nature of self-knowledge when the self-evaluative stakes are quite low. In most research (and probably in life, too), there is little to lose in overclaiming positive self-attributes because there is little cost to doing so and potentially there are substantial benefits (e.g., Taylor & Brown, 1988; but see Kwan et al., 2004, 2008). In a sense, the self-enhancement motive and its influence on self-knowledge might be thought of as the default or resting state of the self-system when it is not being called upon to do something more important or demanding in the way of self-evaluation.

And most of the time, and probably in most research contexts, the self-system is not called upon to do anything that might be called demanding or "high stakes." I return to this point shortly.

When one searches for evidence of self-accuracy, self–other correspondence, and meta-accuracy, the yield is, by comparison, surprisingly low and limited to research on abilities, personality traits, and well-being. To some extent, this reflects the assumption held by many researchers that people must be substantially accurate in their self-views because they have privileged access to much of what stands for self-knowledge, and they have a vested interest in being experts about themselves. More likely, researchers have avoided the accuracy and meta-accuracy questions because of vexing problems in definition and measurement (for discussion, see Schneider & Schimmack, 2009; Vazire, 2010; Vogt & Colvin, 2005; Wilson, 2009; see also in this volume, Back & Vazire, Chapter 9; Carlson & Kenny, Chapter 15). Until recently, most evidence for self-accuracy, self–other correspondence, and meta-accuracy has been rather disappointing and fraught with methodological and conceptual problems (for good discussion of these problems, see Carlson & Furr, 2009; Vazire & Carlson, 2010; Vazire & Mehl, 2008). Recent and more careful analyses show that we are capable of knowing ourselves *to some extent* (Vazire, 2010; Vazire & Carlson, 2010; Vazire & Mehl, 2008), that our self-views can agree *to some extent* with others (e.g., Vazire, 2010; Vazire & Mehl, 2008), and that we are aware *to some extent* of the trait impressions we have on others (Carlson & Furr, 2009). To paraphrase Vazire and Carlson (2010), our self-views are tethered to reality and to others, but the bond is hardly strong or pervasive. Clearly we know stuff about ourselves—others do, too—but the amount we know is apparently not all that impressive, and others know things about us that we apparently don't know ourselves.

Part of the problem is that we shouldn't really expect self-accuracy, self–other correspondence, and meta-accuracy to be particularly robust, at least overall. Vexing measurement problems aside, they should depend in sensible ways on moderators. Emerging evidence is beginning to show this. For example, Vazire (2010) found that self-accuracy relative to other-accuracy depended on whether traits were observable and evaluative. Self–other agreement depended on level of acquaintance as well. Carlson and Furr (2009) found that meta-accuracy was sensitive to context and the nature of the acquaintance whose impressions were in question. In future efforts of this kind, researcher can be guided to some extent by the moderators that have been found to be important in the self-motives area (e.g., trait verifiability, self-attribute centrality, trait modifiability). In summary, although research on the self-knowledge implications of self-motives has been rather limited, it has begun to arrive at some of the same conclusions as the larger self-motives literature—general bias or accuracy should not be expected, moderators matter, and the context in which accuracy and bias are explored is important to consider (see also Funder, 2003; Silvia, 2001).

It would be simple to end at this point and claim that "more research is necessary"—that self-knowledge research is simply in its infancy and needs to grow and develop in much the same way as the self-motives area by mapping the boundary conditions, establishing the relevant moderators, and finding each motive's domain of application and the influence it exerts on what we can know about ourselves. This is surely a large part of it, but I don't think this is entirely the picture. In the next section, I suggest that the manner in which self-evaluation motives have been conceived is limited in an important way and that this has important implications for the way self-knowledge should be studied.

A P-E Fit Perspective

For the most part, research on self-evaluation motives has focused on a particular motive at a time, operating on a single or small number of self-attributes examined in a narrow range of circumstances, under "low impact" conditions. Although this "ground-level" view has been productive, it is rather myopic and may miss much of interest for understanding the nature of self-knowledge, especially as it operates in everyday life. It certainly tends to ignore that we have multiple identities that need to be negotiated *within* the individual, and that these identities exist within a larger social structure (cf. Burke, 2003). It also misses the possibility that self-motives, regardless of their hierarchical relations among themselves, may work in concert for a larger purpose or function.

Rephrasing a question posed earlier, "When the self does what it is designed to do, what does it provide?" One answer is that the self helps bring us into closer relation and better match with the environments we encounter and create. Simply put, what humans seek, and what the self is designed to provide, is P-E fit. When an individual's self-attributes, needs, values, and goals are well matched to the environment—when the individual has found a good "opportunity structure"—successful outcomes are more likely, poor outcomes are more easily overcome, and life generally is experienced as satisfying and fruitful. The P-E fit perspective has been quite popular (e.g., Caplan, 1987; Holland, 1997; Kristof, 1996; Kristof-Brown & Guay, 2011; Pervin, 1968; Walsh, Craik, & Price, 2000) and has been applied in a wide variety of areas, including personality consistency (e.g., Roberts & DelVecchio, 2000; Roberts & Robins, 2004); mental health (Swartz-Kulstad & Martin, 2000); vocational selection and guidance (e.g., Holland, 1997; Nauta, 2010); and job satisfaction, work adjustment, and organizational commitment (e.g., Dawis & Lofquist, 1984; Edwards, Caplan, & Harrison, 1998; Edwards & Shipp, 2007; Wheeler, Buckley, Halbesleben, Brouer, & Ferris, 2005). In the discussion that follows, I outline the basic elements of the P-E fit perspective, suggest how it provides a potentially useful way to view self-evaluation motives, then indicate the particular implications for understanding self-knowledge.

Although particular manifestations of the P-E fit perspective vary, there are several commonalities. First, the P-E fit perspective assumes that individuals seek, construct, and maintain optimal relations of the self with the environment. The environment reflects not only the physical world we inhabit but also the social worlds we traverse and create (e.g., Holland, 1997; Schneider, 2001). We seek environments that match our needs, desires, and values, and within which our abilities allow us to achieve our goals easily. Second, because we inhabit multiple environments, P-E fit is a compromise among them and "best fit" in some absolute sense is illusive. Likewise, we must contend with the P-E fit strivings of others, and these might compete with or assist our own, either benignly or strategically. Consequently, P-E fit changes over time (e.g., Roberts & Robins, 2004). At a particular time, individuals gravitate toward (or actively construct) environments in which they can thrive, *relatively speaking*. Third, P-E fit can arise from proactive or reactive efforts (Lofquist & Dawis, 1991); that is, we might actively seek or construct better fitting environments because the current situation changes and is aversive, or because we desire or believe that a better environment can be found (see, e.g., applications to job mobility; Cable & Judge, 1996; Chatman, 1991). Underlying all of these features is a fundamental assumption: Aspects of the person cannot be defined in the absence of the environments that the person inhabits, and in turn, those environments are defined in part by the people within them.

P-E fit can be conceptualized at different levels, from "atomistic" to "molar" (Edwards, Cable, Williamson, Lambert, & Shipp, 2006). No matter how fit is defined (and the definitions need not agree), a key assumption is that it may make little sense to talk about self-attributes in the abstract, apart from environments. Am I a good driver? Depends on what you are asking me to drive, at what time, under what conditions, and so forth. Only by defining the environment can I begin to answer questions about fit and arrive at a sensible answer. Importantly, if the environmental context is not defined clearly, respondents will make assumptions that may vary considerably and not agree with those held by the researcher. Furthermore, aspects of the person and aspects of the environment can be measured *subjectively* and *objectively*. Subjective assessments are self-reports, from the person's perspective, about the attributes that person possesses and the matching environmental features. Objective assessments represent measures external to the person, often by other people (e.g., peers, coworkers, spouses) who are in a position to know the target person's attributes and the relevant features of that person's environment. Figure 24.1 illustrates the kinds of fit indices that can result. They range from the wholly subjective (Fit_1) to the entirely objective (Fit_4). In each case, the extent to which the person and environment assessments correspond defines *fit* (e.g., a person desiring accurate feedback about quality of performance in a work environment that provides regular performance-based reviews would be in a state of fit; a spouse needing emotional support paired with a partner who instead provides advice and information would be in a state of poor fit).

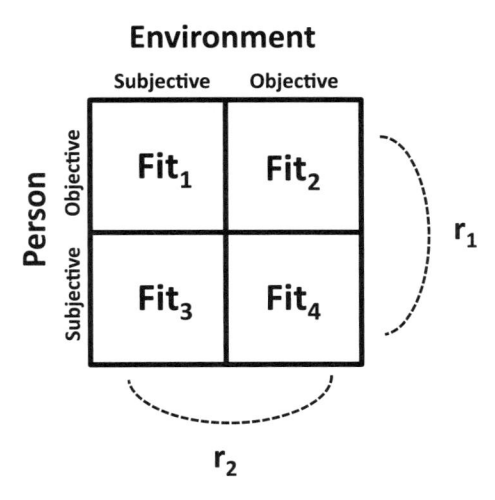

FIGURE 24.1. Indices of fit and self–other correspondence from a P-E fit perspective.

Within this P-E fit framework, the self-evaluation motives operate to identify, maintain, or increase fit, and they can do this by (1) operating on the person or the environment and (2) operating on the subjective or objective dimensions. Depending on the current state of fit (acceptable or not), the goal of the motives can be *fit maintenance* or *fit change*. These goals might be carried out in a multitude of ways, but all are in the service of higher level P-E fit. For example, the self-assessment motive would be valuable for determining accurately what the environment demands (or provides) and whether the attributes of the person provide a reasonable match. If they do not, attempts can be made to change the self in order to bring it into better alignment with the environment (self-improvement, operating on the objective dimension of the person). Alternatively, it might be easier to change the environment, either by altering features of the current environment to provide a better match to the current self, or by identifying a new "opportunity structure" that provides a better match. The former would correspond to the action of the self-verification motive on objective features of the environment; the latter would represent a form of "self-improvement," albeit one that operates to move the individual to a new environment in order to improve the P-E fit. This latter example also indicates how more than two motives might be necessary to achieve the goal of good fit—moving to a new environment would also require the action of the self-assessment motive in order to determine the features of the new environment. Self-verification could likewise operate on the subjective dimension of the environment, in which case the individual alters perceptions of the environment in the service of maintaining perceived fit. Of course, perceived fit cannot deviate too much from objective fit, at least to the extent that we believe objective fit is tied to important consequences for the person.

What about the self-enhancement motive? Surprisingly, its role is rather different in this new perspective compared to its traditional status. Here it operates largely on the subjective dimension of the person to bolster *perceptions* of fit that are biased to appear more favorable than they really are. This would be reflected in deviations between subjective and objective assessments of the self that suggest better self-features than actually possessed (e.g., better than average). But, it could in addition operate on the subjective dimension of the environment to bolster the apparent fit of person to environment. Both are likely to happen when misperceived fit has little consequence or resources are unavailable to produce better actual fit. In the former case, I suspect we harbor these misperceptions in large part because the stakes for being wrong are low in many cases.

One of the most important implications of this P-E fit framework for the present discussion is that other people are key elements of our environments (as we are elements of their environments), and, those others are often not uninterested spectators of our own P-E fit strivings. They often have a vested interest in it and assist it because to do so in turn assists their own P-E fit strivings (e.g., the actions of parents and children, romantic couples, coworkers). In this way, others support, prop up, scaffold, and generally assist the P-E fit strivings for others, often behind the scenes, constituting a "hidden hand" that guides them toward their goals. One important implication is that we may not recognize these efforts on our behalf and, as a consequence, we may believe our P-E fit arises more from our own attributes than is true. Indeed, these helpful others may more truthfully know our limitations because they have been carefully paving the road ahead in ways that skirt our liabilities (e.g., a good defensive driver understands quite well the ineptitude of others on the road and at the same time, by artfully avoiding their mistakes, makes those foolish drivers feel as if they are actually quite skilled). It seems unfair, or at least inaccurate, to label these self-reports as biased in the same manner that we would label brazen attempts at self-aggrandizement.

Space does not permit fleshing out other important details, but brief mention of a few other implications of this model is useful. Clearly, the functioning of the P-E fit system requires a "misfit detector"—a way of knowing that fit is threatened, so that the self-motives can be mobilized in the service of fit maintenance or change. Vigilance of this sort would likely be quite costly and so it likely is served by a threat-monitoring system that is relatively automatic. Previous similar ideas such as Leary's sociometer (Leary & Guadagno, 2011) are useful guides; indeed, in the current framework, the sociometer detects one type of poor fit (low acceptance by others), albeit a quite important one. Likewise, fit should have a discernable phenomenology—we should feel it when we have it and especially when we don't. Previous discussions of *flow* (e.g., Csikszentmihalyi, 1990) provide one avenue for future research, but consistent P-E fit likely correlates well with more common and mundane experiences such as life satisfaction, subjective well-being, and self-esteem. Acute episodes of poor fit likely generate anxiety as customary feelings of control and predictability are challenged. Finally, P-E fit is ultimately self-regulatory, so concerns about limited resources (Vohs & Baumeister, 2011) and the impact that chronic demands have on the ability to achieve fit will be important avenues for future work.

P-E Fit Implications for Self-Knowledge

What does P-E fit have to do with self-knowledge? First, it suggests that people know themselves to the extent that they can easily navigate their environments and achieve good fit. This might be achieved by changing the self or changing the environment, or both, but it ultimately means that self-knowledge has an environment–knowledge referent. Stated differently, self-knowledge is tied to environments, so to know what people know about themselves we need to know what they know about the environments in which they operate—where they apply their self-knowledge. This offers two recommendations for additional measurements in the quest for understanding self-knowledge: (1) Measure the features of the environment in which knowledge is relevant, and (2) measure fit as a proxy for good application of self-knowledge and the degree to which the self-evaluation motives work as part of a coordinated system. Although efforts to measure environments and situations have lagged behind efforts to measure people, recent work (e.g., Funder, 2009; Sherman, Nave, & Funder, 2010; Wagerman & Funder, 2009) is encouraging and suggests the utility of carefully attending to both parts of the P-E relation. By contrast, the utility of P-E fit as an indicator of self-knowledge application remains to be explored. Indeed, agreement among the different forms of fit measurement is an open question.

A second implication of the P-E fit perspective also derives from Figure 24.1, in which there are two representations of correlations. On the right is symbolized (r_1) the correlation between subjective and objective measures of the person. This might be, for example, a correlation of self-reported traits (subjective) and the reports by peers (objective) of those same traits. Or it might be a correlation between self-reported traits (subjective) and directly observed behavioral manifestation of those traits (objective). These kinds of correlations, of course, are commonly calculated and taken as evidence for accuracy or bias. But note that a similar set of correlations can be calculated with reference to environments (r_2). Given the emphasis on environments in the P-E fit perspective, we should be at least as interested in accuracy and bias in the perception of environments as we are for the self. The two are joined at the hip in this view, and complete understanding of self-knowledge will be greatly informed by knowing how people understand the environments in which they operate.

A third implication of the P-E fit perspective derives from an assumption about the outcome of P-E fit striving. When the P-E fit system operates well (and, I would argue, humans are designed so that it does work well most of the time), we are typically in a state of acceptable P-E fit. In this stasis condition, self-knowledge is largely inaccessible because we simply don't need it to be accessible. We operate more from habit than deliberation. To be sure, people will readily answer questions about their self-attributes and environments, but the self-knowledge they purport to have may be largely tacit and not readily open to their inspection. The problem from a P-E fit standpoint is that because they have not had a challenge to their P-E fit, they have not been called upon to think about environment-relevant self-attributes in a careful and deliberate fashion. The implication for self-knowledge measurement is that most assessment situations catch people in these stasis conditions, when the relevance of self-knowledge is low. That won't stop people from reporting what they know, but they may not be able to report much.[5] Accordingly, we can learn much from assessing self-knowledge under conditions when it is relevant—under conditions of active fit maintenance or change.

Conclusion

We don't arrive at our self-conceptions easily or haphazardly, and they can seem to be moved by self-evaluation motives that at times are working at cross purposes. That impression is largely due to viewing self-evaluation motives at the wrong level. When viewed from the perspective of P-E fit, self-evaluation motives can be seen to have important and largely consistent influences on bringing people into closer contact and better commerce with their environments. Importantly, this perspective suggests some ways that self-knowledge should be approached if a clear understanding of accuracy and bias is to be achieved.

NOTES

1. Not surprisingly there is not a complete consensus on the number or nature of self-evaluation motives, their position in a hierarchy, or their relation to other higher or lower motives, drives, or needs. In recent work (Alicke & Sedikides, 2010), for example, the distinction between *self-enhancement* and *self-protection* has been encouraged to highlight that these represent important and distinguishable facets of what has previously been viewed as a

single motive. This may prove to be an important nuance, but in this chapter I refer to both with the term *self-enhancement*. I largely avoid the hierarchy debate as well. Some (e.g., Alicke & Sedikides, 2009; Sedikides & Strube, 1997) have argued that self-enhancement is the more basic and primary motive, with others operating in its service. Others have argued against this hierarchy, according at least as much primacy to consistency or coherence concerns (e.g., Kwang & Swann, 2010; Swann, Rentfrow, & Guinn, 2003). As will become apparent, hierarchy issues will not concern us. Still others have suggested that self-evaluation motives are sometimes supplanted by other motives (e.g., need for communion; Kwang & Swann, 2010) or collectively serve a larger purpose, such as facilitating social relationships (e.g., Leary, 2007, 2008). These nuances, I think, are quite important and suggest the need for a broader context when discussing self-evaluation motives.

2. This does not mean that people know what motives are influencing their self-knowledge—a level of metacognition that seems unlikely, especially given that these motives may operate outside of awareness.

3. Swann (1984; Gill & Swann, 2004) has argued a similar position with regard to person perception accuracy; that is, knowledge of others is likely quite circumscribed, specific to interaction goals in the context of particular relationships.

4. Even here, however, matters may not be as simple as they first appear. Kwan and colleagues (Kwan, John, Kenny, Bond, & Robins, 2004; Kwan, John, Robins, & Kuang, 2008; Kwan, Kuang, & Zhao, 2008) have argued persuasively for the need to delineate self-evaluation into perceiver, target, and unique self-perception components. The *perceiver* component represents the general tendency to view others positively (see also halo bias, Anusic, Schimmack, Pinkus, & Lockwood, 2009; Schimmack, Schupp, & Wagner, 2008) whereas the *target* component represents the general tendency to be viewed positively by others. Both of these components can give rise to apparent self-enhancement bias, without representing a bias unique to self-perceptions in the strict sense. Only self-perceptions that have these general components removed are unique to the self. As Kwan and colleagues show, these distinctions have important implications for the relation of self-enhancement to adjustment.

5. There is one other implication worth mentioning here. If P-E fit is the typical condition for most people, most of the time, then the implication is that correlated markers of well-being should be elevated because most people find their locally optimal opportunity structures. In this sense, most of the time, P-E fit strivings lead most people to believe "all is for the best, in the best of all possible worlds." Available evidence indicates that most people report they are happy (e.g., Biswas-Diener, Vittersø, & Diener, 2005; Diener & Diener, 1996).

REFERENCES

Alicke, M. D., & Sedikides, C. (2009). Self-enhancement and self-protection: What they are and what they do. *European Journal of Social Psychology, 20*, 1–48.

Alicke, M. D., & Sedikides, C. (2010). Self-enhancement and self-protection: Historical overview and conceptual framework. In M. D. Alicke & C. Sedikides (Eds.), *Handbook of self-enhancement and self-protection* (pp. 1–19). New York: Guilford Press.

Anseel, F., & Lievens, F. (2006). Certainty as a moderator of feedback reactions?: A test of the strength of the self-verification motive. *Journal of Occupational and Organizational Psychology, 79*, 533–551.

Anseel, F., & Lievens, F. (2007). The relationship between uncertainty and desire for feedback: A test of competing hypotheses. *Journal of Applied Social Psychology, 37*, 1007–1040.

Anseel, F., Lievens, F., & Levy, P. E. (2007). A self-motives perspective on feedback-seeking behavior: Linking organizational behavior and social psychology research. *International Journal of Management Reviews, 9,* 211–236.

Anusic, I., Schimmack, U., Pinkus, R. T., & Lockwood, P. (2009). The nature and structure of correlations among Big Five ratings: The halo-alpha-beta model. *Journal of Personality and Social Psychology, 97,* 142–156.

Armor, D. A., Massey, C., & Sackett, A. M. (2008). Prescribed optimism: Is it right to be wrong about the future? *Psychological Science, 19,* 329–331.

Arndt, J., & Goldenberg, J. L. (2010). When self-enhancement drives health decisions: Insights from a terror management health model. In M. D. Alicke & C. Sedikides (Eds.), *Handbook of self-enhancement and self-protection* (pp. 380–398). New York: Guilford Press.

Biswas-Diener, R., Vitterso, J., & Diener, E. (2005). Most people are pretty happy, but there is cultural variation: The Inughuit, the Amish, and the Maasai. *Journal of Happiness Studies, 6,* 205–226.

Bosson, J. K., & Swann, W. B., Jr. (2001). The paradox of the sincere chameleon: Strategic self-verification in close relationships. In J. Harvey & A. Wenzel (Eds.), *Close romantic relationships: Maintenance and enhancement* (pp. 67–86). Mahwah, NJ: Erlbaum.

Burke, P. J. (2003). Relationships among multiple identities. In P. J. Burke, T. J. Owens, R. T. Serpe, & P. A. Thoits (Eds.), *Advances in identity theory and research* (pp. 195–214). New York: Kluwer Academic/Plenum Press.

Cable, D. M., & Judge, T. A. (1996). Person–organization fit, job choice decisions, and organizational entry. *Organizational Behavior and Human Decision Processes, 67,* 294–311.

Caplan, R. D. (1987). Person–environment fit theory and organizations: Commensurate dimensions, time perspectives, and mechanisms. *Journal of Vocational Behavior, 31,* 248–267.

Carlson, E. N., & Furr, R. M. (2009). Evidence of differential meta-accuracy: People understand the different impressions they make. *Psychological Science, 20,* 1033–1039.

Chang-Schneider, C., & Swann, W. B., Jr. (2010). The role of uncertainty in self-evaluative processes: Another look at the cognitive–affective crossfire. In R. Arkin, K. C. Oleson, & P. J. Carroll (Eds.), *Handbook of the uncertain self* (pp. 216–231). New York: Psychology Press.

Chatman, J. A. (1991). Matching people and organizations: Selection and socialization in public accounting firms. *Administrative Science Quarterly, 36,* 459–484.

Chen, S., Chen, K. Y., & Shaw, L. (2004). Self-verification motives at the collective level of self-definition. *Journal of Personality and Social Psychology, 86,* 77–94.

Chen, S., Taylor, L. S., & Jeung, K. Y. (2006). Collective self-verification among members of a naturally occurring group: Possible antecedents and long-term consequences. *Basic and Applied Social Psychology, 28,* 101–115.

Chiu, C., Wan, C., Cheng, S. Y. Y., Kim, Y., & Yang, Y. (2010). Cultural perspectives on self-enhancement and self-protection. In M. D. Alicke & C. Sedikides (Eds.), *Handbook of self-enhancement and self-protection* (pp. 425–451). New York: Guilford Press.

Critcher, C. R., Helzer, E. G., & Dunning, D. (2010). Self-enhancement via redefinition: Defining social concepts to ensure positive views of the self. In M. D. Alicke & C. Sedikides (Eds.), *Handbook of self-enhancement and self-protection* (pp. 69–91). New York: Guilford Press.

Csikszentmihalyi, M. (1990). *Flow: The psychology of optimal experience.* New York: HarperCollins.

Dauenheimer, D. G., Stahlberg, D., Spreemann, S., & Sedikides, C. (2002). Self-enhancement, self-verification, or self-assessment?: The intricate role of trait modifiability in the self-evaluation process. *Revue Internationale de Psychologie Sociale, 15,* 89–112.

Dawis, R. V., & Lofquist, L. H. (1984). *A psychological theory of work adjustment*. Minneapolis: University of Minnesota Press.

Diener, E., & Diener, C. (1996). Most people are happy. *Psychological Science, 7*, 181–185.

Edwards, J. R., Cable, D. M., Williamson, I. O., Lambert, L. S., & Shipp, A. J. (2006). The phenomenology of fit: Linking the person and environment to the subjective experience of person–environment fit. *Journal of Applied Psychology, 91*, 802–827.

Edwards, J. R., Caplan, R. D., & Harrison, R. V. (1998). Person–environment fit theory: Conceptual foundations, empirical evidence, and directions for future research. In C. L. Cooper (Ed.), *Theories of organizational stress* (pp. 28–67). Oxford, UK: Oxford University Press.

Edwards, J. R., & Shipp, A. J. (2007). The relationship between person–environment fit and outcomes: An integrative theoretical framework. In C. Ostroff & T. A. Judge (Eds.), *Perspectives on organizational fit* (pp. 209–258). Mahwah, NJ: Erlbaum.

Funder, D. C. (2003). Toward a social psychology of person judgments: Implications for person perception accuracy and self-knowledge. In J. P. Forgas, K. D. Williams, & W. von Hippel (Eds.), *Social judgments: Implicit and explicit processes* (pp. 115–133). New York: Cambridge University Press.

Funder, D. C. (2009). Persons, behaviors, and situations: An agenda for personality psychology in the postwar era. *Journal of Research in Personality, 43*, 120–126.

Gill, M. J., & Swann, W. B., Jr. (2004). On what it means to know someone: A matter of pragmatics. *Journal of Personality and Social Psychology, 86*, 405–418.

Guenther, C. L., & Alicke, M. D. (2010). Deconstructing the better-than-average effect. *Journal of Personality and Social Psychology, 99*, 755–770.

Halliwell, E., & Dittmar, H. (2005). The role of self-improvement and self-evaluation motives in social comparisons with idealised female bodies in the media. *Body Image, 2*, 249–261.

Heine, S. J., & Raineri, A. (2009). Self-improving motivations and collectivism: The case of Chileans. *Journal of Cross-Cultural Psychology, 40*, 158–163.

Hepper, E. G., Gramzow, R. H., & Sedikides, C. (2010). Individual differences in self-enhancement and self-protection strategies: An integrative analysis. *Journal of Personality, 78*, 781–814.

Holland, J. L. (1997). *Making vocational choices: A theory of vocational personalities and work environments* (3rd ed.). Lutz, FL: Psychological Assessment Resources.

Katz, J., & Beach, S. R. H. (2000). Looking for love?: Self-verification and self-enhancement effects on initial romantic attraction. *Personality and Social Psychology Bulletin, 2*, 1526-1539.

Kristof, A. L. (1996). Person–organization fit: An integrative review of its conceptualizations, measurement, and implications. *Personnel Psychology, 49*, 1–49.

Kristof-Brown, A. L., & Guay, R. P. (2011). Person–environment fit. In S. Zedeck (Ed.), *APA handbook of industrial and organizational psychology* (Vol. 3, pp. 3–50). Washington, DC: American Psychological Association.

Kwan, V. S. Y., John, O. P., Kenny, D. A., Bond, M. H., & Robins, R. W. (2004). Reconceptualizing individual differences in self-enhancement bias: An interpersonal approach. *Psychological Review, 111*, 94–110.

Kwan, V. S. Y., John, O. P., Robins, R. W., & Kuang, L. L. (2008). Conceptualizing and assessing self-enhancement bias: A componential approach. *Journal of Personality and Social Psychology, 94*, 1062–1077.

Kwan, V. S. Y., Kuang, L. L., & Zhao, B. X. (2008). In search of the optimal ego: When self-enhancement bias helps and hurts adjustment. In H. A. Wayment & J. Bauer (Eds.), *Transcending self-interest: Psychological explorations of the quiet ego* (pp. 43–51). Washington, DC: American Psychological Association.

Kwang, T., & Swann, W. B., Jr. (2010). Do people embrace praise even when they feel unworthy?: A review of critical tests of self-enhancement versus self-verification. *Personality and Social Psychology Review, 14*, 263–280.

Leary, M. R. (2007). Motivational and emotional aspects of the self. *Annual Review of Psychology, 58*, 317–344.

Leary, M. R. (2008). Functions of the self in interpersonal relationships: What does the self actually do? In J. V. Wood, A. Tesser, & J. G. Holmes (Eds.), *The self and social relationships* (pp. 95–115). New York: Psychology Press.

Leary, M. R., & Guadagno, J. (2011). The sociometer, self-esteem, and the regulation of interpersonal behavior. In K. D. Vohs & R. F. Baumeister (Eds.), *Handbook of self-regulation: Research, theory, and applications* (2nd ed., pp. 339–354). New York: Guilford Press.

Leonardelli, G. J., & Lakin, J. L. (2010). The new adventures of regulatory focus: Self-uncertainty and the quest for a diagnostic self-evaluation. In R. Arkin, K. C. Oleson, & P. J. Carroll (Eds.), *Handbook of the uncertain self* (pp. 249–265). New York: Psychology Press.

Lofquist, L. H., & Dawis, R. V. (1991). *Essentials of person–environment correspondence counseling*. Minneapolis: University of Minnesota Press.

Nauta, M. M. (2010). The development, evolution, and status of Holland's theory of vocational personalities: Reflections and future directions for counseling psychology. *Journal of Counseling Psychology, 57*, 11–22.

Neff, L. A., & Karney, B. R. (2002). Self-evaluation motives in close relationships: A model of global enhancement and specific verification. In P. Noller & J. A. Feeney (Eds.), *Understanding marriage: Developments in the study of couple interaction* (pp. 32–58). New York: Cambridge University Press.

Neiss, M. B., Sedikides, C., Shahinfar, A., & Kupersmidt, J. B. (2006). Self-evaluation in a naturalistic context: The case of juvenile offenders. *British Journal of Social Psychology, 45*, 499–518.

Pervin, L. A. (1968). Performance and satisfaction as a function of individual–environment fit. *Psychological Bulletin, 69*, 56–68.

Pinel, E. C., & Swann, W. B., Jr. (2000). Finding the self through others: Self-verification and social movement participation. In S. Stryker, T. Owens, & R. W. White (Eds.), *Self, identity, and social movements* (pp. 132–152). Minneapolis: University of Minnesota Press.

Reijntjes, A., Thomaes, S., Kamphuis, J. H., de Castro, B. O., & Telch, M. J. (2010). Self-verification strivings in children holding negative self-views: The mitigating effects of a preceding success experience. *Cognitive Therapy and Research, 34*, 563–570.

Roberts, B. W., & DelVecchio, W. F. (2000). The rank-order consistency of personality traits from childhood to old age: A quantitative review of longitudinal studies. *Psychological Bulletin, 126*, 3–25.

Roberts, B. W., & Robins, R. W. (2004). Person–environment fit and its implications for personality development: A longitudinal study. *Journal of Personality, 72*, 89–110.

Schimmack, U., Schupp, J., & Wagner, G. G. (2008). The influence of environment and personality on the affective and cognitive component of subjective well-being. *Social Indicators Research, 89*, 41–60.

Schneider, B. (2001). Fits about fit. *Applied Psychology: An International Review, 50*, 141–152.

Schneider, L., & Schimmack, U. (2009). Self-informant agreement in well-being ratings: A meta-analysis. *Social Indicators Research, 94*, 363–376.

Sedikides, C. (1993). Assessment, enhancement, and verification determinants of the self-evaluation process. *Journal of Personality and Social Psychology, 65*, 317–338.

Sedikides, C. (2007). Self-enhancement and self-protection: Powerful, pancultural, and functional. *Hellenic Journal of Psychology, 4,* 1–13.

Sedikides, C., & Brewer, M. B. (2001). *Individual self, relational self, collective self.* Philadelphia: Psychology Press.

Sedikides, C., & Skowronski, J. J. (2000). On the evolutionary functions of the symbolic self: The emergence of self-evaluation motives. In A. Tesser, R. B. Felson, & J. M. Suls (Eds.), *Psychological perspectives on self and identity* (pp. 91–117). Washington, DC: American Psychological Association.

Sedikides, C., Skowronski, J. J., & Gaertner, L. (2004). Self-enhancement and self-protection motivation: From the laboratory to an evolutionary context. *Journal of Cultural and Evolutionary Psychology, 2,* 61–79.

Sedikides, C., & Strube, M. J. (1995). The multiply motivated self. *Personality and Social Psychology Bulletin, 21,* 1330–1335.

Sedikides, C., & Strube, M. J. (1997). Self-evaluation: To thine own self be good, to thine own self be sure, to thine own self be true, and to thine own self be better. In M. Zanna (Ed.), *Advances in experimental social psychology* (Vol. 29, pp. 209–269). New York: Academic Press.

Seyle, D. C., & Swann, W. B., Jr. (2007). Being oneself in the workplace: Self-verification and identity in organizational contexts. In C. A. Bartel, S. Blader, & A. Wrzesniewski (Eds.), *Identity and the modern organization.* Mahwah, NJ: Erlbaum.

Sherman, R. A., Nave, C. S., & Funder, D. C. (2010). Situational similarity and personality predict behavioral consistency. *Journal of Personality and Social Psychology, 99,* 330–343.

Silvia, P. J. (2001). On introspection and self-perception: Does self-focused attention enable accurate self-knowledge? *Review of General Psychology, 5,* 241–269.

Spencer-Rogers, J., Boucher, H. C., Peng, K., & Wang, L. (2009). Cultural differences in self-verification: The role of naive dialecticism. *Journal of Experimental Social Psychology, 45,* 860–866.

Stets, J. E., & Harrod, M. M. (2004). Verification across multiple identities: The role of status. *Social Psychology Quarterly, 67,* 155–171.

Strube, M. J. (1990). In search of self: Balancing the good and the true. *Personality and Social Psychology Bulletin, 16,* 699–704.

Strube, M. J., & Roemmele, L. A. (1985). Self-enhancement, self-assessment, and self-evaluative task choice. *Journal of Personality and Social Psychology, 49,* 981–993.

Strube, M. J., & Yost, J. H. (1993). Control motivation and self-appraisal. In G. Weary, F. Gleicher, & K. Marsh (Eds.), *Control motivation and social cognition* (pp. 220–254). New York: Springer-Verlag.

Swann, W. B., Jr. (1984). Quest for accuracy in person perception: A matter of pragmatics. *Psychological Review, 91,* 457–477.

Swann, W. B., Jr. (1990). To be adored or to be known?: The interplay of self-enhancement and self-verification. In E. T. Higgins & R. M. Sorrentino (Eds.), *Handbook of motivation and cognition: Vol. 2. Foundations of social behavior* (pp. 408–448). New York: Guilford Press.

Swann, W. B., Jr., & Chang-Schneider, C. (2008). Self-verification in relationships as an adaptive process. In J. V. Wood, A. Tesser, & J. G. Holmes (Eds.), *The self and social relationships* (pp. 49–72). New York: Psychology Press.

Swann, W. B., Jr., Rentfrow, P. J., & Guinn, J. (2003). Self-verification: The search for coherence. In M. Leary & J. Tagney (Eds.), *Handbook of self and identity* (pp. 367–383). New York: Guilford Press.

Swartz-Kulstad, J. L., & Martin, W. E., Jr. (2000). Culture as an essential aspect of person–environment fit. In W. E. Martin Jr. & J. L. Swartz-Kulstad (Eds.), *Person–environment psychology and mental health: Assessment and intervention* (pp. 169–195). Mahwah, NJ: Erlbaum.

Taylor, S. E., & Brown, J. D. (1988). Illusion and well-being: A social psychological perspective on mental health. *Psychological Bulletin, 103,* 193–210.

Taylor, S. E., Neter, E., & Wayment, H. A. (1995). Self-evaluation processes. *Personality and Social Psychology Bulletin, 21,* 1278–1287.

Trope, Y. (1983). Self-assessment in achievement behavior. In J. M. Suls & A. G. Greenwald (Eds.), *Psychological perspectives on the self* (Vol. 2, pp. 93–121). Mahwah, NJ: Erlbaum.

Trope, Y. (1986). Self-enhancement and self-assessment in achievement behavior. In. R. M. Sorrentino & E. T. Higgins (Eds.), *Handbook of motivation and cognition: Vol. 1. Foundations of social behavior* (pp. 350–378). New York: Guilford Press.

Trope, Y., & Pomerantz, E. M. (1998). Resolving conflicts among self-evaluative motives: Positive experiences as a resource for overcoming defensiveness. *Motivation and Emotion, 22,* 53–72.

Trzesniewski, K. H., Kinal, M. P.-A., & Donnellan, M. B. (2010). Self-enhancement and self-protection in a developmental context. In M. D. Alicke & C. Sedikides (Eds.), *Handbook of self-enhancement and self-protection* (pp. 341–357). New York: Guilford Press.

Vazire, S. (2010). Who knows what about a person?: The self–other knowledge asymmetry (SOKA) model. *Journal of Personality and Social Psychology, 98,* 281–300.

Vazire, S., & Carlson, E. N. (2010). Self-knowledge of personality: Do people know themselves? *Social and Personality Psychology Compass, 4,* 605–620.

Vazire, S., & Mehl, M. (2008). Knowing me, knowing you: The accuracy and unique predictive validity of self-ratings and other-ratings of daily behavior. *Journal of Personality and Social Psychology, 95,* 1202–1216.

Vogt, D. S., & Colvin, C. R. (2005). Assessment of accurate self-knowledge. *Journal of Personality Assessment, 84,* 239–251.

Vohs, K. D., & Baumeister, R. F. (Eds.). (2011). *Handbook of self-regulation: Research, theory, and applications* (2nd ed.). New York: Guilford Press.

Wagerman, S. A., & Funder, D. C. (2009). Personality psychology of situations. In P. J. Corr & G. Matthews (Eds.), *The Cambridge handbook of personality psychology* (pp. 27–42). New York: Cambridge University Press.

Walsh, W. B., Craik, K. H., & Price, R. H. (2000). *Person–environment psychology: New directions and perspectives* (2nd ed.). Mahwah, NJ: Erlbaum.

Wayment, H. A., & Taylor, S. E. (1995). Self-evaluation processes: Motives, information use, and self-esteem. *Journal of Personality, 63,* 729–757.

Wheeler, A. R., Buckley, M. R., Halbesleben, J. R. B., Brouer, R. L., & Ferris, G. R. (2005). "The elusive criterion of fit" revisited: Toward an integrative theory of multidimensional fit. In J. J. Martocchio (Ed.), *Research in personnel and human resources management* (Vol. 24, pp. 265–304). New York: Elsevier Science/JAI Press.

Wilson, T. D. (2009). Know thyself. *Perspectives on Psychological Science, 4,* 384–389.

Yost, J. H., Strube, M. J., & Bailey, J. R. (1992). The construction of the self: An evolutionary view. *Current Psychology: A Journal for Diverse Perspectives on Diverse Psychological Issues, 11,* 110–121.

CHAPTER 25

Reducing Egoistic Biases in Self-Beliefs

MARK R. LEARY
KAITLIN TONER

In examining the processes by which people gain knowledge about themselves, many of the authors in this volume have discussed factors that undermine the accuracy of people's self-relevant beliefs. For example, people may rely on information that is incomplete or inaccurate, retrieve self-relevant memories in a biased fashion, draw illogical inferences about themselves from otherwise valid information, or maintain illusions about themselves to ward off negative emotions or lowered self-esteem.

Other authors have discussed such biases in detail (see Campbell & Sedikides, 1999; Dunning, Johnson, Ehrlinger, & Kruger, 2003; Gilovich, 1993; Pronin, 2009; Pronin, Lin, & Ross, 2002; see Hansen & Pronin, Chapter 21, and Helzer & Dunning, Chapter 23, this volume), and we do not review those literatures ourselves. Rather, our goal is to consider ways to minimize egoistic biases in ourselves and others, thereby increasing the validity of people's beliefs about themselves. We acknowledge upfront that little research has explicitly examined methods for decreasing a person's biases—whether those efforts are implemented by the person him- or herself or imposed by others. Yet the literature offers hints regarding the nature and causes of these biases that provide a basis for speculating about how they can be reduced.

Our focus is specifically on egoistic biases. We use the term *egoistic* in its broadest meaning to refer to biases that arise from people's own perspectives, interests, and concerns. There are two general senses in which people's self-views can be egoistic. First, people's perceptions of themselves and their worlds are unavoidably narrow and egocentric, yet people typically believe that those views are correct even in the presence of contradictory information. Second, people's self-views are often more positive or negative than warranted by objective evidence because self-enhancing and self-depreciating self-views can have psychological or interpersonal benefits. After examining these two classes of egoistic biases, we discuss six possible ways to reduce egoistic self-perceptions in the service of improving self-knowledge.

Biases in Perspective: Egocentrism

People are unavoidably egocentric in their views of themselves and their worlds. No one can perceive the world from any perspective other than one's own, and all perceptions are not only biased by one's vantage point but also filtered through one's idiosyncratic experiences, values, personality attributes, motives, and personal concerns. Piaget (1960), who first discussed egocentrism in depth, focused on young children's inability to adopt the spatial perspectives of other people, but later theorists focused more on cognitive perspective taking, demonstrating that children are unable to appreciate the perspectives and thoughts of other people (Thompson, Goodvin, & Meyer, 2006). Although perspective-taking skills improve with age (Selman, 2003), egocentrism persists at least into the late teens or early 20s (Schwartz, Maynard, & Uzelac, 2008), and even after the point at which the extreme egocentric biases of childhood and adolescence have subsided, people nonetheless remain unable to escape their egocentrism entirely (Frankenberger, 2000).

In the realm of self-knowledge, egocentric views are perhaps most obvious when it comes to people's judgments of their own physical appearance and expressive behaviors. None of us can see our physical bodies as other people do, and valid comparisons of ourselves with other people are virtually impossible because we cannot see ourselves from all angles in three dimensions. This constricted view leaves considerable room for distortions in people's judgments of their appearance, along with a good deal of benign misperception.

The same is true of expressive behaviors such as facial expressions, gestures, and body language. People have virtually no access to these aspects of their behavior and thus often infer how they appear to others on the basis of their own intentions and emotions (Malle, 2006; Pronin, 2009). Research shows that people think that they are far more psychologically transparent than they really are, and that other people are able to detect (or should be able to detect) their subjective feelings and reactions (Gilovich, Savitsky, & Medvec, 1998). This point has implications for distortions in self-beliefs. Because people base their self-views heavily on their intentions and feelings (Malle, 2006; Pronin, 2009), they are likely to dismiss feedback about themselves when it diverges from how they intended to be.

The inherent egocentrism of people's physical perspectives is compounded by the fact that people see themselves in a limited array of contexts. Much has been written about the fact that observers often have an exaggerated sense of other people's behavioral stability because they see others in a narrow range of situations (Gilbert & Malone, 1995; Ross, Amabile, & Steinmetz, 1977; Ross & Sicoly, 1979). In many ways, people are in the same situation when it comes to drawing inferences about themselves. People obviously see themselves in a much wider array of situations than other people do, yet the range of contexts in which each person operates is still remarkably constrained. As a result, people cannot fully appreciate how they might respond in situations in which they have never been. A man might firmly believe that he is capable of unhesitatingly and ruthlessly killing someone who threatens his family's safety, but that belief might be quite wrong—yet unlikely to be disconfirmed—because he has never been in a situation that was remotely diagnostic.

Even if people know that their life situation does not provide adequate information about a particular personal characteristic, they may have trouble adjusting their inferences adequately. For example, students with a high grade point average (GPA) at a mediocre college may realize that their courses are not as demanding as those at more rigorous institutions yet not know how much they should adjust estimates of their academic ability. Thus, even when people know that their self-beliefs are influenced by their egocentric perspective and idiosyncratic factors, they may be unable to assess themselves accurately, even if they wish to do so.

Biases in Evaluation: Self-Enhancement and Self-Depreciation

In addition to egocentric biases that render people's self-beliefs narrow, idiosyncratic, and impoverished, egoistic biases are fueled by processes that lead people to evaluate themselves more positively or negatively than evidence suggests that they should. People tend to see the world through valenced eyes, rarely arriving at a conclusion about their personal characteristics without a sense of whether the characteristic is good and desirable or bad and undesirable.

Because self-beliefs carry evaluative connotations and, thus, emotional consequences, people sometimes construe events in ways that reflect on the desirability of their personal characteristics. Animals without the ability to self-reflect can influence their emotions only by taking action—for example, by seeking food, escaping danger, or socializing with conspecifics—but human beings can change their emotions simply by *thinking* about themselves in certain ways (Leary & Buttermore, 2003). Although the ability to regulate emotions through self-thought has benefits, it is accompanied by notable disadvantages in allowing people to feel better about themselves even while in circumstances that are detrimental to their well-being.

Although people's self-views can be biased in both negative and positive directions, social psychologists have focused mostly on self-enhancing beliefs. Many instances of self-enhancement are fueled by people's construal of their relative standing on positive or negative traits, such as when people overestimate their own abilities or good qualities as compared with others (Alicke & Govorun, 2005). In a related vein, some biases are due to unrealistic optimism in which people overestimate the likelihood of experiencing positive events and underestimate the probability of negative events (Armor & Taylor, 2002). Other self-enhancing biases arise when people accept undue responsibility for positive outcomes or downplay responsibility for negative outcomes (Campbell & Sedikides, 1999) to maintain favorable self-views and to avoid anxiety, guilt, and discomfort (Alicke & Sedikides, 2009). People are also egotistical in their judgments of other people's negative traits, overestimating the extent to which others share their undesirable characteristics and behaviors (Monin & Norton, 2003; Mullen & Goethals, 1990; Ross, Greene, & House, 1977) in order to minimize the negative emotions they experience when they contemplate their own negative attributes and behaviors.

Not all self-evaluative biases are positively valenced. Most notably, self-depreciation is a feature of many psychological problems, including depression and chronic shame (Pacini, Muir, & Epstein, 1998). Outside of the clinical domain, many people underestimate and downplay their positive attributes in certain domains (John & Robins, 1994; Owens, 1993; Schriber & Robins, Chapter 8, this volume), and some people steadfastly maintain that they are not as competent as they appear to others (Leary, Patton, Orlando, & Wagoner Funk, 2000). These negative self-views are associated with not only negative emotions but also undesired outcomes such as lower grades, antisocial behavior, interpersonal discord, and relationship dissatisfaction (Kim & Chiu, 2010; Owens, 1993, 1994; Sciangula & Morry, 2009).

We turn our attention in the remainder of the chapter to ways in which people can reduce these egoistic biases and foster more accurate self-beliefs. The recommendations that we offer can be framed at both individual and social levels of analysis; that is, individuals can use these approaches to improve their own or others' self-knowledge, but they can also be implemented at a group or societal level to promote accurate self-assessment more generally. In the remainder of the chapter, we discuss six broad categories of recommendations that involve (1) promoting the value of self-accuracy, (2) adopting a skeptical attitude toward one's self-beliefs, (3) accepting that one is ordinary and fallible, (4) reducing defensiveness, (5) lowering unnecessary self-evaluative thinking, and (6) explicitly challenging others' distorted self-views.

Valuing Accurate Self-Views

The Accuracy–Illusion Debate

This chapter is predicated on the assumption that enhancing the accuracy of people's self-relevant beliefs is often a desired goal because people generally fare better in life when their views of themselves are accurate as opposed to inaccurate and biased. Yet theorists have debated whether accurate self-beliefs are necessarily more adaptive than illusory ones.

Proponents of the merits of self-accuracy argue that accurate information about one's abilities, personality attributes, values, public images, and other personal characteristics is generally, if not universally, beneficial. As Bandura (1986) observed, "A reasonably accurate appraisal of one's capabilities is . . . of considerable value in effective functioning" (p. 393). Successful behavior in any domain requires that people accurately judge their attributes and abilities with respect to the situations they encounter. For example, people who overestimate their ability may tackle tasks on which they are doomed to frustration and failure or engage in unnecessarily risky (or potentially fatal) activities that they are incapable of managing safely. Likewise, students without an appropriate assessment of their strengths, weaknesses, and predilections may make career decisions that ultimately do not suit them well.

Furthermore, insight into one's characteristics may facilitate positive interpersonal interactions and relationships. People who know themselves well have a more accurate view of how they are perceived by other people (Vazire & Carlson, 2010) and can temper personal characteristics that create interpersonal problems. The fact that emotional intelligence is often conceptualized in terms of understanding oneself and others, relating well to people, and adapting to environmental demands suggests that self-knowledge underlies effective social behavior (Kluemper, 2008; Mayer, Salovey, & Caruso, 2008). And virtually all theories of adjustment and psychopathology suggest that psychological health requires an accurate self-view.

In contrast, proponents of the merits of self-illusions have pointed to advantages of maintaining unrealistic beliefs about oneself, particularly ones that are overly favorable (Taylor & Brown, 1988). This perspective suggests that overestimating one's ability promotes confidence and motivation, particularly when a person confronts failures and obstacles, and overestimating one's control over life is associated with indices of psychological health, including lower depression. Positive illusions may be particularly useful when people confront challenging, stressful, or traumatic events such as major failures, life-threatening illnesses, or serious accidents.

Research suggests that both the accuracy and the illusion perspectives are partially correct. People who hold unrealistically positive views of themselves certainly feel better about themselves, experience less negative affect, and persevere on difficult tasks that they might abandon if they had an accurate view of their abilities (Felson, 1984; Isen & Means, 1983; Taylor & Brown, 1988; Taylor, Lerner, Sherman, Sage, & McDowell, 2003; Wright, 2000). On the other hand, the tendency to self-enhance has been associated with maladjustment and relationship problems (Colvin & Block, 1994; Colvin, Block, & Funder, 1995; Kurt & Paulhus, 2008; Kwan, John, Robins, & Kuang, 2008; Robins & Beer, 2001). Furthermore, students who show either a self-enhancing or self-depreciating bias in evaluating their performance had a lower level of academic achievement, as well as lower subjective well-being (Kim, Chiu, & Zou, 2010). In contrast, Knee and Zuckerman (1998) showed that lack of illusions is associated with a nondefensive personality style oriented toward growth and learning. In addition, people's inflated self-beliefs can have consequences for other people and society at large. Excessively positive self-views foster conflict, whether between individuals, groups, or nations. When people, groups, or countries believe that they are more intelligent, moral, or otherwise exceptional than others, they are less likely to compromise. Indeed, many acts of violence—such as terrorism, genocide, and slavery—are fundamentally fueled by overly positive beliefs about one's competence, goodness, or worldview.

Promoting the Value of Accurate Self-Beliefs

The first step toward enhancing self-accuracy is to promote the value of having accurate self-views. Just as most people understand at a deep level that core values of honesty and truthfulness are strongly endorsed by other people and by basic cultural tenets, they should also come to see that having a realistic self-concept is also valued. Of course, people who endorse honesty nonetheless lie from time to time and, likewise, those who believe, in principle, that they should see themselves accurately often fail to do so, owing both to unavoidable biases and to episodes of deliberate self-deception. Indeed, although we suspect that most people claim to value seeing themselves honestly and accurately, evidence suggests that they often behave in ways that do not promote self-knowledge. For example, when given the choice between self-relevant information that is accurate, self-enhancing, or self-consistent, American participants tend to opt for favorable over accurate information (Sedikides, 1993). Even so, getting people to think about the consequences of accurate and inaccurate self-views should be beneficial.

Our suggestion that promoting self-accuracy as a value should enhance the veracity of people's self-views assumes that at least some sources of inaccuracy are under people's control. Research has shown this to be the case. For example, monetary incentives for accurate self-assessment decrease self-evaluation biases (Kim &

Chiu, 2010) and stressing the importance of being accurate increases the correlation between people's actual performance and their self-evaluations (Kim et al., 2010).

People's tendency to prefer accurate versus self-enhancing information about themselves differs across cultures. Although some theorists interpret research findings to indicate that people from East Asian cultures lack a motive to maintain their self-esteem (Heine & Hamamura, 2007), we interpret them differently. Rather than indicating that people in certain cultures do not care whether they feel good or bad about themselves, cultural differences in preferences for accurate versus enhancing feedback appear to reflect differences in cultural values. When their culture values having an accurate, uninflated self-view, people not only seek accurate information about themselves but also feel better about themselves when they believe that their self-views are realistic. These findings show that cultural values can influence the degree to which people prefer and seek out information that fosters accurate self-views.

But how can a culture that presently encourages self-enhancing illusions come to value accuracy? First, children implicitly learn to value accuracy versus positive illusions at an early age through instruction, modeling, and reinforcement for certain patterns of self-beliefs. For example, overpraising children—leading them to believe that a particular accomplishment is far grander than it is, or praising their intelligence or ability rather than their effort—can have detrimental effects on both the accuracy of their self-views and their ability to cope with failure (Mueller & Dweck, 1998). Thus, although teachers and parents may be well meaning in providing positively biased feedback, the positive illusions they instill may cause problems when children later face evidence to the contrary. If, instead, parents and educators model and reinforce accuracy, children will come to value seeing themselves accurately and be prepared for the obstacles and negative feedback they will inevitably confront in life.

Second, accuracy in self-beliefs might be fostered by showing people the detrimental effects of holding inaccurate and egocentric perceptions of oneself (Leary, 2004). Parents, teachers, religious leaders, and others should make an effort to convince people that having biased self-views, while often hedonically pleasant, can undermine their own success, relationships, and happiness in the long run. For example, people must recognize that egoistic beliefs can lead others to mistrust and dislike them, as well as fuel conflicts, whether interpersonal, societal, or international. People who realize the pernicious effects of these biases may become motivated to try to avoid them simply from the recognition that these beliefs compromise their well-being.

Third, cultural and societal messages can promote either illusion or accuracy as a value. Americans in particular seem to be exposed to many excessively positive illusions that stimulate egoistic thinking. For example, much political discourse in the United States is based on the premise of American exceptionalism, a trend that dates back to Puritan settlers who envisioned themselves as a "shining city on a hill" on which the rest of the world should model itself (Winthrop, 1630). Beliefs about national exceptionalism go beyond rational evaluations of the country's many advantages to an irrational minimization of its obvious shortcomings and problems. Indeed, an international study of national pride found that Americans had the highest level of national pride of the 33 nations surveyed (Smith & Kim, 2006). People take great pride in other group affiliations as well, as any sports fan waving a "Number 1" foam finger attests—despite the fact that only one team is actually in first place. Similarly, students and alumni are often very quick to point out the domains in which their school excels, though they may fail to note its less impressive aspects. Whether the group is a bowling league or a nation, its members are often encouraged to believe and endorse positive illusions about the group's qualities, and those who do not do so are often viewed as disloyal.

Promoting the value of nonegoistic self-views is only the first step to improving the accuracy of people's self-beliefs. Once people value seeing themselves accurately, they must take steps that will lead to improved self-knowledge.

Ego Skepticism

Despite overwhelming evidence that people are inclined to view themselves, their beliefs, their loved ones, their groups, and their pursuits in biased ways, most people believe that they see themselves and the world clearly. Indeed, a good deal of human perception is characterized by *naive realism*, the conviction that one sees the world (including oneself) accurately, and that others who do not see things similarly are mistaken (Ross & Ward, 1995). Undermining people's confidence in their self-views requires inculcating a pervasive attitude of *ego-skepticism*, which is the practice of reminding oneself that one's own interpretations and evaluations of events, outcomes, and people—including oneself—are construals rather than objective perceptions, and that those construals are biased in unknown ways. People must regularly acknowledge that their views of themselves are often limited, self-serving, and biased, and that their own views are, on average, no more likely to be correct than other people's. Widespread acceptance that everyone's beliefs about themselves are notoriously inaccurate should, over time, reduce the degree to which people cling too confidently to their beliefs about themselves.

Unfortunately, even when people fully accept the premise that their own views are often biased and commit themselves to practicing ego-skepticism, three factors make it difficult to implement ego-skepticism in practice. First, even if people fully accept that their self-views are often biased, they rightfully assume that many of their self-views and interpretations of events are reasonably correct. Thus, they are in the difficult position of trying to discern when they are and are not biased. Many processes may converge to convince people that their views are valid when they are not. For example, people display a confirmation bias when they test the accuracy of their beliefs, searching for evidence consistent with the hypothesis being tested rather than considering all relevant evidence. As a result, people gather and recall information selectively and interpret it in a biased way (Nickerson, 1998). Confirmation biases appear in particular for emotionally significant issues and for established beliefs, including self-beliefs. In addition, when people receive feedback that conflicts with their self-image, they are less likely to attend to it or remember it than when they receive self-congruent feedback.

Second, even when people recognize that they might be biased, they tend to believe that they are less biased than they actually are. Pronin and her colleagues (Hansen & Pronin, Chapter 21, this volume; Pronin et al., 2002) have studied the *bias blind spot*—the bias to assume that one is not biased (or at least less biased than other people). Thus, although people who endorse ego-skepticism will be skeptical of their self-relevant beliefs, they may nonetheless believe that they are less biased than they are (Hansen & Pronin, 2011). Even if people applied ego-skepticism to an infinite regress of biases about biases, they are still likely to remain somewhat biased. However—and this is the important point—trying to be ego-skeptical should reduce biases even if they are not eliminated, and people who practice ego-skepticism should cling to and defend their self-relevant beliefs less strongly. Merely being aware of their potential biases should lead people to be less insistent that their interpretations of personally relevant events are correct.

Unfortunately, cultural forces sometimes work against an attitude of ego-skepticism. We have already noted that nationalism discourages people from seeing their country and its citizens (including themselves) accurately. In addition, although most religions espouse selflessness as a virtue (see Leary, 2004), many paradoxically promote egoistic biases. The simple fact that most religions proclaim that their teachings are the only true ones fosters followers' beliefs that they are superior by virtue of having a more accurate view of God and the world than those who have other beliefs or none at all. Religious perspectives are particularly immune to externally caused change, but religious leaders who believe in the personal and social value of diminishing egoistic self-views could encourage their parishioners to temper their acceptance of religious doctrine with humility in their conviction that these beliefs are absolutely correct; that is, even highly religious people could potentially accept a particular doctrine as most likely to be correct, without being absolutely certain of their views or disdainful of other viewpoints. In some religions, such a viewpoint even has a scriptural basis (as in Paul's question, "For who has knowledge of the mind of the Lord?"; Corinthians 2:16).

Acceptance of Ordinariness and Fallibility

One reason that people cling to self-enhancing views is that many believe that in order to be a competent, likeable, and good person, they must be nearly perfect, preferably with as little effort as possible. Perfection obviously does not allow for failures or imperfections, so people must actually be free of flaws or else must distort or fail to recognize them. If people wish to reduce egoistic biases, they must accept the fact that they are fundamentally ordinary and fallible.

People should be encouraged to see that they need not be perfect—that flaws, flubs, and failures do not necessarily invalidate a positive self-perception and, in fact, are part and parcel of every well-balanced, successful person. To acknowledge an imperfection does not undermine people's generally positive view of themselves unless they internalize and overgeneralize that imperfection as an indication of pervasive inadequacy. This is not to say that people should never internalize failures or that they should not seek to learn from their mistakes or to improve. Rather, they should be willing to change when necessary, while acknowledging that perfection is impossible. In fact, seeing oneself accurately is a prerequisite for becoming a better person.

Some attempts have been made to promote people's acceptance of their flaws and deficiencies. In many ways, Ellis's (1962) rational-emotive therapy was designed to make people realize that they could relinquish "irrational beliefs" regarding the need always to be right, successful, and acceptable without sacrificing a positive self-image. Ellis argued against what he saw as a universal belief that one must be perfectly adequate, competent, and achieving, and he advocated teaching people to accept imperfection and shades of gray. Although Ellis's views have been applied most often in psychotherapeutic settings, efforts could be made to promote them more broadly.

In a related vein, people should be disabused of the belief that human beings in general are somehow special—a conviction that people often generalize to egoistic perceptions of themselves. In prescientific times, when people believed that Earth was the center of the universe, they could be excused for thinking that human beings are uniquely important in the grand scheme of things. But with the Copernican revolution, geocentric beliefs gave way to the realization that we occupy a small planet in a solar system that lies in the backwaters of an unexceptional galaxy in a universe whose size defies comprehension. Similarly, the Darwinian revolution, combined with advances in paleontology and natural history, knocked human beings off the pedestal on which they had put themselves by showing the evolutionary origins of human life and our place in the natural order. In philosophy, these realizations prompted adoption of the mediocrity principle, which holds that Earth and its inhabitants are not unique or special (Vilenkin, 1995). If we human beings are just another organism on an unremarkable planet, then there is little room for self-aggrandizing interpretations of our place in the universe, or for self-criticism for failing to meet unrealistic standards. Widespread acceptance of the mediocrity principle is thus an important element of reducing inflated self-views.

Without an acceptance of ordinariness, many people cope poorly with unflattering feedback. Instead, they compound the aversiveness of negative self-relevant information by castigating and punishing themselves. Given how harshly people criticize themselves for ordinary failures, problems, and lapses, it is little wonder that they prefer to distort their self-perceptions, thus avoiding self-flagellation. To remove this source of bias, people could learn to be more self-compassionate, treating themselves with kindness and concern in the face of failures, mistakes, rejections, losses, and other negative events (Neff, 2003). Because people who are low in self-compassion beat themselves up for their lapses and failures, they are motivated to distort self-relevant information in ways that minimize self-criticism. In contrast, self-compassionate people do not treat themselves harshly when they fail and thus have less use for self-serving illusions (Leary, Tate, Adams, Allen, & Hancock, 2007). One important feature of self-compassion is the recognition that everyone experiences failures, losses, humiliations, and rejections; thus, such events need not be taken personally (Neff, 2003).

Reducing Defensiveness

The biases that undermine self-knowledge are sometimes intensified when people feel compelled to defend their self-beliefs against information, evaluation, or feedback that challenges or contradicts them. Unlike opportunities for ego-skepticism, which arise from internal questioning, opportunities for defensiveness arise in reaction to external feedback. Two people may hold self-views that are equally colored by egocentric and evaluative biases, but upon receiving information that contradicts a particular self-view, one person may be willing to consider alternative evidence, whereas the other rigidly (and perhaps aggressively) defends his or her viewpoint. Defensiveness shields people from feedback that might otherwise improve the veracity of their self-views; thus, efforts to enhance the accuracy of self-beliefs must consider ways to minimize the degree to which people react defensively.

Such efforts must address four primary sources of defensive reactions. First, people naturally assume that their own beliefs about themselves are true (Ross & Ward, 1995) and certainly more accurate than other people's views of them (Pronin et al., 2002). Thus, when other people offer observations regarding their abilities, motivations, or characteristics that contradict their self-views, people naturally dismiss those observations and defend their views. To combat this tendency, people must be convinced that their views of themselves are not necessarily more accurate than other people's views of them. Simply noting that they can readily see that most other people's views of themselves do not appear to be accurate is a first step toward creating cracks in people's excessive confidence in their self-images. Beyond reminding people that their perceptions of themselves are often suspect, providing them with consensus feedback from a number of people may lower resistance to information that is inconsistent with their self-views. Feedback that might be easily dismissed when coming from an individual may be persuasive when provided by several people. This orchestrated attempt to provide corrective feedback is essentially what occurs in an "intervention," when friends and family members collectively try to convince a troubled individual to seek help for a problem.

Second, self-verification theory maintains that people actively defend their self-views because stable self-views help to guide their behavior and fulfill an epistemic function by providing a basis for understanding and responding to the world (Swann, Stein-Seroussi, & Giesler, 1992). Thus, people may reject information that is inconsistent with their self-views because it would undermine their confidence that they understand themselves and create uncertainty, if not anxiety, regarding how to respond in certain situations. To diffuse the power of self-verification processes that lead people to reject information that is inconsistent with their self-beliefs, people must be assured that revising an aspect of their self-views is not detrimental to their well-being, and that the costs of temporary inconsistency and uncertainty are compensated by the benefits of revising their self-view in ways that make it more accurate and useful. People may not always realize how strongly they are resisting information that does not coincide with their self-views, and recognizing their resistance may be the first step toward understanding and overcoming defensiveness.

Third, people often defensively maintain their positive or negative self-views because such views have benefits for them. Most obviously, people are not motivated to disabuse themselves of overly positive self-views because doing so would deprive them of personal satisfaction and engender negative emotions. But inaccurate negative self-beliefs can also be beneficial in providing excuses for poor performance and avoiding risk by not attempting challenging tasks (Owens, 1993). When this is the case, people must see the long-term value in adopting an accurate self-view that compensates for the loss of whatever benefits are sustaining the inaccurate one.

Fourth, the acknowledgment that one possesses certain characteristics often has implications for one's own, as well as others', expectations for oneself. People who possess positive characteristics are expected to put them to good use, and people who acknowledge problems and deficiencies are often expected to take action to remedy them. In both cases, having a fully accurate view of the self may put pressure on people—whether from themselves or from others—to take actions that they would rather not take. They may find it more desirable to maintain an inaccurate self-view that does not compel them to behave in undesired ways.

Central to most cases of defensiveness is a failure to distinguish real from symbolic threats to one's well-being. Some self-evaluative feedback—such as grades, performance reviews, and accusations of impropriety—can have real consequences for the quality of people's lives. However, a great deal of feedback, although perhaps troubling or inconsistent with people's existing views, has no tangible consequences, but people react as if it portends a real threat. Thus, helping people to distinguish tangible from purely symbolic threats to self would go a long way toward reducing defensiveness. Certain Eastern practices (e.g., Zen), as well as clinical approaches (e.g., dialectical behavior therapy), teach people to take self-relevant information at face value and without defensiveness.

Reducing Unnecessary Self-Evaluative Thinking

People obviously must evaluate themselves in order to make judicious decisions. Yet a great deal of self-evaluation is unnecessary, in that it serves no pragmatic function. And even when a particular self-evaluation is useful, many of people's self-evaluations are stronger and longer-lived than needed to make decisions or correct problems. To the extent that self-illusions and biases often involve self-evaluations that are unnecessary or overblown, egoistic biases might be reduced by lowering the amount of time people spend evaluating themselves.

Reducing illusionary thinking does not necessarily mean reducing self-thoughts as a whole. On the contrary, evidence suggests that increasing self-thoughts can sometimes increase accuracy of self-knowledge. For example, people who are high in private self-consciousness—the tendency to attend to one's own thoughts, feelings, attitudes, and goals—are more accurate in their judgments of true and false personality feedback than those who are low in private self-consciousness (Davies, 1994). Thus, it is not necessarily the overall amount of self-thought that needs to be reduced but rather its content or evaluative nature.

Meditation practices, including mindfulness, lower self-relevant thought, emphasize the deleterious effects of constant evaluation (both of oneself and the world more generally), and teach people to distance themselves from their thoughts about themselves (Shapiro, Schwartz, & Santerre, 2002). Insight meditation, for example, focuses on mindful observation of one's thoughts and feelings. The goal of insight meditation is to experience and accept the flow of sensations and thoughts (including self-thoughts) as they arise, without either getting carried away with them or trying to suppress them. Self-evaluations are noted but then released, and meditation practitioners are taught to respond to negative self-thoughts with kindness rather than judgment. Reflection is encouraged but rumination is not, allowing people to be curious about themselves without berating themselves about their inadequacies.

A related technique to reduce self-evaluation involves *hypoegoic self-regulation*, which occurs when people avoid direct and effortful attempts to control their behavior in favor of responding naturally and spontaneously (Leary, Adams, & Tate, 2006; Leary & Guadagno, 2011). Hypoegoic self-regulation works by both lessening overall self-thinking and increasing the proportion of self-thoughts that are concrete rather than abstract. *Concrete* self-thoughts deal mostly with the immediate situation at hand and with tangible ways to pursue one's goals. In contrast, *abstract* self-thoughts tend to involve more self-judgment and comparisons to higher-order goals and other people. For example, a new mother in a hypoegoic state might evaluate whether her attempts to soothe her infant are working (a concrete self-thought) without transitioning into wondering whether she's a good mother (an abstract self-evaluation). Concrete self-thoughts are more likely to be accurate than abstract thoughts because they involve observable behaviors and outcomes rather than inferences and generalizations.

Explicit Challenges to Egoistic Views

Although people sometimes challenge others' expressed egoistic self-beliefs, they usually let them pass. Norms specify that people refrain from disputing other people's claims about themselves except under special circumstances (Brown & Levinson, 1987). Although the practice of allowing others to save face has much to recommend it, it also has a downside. When egoistic claims go unquestioned, the claimant receives implicit confirmation of his or her biased self-view.

Although we do not recommend that people challenge others' egoistic views as a matter of course, we think that norms should encourage listeners to question others' blatantly egoistic views when they have important implications. If someone's distorted self-views are inconsequential, we can perhaps afford to suffer them in silence. But when a person's inaccurate self-views have consequences (e.g., directly or implicitly disparaging others, implying that one is entitled to be treated in special ways, justifying unfair treatment of other people, or leading to pursuit of dangerous or implausible goals) listeners have the right to question the person's self-beliefs. Of course, rebutting another person's inaccurate self-views is risky, in that doing so may lead to conflict, damaged relationships, and possibly even violence. But when people's self-beliefs have negative consequences for others, rebuttals may be worth the risk.

Some evidence for how to challenge egoistic biases comes from clinical psychology. For example, cognitive-behavioral therapy (CBT) encourages people to treat their thoughts as hypotheses, and to gather and evaluate the evidence for and against these hypotheses. The goal is for clients to learn to consider alternative evaluations of themselves and their lives. The clinical psychologist's role is not so much to tell people that their beliefs are incorrect but rather to train and motivate them to test their assumptions about themselves. CBT has been widely used in the treatment of depression and other disorders with negatively valenced self-perceptions (Dobson, 1989). It has also been used, with more limited success, to treat mania, which is characterized by grandiose self-thoughts (Gregory, 2010).

Applied to everyday life, these approaches might suggest that people should question each other about self-views that seem incorrect and remind each other of the possibility of alternative explanations. Directly criticizing another person's perspective might well lead to defensiveness, but a Socratic method of encouraging self-questioning could promote accurate self-reflection in others.

Conclusions

Despite the benefits of seeing oneself clearly, many psychological and social processes conspire to render people's self-beliefs less than wholly accurate. Some of these processes are coldly cognitive, involving physical perspective, the use of heuristics, and information processing. Others are motivated efforts to maintain certain self-views because they are personally pleasing by virtue of being familiar, consistent, or providing desired hedonic effects. To the extent that accurate self-beliefs promote a higher quality of life than do inaccurate ones, researchers should continue to explore the sources of inaccurate self-beliefs and ways to improve self-knowledge.

REFERENCES

Alicke, M., & Govorun, O. (2005). The better-than-average effect. In M. D. Alicke, D. A. Danning, & J. I. Krueger (Eds.), *The self in social judgment* (pp. 85–106). New York: Psychology Press.

Alicke, M., & Sedikides, C. (2009). Self-enhancement and self-protection: What they are and what they do. *European Review of Social Psychology, 20*, 1–48.

Armor, D., & Taylor, S. (2002). When predictions fail: The dilemma of unrealistic optimism. In T. Gilovich, D. Griffin, & D. Kahneman (Eds.), *Heuristics and biases: The psychology of intuitive judgment* (pp. 334–347). New York: Cambridge University Press.

Bandura, A. (1986). *Social foundations of thought and action: A social cognitive theory.* Englewood Cliffs, NJ: Prentice-Hall.

Brown, P., & Levinson, S. C. (1987). *Politeness: Some universals in language usage.* Cambridge, UK: Cambridge University Press.

Campbell, W., & Sedikides, C. (1999). Self-threat magnifies the self-serving bias: A meta-analytic integration. *Review of General Psychology, 3*, 23–43.

Colvin, C., & Block, J. (1994). Do positive illusions foster mental health?: An examination of the Taylor and Brown formulation. *Psychological Bulletin, 116*, 3–20.

Colvin, C., Block, J., & Funder, D. C. (1995). Overly positive self-evaluations and personality: Negative implications for mental health. *Journal of Personality and Social Psychology, 68*, 1152–1162.

Davies, M. (1994). Private self-consciousness and the perceived accuracy of true and false personality feedback. *Personality and Individual Differences, 17*, 697–701.

Dobson, K. (1989). A meta-analysis of the efficacy of cognitive therapy for depression. *Journal of Consulting and Clinical Psychology, 57*, 414–419.

Dunning, D., Johnson, K., Ehrlinger, J., & Kruger, J. (2003). Why people fail to recognize their own incompetence. *Current Directions in Psychological Science, 12*, 83–87.

Ellis, A. (1962). *Reason and emotion in psychotherapy.* New York: Lyle Stuart.

Felson, R. B. (1984). The effect of self-appraisals of ability on academic performance. *Journal of Personality and Social Psychology, 47*, 944–952.

Frankenberger, K. D. (2000). Adolescent egocentrism: A comparison among adolescents and adults. *Journal of Adolescence, 23*, 343–354.

Gilbert, D. T., & Malone, P. S. (1995). The correspondence bias. *Psychological Bulletin, 117,* 21–38.

Gilovich, T. (1993). *How we know what isn't so: The fallibility of human reason in everyday life.* New York: Simon & Schuster.

Gilovich, T., Savitsky, K., & Medvec, V. H. (1998). The illusion of transparency: Biased assessments of others' ability to read one's emotional states. *Journal of Personality and Social Psychology, 75,* 332–346.

Gregory, V. (2010). Cognitive-behavioral therapy for mania: A meta-analysis of randomized controlled trials. *Social Work in Mental Health, 8,* 483–494.

Hansen, K., & Pronin, E. (2011, January). *Unaffected by bias: Claiming objectivity after knowingly using a biased strategy.* Paper presented at the annual meeting of the Society for Personality and Social Psychology, San Antonio, TX.

Heine, S. J., & Hamamura, T. (2007). In search of East Asian self-enhancement. *Personality and Social Psychology Review, 11,* 1–24.

Isen, A. M., & Means, B. (1983). The influence of positive affect on decision-making strategy. *Social Cognition, 2,* 18–31.

John, O. P., & Robins, R. W. (1994). Accuracy and bias in self-perception: Individual differences in self-enhancement and the role of narcissism. *Journal of Personality and Social Psychology, 66,* 206–219.

Kim, Y. H., & Chiu, C. Y. (2010). *Unaware or unmotivated?: Accuracy motivation in self-assessment of ability.* Unpublished manuscript, University of Illinois.

Kim, Y. H., Chiu, C. Y., & Zou, Z. (2010). Know thyself: Misperceptions of actual performance undermine achievement motivation, future performance, and subjective well-being. *Journal of Personality and Social Psychology, 99,* 395–409.

Kluemper, D. H. (2008). Trait emotional intelligence: The impact of core-self evaluations and social desirability. *Personality and Individual Differences, 44,* 1402–1412.

Knee, C., & Zuckerman, M. (1998). A nondefensive personality: Autonomy and control as moderators of defensive coping and self-handicapping. *Journal of Research in Personality, 32,* 115–130.

Kurt, A., & Paulhus, D. L. (2008). Moderators of the adaptiveness of self-enhancement: Operationalization, motivational domain, adjustment facet, and evaluator. *Journal of Research in Personality, 42,* 839–853.

Kwan, V. Y., John, O. P., Robins, R. W., & Kuang, L. (2008). Conceptualizing and assessing self-enhancement bias: A componential approach. *Journal of Personality and Social Psychology, 94,* 1062–1077.

Leary, M. R. (2004). *The curse of the self: Self-awareness, egotism, and the quality of human life.* New York: Oxford University Press.

Leary, M. R., Adams, C. E., & Tate, E. B. (2006). Hypo-egoic self-regulation: Exercising self-control by diminishing the influence of the self. *Journal of Personality, 74,* 1803–1831.

Leary, M. R., & Buttermore, N. R. (2003). The evolution of the human self: Tracing the natural history of self-awareness. *Journal for the Theory of Social Behaviour, 33,* 365–404.

Leary, M. R., & Guadagno, J. (2011). The role of hypo-egoic self-processes in optimal functioning and subjective well-being. In K. M. Sheldon, T. B. Kashdan, & M. F. Steger (Eds.), *Designing positive psychology: Taking stock and moving forward* (pp. 135–146). New York: Oxford University Press.

Leary, M. R., Patton, K. M., Orlando, A. E., & Wagoner Funk, W. (2000). The impostor phenomenon: Self-perceptions, reflected appraisals, and interpersonal strategies. *Journal of Personality, 68,* 725–756.

Leary, M. R., Tate, E. B., Adams, C. E., Allen, A. B., & Hancock, J. (2007). Self-compassion and reactions to unpleasant self-relevant events: The implications of treating oneself kindly. *Journal of Personality and Social Psychology, 92,* 887–904.

Malle, B. F. (2006). The actor–observer asymmetry in causal attribution: A (surprising) meta-analysis. *Psychological Bulletin, 132,* 895–919.

Mayer, J. D., Salovey, P., & Caruso, D. R. (2008). Emotional intelligence: New ability or eclectic traits? *American Psychologist, 63,* 503–517.

Monin, B., & Norton, M. (2003). Perceptions of a fluid consensus: Uniqueness bias, false consensus, false polarization, and pluralistic ignorance in a water conservation crisis. *Personality and Social Psychology Bulletin, 29,* 559–567.

Mueller, C. M., & Dweck, C. S. (1998). Praise for intelligence can undermine children's motivation and performance. *Journal of Personality and Social Psychology, 75,* 33–52.

Mullen, B., & Goethals, G. R. (1990). Social projection, actual consensus and valence. *British Journal of Social Psychology, 29,* 279–282.

Neff, K. D. (2003). The development and validation of a scale to measure self-compassion. *Self and Identity, 2,* 223–250.

Nickerson, R. S. (1998). Confirmation bias: A ubiquitous phenomenon in many guises. *Review of General Psychology, 2,* 175–220.

Owens, T. (1993). Accentuate the positive—and the negative: Rethinking the use of self-esteem, self-deprecation, and self-confidence. *Social Psychology Quarterly, 56,* 288–299.

Owens, T. (1994). Two dimensions of self-esteem: Reciprocal effects of positive self-worth and self-deprecation on adolescent problems. *American Sociological Review, 59,* 391–407.

Pacini, R., Muir, F., & Epstein, S. (1998). Depressive realism from the perspective of cognitive–experiential self-theory. *Journal of Personality and Social Psychology, 74,* 1056–1068.

Piaget, J. (1960). *The language and thought of the child.* London: Routledge & Kegan Paul.

Pronin, E. (2009). The introspection illusion. In M. P. Zanna (Ed.), *Advances in experimental social psychology* (Vol. 41, pp. 1–67). Burlington, MA: Academic Press.

Pronin, E., Lin, D. Y., & Ross, L. (2002). The bias blind spot: Perceptions of bias in self versus others. *Personality and Social Psychology Bulletin, 28,* 369–381.

Robins, R. W., & Beer, J. S. (2001). Positive illusions about the self: Short-term benefits and long-term costs. *Journal of Personality and Social Psychology, 80,* 340–352.

Ross, L. D., Amabile, T. M., & Steinmetz, J. L. (1977). Social roles, social control, and biases in social-perception processes. *Journal of Personality and Social Psychology, 35,* 485–494.

Ross, L., Greene, D., & House, P. (1977). The false consensus effect: An egocentric bias in social perception and attribution processes. *Journal of Experimental Social Psychology, 13,* 279–301.

Ross, M., & Sicoly, F. (1979). Egocentric biases in availability and attribution. *Journal of Personality and Social Psychology, 37,* 322–336.

Ross, L., & Ward, A. (1995). Psychological barriers to dispute resolution. In M. Zanna (Ed.), *Advances in experimental social psychology* (pp. 255–304). San Diego, CA: Academic Press.

Schwartz, P. D., Maynard, A. M., & Uzelac, S. M. (2008). Adolescent egocentrism: A contemporary view. *Adolescence, 43,* 441–448.

Sciangula, A., & Morry, M. (2009). Self-esteem and perceived regard: How I see myself affects my relationship satisfaction. *Journal of Social Psychology, 149,* 143–158.

Sedikides, C. (1993). Assessment, enhancement, and verification determinants of the self-evaluation process. *Journal of Personality and Social Psychology, 65,* 317–338.

Selman, R. L. (2003). *The promotion of social awareness: Powerful lessons from the partnership of developmental theory and classroom practice.* New York: Russell Sage Foundation.

Shapiro, S. L., Schwartz, G. E. R., & Santerre, C. (2002). Meditation and positive psychology.

In C. R. Snyder & S. J. Lopez (Eds.), *Handbook of positive psychology* (pp. 632–645). New York: Oxford University Press.

Smith, T. W., & Kim, S. (2006). National pride in comparative perspective: 1995/96 and 2003/04. *International Journal of Public Opinion Research, 18,* 127–136.

Swann, W. B., Jr., Stein-Seroussi, A., & Giesler, R. B. (1992). Why people self-verify. *Journal of Personality and Social Psychology, 62,* 392–401.

Taylor, S. E., & Brown, J. D. (1988). Illusion and well-being: A social psychological perspective on mental health. *Psychological Bulletin, 103,* 193–210.

Taylor, S. E., Lerner, J. S., Sherman, D. K., Sage, R. M., & McDowell, N. K. (2003). Portrait of the self-enhancer: Well adjusted and well liked or maladjusted and friendless? *Journal of Personality and Social Psychology, 84,* 165–176.

Thompson, R. A., Goodvin, R., & Meyer, S. (2006). Social development: Psychological understanding, self-understanding, and relationships. In J. L. Luby (Ed.), *Handbook of preschool mental health: Development, disorders, and treatment* (pp. 3–22). New York: Guilford Press.

Vazire, S., & Carlson, E. N. (2010). Self-knowledge of personality: Do people know themselves? *Social and Personality Psychology Compass, 4,* 605–620.

Vilenkin, A. (1995). Predictions from quantum cosmology. *Physical Review Letters, 74,* 846–849.

Winthrop, J. (1630). *A modell of Christian charity* [Sermon to the Massachusetts Puritans]. Collections of the Massachusetts Historical Society (Coal Bin Serials Old South No. 207), Boston.

Wright, S. S. (2000). Looking at the self in a rose-colored mirror: Unrealistically positive self-views and academic performance. *Journal of Social and Clinical Psychology, 19,* 451–462.

Author Index

Aarts, H., 23
Abelson, R. P., 169, 380
Ablow, J. C., 96
Abramson, L., 93
Abramson, L. Y., 108, 117
Achenbach, T. M., 265
Acitelli, L. K., 225, 226, 227, 228, 229, 250
Acker, F., 189
Adams, C. E., 421, 424
Adler, J. M., 9, 18, 293, 327, 329, 330, 337
Agatstein, F., 242
Agerström, J., 316
Ahadi, S., 134
Aharon, I., 212
Ainslie, G., 363
Ajzen, I., 317
Akert, R. M., 97
Alba, J. W., 163
Albarracín, D., 173
Albers, L. W., 158
Albright, L., 91, 242, 243, 245, 248, 249
Albright, M. D., 96
Aldridge, J. W., 213
Alea, N., 295
Alenius, M., 258
Alessandri, G., 373
Alexander, R. A., 97
Alhakami, A., 181
Alicke, M., 415
Alicke, M. D., 93, 345, 347, 385, 386, 398, 400, 406, 407

Allen, A., 310
Allen, A. B., 421
Alloy, L. B., 117
Allport, G. W., 106, 113
Allyn, J., 170
Alnaes, R., 268
Alonso, P., 260
Alvarez, G., 12
Amabile, T. M., 414
Amador, X. F., 258, 263
Ames, D. R., 99, 118, 250
Amsterdam, B., 16
Andersen, S. M., 97
Anderson, C., 92, 96, 99, 100, 118
Anderson, C. P., 99, 100
Anderson, K., 332
Anderson, R. D., 245
Andrade, E. B., 219
Angleitner, A., 133
Anseel, F., 399
Anthony, J. C., 259
Antonucci, T. C., 228
Anusic, I., 407
Anyan, W. R., 260
Apanovitch, A. M., 382
Arango, C., 258
Ariely, D., 184, 218, 220, 249, 323
Arkes, H. R., 185, 389
Armitage, C. J., 160
Armor, D. A., 117, 387, 391, 400, 415
Arndt, J., 399

Arnold, L., 388
Aron, A., 225, 229, 230, 231
Aron, A. P., 217, 218
Aron, E. N., 225, 229, 230
Aronson, E., 96
Aronson, J., 389
Asch, S. E., 310
Asendorpf, J. B., 132, 134, 135, 136
Asher, T., 98
Ashton-James, C., 279, 285, 288
Asneel, F., 84
Atance, C. M., 220
Attia, E., 264
Atwater, L. E., 93, 106
Austin, S. N., 280
Ausubel, D. P., 9, 10, 11, 15
Axsom, D., 279
Ayton, P., 278

B

Back, M. D., 3, 113, 119, 131, 132, 134, 135, 136, 137, 138, 139, 140, 141, 142, 146, 401
Baddeley, A., 303
Baeyens, F., 24, 25, 26
Bagby, R. M., 53
Bahrick, H. P., 299, 300
Bailey, J. R., 397
Bailey, S., 332
Baird, B., 82
Bakan, D., 331
Baker, H., 4
Balcetis, E., 390
Baldwin, E., 108
Baldwin, J. M., 9, 10, 11, 15
Baldwin, M. W., 97, 98, 111, 316
Balkin, J., 112
Balter, J. M., 264
Banaji, M., 159, 165, 196
Banaji, M. R., 28, 33, 63, 69, 132, 135, 136, 144, 158, 294, 352
Bandettini, P. A., 25
Bandura, A., 416
Banfield, J. F., 63
Banner, M. J., 159
Banse, R., 28, 31, 132, 135, 136
Bar-Anan, Y., 27, 30
Barden, J., 165, 166
Bargh, J. A., 23, 25, 26, 27, 33, 92, 98, 133, 142, 157, 158, 160, 353, 390
Barndollar, K., 26
Baron, J., 182, 185
Barron, E., 261
Bartlett, F. C., 197
Baruch, E., 264

Bassili, J. N., 165
Bassis, S., 230
Bauer, J. J., 337
Baumann, N., 40, 54, 56
Baumeister, R. F., 93, 110, 117, 132, 145, 146, 168, 293, 365, 381, 405
Baumert, J., 17
Bazerman, M. H., 319
Beach, E., 81
Beach, S. R. H., 398
Beaver, J. D., 214
Bechara, A., 66
Beck, A. T., 264
Becker, G. S., 212
Beckman, L., 380
Beer, J., 248
Beer, J. S., 64, 92, 94, 98, 99, 107, 108, 109, 114, 115, 117, 118, 141, 142, 348, 417
Bekker, H. L., 188
Belding, J., 163
Belezza, F. S., 189
Bell, D. E., 160
Bem, D., 98
Bem, D. J., 29, 68, 84, 141, 143, 144, 167, 310, 320
Bender, D. S., 268
Benet-Martinez, V., 149
Benjamin, A. S., 296
Berdahl, J. L., 99
Berger, J. A., 346
Berger, S. A., 299
Berkman, E. T., 70
Berridge, K. C., 40, 211, 212, 213, 214, 215, 216, 219
Berry, C. M., 373
Berscheid, E., 98
Best, R., 162
Bettman, J. R., 181, 183, 188
Betz, A. L., 25
Bezmenova, I., 373
Biek, M., 165
Biernat, M., 41
Biesanz, J. C., 98, 139, 250, 278
Bigbee, L., 261
Bisanz, G. L., 169
Bishara, A. J., 300, 301
Biswas-Diener, R., 407
Björklund, F., 316
Black, J., 184
Black, J. J., 278
Blackman, M. C., 139, 248
Blackstone, T., 233
Blakemore, S.-J., 67
Blank, H., 24
Blanton, H., 27, 40, 135
Bleeker, M. M., 107

Bless, H., 185
Block, J., 107, 417
Bluck, S., 95, 295, 329
Blumberg, H. H., 146, 247
Blumberg, S. J., 278, 349
Boals, A., 298
Boden, J. M., 110
Bodenhausen, G. V., 3, 4, 22, 24, 28, 31, 133, 142, 144, 158, 367
Bodner, R., 84
Bogdan, R., 297
Bohus, M., 95
Bolger, N., 70
Bonanno, G. A., 117, 373
Boncimino, M., 231
Bond, M. H., 116, 117, 142, 407
Bongers, K. C. A., 158
Bons, T., 52
Borkenau, P., 114, 132, 137, 139
Borkovec, T. D., 56, 204
Bornemann, B., 216
Bos, M. E., 181
Bos, M. W., 3, 187, 188, 189
Bosson, J. K., 112, 135, 136, 141, 399
Bouchard, M., 330
Boucher, E. M., 250
Boucher, H. C., 97, 399
Bowlby, J., 95
Boyd, J. H., 111
Brackett, M. A., 285
Bradley, G. W., 93
Bradley, M. M., 49
Brainerd, C. J., 18
Brandstätter, V., 40, 43
Braverman, J., 172
Breckler, S. J., 164
Brekke, N., 30, 32, 166, 351
Bremner, A. J., 12
Brendel, D. H., 338, 339
Brett, J. F., 93
Brewer, M. B., 399
Brewer, W. F., 294
Brewin, C. R., 56, 57
Brickman, P., 83
Briñol, P., 3, 4, 157, 158, 159, 160, 161, 163, 165, 166, 171, 172
Brock, T. C., 165
Brooks, K., 185
Brooks-Gunn, J., 16
Brouer, R. L., 402
Broverman, D. M., 44, 45
Brown, J., 106, 109, 117, 300
Brown, J. D., 114, 132, 142, 246, 348, 363, 380, 400, 417
Brown, K. W., 199, 250
Brown, P., 424

Brown, R., 247
Brown, R. P., 112
Brown, T. J., 134
Brownell, C. A., 16
Bruce, M. N., 115, 144, 372
Brucks, M., 163
Brunell, A. B., 118
Bruner, J., 328, 329
Brunstein, J. C., 40, 41, 43, 54, 57, 58
Brunswik, E., 141
Buber, M., 72
Bucci, W., 42, 44, 45, 46, 47, 52, 53, 54, 57
Buckels, E., 3, 110, 144, 363, 370, 389
Buckley, M. R., 402
Buckner, R. L., 70
Buehler, R., 278, 281, 284, 388
Bufferd, S. J., 263
Buhrmester, M. D., 27, 135
Burger, J. M., 357
Burke, P. J., 402
Burrows, L., 26, 92
Burt, C., 298
Busch, H., 55
Bushman, B. J., 93
Buss, D. M., 114, 233
Butler, J., 66
Butsch, S., 357
Buttermore, N. R., 415
Buunk, B. P., 229
Bybee, J. A., 164

C

Cabanac, M., 211
Cable, D. M., 403
Cacioppo, J. T., 161, 163, 165, 170, 171, 172
Calkins, E. V., 388
Camerer, C., 283
Cameron, J. J., 249
Cameron, K. A., 170, 171
Campbell, J. D., 245
Campbell, M. C., 169
Campbell, W., 413, 415
Campbell, W. K., 93, 107, 109, 110, 111, 118
Campos, D., 40
Cantor, N., 40
Caplan, R. D., 402
Carlsmith, K. M., 281
Carlson, C., 228
Carlson, E., 265, 266
Carlson, E. N., 3, 91, 121, 131, 133, 135, 137, 138, 139, 140, 146, 148, 149, 242, 243, 245, 246, 247, 248, 249, 250, 251, 259, 261, 266, 357, 401, 416
Carlson, T. A., 12

Carr, T. H., 284
Carroll, L., 111
Caruso, D. R., 416
Carver, C., 29
Carver, C. S., 95
Caspi, A., 94
Castel, A. D., 303
Catapano, F., 260
Ceci, S. J., 18
Chaiken, S., 98, 157, 158, 160, 315, 317, 367
Chambers, J. R., 115, 249
Chang, E. C., 318
Chang-Schneider, C., 399
Chartrand, T. L., 133, 353
Chasiotis, A., 40, 55
Chatman, J. A., 99, 118, 403
Chelminski, I., 268
Chen, K. Y., 399
Chen, M., 26, 92, 98
Chen, S., 97, 399
Cheng, J. T., 110, 112
Cheng, S. M., 28
Cheng, S. Y. Y., 399
Cheung, I., 284
Cheung, J. C. H., 188, 189
Chin, E. D., 330
Chin, J., 3, 77, 79
Chin, J. M., 87
Chiu, C., 399
Chiu, C. Y., 416, 417, 418
Chiu, C.-Y., 115, 121
Choudhury, S., 67
Christensen, A., 229
Christensen, C., 185
Christensen-Szalanski, J. J., 280
Christian, C., 47
Christoff, K., 81
Chua, H. F., 70
Cialdini, R. B., 168, 288
Civettini, A. J. W., 379
Clancy, S. A., 297
Clark, J. K., 160
Clark, J. M., 52
Clark, L. A., 288
Clark, M. S., 72, 251
Clifton, A., 265
Clore, G. L., 3, 34, 43, 194, 196, 197, 199, 200, 201, 202, 203, 205, 206, 217, 218
Cohen, G. L., 383, 389
Cohen, M. X., 214
Coifman, K. G., 373
Cole, D. A., 92
Colvin, C., 135, 417
Colvin, C. R., 107, 115, 117, 133, 139, 401
Combs, B., 185
Cone, J., 182

Connelly, B. S., 247
Conner, M., 160
Conner, T. S., 205, 206
Connolly, J. J., 139
Constable, G., 263
Constantino, M. J., 107
Conway, M., 168, 298, 299, 321
Conway, M. A., 294, 295, 296
Cooley, C. H., 91, 146, 247
Correll, J., 93, 111, 373
Cousins, A. J., 211
Cowan, C. P., 96
Cowan, P. A., 96
Craig, J. A., 41
Craik, F. I. M., 64
Craik, K. H., 114, 134, 249, 331, 402
Cramer, P., 111
Craven, R. G., 17
Creighton, L. A., 22, 33
Creswell, J. D., 66
Crimins, M., 47
Critcher, C. R., 383, 387, 388, 391, 400
Crites, S., 164
Crocker, J., 95, 109
Crombez, G., 24
Cronbach, L. J., 250, 372
Cronk, R., 197
Cross, P., 347
Crow, D. M., 138
Crowell, J. A., 55
Csikszentmihalyi, M., 405
Cuesta, M. J., 258
Curry, T., 245
Custers, R., 23
Cuthbert, B. N., 49

D

Dabbs, J., 138
Dalgleish, T., 56
Damasio, A. R., 185
Dapretto, M., 11, 67
Dare, P. A. S., 259
D'Argembeau, A., 66
Darley, J. M., 353
Dauenheimer, D. G., 399
David, A. S., 263
Davidson, D., 9
Davies, M., 423
Davies, R. F., 117
Davis, A. Q., 40
Davis, J. L., 316
Davis, M. H., 226
Davis, P. J., 195
Dawes, R. M., 183, 185, 282

Dawis, R. V., 402, 403
Dawson, E., 382
De Boeck, P., 181
de Castro, B. O., 399
De Courville, N., 388
De Dreu, C. K., 318
de Gelder, B., 215
De Houwer, J., 23, 24, 25, 28, 136
De La Ronde, C., 97, 231
de Liver, Y. N., 160
de Schonen, S., 16
Debner, J. A., 300
Dechesne, M., 380
Deci, E. L., 54
DeCoster, J., 159
Dekel, S., 117
Delaney, P. F., 304
DelVecchio, W. F., 402
DeMarree, K. G., 159, 160, 163, 164, 168, 172
den Ouden, H., 67
Denissen, J. J. A., 146
Dennett, D. C., 363
Denton, K., 365
DePaulo, B. M., 92, 139, 145, 242, 243, 245, 246, 247, 248, 249, 261
Derigne, L., 259
Descartes, R., 184, 185
DeSteno, D., 172
Deutsch, R., 28, 31, 133, 142, 143
Devine, P. G., 25, 352
Dickey, A. S., 135
Dickinson, K. A., 121
Diener, C., 407
Diener, E., 134, 195, 202, 214, 407
Digdon, N., 52
Digman, J. M., 310
Dijksterhuis, A., 3, 25, 133, 158, 181, 182, 186, 187, 188, 189, 316
Dirlikov, B., 47
Dittmar, H., 399
Ditto, P. H., 220, 367, 373, 380, 382
Dobson, K., 424
Dobson, K. S., 259
Dolan, P., 286
Donahue, E. M., 313
Donnellan, M. B., 107, 399
Doughtery, D. M., 266
Douglas, C. J., 262
Douglas, K. M., 170
Dovidio, J. F., 30, 159, 162, 283, 316, 353
Downing, J., 165
Downs, D. L., 94
Driver-Linn, E., 283
Druss, R. G., 262
Dumenci, L., 265
Duncan, B. L., 31

Dunn, D. S., 23, 164
Dunn, E., 282, 283
Dunn, E. W., 3, 22, 132, 142, 219, 251, 277, 278, 279, 280, 281, 282, 284, 285, 287, 288
Dunning, D., 3, 92, 107, 132, 142, 163, 171, 184, 283, 287, 345, 347, 349, 359, 367, 379, 380, 381, 383, 385, 387, 388, 390, 391, 398, 400, 413
Dunning, D. A., 219
Dunton, B. C., 28, 31, 158
Dutton, D. G., 217, 218
Dweck, C. S., 418
Dywan, J., 298

E

Eastwick, P. W., 249
Eaton, L. G., 137
Ebert, J. E. J., 278
Edelstein, R. S., 112
Edwards, J. R., 402, 403
Edwards, W., 183
Eelen, P., 24, 26
Egan, V., 373
Egloff, B., 119, 132, 134, 135, 136, 137, 139, 143, 149
Ehrlinger, J., 350, 388, 413
Ehrsson, H. H., 12
Eibach, R. P., 66, 321
Eich, E., 294
Eisen, J. L., 264
Eisenberg, N., 196
Eisenberger, N. I., 66
Elliot, A. J., 54, 55, 109, 111
Ellis, A., 420, 421
Ellis, B. J., 146
Elster, J., 66
Elwakili, N., 278
Emmerson, K. M., 379
Emmons, R. A., 56
Ende, J., 270
Enns, V., 97
Epler, A. J., 259, 270
Epley, N., 249, 287, 349, 359, 388
Epstein, E. B., 220
Epstein, S., 22, 133, 137, 161, 279, 415
Erbs, J., 134, 265
Ericsson, K. A., 162
Erikson, E., 90
Ersner-Hershfield, H., 66
Esses, V. M., 160
Evans, J. S. B. T., 133
Eyal, T., 315
Eyre, R. N., 285
Eyssell, K. M., 196

F

Faber, R., 54
Fabrigar, L., 164
Fabrigar, L. R., 160, 163, 164
Falk, C. F., 281
Falk, E. B., 70
Farb, N. A. S., 66
Farnham, S. D., 56
Fasolo, B., 134
Faust, D., 389
Fazio, R. H., 22, 26, 28, 31, 34, 133, 142, 158, 162, 165, 166
Feeney, B. C., 251
Fehr, B., 97, 245
Feldman Barrett, L., 121, 195, 196, 199, 205
Feldt, T., 373
Felson, R., 92, 96
Felson, R. B., 117, 146, 247, 248, 417
Fennis, B. M., 170
Ferguson, M. J., 25, 26, 33
Fernbach, P. M., 367
Ferris, G. R., 402
Festinger, L., 90, 98, 142, 160, 166, 170, 380
Fetterman, A. K., 203
Fiedler, E. R., 114, 267
Fiedler, K., 170
Field, A. P., 244
Fillo, J., 3, 225, 251
Fingarette, H., 363, 366
Finkel, E. J., 118, 249
Finn, S., 278
Finucane, M. L., 181
Fischhoff, B., 389
Fishbach, A., 323
Fishbein, M., 317
Fishman, D., 82
Fiske, S. T., 72
Fivush, R., 14, 335
Fleeson, W., 150, 205
Fleming, J. J., 355, 356
Fletcher, G. J. O., 167, 226, 232, 233, 234, 243
Florack, A., 28
Flyer, E. S., 261
Fodor, J., 367
Fogel, A., 11
Fong, G. T., 381
Forest, C., 242
Forrin, N., 279
Fournier, J. C., 268
Fox, M. C., 162
Fragale, A. R., 99
Fraisse, P., 44
Fraley, R. C., 55
Frank, S. A., 217
Frankenberger, K. D., 414
Franzoi, S., 226
Fredrickson, B. L., 285
Fredrickson, R., 298
Freedman, N., 42, 44, 45, 46, 53, 57
Freeman, M., 329, 330, 331
Freitas, A. L., 319
Frenkel-Brunswik, E., 372
Frey, D., 380
Frey, F. E., 243
Freytag, P., 170
Fridhandler, B., 366, 372
Friedman, J. N. W., 119
Friedman, M., 238
Friedrich, J., 347
Friese, M., 31
Friestad, M., 169
Frith, C. D., 67, 70, 81
Frith, U., 70
Fritz, U., 134, 265
Fröhlich, S. M., 40
Frost, R. O., 181
Fuhrman, R. W., 65
Fujita, K., 319
Fukuno, M., 245
Fuller, V. A., 32
Funder, D. C., 91, 94, 97, 107, 109, 112, 113, 132, 133, 134, 135, 137, 139, 141, 146, 147, 148, 150, 248, 251, 261, 401, 405, 417
Furr, R. M., 132, 133, 140, 150, 242, 243, 245, 246, 248, 250, 266, 401

G

Gabbard, G. O., 270
Gaertner, L., 110, 121, 397
Gaertner, S. L., 30, 353
Gage, P., 121
Galak, J., 220
Galinsky, A. D., 99, 284
Gallagher, H. L., 81
Gallardo, I., 163
Gallo, D. A., 297
Gallup, G. G., Jr., 69
Gangestad, S. W., 211
Garb, H. N., 265
Garon, N., 16
Garry, M., 297
Garver-Apgar, C. E., 211
Gawronski, B., 3, 4, 22, 23, 24, 25, 28, 29, 30, 31, 33, 34, 56, 133, 136, 142, 143, 144, 158, 367
Gazzaniga, M. S., 55
Geise, A. C., 336
Gerbasi, M., 351
Gerberding, J. L., 282

Gergen, K. J., 366
Germeijs, V., 181
Geschke, D., 31
Ghaderi, A., 54
Giacomantonio, M., 318
Giesler, R. B., 422
Gigerenzer, G., 218
Giladi, E. E., 385
Gilbert, D. T., 197, 199, 218, 219, 277, 278, 279, 280, 281, 282, 283, 285, 287, 288, 289, 322, 349, 351, 414
Gilbertson, M. W., 57
Gilboa, I., 210
Gill, M. J., 279, 407
Gillet, R., 244
Gillis, R., 282
Gilovich, T., 96, 182, 249, 350, 355, 356, 382, 392, 413, 414
Gladwell, M., 181
Gleason, M. E., 266, 267
Gleason, M. E. J., 114, 119
Godden, D. R., 303
Goethals, G. R., 166, 167, 415
Gold, D. B., 82
Gold, J. M., 196
Goldberg, L. R., 149, 313
Goldenberg, J. L., 399
Goldman, B. M., 374
Goldstone, R. L., 185
Gollwitzer, P. M., 26, 117
Gonzalez-Vallejo, C., 189
Goodvin, R., 414
Gordon, A. M., 81
Gordon, K. H., 203
Gosejohann, S., 28
Gosling, S., 114
Gosling, S. D., 99, 118, 119, 132, 133, 134, 135, 139, 248, 249, 278, 279
Govender, R., 157, 160
Govorun, O., 28, 93, 385, 415
Gramzow, R. H., 112, 117, 118, 399
Grande, T., 54
Grannemann, B. D., 95
Grässmann, R., 40
Grawe, K., 57
Greco, J., 334
Greenberg, J., 380, 382
Greene, D., 415
Greenfeld, D. G., 260
Greenleaf, E. A., 181
Greenwald, A. G., 22, 28, 33, 34, 56, 63, 106, 132, 133, 135, 136, 144, 158, 159, 162, 165, 294, 352, 363, 367
Gregg, A. P., 106, 111, 112
Gregory, V., 424
Greve, W., 386, 387, 388

Grich, J., 237, 251
Griffin, D., 388
Griffin, D. W., 160, 231
Griffin, K. M., 184, 278
Gromet, D. M., 356
Gross, J. J., 55, 217, 373
Gruenfeld, D. H., 99
Grumm, M., 136
Gschwendner, T., 28, 30, 56, 136, 137, 141, 142, 143
Guadagno, J., 405, 424
Guay, R. P., 402
Guenther, C. L., 385, 386, 400
Guglielmo, S., 248
Guilmette, T. J., 389
Guinn, J., 407
Guinn, J. S., 83
Gupta, S., 117
Gur, R. C., 368, 369, 371, 372
Gyurak, A., 87

H

Habermas, T., 95, 295, 329
Habib, R., 67
Haddock, G., 166
Hagen, L., 297
Hagmayer, Y., 367
Halberstadt, J. B., 185
Halbesleben, J. R. B., 402
Hale, J. A., 40
Hall, D. L., 30
Hall, J., 97
Hall, J. A., 249
Hall, L. K., 299
Halliwell, E., 399
Halperin, K., 96
Halpern, D. V., 79
Ham, J., 188
Hamamura, T., 121, 418
Hamm, A. O., 215
Hammack, P. L., 329
Hammarlund-Udenaes, M., 258
Hammond, S., 148
Hancock, J., 421
Hancock, J. T., 250
Handy, T. C., 81
Hankin, B. L., 93, 108
Hannover, B., 30, 31, 32
Hansen, K., 420
Hansen, K. E., 3, 87, 96, 132, 140, 249, 345, 351, 413, 419
Hansenne, M., 285
Hansford, B. C., 347
Hardin, C., 99

Hardin, C. D., 99, 310
Harms, P., 248
Harms, P. D., 115, 372
Harris, L. T., 72
Harris, M. J., 98
Harris, P. R., 160
Harrison, B., 70
Harrison, R. V., 402
Harrod, M. M., 399
Harrow, M., 259
Hart, D., 3, 7, 17
Hart, K., 389
Harter, S., 92, 96
Hartshorn, K., 18
Hartvig, P., 258
Harvey, J. H., 225, 226, 228, 229, 231
Haselton, M. G., 233
Hashtroudi, S., 297
Hassin, R. R., 27
Hastie, R., 66, 181, 277
Hattie, J. A., 347
Hau, K. T., 17
Haugtvedt, C. P., 165, 171
Havenstein, N. M., 97
Haviland, J. M., 196
Hay, J. F., 300
Hayes, S., 366, 372
Hayes, S. C., 203, 206
Hayne, H., 14
Hazan, C., 231
Healy, H., 204
Heath, C., 163, 349, 385
Heatherton, T. F., 63, 68, 117
Hebert, B. G., 243
Heider, F., 142, 160, 380, 391
Heine, S. J., 121, 399, 418
Helmreich, R., 195
Helson, R., 96
Helweg-Larson, M., 348
Helzer, E. G., 3, 92, 107, 132, 142, 367, 379, 383, 387, 398, 400, 413
Henderson, M. D., 317
Hendrickx, H., 25
Hepper, E. G., 112, 399
Hespos, S. J., 12
Hessels, S., 300, 301
Higgins, E. T., 99, 168, 311, 316
Higgins, N., 365
Hilton, J. L., 137
Hintzman, D. L., 303
Hixon, J. G., 97, 231
Hobart, M., 260
Hoch, S. J., 389
Hodges, S. D., 97, 162, 204, 280, 346, 358
Hoerger, M., 284
Hofer, J., 40, 55

Hoffmann, L., 47
Hofmann, W., 23, 24, 25, 27, 28, 29, 30, 31, 56, 134, 136, 137, 141, 142, 143, 144, 148
Hofree, G., 3, 34, 210
Hofstee, W. K. B., 132, 134, 265
Hogan, R., 93, 132
Holbrook, A. L., 165
Holland, J. L., 402
Holleran, S. E., 139
Holmberg, D., 227, 228
Holmes, J. G., 231, 316
Holmes, N. P., 12
Holt, K., 380
Holzberg, A. D., 345, 383
Honkaniemi, L., 373
Hooley, J. M., 111
Hoorens, V., 373
Horcajo, J., 163, 172
Horowitz, M. J., 270
Horton, R. S., 106
Horvath, S., 112
Hoshino-Browne, E., 93, 111, 373
House, P., 415
Houston, B. K., 96
Houston, C. E., 167
Howard, A., 159
Hoyer, S., 41
Hsee, C. K., 277, 280, 391
Hubbard, B., 139
Huber, D. E., 219
Hugenberg, K., 31, 170
Hughes, A., 300
Huh, Y. E., 219
Hull, C. L., 211
Human, L. J., 278
Hunt, T., 77
Huntsinger, J., 99
Huntsinger, J. R., 217, 218
Hutchinson W., 163
Hyde, J. S., 93, 108
Hydén, L. C., 329
Hyman, D. B., 164
Hyman, I. E., Jr., 297
Hymes, C., 158
Hyvärinen, M., 329, 330

I

Iacoboni, M., 11
Ickes, W., 97, 226, 228, 233, 234, 235, 237, 238, 251
Igou, E. R., 185
Iliev, R., 86, 384
Inbar, Y., 182
Inman, C., 228

Inz, J., 56
Irwin, K. R., 219
Isarida, T. K., 303
Isen, A. M., 417
Ivanova, M. Y., 265

J

Jablonsky, A., 258
Jaccard, J., 27, 162
Jacks, J. Z., 170, 171
Jackson, D. N., 40
Jackson, J. R., 28, 158
Jacobs, J. E., 107
Jacobson, J. A., 220
Jacobson, L., 98
Jacobson, N. S., 229
Jacoby, L. L., 3, 9, 293, 298, 299, 300, 301, 302, 303
James, W., 8, 67, 68
Janis, I. L., 171, 183
Janiszewski, C., 26
Janowski, C. L., 243, 245
Janssen, L., 170
Jarcho, J. M., 65
Jarvis, W. B. G., 157, 160
Jasechko, J., 300
Jensen, A. R., 202
Jepson, C., 284
Jeung, K. Y., 399
Job, V., 40, 43
John, O. P., 64, 106, 107, 108, 109, 110, 113, 114, 115, 116, 117, 119, 121, 131, 132, 134, 142, 149, 247, 248, 249, 313, 372, 373, 407, 415, 417
Johnson, B., 159
Johnson, C., 159
Johnson, E. A., 373
Johnson, E. J., 181
Johnson, J. T., 195, 196
Johnson, K., 413
Johnson, M. K., 297
Johnson, S. C., 64
Johnson, S. M., 181
Johnson, T., 373
Jones, E. E., 29, 71
Jones, N. M., 40
Jones, S. E., 261
Jones, T. S., 233
Jordan, A. H., 383
Jordan, C. H., 93, 95, 111, 159, 373
Joseph, S., 56
Josselson, R., 331, 333
Judd, C. M., 25
Judge, T. A., 403

Judice, T. N., 98
Jussim, L., 92, 247
Jussim, L. J., 25

K

Kabasakalian-McKay, R., 45, 52
Kagan, J., 13, 17
Kahn, M., 233
Kahneman, D., 184, 185, 197, 199, 201, 204, 205, 218, 279, 285, 302
Kaikati, A. M., 315
Kamphuis, J. H., 399
Kane, J., 218
Kanouse, D., 184
Kaplan, G. B., 264
Kaplan, K. J., 160
Kaplan, S. A., 247
Karali, A., 260
Kardes, F. R., 158
Karmali, F., 283
Karney, B. R., 226, 232, 399
Karniol, R., 71
Karpinski, A., 137
Kaschel, R., 40
Katz, J., 398
Kavanagh, E. J., 139
Kavanagh, P. S., 146
Kawahara, T. N., 64
Kawakami, K., 159, 283, 286, 316, 353
Keating, C .F., 365, 373
Keelan, J. P. R., 97
Kellerman, J., 163
Kelley, C., 304
Kelley, C. M., 3, 9, 293, 298, 299, 300, 302, 303, 304
Kelley, W. M., 63, 68
Kelley, W. M. C., 64
Kemp, R., 263
Kemp, S., 296, 298
Kennedy, K., 357
Kennedy, K. A., 357, 358, 359
Kennedy, L. A., 318
Kenny, D. A., 3, 91, 92, 114, 116, 117, 134, 135, 139, 140, 141, 142, 145, 146, 242, 243, 245, 246, 247, 248, 249, 250, 252, 259, 261, 401, 407
Kenrick, D. T., 134, 137
Kermer, D. A., 283
Kernberg, O., 111
Kernis, M. H., 95, 107, 112, 374
Kerr, P. S. G., 226, 232, 233, 243
Kessler, R. C., 263
Khan, U., 214
Kiesler, C. A., 165

Kiessling, F., 55
Kihlstrom, J. F., 65, 108, 365, 366
Killingsworth, M. A., 285
Kim, A. S. N., 14, 67
Kim, S., 418
Kim, Y., 399
Kim, Y. H., 416, 417, 418
Kim, Y.-H., 115, 121
Kinal, M. P.-A., 107, 399
Kinch, J. W., 91, 92
King, B. T., 171
King, L. A., 40, 56, 334, 336, 337
Kirker, W. S., 64
Kirmani, A., 169
Kivetz, Y., 315
Klar, Y., 385
Klauer, K. C., 149
Klein, C., 348
Klein, D. N., 263, 267
Klein, K. J. K., 204
Klein, S. B., 65, 108
Kley, C., 40
Klinger, E., 40
Klonsky, E. D., 114, 265, 266
Kluemper, D. H., 416
Knee, C. R., 228, 417
Knight, D. C., 25
Knight, R. T., 64, 108
Knutson, B., 66, 220
Ko, S. J., 139
Kobak, R., 231
Koehler, D. J., 388
Koestler, A., 185
Koestner, R., 40, 41
Kohlhepp, K., 247
Kohn, M., 169
Koh-Rangarajoo, E., 97
Kohut, H., 111
Kolar, D. C., 139, 248
Kolar, D. W., 135, 137
Kolisetty, A. P., 330
Köller, O., 17
Köllner, M., 41
Kong, C. K., 17
Koriat, A., 303, 389
Kotov, R., 263
Kraft, D., 23, 218
Kramer, J. H., 108
Krause, S., 146
Krebs, D. L., 365
Krienen, F. M., 70, 71
Kring, A. M., 195
Kristof, A. L., 402
Kristof-Brown, A. L., 402
Krosnick, J. A., 25, 165
Krueger, R. F., 260

Kruger, J., 140, 345, 347, 348, 354, 385, 392, 413
Kruglanski, A. W., 23, 170, 181, 380
Krukowski, R. A., 265
Krull, D. S., 94
Kuang, L., 417
Kuang, L. L., 107, 116, 407
Küfner, A. C. P., 139
Kugler, M. B., 346, 350, 354, 358, 392
Kuhl, J., 40, 54, 57
Kuhnen, C. M., 220
Kuiper, N. A., 64, 314
Kulik, J., 357
Kunak, J., 230
Kunda, Z., 363, 367, 380, 381, 391
Kupersmidt, J. B, 399
Kurt, A., 117, 119, 417
Kurtz, J., 282
Kushlev, K., 3, 277
Kushnir, T., 13
Kutzner, F., 170
Kwan, V. S. Y., 107, 108, 116, 117, 119, 121, 142, 400, 407
Kwan, V. Y., 417
Kwang, T., 94, 97, 247, 251, 407

L

Labouvie-Vief, G., 96
Labov, W., 329
Lachendro, E., 348, 385
LaFleur, S. J., 346, 358
LaFrance, M., 196
Lagattuta, K. H., 107
Laing, R. D., 242
Laird, J. D., 163
Lakin, J. L., 363, 399
Lalwani, A. K., 373
Lam, K. C. H., 281, 284, 287
Lamb, R. J., 213
Lambert, L. S., 403
Lane, R. D., 195
Lang, P. J., 49
Lange, C., 234
Langer, E. J., 348
Langer, T., 24
Larsen, R. J., 196, 199, 214
Larson, J., 195
Lassiter, G. D., 189
Latane, B., 353
Lau, K. S.-L., 370
Lawton, E. M., 268
Le, H., 28, 56, 136
Leary, M. R., 3, 94, 117, 142, 146, 149, 251, 374, 405, 407, 413, 415, 416, 418, 420, 421, 424

LeBel, E. P., 25, 28, 34
Ledgerwood, A., 317
LeDoux, J., 215
LeDoux, J. E., 40
Lee, A., 163
Lee, A. R., 242
Lee, S. S., 67
Lee-Chai, A., 26
Lehmann, D. R., 181
Leibold, J. M., 31
Leising, D., 54, 134, 135, 249, 265
Lemay, E. P., Jr., 251, 252
Lennon, R., 196
Lenton, A. P., 134
Lenzenweger, M. F., 297
Leonardelli, G. J., 399
Lepper, M. R., 389
Lerner, J. S., 117, 348, 417
Lerouge, D., 188
Levenson, R. W., 55, 87, 217
Levesque, M. J., 139
Levi, A., 121
Levine, B., 14, 67
Levine, G. M., 185, 186
Levin-Sagi, M., 319
Levinson, S. C., 424
Levy, P. E., 96, 399
Lewandowski, G. W., Jr., 230
Lewis, M., 11, 16, 17
Ley, J., 247
Libby, L. K., 66, 321
Liberman, M. D., 247
Liberman, N., 3, 310, 311, 312, 313, 315, 317, 318, 319
Liberzon, I., 70
Lichtenstein, S., 389
Lieb, K., 95
Lieberman, M. D., 3, 63, 64, 65, 66, 67, 68, 69, 70
Liebler, A., 114, 139
Lieblich, A., 331, 333
Lievens, F., 84, 399
Ligon, E. M., 44
Lin, D. Y., 87, 332, 347, 392, 413
Lin, J., 216
Lindberg, M., 189
Lindberg, M. J., 189
Linden, W., 117
Lindsay, D. S., 297, 298, 302, 303, 305
Lindsey, S., 31, 52, 132, 159
Lindström, L., 258
Linehan, M. M., 95
Linville, P. W., 313
Lisle, D. J., 23
Litt, A., 214
Livingston, J., 250

Lockard, J. S., 365
Locke, J., 65, 66
Lockhart, L. K., 382
Lockie, R., 366
Lockwood, N., 160
Lockwood, P., 407
Lodi-Smith, J., 336
Loersch, C., 158
Loevinger, J., 330, 336
Loewenstein, G., 66, 184, 218, 220, 278, 280, 282, 283, 284, 287, 289
Lofquist, L. H., 402, 403
Loftus, E. F., 297
Loftus, J., 65, 108
Logan, G. D., 198
Lönnqvist, J. E., 373
Lopez, D. F., 367, 373, 380, 382
Lopez-Ibor, I., 263
Lord, C. G., 389
Lowery, B., 99
Lowery, B. S., 310, 316
Lu, Z.-L., 66
Lucas, R. E., 202, 284
Luce, M. F., 183, 188
Luo, S., 231
Luus, B., 81
Lynam, D. R., 261, 268
Lynn, A. R., 25
Lysaker, J. T., 330
Lysaker, P. H., 330
Lysy, D. C., 115, 372

M

Ma'ayan, H., 303
Mabe, P. A., III, 347
MacDonald, T. K., 220
MacDougall, B. L., 163
Machilek, F., 139
Machon, D., 249
Mackie, D. M., 25, 159, 162
Macrae, C. N., 63, 69
Maddux, W. W., 284
Magee, J. C., 99
Mahler, H., 357
Mahler, S. V., 213
Maier, G. W., 40, 41
Maio, G. R., 160, 168
Malle, B. F., 249, 414
Mallett, R. K., 282
Malloy, T. E., 242, 243, 245, 248
Malone, P. S., 414
Mandler, J. M., 329
Manis, M., 117
Mann, L., 183

Mann, T., 70
Mannarelli, T., 139
Mannetti, L., 318
Manstead, A. S. R., 196
Mar, R. A., 14
Marcus, B., 139
Marin, K. A., 335
Marks, J. S., 282
Markus, H., 64, 91, 168, 312, 314
Marsh, D. M., 266
Marsh, H. W., 17
Marshall, R. D., 335
Martens, J. P., 110
Martin, A. M., 238
Martin, L. L., 143, 371
Martin, W. E., Jr., 402
Mashek, D. J., 231
Maskit, B., 47
Massey, C., 400
Mast, M. S., 249
Mathias, C. W., 266
Mathieu, M. T., 278, 279
Mathis, L. C., 95
Matsuba, M. K., 3, 7, 17
Matute, H., 348
Mauer, N., 132
Mauss, I. B., 55, 79, 87, 217
Mayer, J. D., 416
Mayer, L., 264
Mayman, M., 117
Maynard, A. M., 414
McAdams, D. P., 56, 95, 96, 293, 328, 329, 330, 332, 335, 337
McCarter, L., 55, 217
McCarthy, K., 348
McCaslin, M. J., 158, 171
McClelland, D. C., 40, 41, 42
McClelland, J. L., 71, 197, 199, 201
McClintic, S., 17
McConnell, A. R., 25, 28, 31, 158, 159, 162, 170, 280, 296, 306
McConnell, H. K., 167
McCrae, R. R., 149
McDowell, N. K., 117, 348, 417
McElwee, R. O., 383
McFarland, C., 167, 278, 281, 284, 388
McGhee, D. E., 28, 136, 158
McKay, R. T., 363
McLean, K. C., 95
McLeod, J., 328, 329
McNally, R. J., 297
McNaughton, B. L., 71, 197
McNulty, S. E., 247
McSpadden, M. C., 81
Mead, G. H., 10, 14, 15, 91, 146, 247
Mealiea, J., 16

Means, B., 417
Measelle, J. R., 96
Medin, D. L., 86, 384
Medvec, V. H., 249, 355, 414
Mehl, M. R., 3, 114, 132, 133, 134, 135, 137, 138, 139, 148, 248, 249, 332, 338, 359, 401
Mele, A. R., 363, 367, 390
Meltzoff, A. N., 11, 220
Mendoza-Denton, R., 281
Mergenthaler, E., 46
Merikangas, K. R., 263
Messick, D. M., 363
Metcalfe, J., 319
Metcalfe, R., 286
Mettee, D. R., 96
Meurs, T., 188
Meyer, S., 414
Meyerowitz, J. A., 345, 383
Meyers, J., 285
Meyers, J. M., 167, 279
Meyersburg, C. A., 297
Meyvis, T., 220
Mezulis, A. H., 93, 108
Michalak, J., 40
Mierke, J., 149
Mijovic-Prelec, D, 363
Mikolajczak, M., 285
Mikulincer, M., 238
Milgram, S., 310
Miller, B. L., 108
Miller, D. T., 107, 384
Miller, J. D., 261, 265, 268, 269
Millevoi, A., 139, 250
Millon, T., 111
Mills, J., 72
Mintz, A. R., 259
Mischel, W., 137, 281, 295, 313, 319
Mitchell, A. L., 173
Mitchell, J. P., 69, 70, 71
Mitchell, T. R., 197, 204
Mittal, V., 181
Moffitt, T. E., 305
Mokdad, A. H., 282
Molouki, S., 346
Monahan, J., 183
Monin, B., 383, 384, 415
Moore, C., 16
Moore, D. A., 348
Moors, A., 23, 28
Moran, J. M., 63, 68
Morelli, S. A., 70
Morewedge, C. K., 219, 283, 285
Morf, C. C., 110, 112, 373
Morgan, C., 40
Morgan, R., 12
Morris, M. E., 139

Morry, M., 416
Mortazavi, M., 54
Moskowitz, D. S., 199
Moulin, C. J. A., 295
Mrazek, M. D., 3, 77, 82, 87
Mücke, D., 132
Muckli, L., 197
Mueller, C. M., 418
Mueller, P., 352
Muir, F., 415
Mullen, B., 415
Munro, G. D., 382
Muris, P., 181
Murphy, K. M., 212
Murphy, M. A., 233
Murphy, N. A., 249
Murphy, S. T., 215
Murray, H. A., 40, 136
Murray, S. L., 231
Mussweiler, T., 382, 389
Myers, J., 3, 225, 251

N

Nagengast, B., 26
Nagin, D., 184, 278
Narrow, W. E., 263
Nathanson, C., 370
Naumann, L. P., 119, 139, 149
Nauta, M. M., 402
Nave, C. S., 405
Neale, J. M., 195
Neff, K. D., 421
Neff, L. A., 226, 232, 399
Neiss, M. B., 399
Neisser, U., 8, 11, 91
Nelis, D., 285
Nelson, G., 230
Nelson, K., 14
Nelson, L. F., 220
Nelson, R. E., 166
Ness, D. E., 270
Nestler, S., 139
Neter, E., 398
Neuberg, S. L., 98
Neumann, R., 143
Neumark, Y. D., 259
Newcomb, T. M., 249
Newell, B. R., 188, 189
Newman, E. J., 297, 298
Newman, L. S., 381
Newsome, J. T., 168
Nguyen, H. T., 25
Nicholls, L., 65
Nichols, S. R., 16

Nickerson, R. S., 419
Nisbett, R. E., 29, 33, 55, 132, 137, 162, 182, 183, 184, 217, 345, 353, 358
Noftle, E. E., 150
Nolen-Hoeksema, S., 195, 203
Noller, P., 233
Nordgren, L. F., 133, 182, 184, 186, 187, 188
Norenzayan, A., 281
Norman, C., 225
Norton, M., 415
Nosek, B. A., 28, 135, 136, 137, 159
Novacek, J., 93
Nurius, P., 168
Nussbaum, S., 313, 318, 322
Nussinson, R., 303
Nyberg, L., 67

O

Ochsner, K., 70
Ode, S., 203
Oettingen, G., 117
Ohlsson, S., 185
Ohtsubo, Y., 245, 246, 249
Oishi, S., 196, 199, 202, 203, 205
O'Leary, J., 112
Oliver, P. V., 245
Olivola, C. Y., 358, 359
Olson, M. A., 26, 34, 142, 158, 162
Oltmanns, T. F., 3, 114, 119, 121, 251, 258, 261, 265, 266, 267, 268, 269, 330, 357
Omarzu, J., 225, 226, 228, 229, 231
Ones, D. S., 247
Orehek, E., 380
O'Reilly, R. C., 71, 197
Oriña, M. M., 238, 251
Orlando, A. E., 416
Ostendorf, F., 139
Otter, Z., 373
Otway, L. J., 111
Owens, T., 415, 416, 422
Ozdemir, O., 260
Ozer, D. J., 149

P

Pace-Savitsky, C., 108
Pacini, R., 415
Page, R. C., 373
Paivio, A., 42, 44, 51, 52, 53, 56, 58
Palmer, M., 357
Pals, J. L., 95, 329, 330
Pang, J. S., 40
Panter, A. T., 97

Paris, J., 263
Paris, M., 230
Park, B., 25, 66
Park, K., 160
Parker, J. D., 53
Parker, L., 195
Parks, C. D., 318
Parling, T., 54
Passingham, R. E., 12
Pasupathi, M., 95
Patalakh, M., 56
Paternoster, R., 184, 278
Patton, K. M., 416
Paulhus, D. L., 3, 106, 110, 115, 117, 119, 121, 144, 363, 365, 366, 370, 372, 373, 389, 417
Pauwels, B. G., 228
Payne, B. K., 28, 29, 30
Payne, J. W., 181, 182, 183, 188
Pearce, B. E., 249
Pears, D., 363
Peciña, S., 213
Pelham, B. W., 94
Peng, K., 399
Penke, L., 134, 146
Pennebaker, J. W., 3, 58, 133, 135, 138, 199, 202, 248, 366
Pentland, J., 297
Peoples, L. L., 213
Peralta, V., 258
Perie, M., 383
Perrino, A. L., 282
Perugini, M., 24, 31, 135
Pervin, L. A., 402
Peters, K. R., 34, 143
Peterson, E., 197
Petty, R. E., 3, 4, 30, 32, 157, 158, 159, 160, 161, 163, 164, 165, 166, 167, 168, 170, 171, 172
Pfeifer, J. H., 67, 92, 96
Pfeiffer, T., 389
Phillips, N. D., 189
Phillipson, H., 242
Piaget, J., 414
Pickrell, J. E., 297
Pierro, A., 380
Pietromonaco, P., 25
Pietromonaco, P. R., 196
Pike, G. R., 233
Pilkonis, P. A., 265, 269
Pincus, A. L., 121
Pinel, E. C., 278, 349, 399
Pinkus, R. T., 407
Pitman, R. K., 297
Pizarro, D. A., 220
Plantes, M., 260
Pleydell-Pearce, C. W., 296
Poehlman, T. A., 158

Pöhlmann, K., 40
Pomerantz, E. M., 398
Poon, C. S. K., 388
Pope, A., 242
Popper, K., 339
Pott, A., 278
Pourtois, G., 215
Povinelli, D. J., 16
Powell, M. C., 158
Powers, A. D., 3, 258
Pratto, F., 157, 160
Prelec, D., 84, 363
Prelec, E., 389
Price, J. H., 138
Price, R. H., 402
Priel, B., 16
Priester, J. M., 160, 168
Pronin, E., 3, 71, 87, 96, 132, 140, 249, 332, 345, 346, 347, 348, 349, 350, 351, 352, 353, 354, 355, 356, 357, 358, 359, 392, 413, 414, 419, 420, 422
Pruyn, A. T. H., 170
Pueschel, O., 40, 57
Pyszczynski, T., 380, 382

Q

Quas, J. A., 112
Quattrone, G. A., 84, 368, 369, 370, 371, 374
Quinlan, D. M., 260
Quirk, S. W., 284
Quoidbach, J., 219, 281, 285, 288

R

Rachmiel, T. B., 195
Radecki, C. M., 162
Rae, D. S., 263
Raineri, A., 399
Rakow, T., 188, 189
Ramani, G. B., 16
Rameson, L. T., 68, 70
Ramsey, C., 336
Ranganath, K. A., 28, 159
Rankin, K. P., 108
Raskin, R. N., 93
Raspin, C., 336
Rassin, E., 181
Ratliff, A., 181
Rathbone, C. J., 295, 296
Rattenbury, F., 259
Rawn, C. D., 280
Rawolle, M., 56
Ray, R. D., 373

Raymond, P., 158
Read, D., 184, 278, 349
Read, J. D., 297, 303, 305
Read, S. J., 94
Reber, E., 381
Reber, R., 166
Recchia, S., 17
Reckman, R. F., 167
Redlawsk, D. P., 379, 380
Reeder, G., 109, 111
Regan, D. T., 382
Regier, D. A., 263
Rehbein, D., 249
Reichle, E. D., 79, 80
Reid, D. B., 144, 372
Reijntjes, A., 399
Reineberg, A. E., 80
Reiseter, K., 242
Rempel, J. K., 164
Rennicke, C., 117
Reno, R., 245
Rentfrow, P. J., 83, 119, 139, 407
Rettinger, D. A., 181
Reyna, V. F., 18
Rhodes, M. G., 298, 302, 303
Rhodes, N., 165
Rhodewalt, F., 110, 373
Rholes, W. S., 238, 316
Richetin, J., 31
Richman, C. L., 13, 17
Riemann, R., 132
Riessman, C. K., 335
Robart, S. Y., 87
Roberts, B. W., 94, 132, 313, 336, 402
Robertson, D. A., 195
Robin, L., 196
Robins, L. N., 263
Robins, R. W., 3, 93, 105, 106, 107, 108, 109, 110, 111, 112, 113, 114, 115, 116, 117, 118, 131, 134, 142, 149, 247, 248, 249, 313, 336, 348, 402, 407, 415, 417
Robins, S. C., 146
Robinson, M. D., 3, 34, 117, 194, 195, 196, 197, 199, 200, 201, 202, 203, 205, 206, 367
Robinson, T. E., 40, 211, 212, 213, 219
Rochat, P., 12
Rodriguez, M. L., 319
Rodriguez, S., 348
Roemmele, L. A., 398
Rogers, 64
Rogers, S., 228
Rogers, T., 318
Rolls, B. J., 211
Rolls, E. T., 40, 211
Romney, D. M., 259
Rosen, S., 146

Rosenthal, R., 98, 247, 279
Rosenthal, S. A., 110
Roser, M., 55
Roskos-Ewoldsen, D. R., 169
Rosnow, R. L., 279
Ross, B. H., 296
Ross, B. M., 8
Ross, L., 87, 96, 140, 332, 345, 347, 350, 353, 354, 356, 392, 413, 415, 419, 422
Ross, L. D., 414
Ross, M., 107, 167, 168, 284, 298, 299, 306, 388, 414
Rothman, A. J., 166
Rothschild, L., 268
Rotondo, J. A., 164
Rowe, E. A., 211
Rowley, H. A., 64
Rubin, D. C., 294, 295, 296, 298
Ruby, M. B., 282, 287, 288
Rucker, D. D., 163, 164, 165, 166, 172
Rudich, E., 107
Rule, B., 169
Rule, B. G., 169
Rusbult, C. E., 316
Ruscher, J. B., 247
Rutledge, T., 117
Ryan, R. M., 54, 250
Rydell, R. J., 25, 28, 158, 159, 161, 162, 170
Ryff, C. D., 117, 367
Ryle, G., 68

S

Saarenheimo, M., 329
Sachdeva, S., 86, 384
Sackeim, H. A., 366, 368, 369, 371, 372
Sackett, A. M., 400
Sackett, P. R., 373
Sagar, H. A., 31
Sage, R. M., 117, 348, 417
Sagristano, M. D., 315
Sahakyan, L., 304
Sakaeda, A. R., 337
Sakellaropoulo, M., 111
Salancik, G. R., 321
Salovey, A. P., 295
Salovey, P., 285, 319, 416
Saltzberg, J. A., 195
Samper, A., 188
Samuelson, W., 283
Sanbonmatsu, D. M., 158
Sanders, A. F., 202
Sanitioso, R., 381
Sanna, L. J., 318
Santerre, C., 423

Santuzzi, A. M., 247
Sanz, M., 263
Saravanan, B., 258
Sartorius, N., 258
Sartre, J.-P., 363, 366
Satpute, A. B., 65, 68
Savitsky, K., 140, 249, 354, 355, 414
Sayette, M. A., 80, 184, 278
Scabini, D., 64, 108
Scarabis, M., 28
Scarpati, S., 243
Scepansky, J. A., 382
Schachter, S., 217
Schacter, D. L., 297
Schad, D. J., 47
Schank, R. C., 169
Schapiro, S. J., 135
Scheffler, I., 7, 8
Scheier, M. F., 29, 95
Schimmack, U., 401, 407
Schkade, D. A., 197, 199, 279, 280, 287
Schlenker, B. R., 117
Schmahl, C., 95
Schmeichel, B. J., 316
Schmitt, C. H., 41
Schmitt, D. P., 146
Schmitt, M., 28, 30, 31, 56, 136, 143
Schmitz, T. W., 64
Schmukle, S. C., 119, 132, 134, 135, 136, 137, 138, 139, 140, 141, 142, 149
Schnabel, K., 135, 136
Schneider, B., 402
Schneider, L., 401
Schneider, S. L., 387, 388
Schneiderman, E., 285
Schnyer, D. M., 64
Schoeneman, T. J., 92, 146
Schofield, J. W., 31
Schooler, J. N., 77
Schooler, J. W., 3, 23, 77, 78, 79, 80, 81, 82, 83, 84, 87, 182, 185, 186, 217, 218
Schooler, T. Y., 31, 52, 132, 159
Schriber, R. A., 3, 93, 105, 108, 142, 149, 415
Schryer, E., 168
Schüler, J., 40
Schulte, D., 40
Schultheiss, O. C., 3, 4, 39, 40, 41, 42, 43, 46, 47, 48, 49, 50, 51, 53, 54, 55, 56, 57, 58, 137, 142, 143, 144
Schulze König, S., 136
Schupp, J., 407
Schutz, A., 139
Schwartz, B., 181
Schwartz, G. E., 195
Schwartz, G. E. R., 423

Schwartz, J. L. K., 28, 136, 158
Schwartz, P. D., 414
Schwarz, N., 43, 166, 195, 199, 216, 217
Schwerdtfeger, A., 135
Sciangula, A., 416
Scollon, C. K., 336
Seaton, M., 17
Sechrest, L., 195
Sedikides, C., 93, 106, 107, 109, 110, 111, 112, 121, 199, 397, 398, 399, 406, 407, 413, 415, 417
See, Y. H. M., 164
Seidlitz, L., 195
Seise, J., 28
Selman, R. L., 414
Semendeferi, K., 69
Semin, G. R., 159
Seyle, D. C., 399
Shaeffer, E. M., 321
Shahinfar, A., 399
Shakarchi, R. J., 363
Shanks, D. R., 188
Shapiro, R., 258
Shapiro, S. L., 87, 423
Sharpless, B., 204
Shaver, P. R., 55, 111, 238
Shavitt, S., 373
Shaw, L., 399
Shechtman, Z., 247
Shedler, J., 117
Sheen, M., 296
Shenkel, R. J., 96
Sher, K. J., 259, 270
Sherman, D. K., 117, 348, 389, 417
Sherman, R. A., 405
Shields, A. J., 268
Shields, S. A., 196
Shipp, A. J., 402, 403
Shiv, B., 214
Shoda, Y., 281, 313, 319
Shows, D. L., 181
Shrauger, J. S., 92, 146
Shu, L. L., 283
Sicoly, F., 414
Sieff, E. M., 282
Sifneos, P. E., 52, 53
Sigman, M., 67
Sillars, A. L., 233
Silvia, P. J., 401
Simpson, J. A., 3, 211, 225, 226, 233, 234, 235, 236, 237, 238, 239, 251
Sinclair, S., 99, 310
Singer, J., 217
Singer, J. A., 295
Singer, J. L., 373

Author Index

Skalina, L. M., 337
Skodol, A. E., 268
Skorinko, J. L., 99
Skowronski, J. J., 397
Slemmer, J. A., 321
Sloman, S. A., 367, 369, 372, 375
Slovic, P., 181, 185
Small, D. A., 348
Smallwood, J., 79, 81, 82, 84, 87
Smart, L., 110
Smith, C. P., 40
Smith, C. T., 28, 159
Smith, D. A., 195
Smith, D. M., 98
Smith, E. R., 159
Smith, F. W., 197
Smith, H. L., 202
Smith, J. L., 97
Smith, K. S., 213
Smith, N. G., 336
Smith, R., 81
Smith, S. H., 367
Smith, S. M., 163, 165, 304
Smith, T. W., 418
Sneed, C. D., 248
Snell, J., 218
Snider, A. G., 231
Snodgrass, S. E., 245, 251
Snook, A., 250
Snyder, C. R., 96
Snyder, M., 92, 98, 381
Socrates, 119
Soffin, S., 247
Soto, C. J., 149
Spain, J. S., 137
Spangler, W. D., 41, 43
Sparks, P., 160
Sparrow, B., 32
Spataro, S. E., 99, 118
Spence, C., 12
Spence, D. P., 333, 339
Spence, J. T., 195
Spencer, S. J., 93, 111, 373
Spencer-Rogers, J., 399
Spinath, F. M., 132
Sporberg, D., 249
Spreemann, S., 399
Spreng, R. N., 14
Spruyt, A., 28
Spyropoulos, V., 281
Squire, L. R., 40, 57
Srivastava, S., 3, 14, 90, 92, 94, 96, 98, 99, 100, 118, 132, 141, 248
Srull, T. K., 310
Stahlberg, D., 399

Stanton, S. J., 40
Stapley, J. C., 196
Stapp, J., 195
Starek, J. E., 365, 373
Starr, M. J., 216
Stathi, S., 170
Steele, C. M., 380, 389
Steer, R. A., 264
Steffel, M., 355, 356
Steffens, M. C., 136
Steiner, I. D., 251
Steiner, J. E., 216
Steinglass, J. E., 264
Steinman, R. B., 137
Steinmetz, J. L., 414
Stein-Seroussi, A., 247, 422
Stepper, S., 143
Stern, D., 11
Stets, J. E., 399
Steup, M., 7, 8
Stewart, B. D., 28
Stipek, D., 17
Stoll, F., 259
Stone, A. A., 195
Stopfer, J. M., 139
Storebeck, J., 217
Story, A. L., 383, 388
Strack, F., 28, 30, 31, 32, 133, 142, 143, 382, 389
Strain, L. M., 25, 159
Strasser, A., 3, 4, 39, 137, 142, 143, 144
Strathman, A. J., 172
Strauss, G. P., 196
Strecher, V. J., 70
Strick, M., 188
Stroop, J. R., 44
Stroup, D. F., 282
Strube, M. J., 3, 93, 397, 398, 399, 407
Stukas, A. A., 98
Suedfeld, P., 363
Suh, E., 202
Suls, J., 385
Suls, J. M., 163, 349
Sun, C. R., 107
Sutin, A. R., 108
Sutton, R. M., 170
Svetlova, M., 16
Swann, W. B., 27, 135, 231, 247, 381
Swann, W. B., Jr., 83, 92, 94, 96, 97, 112, 114, 141, 145, 247, 251, 398, 399, 407, 422
Swartz-Kulstad, J. L., 402
Sweeny, P. D., 332
Sweldens, S., 26
Swets, J. A., 183
Syty, N. A., 195

Szabados, B., 363, 366
Sze, J. A., 87

T

Tajfel, H., 90
Takezawa, M., 245
Tambor, E. S., 94
Tamboukou, M., 329
Tangney, J. P., 195
Tanke, E. D., 98
Tapias, M. P., 97
Tate, E. B., 421, 424
Taylor, G. J., 53
Taylor, L. S., 399
Taylor, S., 415
Taylor, S. E., 106, 109, 117, 132, 142, 246, 348, 363, 380, 387, 398, 400, 417
Teasdale, J. D., 204
Teige-Mocigemba, S., 28
Telch, M. J., 399
Tellegen, A., 288
Tenbrunsel, A. E., 363
Tennen, H., 205
Terdal, S. K., 94
Tesser, A., 146, 371
Tetlock, P. E., 121
Thomaes, S., 399
Thomas, C., 266
Thomas, G., 168, 234
Thompson, L., 197
Thompson, M. M., 160
Thompson, R. A., 107, 414
Thrash, T. M., 54, 55
Tice, D. M., 92, 117
Tiedens, L. Z., 99
Tindell, A. J., 213
Toates, F. M., 211
Todd, P. M., 134
Todorov, A., 351
Toguchi, Y., 110
Toner, K., 3, 142, 149, 251, 374, 413
Torelli, C. J., 315
Torgersen, S., 268
Tormala, Z. L., 160, 163, 165, 166, 170, 172
Toth, J. P., 301
Tracy, J. L., 110, 111, 112
Trafton, J. G., 65
Tran, S., 238
Trapnell, P. D., 144
Trivers, R., 365
Trope, Y., 3, 83, 310, 311, 312, 313, 315, 316, 317, 318, 319, 323, 367, 398
Tropp, L. R., 243
Trost, M. R., 168

Trötschel, R., 26
Trzesniewski, K. H., 107, 112, 399
Tsiros, M., 181
Tu, P. C., 70
Tudor, M., 230
Tükel, R., 260
Tulving, E., 67, 195, 304
Turkheimer, E., 114, 119, 261, 265, 266, 267, 269
Türksoy, N., 260
Turner, J. C., 90
Tversky, A., 84, 184, 185, 285, 302, 368, 369, 370, 371, 374
Tyler, T. R., 315

U

Ubel, P. A., 284
Uhlmann, E. L., 158
Uzelac, S. M., 414

V

Van Aken, M. A. G., 146
Van Baaren, R. B., 187, 188
Van Boven, L., 184, 201, 218, 219, 283
Van den Bergh, O., 24, 26
Van den Bos, K., 188
van den Brink, W., 203
Van der Leij, A., 187
Van der Linden, M., 66
van der Meer, E., 216
van der Pligt, J., 160, 184
Van Doorn, E., 188
Van Etten, M. L., 259
van Harreveld, F., 160, 184
van Leeuwen, B., 184, 278, 349
Van Olden, Z., 187, 188, 189
Van Osselaer, S., 26
van Overwalle, F., 64, 70
van Raamsdonk, M., 215
Van Yperen, N. W., 229
Vandereycken, W., 260
Vazire, S., 1, 3, 14, 91, 94, 97, 112, 113, 114, 119, 121, 131, 132, 133, 134, 135, 137, 138, 139, 140, 141, 145, 148, 149, 242, 245, 246, 247, 248, 249, 250, 251, 261, 265, 266, 267, 331, 332, 338, 340, 357, 359, 401, 416
Vecchione, M., 373
Venier, I. L., 212
Verfaellie, M., 65
Verheul, R., 203
Verkasalo, M., 373
Verstraten, F. A., 12

Vevea, J. L., 121
Viel, S. C., 282
Vignoles, V. L., 111
Vilenkin, A., 421
Visser, P. S., 165
Viswesvaran, C., 139
Vitousek, K., 270
Vittersø, J., 407
Vogel, T., 170, 171
Vogt, D. S., 401
Vohs, K. D., 132, 316, 405
von Collani, G., 136
von Hippel, W., 363, 365, 373
Vorauer, J. D., 243, 249
Vosgerau, J., 219
Vroomen, J., 215

W

Wade, K. A., 297
Wagerman, S. A., 405
Wagner, B. C., 166
Wagner, G. G., 407
Wagner, J. W., 330
Wagoner Funk, W., 416
Wakslak, C. J., 3, 310, 313, 316, 317, 320, 321
Wallace, A. B., 87
Wallace, H. M., 92
Walsh, B., 264
Walsh, W. B., 402
Walther, E., 24, 26
Wan, C., 399
Wan, X., 213
Wang, A. T., 67
Wang, L., 399
Wang, P. S., 263
Wang, Q., 18
Ward, A., 96, 357, 419, 422
Warman, D. M., 264
Watson, D., 139, 199, 202, 288
Watson, S., 270
Way, B. M., 66
Wayment, H. A., 398
Weber, J., 70
Webster, D., 181
Webster, D. M., 170
Weck, F., 137
Wegener, D. T., 30, 32, 160, 165, 166, 167, 172
Wegner, D. M., 32, 79, 82, 348, 366
Weinberger, D. A., 373
Weinberger, J., 40, 41, 42
Weiner, B., 210
Weinstein, N. D., 348, 385
Weiskrantz, L., 215
Wellman, H. M., 13

Wells, G. L., 165
Welsh, R. C., 70
Wentura, D., 386, 387, 388
Wenzlaff, R. M., 79, 94
Wertenbroch, K., 323
West, S. G., 134, 139, 250, 347
West, T. V., 242
Westen, D., 364, 366
Wheatley, T., 32, 279, 282
Wheatley, T. P., 278, 349
Wheeler, A. R., 402
Wheeler, C., 160
Wheeler, S. C., 161, 164, 169
White, P., 167
Whitehead, G. I., 367
Whitehouse, K., 302
Whitfield, M., 159
Wicklund, R. A., 29
Widiger, T. A., 203, 268
Wiese, D., 139
Wiesentahl, N. L., 163
Wilbarger, J. L., 216
Wilbur, C. J., 23
Wilhelm, F. H., 55, 217
Willard, G., 117, 118
Williams, B., 7
Williams, C. J., 28, 158
Williams, J. M. G., 204
Williams, T., 336
Williamson, I. O., 403
Williamson, R. A., 11
Willis, T. A., 380
Willoughby, T. L., 388
Wilson, A., 119
Wilson, A. E., 299
Wilson, G. T., 270
Wilson, T., 219
Wilson, T. D., 1, 22, 23, 27, 29, 30, 31, 32, 33, 52, 55, 132, 133, 134, 136, 137, 141, 142, 144, 149, 159, 162, 164, 166, 167, 168, 171, 182, 183, 185, 186, 187, 188, 189, 197, 199, 217, 218, 251, 277, 278, 279, 280, 281, 282, 283, 284, 285, 288, 289, 322, 333, 345, 346, 349, 351, 353, 358, 363, 365, 401
Wimmer, G. E., 66, 220
Windschitl, P. D., 115, 249
Winerman, L., 32
Wink, P. M., 118
Winkielman, P., 3, 34, 79, 210, 212, 216, 217, 219, 220
Winquist, L., 242, 252
Winthrop, J., 418
Wittenbrink, B., 25, 28
Wolfe, C. T., 95, 109
Woloshyn, V., 299
Wong, K. Y., 188, 189

Wood, D., 248
Wood, J. T., 228
Wood, W., 162, 165, 195
Worth, M., 47
Wright, F., 112
Wright, P., 169
Wright, S. S., 114, 417
Wu, D., 12
Wurf, E., 312
Wyer, R. S., 310, 380
Wyvell, C. L., 213

X

Xenophon, 116
Xu, F., 13
Xu, J., 195, 199
Xue, G., 66

Y

Yammarino, F. J., 106
Yang, Y., 399
Yankova, D., 47

Yim, I. S., 112
Yost, J. H., 397, 399
Young, R. D., 226
Yuan, J. W., 87

Z

Zajonc, R. B., 215, 216, 363, 367
Zaki, J., 70
Zanarini, M. C., 95
Zanna, M. P., 93, 111, 160, 164, 165, 166, 373
Zarzuela, A., 258
Zeckhauser, R., 283
Zeigler-Hill, V., 111, 112, 159
Zerbes, N., 28
Zerwas, S., 16
Zhang, J., 280
Zhao, B. X., 407
Zickmund, S., 228
Zimmerman, C. A., 304
Zimmerman, M., 268, 269
Zogmaister, C., 31
Zou, Z., 115, 417
Zuckerman, M., 417
Zuroff, D. C., 41

Subject Index

Page numbers followed by *f* indicate figure; *n*, note; and *t*, table

Ability, task characteristics and, 318
Abstract and concrete self-guides. *See also* Self-representation
  context and, 314–319
  distance and, 313–314
  overview, 311–313, 323–324
Academic achievement, 17
Acceptance
  egoistic biases and, 420–421
  relationship knowledge and, 229
Acceptance therapy, 229
Accessibility bias, 294, 300–301. *See also* Memory
Accessibility model of emotion reporting, 197–201, 198*f*, 200*f*. *See also* Emotions
Accuracy
  affective forecasting and, 287
  autobiographical memories and, 296–299
  defensiveness and, 421–423
  empathic accuracy, 233–238, 235*f*
  epistemological traditions and, 331–333
  forecasting accuracy, 278–279
  mental disorders and, 261, 264–265
  motivated reasoning and, 386–389
  relationship knowledge and, 226, 232–233
  self-views and, 416–419
  study of self-knowledge and, 2
  See also Illusions of self-knowledge; Meta-accuracy
Accuracy bias, 231–232. *See also* Biases
Accuracy criterion
  assessing individual differences in self-enhancement and, 113–115
  relationship knowledge and, 231–233
Action orientation after failure (AOF), 54–55
Activation of mental associations, 25. *See also* Mental associations
Actual–desired attitude discrepancies, 168–169. *See also* Attitudes
Addiction
  self-deception and, 364
  wanting and liking and, 212–214
  See also Alcoholism; Substance use disorders
Adjustment, 137
Adult development, 96–97
Affect Intensity Measure (AIM) scale, 214
Affective blindsight, 215
Affective forecasting
  forecasting errors and, 278, 281–283, 349
  improving, 284–285
  limited self-knowledge and, 279–281
  methodological issues and, 285–288
  overview, 277–279, 289
  prediction illusions and, 349
  study of self-knowledge and, 2
  See also Emotions; Prediction
Affective origins of attitudes, 164–165. *See also* Attitudes
Affective response, 215–217. *See also* Emotions
Affiliative social tuning hypothesis, 99

Age, 95–96
Alcohol intoxication, 80. *See also* Substance use disorders
Alcoholism, 259, 364. *See also* Addiction; Substance use disorders
Alexithymia, 53–54
Ambivalence, 159–162, 173–174
Analytic processes, 279–281
Ancient Greeks, 64–65
Anorexia nervosa, 260. *See also* Mental disorders
Anxiety disorders
　autobiographical memories and, 305
　referential processing and, 56
Assessment
　emotions and, 206
　epistemological traditions and, 332
　individual differences in self-enhancement and, 113–116
　mental disorders and, 263–264
　personality self-knowledge (PSK) and, 132–136, 133f, 140
　person–environment (P-E) fit and, 403–405
　self-deception and, 372–374
　See also Measures; Self-assessment
Associations, mental, 280–281. *See* Mental associations
Associative learning, 24–25, 212–214
Assumed reciprocity, 249–250
Assumed similarity, 249–250
Attitudes
　changes in, 167–173
　consequences of, 165–166
　correcting for presumed biases and, 166–167
　ideologies and, 316–317
　measures of, 158–167
　origins of, 164–165
　overview, 157–158, 173–174
　social judgment and, 317
　study of self-knowledge and, 1
　See also Evaluation
Attributional theory, 332
Attributions
　autobiographical memories and, 294
　false memories and, 300
　self-enhancement and, 93–94
Autism spectrum disorders (ASDs), 108
Autobiographical memories
　accuracy and, 296–299
　emotions and, 204
　false memories and, 296–302
　fluency heuristic and, 302–303
　memory retrieval and, 303–305
　models of the self and, 295–296
　nature of the self and, 8
　overview, 293–295, 306
　See also Memory; Past selves

Automaticity, 23, 28–29
Availability heuristic, 184–185
Avoidance, 203–204
Awareness
　of capabilities, 13
　insight into the contents of one's mental associations, 28–29

B

Balance theory, 160
Beck Cognitive Insight Scale (BCIS), 264. *See also* Measures
Behavior
　attitudes and, 165–166
　blind spots in self-knowledge and, 144–145
　distance and, 319–321
　epistemological traditions and, 332
　ideologies and, 316–317
　illusions of self-knowledge and, 358, 359f
　insight into the effects of one's mental associations, 30–32
　introspection illusion and, 346–347
　mental disorders and, 263
　meta-accuracy and, 247, 248–249
　motivated reasoning and, 383–384
　personality self-knowledge (PSK) and, 131, 134, 137, 141f, 144–145
　prediction and, 144–145
　referential competence and, 55–57
　self-deception and, 369–372, 372t
　social mechanisms and, 98–99
　unawareness of, 31
　values and, 315–316
Behavioral confirmation, 98–99
Behavioral observations, 3. *See also* Measures
Behavioral prediction domain in PSK
　blind spots in self-knowledge and, 146–147
　overview, 133f, 134, 144–145
Behavioral resistance, 93–94
Beliefs
　acceptance of ordinariness and fallibility and, 420–421
　changes in attitudes and, 169–173
　defensiveness and, 421–423
　emotions and, 194–197, 204–205
　See also Illusions of self-knowledge
Believability, 332–333
Bias protection procedures, 351–352. *See also* Biases; Blind spots in self-knowledge; Introspection illusion
Biases
　affective forecasting and, 287
　assessing individual differences in self-enhancement and, 115–116

Subject Index

   correcting attitudes for, 166–167, 173–174
   forecasting errors and, 278
   individual differences and, 105–106
   motivational–affective accounts and, 109–113
   overview, 413
   personality self-knowledge (PSK) and, 137
   relationship knowledge and, 226, 231–233
   self-enhancement and, 107–109
   social conflict and, 356–357
   See also Blind spots in self-knowledge; Egoistic biases
Big Five personality traits
   empirical findings, 136–137
   generalized meta-accuracy (GMA) and, 243–245, 244t–245t
   overview, 149n
   self-representation and, 314
   See also Five-factor model of personality
Blind spots in self-knowledge
   awareness of contents of thoughts and, 78–81
   egoistic biases and, 420
   introspection illusion and, 350–354, 352f
   motivation and, 81–83
   overview, 77–78, 86–87
   personal traits and, 83–86
   personality self-knowledge (PSK) and, 141–149, 141f
   social conflict and, 356–357
   wanting and liking and, 215, 221
   See also Biases
Blindsight phenomenon, 215
Bolster-Counterargue Scale (BCS), 172–173
Brain imaging studies, 11. *See also* Neuroscience
Brain structures, 213–214. *See* Neuroscience
Broadening of the self, 230. *See also* Self-expansion model
Brown Assessment of Beliefs Scale (BABS), 264. *See also* Measures

C

Capabilities, 17
Capacities, awareness of, 13
Catastrophic interference, 72
Causal coherence, 329
Causal explanations, 338–339
Causal link, 31–32
Change
   in attitudes, 167–173
   conditions under which people might be open to contributions to self-knowledge from others, 97
   resistance to, 95, 97
Cheating, self-deception and, 369–372, 372t
Childhood, 16, 17

Choice
   decision making and, 181–189
   forecasting errors and, 278
   introspection illusion and, 353–354
   wanting and liking and, 218–221
   See also Preferences
Cigarette cravings, 80
Clinical psychology, 1
Cognitive biases, 93–94
Cognitive developmental theory, 9–11
Cognitive origins of attitudes, 164–165. *See also* Attitudes
Cognitive psychology, 366–367
Cognitive-behavioral therapy (CBT), 424–425
Cognitive–experiential self-theory (CEST), 279–281
Cognitive–informational accounts, 107–109
Coherence, 329–330, 332–333
Coherent positive resolution, 330
Collaborative Longitudinal Personality Disorders Study (CLPS), 268–269
Color-naming task
   referential activity (RA) scales and, 44–47, 46t
   referential competence and, 51f, 52
   referential processing and, 44–45
Communication, 10
Comorbidity, 263. *See also* Mental disorders
Comparison processes, 142
Competitive bargaining, 318
Computerized RA (CRA) measure, 46–47, 46t. *See also* Measures
Concrete self-guide. *See* Abstract and concrete self-guides
Conditioned stimulus, 24–27
Confidence, 348–349, 349
Confirmatory behavior, 98–99
Confirmatory biases, 419
Confirmatory evidence, 385–386
Conflict, social, 356–357
Congenial conclusions, 385–386
Conscious desire, 211. *See also* Wanting
Conscious pleasure, 211. *See also* Liking
Conscious processes
   awareness of contents of thoughts and, 78–81
   decision making and, 181–189
   introspection illusion and, 346–347
   overview, 184
   wanting and liking and, 214–218
Consensual behavior observation approach, 145–146
Considering the opposite, 389
Consistency processes
   affective forecasting and, 288
   autobiographical memories and, 295–296
   personality self-knowledge (PSK) and, 142
Construals, 322–323

Context, 303, 314–319
Continuity
  autobiographical memories and, 295
  relationship knowledge and, 229
Control, 23, 29
Control illusion, 348–349. *See also* Illusions of self-knowledge
Controlled recollection, 301–302. *See also* Autobiographical memories
Convergent validity, 49–55, 50t, 51f. *See also* Validity
Cooperative bargaining, 318
Criterion measures, 2–3, 332. *See also* Measures
Cued recall, 302, 304
Cultural concept of biography, 329–330
Cultural factors
  egoistic biases and, 418–419
  narratives and, 333

D

Daydreaming, 78–83
Decision making
  conscious thought in, 184–186
  meta-accuracy and, 251
  normative strategies for, 182–183
  overview, 181–182
  prediction and, 218–221
  self-knowledge and, 186–187
  unconscious thought and, 187–189
  wanting and liking and, 218–221
Defensiveness, 421–423. *See* Motivated reasoning
Degree of regulatory scope, 311. *See also* Regulatory scope
Dehumanization, 72
Depression
  autobiographical memories and, 305
  referential processing and, 56
Development of self-knowledge
  contemporary directions of, 11–15
  nature of the self and, 7–11
  overview, 7, 15–19
Developmental perspectives, 1, 9–11
Developmental processes
  conditions under which people might be open to contributions to self-knowledge from others, 95–97
  developmental sequencing, 15
  narcissism and, 111
Diagnosis, 258. *See also* Mental disorders
Diagnostic and Statistical Manual of Mental Disorders (DSM-IV), 258
Diagnostic utility, 84
Direct self-appraisal, 91–92

Directional thought, 380
Disclosure, 355–356
Discounting effect, 358, 359f
Discrepancies, attitudes and, 159–162, 168–169
Discriminant validity, 53–55. *See also* Validity
Dissociations, wanting and liking and, 214
Distance
  behavior and, 319–321
  self-knowledge and, 321–323
  self-representation and, 313–319
  See also Psychological distance points
Distortions in self-perception, 110–113
Dominance, emotions and, 198t
Dopaminergic pathway, wanting and liking and, 213
Dorsomedial prefrontal cortex (DMPFC)
  overview, 73–74
  philosophy and, 64–65
  theories of MPFC and DMPFC function and, 70–73
Drug addiction. *See* Addiction
Dual-attitudes approach, 159. *See also* Attitudes
Dual-process theories
  automaticity and control and, 23
  insight into the contents of one's mental associations, 27–30
  insight into the effects of one's mental associations, 30–32
  overview, 22–23, 33
  study of self-knowledge and, 1
Dyadic or differential meta-accuracy (DMA)
  impressions on others, 245–246
  overview, 243, 244t–245t
  self-observations of behavior and, 248–249
  See also Meta-accuracy; Metaperception

E

Eating disorders, 260. *See also* Mental disorders
Economic problems, 283
Education, 357–358
Ego development, 330
Ego involvement, 109–110
Egocentrism, 413–414
Egoistic biases
  acceptance of ordinariness and fallibility and, 420–421
  accuracy and, 416–419
  challenging, 424–425
  defensiveness and, 421–423
  overview, 413–415, 425
  self-enhancement and self-depreciation and, 415–416
  self-evaluative thinking and, 423–424

skepticism, 419–420
    See also Biases
Ego-skepticism, 419–420. *See also* Egoistic biases; Skepticism
Electronically Activated Recorder (EAR), 138
Emotional intelligence, 285
Emotions
    accessibility model of reporting, 197–201, 198f, 200f
    overview, 194, 205–206
    self-stereotyping and, 201–205, 203f
    sources of information about, 194–197
    wanting and liking and, 215–217
    See also Affective forecasting; Affective response
Empathic accuracy, 233–238, 235f. *See also* Accuracy; Empathy
Empathy
    empathy gaps, 278, 289n
    gender and, 195–196
    medial prefrontal context (MPFC) and, 70
    transactional social experience and, 73
Endowment effect, 283
Enhancement, self. *See* Self-enhancement
Enhancement illusions, 347–348. *See also* Illusions of self-knowledge; Self-enhancement
Enlightenment, 65–67
Environment, person–environment (P-E) fit and, 397–398, 402–406, 403f
Episodic memory
    neuroscience and, 65–66
    overview, 14
    theories of MPFC and DMPFC function and, 71–72
    See also Memory
Epistemological pluralism, 333–339
Epistemological traditions
    accuracy and, 331–333
    epistemological line and, 333–338
    narrative model, 328–331, 333–335
    overview, 327, 338–339
    paradigmatic model, 328, 333–335
    self-knowledge and, 335–338
    See also Narrative model
Equal weight heuristic (EQW), 182–183
Errors
    decision making and, 184–185
    egoistic biases and, 416–419
    forecasting errors, 278, 281–283, 289n, 349
    motivated reasoning and, 386–389
    See also False memories; Illusions of self-knowledge
Evaluation, 2–3. *See also* Attitudes; Measures
Evaluative associations, 31–32
Evaluative conditioning, 24–27

Evanescence, 198t
Evidence seeking, 382, 385–386
Evolutionary perspectives, self-deception and, 365
Expansion of the self. *See* Self-expansion model
Experience, 357–358
Experience-sampling methodology, 80–81
Experiential systems, 279–281
Experimental avoidance, 203–204
Expertise, 96
Explicit attitudes, 158–162. *See also* Attitudes
Explicit measures
    insight into the contents of one's mental associations, 29
    personality self-knowledge (PSK) and, 136
    See also Measures
Explicit motivation, 40–41, 41f, 47–49, 48f. *See also* Motivation
Explicit personality, 141f. *See also* Personality
Explicit–implicit consistency domain in PSK
    blind spots in self-knowledge and, 146–147
    overview, 133–134, 133f, 142–143
Exploratory processing, 330
Exposure control, 351–352
Extraversion
    emotions and, 202–203, 203f
    generalized meta-accuracy (GMA) and, 243–245, 244t–245t
Extremity, 287

F

Fallibility, acceptance of, 420–421
False fame experiments, 299–302
False memories, 296–302. *See also* Autobiographical memories; Errors; Illusions of self-knowledge
Feedback
    integration of, 146
    from others, 246–247
    self-serving bias and, 93–94
Feelings. *See* Affective response; Emotions
Feelings-as-information hypothesis, 217–218
Five-factor model of personality, 149n. *See also* Big Five personality traits
Fluency heuristic, 302–303
Focalism, 279–280, 284
Folk perceivers, 96
Forebrain, wanting and liking and, 213–214
Forecasting, affective. *See* Affective forecasting
Forgetting, 303–305. *See also* Memory
Formation of mental associations, 25. *See also* Mental associations
Free will, introspection illusion and, 354
Frontotemporal dementia (FTD), 108

Functional magnetic resonance imaging (fMRI)
ME and I and, 67–68
overview, 64
transactional social experience and, 73
Future behaviors, 320. *See also* Behavior

G

Gender
emotions and, 195–196, 199
relationship knowledge and, 228
Generalized anxiety disorder (GAD), 56
Generalized meta-accuracy (GMA), 243, 243–245, 244t–245t. *See also* Meta-accuracy; Metaperception
Generic representations of people, 70–72
German Observational Study of Adult Twins (GOSAT), 137–138, 139
Gifted scholarship, 383
Global bias, 232. *See also* Biases
Goal imagery, 58
Goal priming, 33
Goal pursuit
evaluative conditioning and, 26
insight into the effects of one's mental associations, 30–32
overview, 33
referential processing and, 43–55, 46t, 48f, 50t, 51f
resistance to change and, 95
wanting and liking and, 214
Grandiosity, 110–113
Guilt
gender and, 195–196
representations of capabilities and, 17

H

Happiness, 278, 281–282
Health
autobiographical memories and, 305
forecasting errors and, 282
Heuristics
autobiographical memories and, 302–303
meta-accuracy and, 249–250
Holistic processes, 279–281
Hypoegoic self-regulation, 424

I

Ideal self, 168–169
Identity definition, 295
Identity development, 96–97

Identity negotiation theory, 141–142
Ideologies, 316–317
Idiosyncratic representations of people, 70–72
Illusion of control, 348–349. *See also* Illusions of self-knowledge
Illusions of self-knowledge
challenging, 424–425
egoistic biases and, 416–419
introspection illusion, 346–349
overcoming, 357–359, 359f
overview, 345–346
reducing, 423–424
research support of, 347–349
social interactions and, 354–357
things we cannot know, 350–354, 352f
See also Accuracy; Errors; False memories; Self-perception
Imaging to words, referential competence and, 49–53, 50t, 51f
Imitation, 9–10, 11
Immersive social experience, 72–73
Immoral behavior, 315–316. *See also* Behavior
Immune neglect, 280, 284
Impact bias, 278. *See also* Biases
Implicit Association Test (IAT)
overview, 149n
personality self-knowledge (PSK) and, 132–133, 136, 143–144
referential processing and, 56
See also Measures
Implicit associations, 280–281
Implicit attitudes
introspection illusion and, 353
overview, 158–162
study of self-knowledge and, 1
See also Attitudes
Implicit cognition, 2
Implicit measures
insight into the contents of one's mental associations, 29
personality self-knowledge (PSK) and, 136
study of self-knowledge and, 3
See also Measures
Implicit memory, 294. *See also* Memory
Implicit motivation, 1, 40–41, 41f, 47–49, 48f. *See also* Motivation
Implicit personality
personality self-knowledge (PSK) and, 141f
study of self-knowledge and, 1
See also Personality
Implicit self, 8
Impressions on others, 245–246. *See also* Metaperception; Other people and self-knowledge
Impulse control
autobiographical memories and, 301–302
narcissism and, 112–113

narcissists and, 94
personality self-knowledge (PSK) and, 141f
Inaccuracy in self-views, 2
Inaccurate theories, 278
Incentive salience hypothesis, 212–214
Individual differences
  assessing in self-enhancement, 113–116
  autobiographical memories and, 297, 301–302
  emotions and, 196–197, 202–203
  false memories and, 297
  overview, 105–106, 120
  personality and, 55
  positive illusions, 116–119
  referential processing and, 43–55, 46t, 48f, 50t, 51f
  self-deception and, 372–374
  self-enhancement and, 106–113
Infancy, 16
Inference, 13
Information processing, 165–166
Information seeking, 381–382
Information-processing perspective
  overview, 39
  referential processing and, 42–43, 42f, 57–58
  self-deception and, 363–364, 366–367
  two-systems model of motivation and, 39–41, 41f
Insight
  into the contents of one's mental associations, 27–30
  into the effects of one's mental associations, 30–32
  mental associations and, 23–27, 24f
  study of self-knowledge and, 2
  substance use disorders and, 259
  unnecessary self-evaluative thinking and, 423–424
  See also Self-insight
Integrative model, 141, 141f
Intentionality, 29
Interdisciplinary focus, 2
Intergroup relations, 282–283. See also Relationship knowledge
Interpersonal factors, 160
Interpersonal outcomes, 117–118
Intimacy, illusions of self-knowledge and, 355–356
Intrapersonal discrepancy, 160
Intrapersonal empathy gaps, 278
Intrapsychic outcomes, 117–118
Introspection illusion
  overcoming, 357–359, 359f
  overview, 346–347
  research support of, 347–349
  things we cannot know, 350–354, 352f
  See also Illusions of self-knowledge

J

Judgment
  attitudes and, 317
  decision making and, 186–187
  personality self-knowledge (PSK) and, 147–148

K

Knowledge acquisition processes, 15

L

Lateral parietal regions, 66–67
Learning processes
  affective forecasting and, 284–285
  insight into the causes of mental associations and, 24–25
Liking
  awareness of, 214–218
  overview, 210–214, 221
  prediction and, 218–221
Limitations, narcissism and, 112–113
Limits in self-knowledge. see Blind spots in self-knowledge
Loss aversion, forecasting errors and, 283
Luxury, emotions and, 195
Lying to oneself. see Self-deception

M

Magical thinking, 348–349
Mainz Observation of Behavior Study, 138
ME and I, 67–69
Meaningful explanations, 338–339
Mean-level bias, 232–233. See also Biases
Measures
  affective forecasting and, 288
  alexithymia and, 53–54
  attitudes and, 158–167
  autobiographical memories and, 295
  emotions and, 206
  epistemological traditions and, 332
  insight into the contents of one's mental associations, 29
  mental disorders and, 263–264, 266–267
  motivational congruence and. see also Measures
  personality self-knowledge (PSK) and, 132–136, 133f, 136, 138–139, 140
  referential activity (RA) scales and, 45–47, 46t
  resisting influence and, 172–173
  self-deception and, 372–374

Measures *(cont.)*
 of self-enhancement, 119
 study of self-knowledge and, 2–3
 two-systems model of motivation and, 39–41, 41f
 See also Assessment; Evaluation; *individual measures*
Medial prefrontal context (MPFC)
 ME and I and, 67–69
 overview, 63, 73–74
 philosophy and, 64–65
 psychology and, 69–73
 theories of MPFC and DMPFC function and, 70–73
 See also Neuroscience
Medial temporal lobe, 65–66
Meditation practices
 blind spots in self-knowledge and, 87
 unnecessary self-evaluative thinking and, 423–424
Memory
 blind spots in self-knowledge and, 87
 emotions and, 204
 memory maturation, 13–14
 nature of the self and, 8
 neuroscience and, 65–66
 personal memories, 17–18
 retrieval, 303–305
 theories of MPFC and DMPFC function and, 71–72
 See also Autobiographical memories
Memory fluency, 294. *See also* Memory
Memory maturation, 13–14. *See also* Memory
Mental associations
 causes of, 23–27, 24f
 contents of, 27–30
 effects of, 30–32
Mental disorders
 autobiographical memories and, 305
 epistemological traditions and, 336–337
 lack of self-knowledge for, 268–269
 methodological challenges and, 262–265
 overview, 258–262, 269–270
Meta-accuracy
 causes of, 246–250
 improving, 250–252
 overview, 242–246, 244t–245t, 252
 self-observations of behavior and, 248–249
 See Accuracy
Meta-accuracy domain in PSK, 133f, 135, 139–140, 141
Meta-awareness
 awareness of contents of thoughts and, 79–81
 motivation and, 81–83
Metacognition, 2
Meta-insight, 248–249

Metaperception
 causes of, 246–250
 heuristics and, 249–250
 improving, 250–252
 mental disorders and, 266
 overview, 242–246, 244t–245t
 personality self-knowledge (PSK) and, 141f
 reflected appraisals and, 91–92
 study of self-knowledge and, 2
 See also Meta-accuracy; Other people and self-knowledge; Perceptions of others
Metaperception enhancement (MPE), 243, 246. *See also* Metaperception
Mind wandering
 awareness of contents of thoughts and, 78–81
 blind spots in self-knowledge and, 77–78
 motivation and, 81–83
Mindfulness
 blind spots in self-knowledge and, 87
 meta-accuracy and, 250–251
 unnecessary self-evaluative thinking and, 423–424
Minding model, 228–229
Minnesota Multiphasic Personality Inventory (MMPI), 372
Mirror neurons, 11
Mirror self-recognition task, 16
Model of attitude structure (MCM), 159–162
Moral behavior, 315–316. *See also* Behavior
Moral licensing, 384
Moralistic bias, 110
Motivated accuracy/inaccuracy, 236–238, 238–239
Motivated blind spots, 142
Motivated cognition, 367
Motivated reasoning
 overview, 379–381, 389–392
 strategies for, 381–384
 theory and research regarding, 385–389
Motivated skepticism, 382
Motivation
 ambivalence and, 160
 blind spots in self-knowledge and, 81–83, 146–147
 overview, 398–402
 personality self-knowledge (PSK) and, 146–147
 referential processing and, 42–43, 42f
 self-deception and, 369–372, 372t
 self-enhancement and, 93–94
 self-verification and, 94
 status and, 100
 two-systems model of, 40–41, 41f
 wanting and liking and, 211, 216–217
Motivational congruence
 correlates of, 54–55
 referential competence and, 47–49, 48f, 49–53, 50t, 51f, 54–55

Motivational–affective accounts, 107, 109–113
Multi-attribute utility theory (MAUT), 183
Multiple-contextualized selves, 305

N

Naive realism
  conditions under which people might be open to contributions to self-knowledge from others, 96
  egoistic biases and, 419–420
  epistemological traditions and, 332
Naming, 44–45
Narcissism, 110–113
Narcissistic personality disorder, 261. *See also* Mental disorders
Narcissists
  distortions in self-perception and, 110–113
  self-serving bias and, 93–94
  status and, 100
Narrative model
  accuracy and, 331–333
  overview, 327, 328–331, 338–339
  paradigmatic model and, 333–335
  self-knowledge and, 335–338
  See also Epistemological traditions
Nature of the self, 7–11
Need-based modulation of value, 211
NEO Five Factor Inventory (NEO-FFI), 139
NEO Personality Inventory, 268
Neopsychoanalytic theories, 9
Neuroscience
  imitation and, 11
  incentive salience hypothesis and, 212–214
  individual differences and, 108
  neural basis to the self, 14
  overview, 63, 73–74
  from philosophy to, 64–69
  to psychology, 69–73
  self-enhancement and, 121*n*
  study of self-knowledge and, 1
  wanting and liking and, 211–212, 212–214
  See also Brain imaging studies
Neuroticism, 202–203, 203*f*
Nonconscious thought, 1
Nonverbal system, 42, 57–58. *See also* Referential processing
Normativeness, 250

O

Objective assessments, 403–405. *See also* Assessment
Objective criteria, 114

Objective knowledge
  of attitudes, 163
  introspection illusion and, 351
Obsessive–compulsive disorder (OCD), 260, 264. *See also* Mental disorders
Operationalizing bias, 115–116
Optimism, 348–349
Orbitofrontal cortex, 108
Ordinariness, acceptance of, 420–421
Other people and self-knowledge
  conditions under which people might be open to contributions to self-knowledge from others, 95–98
  example of, 99–100
  illusions of self-knowledge and, 354–357, 359
  mechanisms of, 98–99
  motivated reasoning and, 392
  overview, 90–91, 100
  personality self-knowledge (PSK) and, 134–135, 139, 141*f*
  reflected appraisals and, 91–92
  self-perception and, 92–95
  social consensus and, 113–115
  status and, 99–100
  See also Meta-accuracy; Metaperception
Other-stereotyping, 201–205, 203*f*. *See also* Stereotypes

P

Pain paradigm, 369
Paradigmatic model
  accuracy and, 331–333
  narrative model and, 333–335
  overview, 328, 331, 338–339
  self-knowledge and, 335–338
Partner knowledge
  empathic accuracy and, 233–238, 235*f*
  outcomes related to, 229–231
  overview, 225–226, 238–239
  See also Other people and self-knowledge; Relationship knowledge
Partner-oriented thoughts and discussions, 228–229
Past selves
  fluency heuristic and, 302–303
  memory retrieval and, 303–305
  overview, 293–294, 306
  See also Autobiographical memories
Pathology. *See* Mental disorders
Peer Nomination Study, 265–266
Perceived knowledge, 163
Perception
  attitudes and, 165–166
  distance and, 321

Perception *(cont.)*
    egocentrism and, 413–414
    fluency heuristic and, 302–303
    of knowledge, 162–164
    mental disorders and, 261
    motivated reasoning and, 392
    person–environment (P-E) fit and, 404
    See also Perceptions of others; Self-perception
Perceptions of others
    affect on self-knowledge, 90–100
    conditions under which people might be open to contributions to self-knowledge from others, 96
    personality self-knowledge (PSK) and, 141*f*
    See also Perception
Perceptual mechanisms, 12
Perfection, 420–421
Personal memories, 8, 17–18. *See also* Memory
Personal traits and predispositions, 83–86
Personality
    autobiographical memories and, 295–296
    emotions and, 201–202
    epistemological traditions and, 335–336
    meta-accuracy and, 247–247
    overview, 131–132
    referential processing and, 55–57
    self-enhancement and, 108
    See also Personality self-knowledge (PSK)
Personality disorders
    lack of self-knowledge for, 268–269
    overview, 260–262, 269–270
    self-knowledge and, 265–268
    self–other agreement and, 265–266
    See also Mental disorders
Personality neglect, 281
Personality psychology, 1
Personality self-knowledge (PSK)
    adaptiveness of, 148–149
    blind spots in self-knowledge and, 141–149, 141*f*
    empirical findings, 136–140
    improving, 148
    meta-accuracy and, 247–248
    overview, 131–136, 133*f*
    See also Personality; Trait uncertainty
Person–environment (P-E) fit
    overview, 397–398, 402–406, 403*f*
    self-knowledge and, 405–406
Perspective, 413–414
Persuasion, 169–173
Persuasion knowledge model, 169–173
Persuasion schema notion, 169
Philosophy, 63, 64–69
Physical representations of self, 15–16. *See also* Representations

Picture Story Exercise (PSE)
    referential competence and, 47–49, 48*f*
    two-systems model of motivation and, 40–41, 41*f*
Pleasure, emotions and, 195
Positive and Negative Affect Schedule (PANAS), 288
Positivity bias, 231–232. *See also* Biases; Self-enhancement
Posttraumatic stress disorder (PTSD), 56–57
Practical assessment perspective, 140
Pragmatic accuracy, 114
Praise, egoistic biases and, 418
Precision, 322–323
Prediction
    blind spots in self-knowledge and, 144–145
    illusions of self-knowledge and, 349
    overview, 95
    personality self-knowledge (PSK) and, 133*f*, 134, 141, 144–145, 146–147
    wanting and liking and, 218–221
    See also Affective forecasting
Prediction illusions, 349. *See also* Illusions of self-knowledge
Preferences, 353–354. *See also* Choice
Prejudice, 22–23, 352–353
Pride
    gender and, 195–196
    representations of capabilities and, 17
Priming effects, 26–27
Procrastination, 365
Projective stage, 10
Propositional learning, 24–25
Psychoanalytic theory, 366–367
Psychological distance points, 311–312. *See also* Distance
Psychological factors, 214
Psychology, from neuroscience to, 69–73
Psychopathology. *see* Mental disorders
Psychotherapy, epistemological traditions and, 337
Psychotic symptoms, 259. *See also* Mental disorders

R

Race models, emotions and, 198
Racism, forecasting errors and, 282–283
Rational systems, 279–281
Rational–emotive therapy, 420–421
Rationalization. *See* Motivated reasoning
Reading
    blind spots in self-knowledge and, 77–78
    referential processing and, 43–55, 46*t*, 48*f*, 50*t*, 51*f*

Subject Index

Realistic accuracy model
   meta-accuracy and, 251
   personality self-knowledge (PSK) and, 147–148
Reality constraints, 391–392
Reciprocity
   assumed reciprocity, 249–250
   relationship knowledge and, 229
Recollection, 294. *See also* Autobiographical memories
Referential activity (RA) scales, 45–47, 46t. *See also* Measures
Referential competence (RC)
   measures of, 45–47, 46t
   overview, 44
   personality and, 55–57
   reliability and validity of, 47–49, 48f
Referential processing
   individual differences in, 43–55, 46t, 48f, 50t, 51f
   overview, 57–58
   personality and, 55–57
   role of in motivational congruence, 42–43, 42f
Reflected appraisals
   meta-accuracy and, 247–248
   overview, 91–92
   personality self-knowledge (PSK) and, 141f
Regulatory scope
   abstract and concrete self-guides and, 311–313
   distance and, 313–314
   overview, 310–311
   See also Self-regulation
Relationship knowledge
   accuracy and bias in, 231–233
   acquiring, 226–229, 227f
   forecasting errors and, 282–283
   illusions of self-knowledge and, 354–357
   meta-accuracy and, 251
   outcomes related to, 229–231
   overview, 225–226, 238–239
   See also Other people and self-knowledge; Partner knowledge
Relationship-enhancing attributions, 228–229. *See also* Relationship knowledge
Relationship-oriented thoughts and discussions, 228–229
Relative accessibility, 198t
Reliability
   construals and, 322–323
   referential competence and, 47–49, 48f
Representations, 15–17
Representations of capabilities, 17. *See also* Capabilities; Representations
Reputations, personality self-knowledge (PSK) and, 141f
Residualized difference score, 115
Resistance to Persuasion Scale (RPS), 172–173
Resisting influence, 170–173. *See also* Persuasion
Respect, relationship knowledge and, 229
Rewards
   overview, 210–211
   self-deception and, 372t
Risk-taking behavior, 220
Role prescriptions, 251
Romantic relationships. *See* Relationship knowledge
Rostral anterior cingulate cortex (rACC), 69
Rumination, emotions and, 203–204

S

Sampling, mental disorders and, 263
Scale to Assess Unawareness of Mental Disorder (SUMD), 263–264. *See also* Measures
Self, nature of, 7–11
Self-affirmation, 389. *See also* Motivated reasoning
Self-aggrandizing, 110–113
Self-assessment, 1, 398–402. *See also* Assessment
Self-catching procedure, 82
Self-caught/probe-caught methodology
   awareness of contents of thoughts and, 79–80
   motivation and, 82
Self-concepts
   explicit and implicit distinctions, 143–144
   overview, 22–23
   study of self-knowledge and, 2
Self-conscious emotions, 17
Self-control, 318–319
Self-deception
   experimental evidence and, 367–372, 372t
   individual differences in, 372–374
   motivated reasoning and, 389–391
   overview, 363–367, 374
   study of self-knowledge and, 2
   See also Accuracy; Errors
Self-Deception Scale, 372–374
Self-Deceptive Denial (SDD) scale, 372–374
Self-Deceptive Enhancement (SDE) scale, 372–374
Self-depreciation, 415–416
Self-determination, 54–55
Self-Determination Scale (SDS), 55. *See also* Measures
Self-diminishing tendencies, 106–107
Self-disclosure, illusions of self-knowledge and, 355–356
Self-enhancement
   assessing individual differences in, 113–116
   cognitive–informational accounts and, 107–109

Self-enhancement *(cont.)*
conditions under which people might be open to contributions to self-knowledge from others, 95–98
domains of, 118
egoistic biases and, 415–416
individual differences and, 106–113
measurement of, 119
motivated reasoning and, 386–388
motivational–affective accounts and, 109–113
outcomes related to, 116–119
overview, 92, 93–94, 120, 120n–121n, 398–402, 406n–407n
personality self-knowledge (PSK) and, 142
positive illusions, 116–119
resistance to change and, 95
self-deception and, 369–372, 372t
study of self-knowledge and, 2
See also Self-perception

Self-esteem
narcissism and, 110–113
overview, 22–23
self-deception and, 368
self-serving bias and, 93–94
study of self-knowledge and, 2

Self-evaluative thinking, 423–424

Self-expansion model, 229, 230–231. *See also* Self-improvement

Self-expression
behavior and, 144–145
personality self-knowledge (PSK) and, 141f

Self-guides. *See* Abstract and concrete self-guides

Self-identification, 8

Self-illusions. *See* Illusions of self-knowledge

Self-immunization, 386–388

Self-improvement, 398–402. *See also* Self-expansion model

Self-insight
blind spots in self-knowledge and, 83–86
improving, 148–149
mental associations and, 23–27, 24f
overview, 22–23, 33
relations between different components of, 32–33
See also Insight; Self-knowledge overview

Self-knowledge, development of. *See* Development of self-knowledge

Self-knowledge overview, 1–2

Self-observations of behavior, 247, 248–249

Self–other agreement domain in PSK
blind spots in self-knowledge and, 145–147
overview, 133f, 134–135, 139

Self–other agreement, mental disorders and, 265–268

Self–other knowledge asymmetry model (SOKA), 138, 141

Self-perception
cognitive–informational accounts and, 107–109
distance and, 321
mental disorders and, 261
motivated reasoning and, 392
motivational–affective accounts and, 109–113
narcissism and, 110–113
other people and, 92–95
of personality traits, 247–248
relationship knowledge and, 229
self-enhancement and, 93–94
self-representation and, 320–321
See also Illusions of self-knowledge; Perception; Self-enhancement

Self-perception theory, 141–142

Self-perceptions of personality, 247–248

Self-prediction, 218–221. *See also* Prediction

Self-projection system, 14

Self-protection, 406n–407n. *See also* Self-enhancement

Self-reflection
nature of the self and, 10
physical representations of self and, 16

Self-regulation
context and, 314–319
distant and near contexts and, 314–319
overview, 310–311, 323–324
study of self-knowledge and, 2
See also Regulatory scope

Self-report measures
epistemological traditions and, 332
mental disorders and, 266–267
personality self-knowledge (PSK) and, 136, 138–139
study of self-knowledge and, 3
See also Measures

Self-representation
context and, 314–319
distant behavior and, 319–321
effect of distance on, 313–314
overview, 310–311, 311–313, 323–324
See also Abstract and concrete self-guides

Self-schemas, 2

Self-self-knowledge, 2

Self-serving attributional bias
cognitive–informational accounts and, 107–109
motivated reasoning and, 383–384
overview, 93–94
self-deception and, 373

Self-signaling theory
blind spots in self-knowledge and, 87
overview, 83–86
trait uncertainty and, 84–86

Self-stereotyping, 201–205, 203f. *See also* Stereotypes
Self-verification
   blind spots in self-knowledge and, 145–146
   conditions under which people might be open to contributions to self-knowledge from others, 95–98
   defensiveness and, 422
   overview, 92, 94, 120, 398–402
   personality self-knowledge (PSK) and, 145–146
   resistance to change and, 95
Self-views
   accuracy and, 416–419
   egoistic biases and, 415–416
   study of self-knowledge and, 2–3
Semantic memory
   emotions and, 199–201, 200f
   overview, 14
   theories of MPFC and DMPFC function and, 71–72
   See also Memory
Sensory integration, 12
Shame
   gender and, 195–196
   representations of capabilities and, 17
   self-enhancement and, 112–113
Shape naming, 49–53, 50t, 51f
Similarity, assumed, 249–250
Similarity bias, 231–232. *See also* Biases
Simple difference score, 115
Single attitude approach, 158–159. *See also* Attitudes
Skepticism
   egoistic biases and, 419–420
   motivated reasoning and, 382
   self-deception and, 366
Social attunement, 10, 14–15
Social cognition
   medial prefrontal context (MPFC) and, 69–70
   transactional social experience and, 72–73
Social concepts, 383–384
Social conflict, 356–357
Social consensus, 113–115
Social experience, 10–11
Social feedback, 141f
Social influence, 353
Social input
   conditions under which people might be open to contributions to self-knowledge from others, 97–98
   overview, 100
   status and, 99–100
Social interaction, 354–357
Social judgment, 317
Social mechanisms, 98–100
Social perception, 261

Social psychology
   epistemological traditions and, 332
   introspection illusion and, 353
   study of self-knowledge and, 1
   wanting and liking and, 218–221
Social rejection, 99–100
Social self
   conditions under which people might be open to contributions to self-knowledge from others, 95–98
   other people and, 90–100
Social value orientation, 318
Sociocultural factors
   egoistic biases and, 418–419
   relationship knowledge and, 226–228, 227f
SPAN Study, 267–268
Stanislavski method, 73
Statistical sensitivity, 13
Status, 99–100
Stereotypes
   emotions and, 199, 201–205, 203f, 204–205
   evaluative conditioning and, 26
   gender and, 196
   overview, 22–23
Strengths, narcissism and, 112–113
Stroop task, 44–45
Subjective assessments, 403–405. *See also* Assessment
Subjective knowledge, of attitudes, 163
Subjective stage, 10
Subliminal stimuli, wanting and liking and, 216
Substance use disorders, 259, 305. *See also* Alcohol intoxication; Alcoholism; Drug addiction; Mental disorders
Suggestibility, false memories and, 297
Symbolic interactionism
   nature of the self and, 10
   reflected appraisals and, 91–92
Sympathy, transactional social experience and, 73
Symptoms, 259. *See also* Mental disorders

T

Task characteristics, 318
Temporal coherence, 329
Temporality of the self, 65–67
Thematic Apperception Test (TAT)
   personality self-knowledge (PSK) and, 136
   two-systems model of motivation and, 40–41
Thematic coherence, narratives and, 329
Theoretical perspective, 140
Thinking about Life Experiences (TALE) measure, 295
Thoughts
   awareness of the contents of, 78–81
   motivated reasoning and, 380

Thoughts *(cont.)*
  personality self-knowledge (PSK) and, 131
  unnecessary self-evaluative thinking, 423–424
Time-course matters, 118–119
Toronto Alexithymia Scale (TAS), 53–54. *See also* Measures
Tracking accuracy, 232–233. *See also* Biases
Trait uncertainty, 83–87, 383. *See also* Blind spots in self-knowledge; Personality self-knowledge (PSK)
Traits, Big Five personality traits, 136–137
Transactional social experience, 72–73
Transitions, epistemological traditions and, 336–337
Treatment outcomes, 268–269
Two-process model, 201–205, 203f
Two-systems model of motivation, 39–41, 41f. *See also* Motivation

U

Unattended stimuli, wanting and liking and, 215
Unconscious bias
  introspection illusion and, 350–353, 352f
  self-deception and, 390
  See also Biases
Unconscious thought theory, 187–188
Unconsciousness
  decision making and, 181–189
  wanting and liking and, 215
Unrealistic optimism illusion, 348–349. *See also* Illusions of self-knowledge

V

Valence judgments, 49–53, 50t, 51f
Validity
  affective forecasting and, 288
  of attitudes, 163
  correcting attitudes for presumed biases and, 166–167
  referential competence and, 47–49, 48f, 49–55, 50t, 51f
  self-assessment, 1
  two-systems model of motivation and, 40
Values
  as behavioral guides, 315–316
  egoistic biases and, 416–419
  illusions of self-knowledge and, 355–356
  wanting and liking and, 211
Verbal system, referential processing and, 53, 57–58

W

Wanting
  awareness of, 214–218
  overview, 210–214, 221
  prediction and, 218–221
Weighted adding strategy (WADD), 183
Wishful thinking. *See* Motivated reasoning
Worry
  emotions and, 203–204
  motivated reasoning and, 384